May '89   Co   sby

DIAGNOSTIC HEMATOLOGY

Clinical and Technical Principles

DIAGNOSTIC HEMATOLOGY

Clinical and Technical Principles

LAWRENCE W. POWERS, Ph.D.

Associate Professor and Chairman
Department of Medical Technology
University of South Alabama
Mobile, Alabama

with 225 illustrations and 8 color plates
Cover art and illustrations by Don O'Connor

THE C. V. MOSBY COMPANY

ST. LOUIS • PHILADELPHIA • BALTIMORE • TORONTO   1989

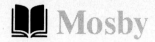 Mosby

Editor: Stephanie Bircher
Assistant Editor: Anne Gunter
Project Manager: Mark Spann
Designer: Liz Fett

Printed in the United States of America

The C.V. Mosby Company
11830 Westline Industrial Drive, St. Louis, Missouri 63146

Library of Congress Cataloging-in-Publication Data

Powers, Lawrence W.
    Diagnostic hematology: clinical and technical principles
Lawrence W. Powers.
      p. cm.
    Includes bibliographies and index.
    ISBN 0-8016-4042-3
    1. Hematology. 2. Blood—Examination. 3. Blood—Diseases—
—Diagnosis. I. Title.
    [DNLM: 1. Blood Cells. 2. Hematologic Diseases—diagnosis.
3. Hematologic Tests. WH 100 P888d]
    RB45.P68 1989
    616.1'5—dc19   89-3092
    DNLM/DLC
    for Library of Congress   CIP

C/D/D 9 8 7 6 5 4 3 2 1

Contributors

SUSAN AYCOCK, B.S., M.T. (ASCP)
Laboratory Coordinator
Department of Medical Technology
University of Mississippi Medical Center
Jackson, Mississippi

RODGER L. BICK, M.D., FACP
Associate Clinical Professor of Medicine
UCLA School of Medicine
Los Angeles, California;
Medical Director
Regional Cancer and Blood Disease Center
 of Kern
Bakersfield, California

CHERYL LEE DRENNAN, B.S., M.T. (ASCP)
Chief Medical Technologist
Adult Special Hematology
University of Mississippi Medical Center
Jackson, Mississippi

CHERYL DAHL McROYAN, B.S., M.T.
 (ASCP), C.L.S. (NCA)
Clinical Instructor and Assistant Chief
 Technologist
Department of Medical Technology
University of South Alabama Medical Center
Mobile, Alabama

For *Molly*,
for being there

Preface

The field of hematology is represented by a number of different textbooks, some designed as brief introductions or reviews, some as comprehensive reference works. Contents also differ, emphasizing hematopathology for medical students and procedural principles for laboratory technicians and technologists. Until recently it was difficult to obtain, in a single volume, a balanced treatment of normal blood cell morphology and function, blood diseases, and technical principles. It would be marvelous indeed if the perfect textbook could be written, one that meets the needs of all potential users or that reflects the organizational criteria of all educators. Since dissatisfaction is the real mother of creation, *Diagnostic Hematology* was designed as an intermediate level presentation for clinical laboratory technologists and other laboratory scientists who may need a background in blood cell morphology or function. This book may also be useful to other practitioners in the medical field, including nurses and members of the allied health professions.

Normal blood cell features are presented first so that the student has a basis for understanding pathological changes. Educators that prefer to combine normal physiology and pathology for each cell series can reorder the chapters appropriately (e.g., Chapter 4 followed by Chapter 18); reference is made throughout the text to related material in other sections of the book. Methodological information is selective, with regard to both the detail presented and the types of procedures. Most hematology courses utilize a laboratory procedure manual that accommodates the available materials and instruments; therefore only a general synopsis of the procedure is provided. Blood cell collection is presented as a reference for those without formal phlebotomy training, but this skill, like many others, can only be learned by experience.

Hematopathology is presented with two points of emphasis: pathophysiological mechanisms underlying the disease and diagnostic approaches utilizing laboratory analyses. Selected case histories illustrate typical laboratory results and the progression of the disorder.

There is no adequate way to express my gratitude to all of my friends and colleagues, the many people that have answered questions, offered advice or provided critical feedback during preparation of the manuscript. This project was initiated at the University of Mississippi Medical Center, and I would like to acknowledge Mrs. Frances Freeman, Chair of the Department of Medical Technology, for her encouragement. Susan Aycock contributed the information on blood collection, and Cheryl Drennan wrote the material on special stains and provided data on leukemia protocols.

Edward North III and Tiffany Hefferman (Cytogenetics Laboratory, Department of Preventive Medicine) provided the leukemia karyotypes in Chapter 20. Ed North and Zelma Cason (Chair, Cytotechnology) generously permitted me the use of their photomicrographic equipment for the color illustrations. Dr. William Lushbaugh (Pre-

viii   Preface

ventive Medicine) provided slides of malaria, and Dr. Joe Files (Medicine) contributed early drafts of case histories. My Medical Technology students at UMMC, especially the class of 1989, served as critics for several of the chapters. David McAllister and Mary Barry posed as phlebotomy patients.

I wish to express special gratitude to Cheri McRoyan for the chapter on fibrinolysis and to Dr. Rodger Bick for the chapter on coagulopathies as well as the case histories used in Chapters 17-24. Mary Louise Turgeon contributed to the glossary. Typing and other secretarial assistance, especially during the last hectic weeks, was provided by Marcy Merrill (Medical Technology, University of South Alabama).

Finally, I wish to express my appreciation to the many editors, artists and photographers at The C.V. Mosby Company. Their patience (how many missed deadlines?), encouragement, and professionalism made this project a reality. Any remaining errors are to be laid at my feet, as I hope the readers of this book will do without hesitation.

Lawrence W. Powers

Contents

COLOR PLATES

SECTION I
Introduction

1

The Science of Hematology

For ancient peoples, the blood and heart were the very essence of the living spirit. Trauma followed by sustained bleeding usually led to shock and death. The heartbeat was regarded as synonymous with life, a vital sign that has been superseded by evidence of brain activity only in recent times. Drinking animal or human blood was thought by peoples of many cultures to impart strength and other virtues, a belief that is not entirely without justification. Blood continued to be a topic of vital interest, a continuing source of fable and mystery, to be sure, but also a prominent subject of inquiry for Renaissance-era physiologists. A renewed interest in investigations based on experimental methodology set the stage for the many advances made during the nineteenth and early twentieth centuries.

Progress in any field of science requires the activities of dedicated individuals whose work is founded on the observations and results of numerous other scientists. Specific technological developments arise as a result of earlier experiments; new equipment and methods then provide the foundation for further advances. For example, knowledge of cellular and subcellular morphology advanced rapidly as improvements in the optical qualities of microscopes and the chemical properties of biological stains proceeded. Particularly during the nineteenth century, advances in other fields of biology, such as genetics, embryology, and biochemistry, had major impacts

on the field of hematology. Similarly, progress in this century has been greatly influenced by discoveries in molecular biology and immunology, the use of electron microscopes and radiobiological tracers, and advances in tissue culturing techniques. The events and persons listed on page 4 indicate, in a very cursory manner, some of the discoveries that were especially important for the development of hematology. Wintrobe (1980) provides excellent accounts of these historical developments. He also describes the personal and professional attributes of the scientists, physicians, and other individuals who made these events possible (Wintrobe, 1985). The purpose of this book is to present a sample of this knowledge: what blood is, how it functions, what can go wrong in various diseases and disorders, and some of the methods used in clinical laboratories to investigate blood properties.

BLOOD, THE TRANSPORT SYSTEM

Blood is the fluid that bathes the body, bringing to the tissues nutrients, chemical messages, and oxygen. Blood also transports most of the wastes produced by the tissues: carbon dioxide and byproducts of protein, carbohydrate, and lipid metabolism. Contained within this fluid are diverse populations of cells with functions that include sentry duty (cells that recognize substances that are foreign to the body), active defense (cells that produce proteins that neutralize the foreign material and phagocytic cells

SELECTED SCIENTIFIC DEVELOPMENTS RELEVANT TO HEMATOLOGY

1628 Blood circulation described by William Harvey (1578-1657) in England

1674 First description of red blood cells, by Antonj van Leeuwenhoek (1623-1723) in Holland

1772 Plasma clotting factors described by William Henson (1739-1774)

1773 First descriptions of white blood cells, by William Henson in England

1830 Compound microscope developed

1843 First hematology monograph published, in France by Gabriel Andral (1797-1876)

1845 Leukemia described as a distinct disease by Rudolf Virchow (1821-1902) in Germany and John Bennett (1812-1875) in Scotland

1851 Hemoglobin discovered by Otto Funke in Germany; first blood cell counts published, by Karl Vierordt in Germany

1858 Fibrinogen isolated by Denis de Commercy in France and Olaf Hammarsten in Uppsala

1865 Red blood cell function described by Felix Hoppe-Seyler (1825-1895) in Germany

1869 Bone marrow identified as source of blood cells by Ernst Neumann (1834-1918) in Germany and Giulio Bizzozero (1846-1901) in Italy

1870 Leukemia identified as a disease of the bone marrow by Neumann

1879 Paul Ehrlich (1854-1915) in Germany develops white blood cell differential count and tri-acid staining technique

1886 Phagocytosis described by Ilya Metchnikov (1845-1916), a Russian

1890 Anticoagulants based on calcium removal described by Arthus and Pages in Switzerland

1900 ABO blood groups discovered by Karl Landsteiner (1868-1943) in Austria

1902 May-Grünwald stain and Wright stain (1906) introduced for blood smears

1905 Common coagulation pathway proposed by Paul Morawitz (1879-1936) in Germany

1906 Platelets accurately characterized by James Wright (1869-1938) in Boston

1910 Sickle-cell anemia presented as a disease by James Herrick in Chicago

1925 Thalassemia described by Thomas Cooley in Detroit

1926 Studies on lymphocytes and cell-mediated immunity by James Murphy in New York

1927 Sternal puncture technique utilized by Mikhail Arinkin (1876-1948) in Russia; makes possible routine bone marrow examination

1929 Closed-tube hematocrit introduced by Maxwell Wintrobe in the United States

1931-1949 Red cell metabolism and enzymes detailed by Otto Warburg (1883-1970), Gustav Embden (1874-1933), and Otto Meyerhof (1884-1951) in Germany

1936 Prothrombin assays introduced; expand understanding of coagulation mechanism

1950 Ferrokinetic studies used to study iron turnover

1957 Introduction of automated cell counters to the clinical laboratory

1961 Hematopoietic stem cell demonstrated by transplantation and irradiation techniques; platelet aggregation with ADP studied in Sweden

1969 T and B lymphocytes characterized

1975 Kohler and Milstein describe the production of monoclonal antibodies by cells in tissue culture

that ingest the invader), transport of respiratory gases to and from the tissues, and the prevention of blood loss (cells that participate in hemostasis and coagulation). A drop of blood, spread thinly on a glass microscope slide and stained with a biological dye, reveals this remarkable variety of cell types (Fig. 1-1). The circulatory system, consisting of the heart and blood vessels, contains and controls distribution of this fluid, routing it to meet the needs of various body activities, such as heat conservation, strenuous exercise, and digestion. Other organs and tissues, such as liver, spleen, kidney, bone marrow, and lymph nodes, participate in the formation and function of blood elements.

Blood can be easily separated into its liquid and cellular components by centrifugation. Blood is rotated in tubes at high speed so that the heavier cells are forced to the bottom of the tube, leaving a relatively clear fluid at the top. If blood is allowed to clot completely before centrifugation, the fluid portion is defined as **serum** (plural: sera). Chemical substances that prevent clotting, **anticoagulants,** can be added to the

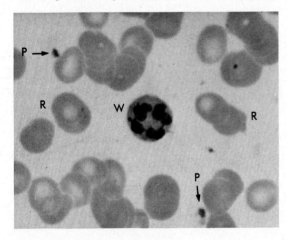

Fig. 1-1. Normal blood cells.
Smear stained with Wright's stain (970X). *R*, red blood cell (erythrocyte); *W*, white blood cell (leukocyte); *P*, platelet.

blood immediately after it is drawn from the body. Centrifugation of anticoagulated blood results in a fluid layer that is defined as **plasma.** The difference between serum and plasma is the presence of various proteins in plasma that participate in the coagulation process; these have been removed from the serum as a result of coagulation (Fig. 1-2). Coagulation also produces changes in the cellular component, since certain cells participate in the formation of the blood clot. As one would expect, a substance containing many different substances and diverse cellular elements has complex physical and chemical properties. Studies of the blood involve measuring these properties in health and disease, through the use of many methods and approaches.

HEMATOLOGY AS A LABORATORY SCIENCE

Hematology is defined as the study of the blood (from the Greek word for blood, *hemo* or *hemato*), but the modern practice of hematology emphasizes studies of the blood cells, or hematocytes. Constituents of the fluid portion (serum or plasma), except for the soluble substances involved in blood clotting, are primarily the concern of physiological and clinical chemists. The blood cells include leukocytes (white blood cells or WBCs), erythrocytes (red blood cells or RBCs) and thrombocytes (platelets). Hematologists study the morphology of blood cells, events of cellular reproduction and maturation, distribution of different blood cells within various tissues of the body, their physiological functions, and the various disorders that involve hematopoietic tissue. Several types of blood cells interact in host defense, including phagocytes that engulf invading microorganisms and lymphocytes that provide immunological defenses. Thus, there are topics in hematology that overlap with the science of **immunology** in content and methodology. Studies of

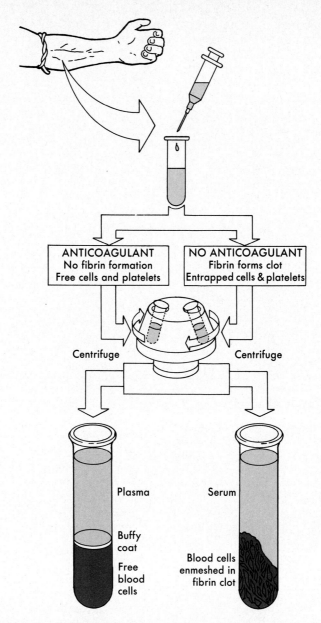

Fig. 1-2. Liquid and cellular blood components.
When blood is drawn and mixed immediately with an anticoagulant, fibrin formation is prevented. Most cellular studies are done with anticoagulated blood. Centrifugation provides an upper liquid layer of plasma and a lower layer of free cells and platelets. A buffy coat, composed mainly of white blood cells, may appear between the plasma and red cell layers. Serum results if the blood is allowed to coagulate; fibrinogen is converted to a fibrin clot in which platelets and cells adhere.

red blood cells may also be included in the field of **immunohematology,** the applied science of blood transfusion and compatability testing. The mechanisms of clotting and hemostasis, which involve both cellular and soluble elements of the plasma, constitute a specialized subdiscipline within hematology.

Hematology is also a definable specialty of internal medicine in which physicians acquire additional knowledge and skills to diagnose and treat blood disorders. Clinical hematologists may serve as a patient's primary or attending physician or they may serve as consultants to a patient's personal physician and other members of the medical team, such as pathologists, radiologists, and surgeons. Since malignancies or cancers are among the more commonly encountered blood diseases, some clinical hematologists are also oncologists, specialists in abnormal tissue growths or neoplasms. Pathologists study the disease processes directly in tissues, such as bone marrow or spleen; some specialize in hematology. Some pathologists may focus primarily on anatomical sources, such as autopsy and surgical materials, whereas others are primarily clinical, using the laboratory as a diagnostic tool. Radiologists, in addition to various diagnostic duties using x-rays, direct radiation therapy for some types of blood cell cancers.

Hematological research is conducted at universities, medical schools, hospitals, pharmacological companies, instrument manufacturers, and other institutions to provide the theoretical and methodological data base for practitioners. The results of this research are published in scholarly journals and books and disseminated through professional societies (see Appendix C).

Laboratory hematology: technology and training

The methodological application of hematology (technical hematology) occurs primarily in clinical laboratories and is performed by medical technologists and technicians. Some routine procedures are performed in doctor's offices and small clinics by nurses, medical assistants, or physicians, but these tests are usually intended to screen patients as part of routine physical examinations or to provide therapeutic monitoring over extended periods of time. Additional testing often requires specialized instruments and procedures that are only available in a laboratory staffed by trained professionals. Laboratories range in size from small clinic and hospital units with one or a few employees to reference laboratories with a large staff of specialists. Large medical centers may contain several different laboratories, each providing unique testing services. The main clinical laboratory may be supplemented by outpatient facilities, a newborn laboratory near a nursery, an acute care laboratory near an emergency room or intensive care ward, a surgery laboratory to provide results during critical operations, and laboratories designated for pediatrics, oncology, gynecology, fertility, and other specialized areas of medical practice.

Training, including formal education and experience, varies greatly among laboratory workers. Requirements for employment depend on the function of the laboratory, its institutional affiliation, and the laws and licensing requirements of various geographical regions. A license based on passing a written examination is required in order to work in some states (e.g., California, Florida, and Tennessee), and most other states either require, or recognize as a qualification, certification in medical technology by a recognized professional organization, such as the Board of Registry of the American Society of Clinical Pathologists (ASCP), the American Medical Technologists (AMT), or the National Certifying Agency (NCA). Federal laboratories (public health, military, Veterans Administration) may be exempt from state licensing requirements. Certification is based on the completion of a didactic program of study at a college, university, or hospital, plus a period of supervised clinical experience (practicum). After passing a comprehensive written examination, an applicant can be certified by the ASCP as a medical technologist (MT) or a medical laboratory technician (MLT) or by the NCA as a clinical laboratory scientist (CLS) or technician (CLT). There are several other certification catagories available, including advanced levels of specialization based on experience, advanced study, and/or graduate work. Further information on each examination can be obtained from the appropriate organization, listed in Appendix C.

Laboratory technology, including hematology, has changed dramatically during the last three decades. For most of this century the microscope played a central role in evaluating blood samples. At the turn of the century, numerical values and criteria for cell appearance were established in normal patients and those with various disorders as counting and staining methods were standardized. A physician or laboratory technician diluted the blood, counted the number of red and white blood cells on a marked slide or counting chamber, then prepared smears of the cells for staining various features. Hemoglobin was quantitated by colorimetry, the measuring of the intensity of color imparted by lysed red blood cells to a solution. Measures of plasma clotting capability utilized test tubes and a few simple reagents; the technician tilted the tubes and noted the time required for a clot to form. During the 1940s, a revolution in biochemistry introduced new approaches to the measuring of blood constituents. The 1950s saw the widespread replacement of vacuum tubes by transistors and the introduction of semi-automated analytical equipment to the chemistry and hematology laboratories. Complete blood counts could be performed faster, with greater accuracy and precision, and more economically. The microscope remained prominent, as new staining techniques with enzymatic and fluorescent re-

agents supplemented the traditional dyes. Rapid advances in electronics and computer technology during the 1960s, particularly the introduction of solid-state circuitry, ushered in the era of laboratory automation and made possible an extensive program of quality assurance for procedures, reagents, and results. Radioisotopes served as tracers to measure blood volume, iron metabolism, and red blood cell survival. Advances in immunology had a great impact in the 1970s, providing techniques for marking and identifying specific populations of blood cells, characterizing leukemias and other malignancies, and yielding further knowledge of blood cell function and interactions. During the 1980s, computers and analytical instruments have increased in complexity and diversity of application. Laser technology is being used for cell counting and sorting. Immunologically linked medications are being tested as therapeutic tracers. To match this expanding technology, additional skills and continuous re-education will be required in order to evaluate the data generated by these instruments and to assess the clinical

Table 1-1. Système International d'Unités (SI)

SI units		
length	meter	m
mass	kilogram	kg
time	second	s
amount	mole	mol
temperature	kelvin	K
SI prefixes		
kilo-	k	$\times 10^3$
milli-	m	$\times 10^{-3}$
micro-	μ	$\times 10^{-6}$
nano-	n	$\times 10^{-9}$
pico-	p	$\times 10^{-12}$
femto-	f	$\times 10^{-15}$

status of patients; close communication and cooperation among all members of the medical team, clinical and technical, is mandatory.

MEASUREMENT AND TERMINOLOGY

A standardized, precise system of measurement is critical to communication and progress in any science. Laboratory scientists utilize the *Système International d'Unités* (SI), the current form of the metric system, for measurement of length, area, volume, and mass (Table 1-1). A thorough understanding of metric system nomenclature and of the relationships between various units of measure is essential. Appendix A contains useful conversion factors and equivalents. Students should also be comfortable with the use of exponents and be able to manipulate variables in simple mathematical formulas.

Units of measure

Historically, linear distances in cellular biology have been expressed in micrometers, or "microns," symbolized by the greek letter μ. The preferred symbol is μm. A micrometer is a distance of 0.001 millimeters or 10^{-6}m. A red blood cell is about 7 μm in diameter, and most other cells have diameters between 1 and 100 μm. In the past, ultrastructural features and radiation wavelengths were often cited in angstroms (Å), 1 Å being equivalent to 10^{-10} m or 0.0001 μm (1Å = 10,000 μm); modern usage is to cite such measurements in nanometers (1 nm = 10^{-9}m) and picometers (1 pm = 10^{-12} m). Area measurements, employed in manual counting methods and in descriptions of skin surface area, are expressed in square millimeters (mm^2) and square centimeters (cm^2), respectively. Since there are 10^3 μm in each millimeter, there are 10^6 μm ($10^3 \times 10^3$) in each square millimeter (Fig. 1-3). In formal scientific practice, the prefixes *deci-* and *centi-* are not used (only prefixes in multiples of three, such as *milli-* and *micro-* are recognized), but their widespread use in clinical practice justifies their inclusion in this textbook.

Cell volumes were formerly given in cubic microns (μ^3), but these are now cited in

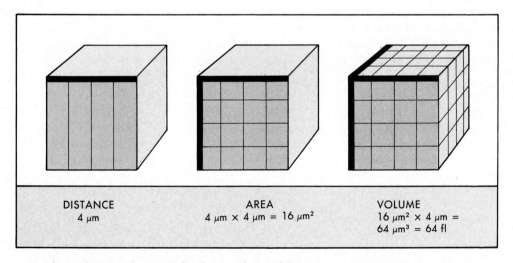

DISTANCE
4 μm

AREA
4 μm × 4 μm = 16 μm²

VOLUME
16 μm² × 4 μm =
64 μm³ = 64 fl

Fig. 1-3. Distance, area, and volume relationships.
Exponential multiplication of a linear measure to illustrate the relationship between a micrometer (e.g. cell diameter) and femtoliter (cell volume).

femtoliters (1 fL 10^{-15} L). The liter (L) is a non-SI unit, equal to a cubic decimeter (dm^3), which has been retained for clinical practice. One milliliter (mL) is equivalent to a cubic centimeter (cc or cm^3), and chemical constituents in blood are often expressed in deciliters (dL) or microliters (μL). Liter is abbreviated "L" (capitalized) in North America in order to avoid confusion with the number "1," which is often typed as "1" (lower case "L"). Cell counts are expressed as a number per liter or microliter: 7000/μL, $7.0 \times 10^3/\mu$L, or 7.0×10^9/L. Expressing cell counts in numbers per cubic millimeter is discouraged. To avoid the use of large exponents, it is preferred that SI units be used with prefixes so that numbers preceding the unit do not have to be greater than 1000 or less than 0.001.

The base unit for mass in the SI is the kilogram (kg), but most applications in hematology use substantially smaller amounts: picograms (pg) of hemoglobin in an average red blood cell or micrograms (μg) and milligrams (mg) in reagent preparation. Substance concentration can be expressed in moles (mol) (gram molecular weights), as mol/L, mmol/L, or μmol/L, instead of mass concentration (kg/L). A concise review and discussion of conventional metric and SI units, along with tables of clinical laboratory values, is presented by Lehmann and Henry (Henry, 1984) and by Bermes and Young (Tietz, 1986).

Terminology

Developments in a science occur over an extended period of time and in many places. Terminology reflects the geographical isolation and divergent investigational approaches of scientists. Add to this the delays and confusion that result from publication in various languages, and one can readily understand how two or more sets of names may be applied to the same cell types or why there may be disagreement about the interpretation of research or clinical data. This often results in differences in normal values or in the interpretation of a metabolic pathway. In some cases (e.g., red blood cell stages) more than one name is used in this book for a cell or disorder because the alternate terms are well known. In other cases, alternate terms are abandoned as either antiquated or inappropriate. This has been done with regard to the names of many diseases, for which a descriptive term has frequently replaced a name based on the name of the scientist or physician who studied the disease (e.g., thalassemia for Cooley's anemia). Since science is a dynamic process, constantly presenting new findings and permitting new interpretations, it is to be expected that the terminology applied to these topics will change accordingly. Hopefully (despite the confusion that temporarily results), most of these changes are indications of scientific progress.

SUGGESTED READINGS—SECTION I

Henry, JB, ed: Todd, Sanford, and Davidsohn. Clinical diagnosis and management by laboratory methods, ed 17, Philadelphia, 1984, WB Saunders Co.

Tietz, NW, ed: Textbook of clinical chemistry, Philadelphia, 1986, WB Saunders Co.

Wintrobe, MM: Blood, pure and eloquent, New York, 1980, McGraw-Hill Book Co.

Wintrobe, MM: Hematology, the blossoming of a science: a story of inspiration and effort, Philadelphia, 1985, Lea & Febiger.

The Normal Erythrocyte

2

Introduction to the Erythron

DEFINING THE ERYTHRON

The red blood cells or erythrocytes (*erythros*, red) contain an oxygen-binding protein, **hemoglobin,** which transports oxygen from the lungs to the various tissues. A typical adult has four to five trillion (4 to 5 $\times 10^{12}$) red blood cells (RBC) in each liter of blood and a blood volume of about 4 to 6 liters, which accounts for about 3.5% of the total body weight. The entire population of red cells (the **erythron**) constitutes a dispersed tissue that includes the immature RBC precursors of the bone marrow, the red cells circulating through the blood, and RBCs present in various organs and tissues (Table 2-1). The circulating RBC component is easily sampled from capillaries by dermal puncture (fingerstick or heelstick in infants) and from veins by venipuncture (phlebotomy). The circulating or peripheral erythron is measured and evaluated in two different, but complementary ways: (1) The total red cell mass or red cell volume is an absolute value that can be expressed as milliliters of RBCs or as milliliters per kilogram of body weight. (2) The quantity of red cells can be expressed as a fraction of the total blood volume, either as a red blood cell count (RBCs per microliter of whole blood) or as the hematocrit (ratio of volume of RBCs to volume of whole blood, expressed as a decimal or percentage). Fig. 2-1 compares the normal values for and relationships between these measures of red cell quantity.

The total red cell content of the body is regulated by complex physiological mechanisms that monitor the oxygen demand of the body's tissues and stimulate RBC production to meet the demand. Red blood cells are formed by the division of mitotically active precursor cells in the bone marrow, and they exist as mature hemoglobin-carrying units for about 120 days after their release from the marrow. These circulating cells are nonnucleated and have limited capabilities for membrane repair. As the red cells circulate and sustain minor damage from distortion and contact with small vessels, they are removed by macrophages in the spleen. Some of the hemoglobin components are recycled for incorporation into new red cells. Thus, a constant turnover of red blood cells occurs, and the total quantity of RBCs present at any time is a function of marrow production (**erythropoiesis**) and of loss, either by bleeding (**hemorrhage**) or cell aging (**senescence**). Conditions in which insufficient red cells are available to meet the oxygen consumption requirements of the body are termed **anemias.** There are also some conditions in which excess red blood cells are manufactured (**polycythemia**), either as a physiological response to metabolism (high-altitude adaptation or increased exercise) or as a disease of uncontrolled production.

FUNCTION OF RED BLOOD CELLS

The primary function of erythrocytes is to efficiently transport oxygen to tissues throughout the body and to transport car-

13

Table 2-1. The numerical erythron (normal values)

Individual erythrocytes
Diameter: 7.4 to 8.2 μm
Thickness (biconcave disk): 1.5 to 1.8 μm
Surface area: 130 to 150 μm^2
Volume: 85 to 95 fL
Mass: 90 to 100 pg
Hemoglobin content: 27 to 31 pg

Erythrocyte turnover
Production rate: 2.5 million/sec; 200 billion/day
Life span: 110 to 130 days

Erythrocytes in circulation	Male	Female
Density in blood (million/μL)	4.2-5.4	3.6-5.0
Total red cell volume (mL/kg)	25-31	22-28
Hemoglobin (g/dL)	14-16	13-15
Hematocrit (%)	41-48	38-45

---

bon dioxide to the respiratory organs for elimination. Actually, hemoglobin does the work of binding, carrying, and releasing respiratory gases, and the red cell serves as the manufacturer and the "package" for hemoglobin. In most invertebrates, oxygen is distributed to the tissues without specialized cells: a blood pigment that binds oxygen is present as a diffuse protein in the circulatory fluid. Animals with higher rates of metabolism and larger masses of tissue require a more efficient distribution system. In humans, Bowman's capsule of the kidney and the endothelial cell linings of the capillaries are "leaky." As a result, hemoglobin, when free in the plasma, is lost to the nephron and into the tissues, respectively. The red cell membrane serves as a retaining barrier for hemoglobin while permitting oxygen and carbon dioxide to pass freely.

Since oxygen-carrying capacity of the blood is a function of hemoglobin, it fol-lows that the amount of oxygen delivered is a function of the red blood cell count *and* the average hemoglobin content of erythrocytes. If a specified volume of red blood cells is exposed to a chemical that destroys the red cell membrane (**cell lysis**), the hemoglobin is released and the color imparted to the solution can be measured. By comparison with standard solutions, a value for hemoglobin is calculated and expressed as grams of hemoglobin per deciliter of whole blood (g/dL). In a normal individual, the hemoglobin value corresponds to the hematocrit (%) by a ratio of approximately one to three; significant deviations from this ratio indicate one or more erythrocyte abnormalities. In clinical practice, the hematocrit, the hemoglobin, or both can be used as screening tests to determine RBC sufficiency.

ERYTHROCYTE CONTENTS: RBC INDICES

A low red blood cell count would obviously yield a correspondingly low hemoglobin value, but it is also possible for each red blood cell to be deficient in hemoglobin. In this case, a relatively normal red cell count (or a relatively normal hematocrit) could yield a low hemoglobin value. The average amount of hemoglobin contained within an erythrocyte, the **mean corpuscular hemoglobin (MCH)**, is calculated by dividing the hemoglobin value (g/dL) by the red blood cell count (millions/μL) and multiplying by 10 to obtain the average number of picograms of hemoglobin per RBC. This can also be expressed as an average concentration by dividing the hemoglobin value (g/dL) by the hematocrit and multiplying by 100 to obtain the **mean corpuscular hemoglobin concentration (MCHC)**, which is a percentage representing the ratio of the weight of hemoglobin to the volume of the average RBC.

The average erythrocyte has a diameter of 7.4 to 8.2 μm. When suspended freely in a

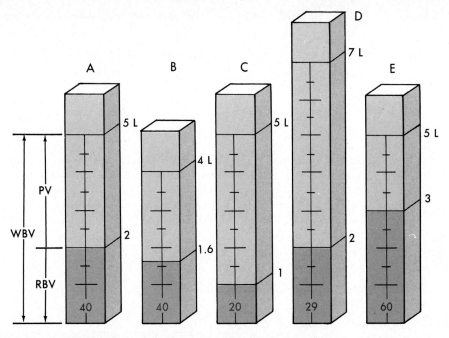

Fig. 2-1.   Relative and absolute measures of red cell quantity.
The height of each column represents the total whole blood volume *(WBV)* of an adult, in liters, separable into a plasma volume *(PV)* and a red blood cell volume *(RBV)*, each an absolute measure of blood quantity that is independent of other measurements. The number in each column is the packed cell volume or hematocrit, expressed as a percentage of the total blood volume, a relative measure that is dependent on other quantitative parameters. The normal state of volume and hematocrit (**A**) is compared with other conditions. Acute hemorrhage (**B**), such as from trauma, results in a rapid decrease in total volume, but the hematocrit remains proportionately the same until the plasma volume expands 24 to 48 hours later. Chronic anemia (**C**), due to a production failure or ongoing destruction of red cells, results in a low hematocrit in the presence of a compensated, normal total volume. An expanded plasma volume, as in hyperproteinemia or after excessive administration of fluids, can produce an apparently low hematocrit (**D**), despite a normal red cell mass. Polycythemia, due to increased red cell production (**E**), can result in an elevated hematocrit and a normal total blood volume.

solution, RBCs form biconcave disks that are about 1.5 to 1.8 μm thick. A total membrane surface area of 130 to 150 μm² encloses a volume of 85 to 95 fL of intracellular contents. In some disease states, the average erythrocyte volume can be decreased or increased from the normal range. Large RBCs occupy a greater volume of space, so that the hematocrit will be correspondingly increased. Conversely, small RBCs yield a low hematocrit, even though the actual cell count might be normal. Dividing the hematocrit, expressed as a decimal, by the RBC count in millions and multiplying by 10 results in a value for average RBC content, **mean cellular volume (MCV)**, expressed in femtoliters.

Each of these RBC values, or **indices**, represents a calculated measurement of the average cell, based on determinations of average cell count, cell size (hematocrit volume), and hemoglobin content. Red cell indices are helpful in determining the causes and severity of anemic disorders. Calculations and methods of determination are discussed further in Chapter 26.

COMPONENTS OF THE ERYTHRON

The erythron consists of production, circulation, and extravascular components (Fig. 2-2). More than 90% of the red cell mass is found in the circulating compartment as mature erthrocytes. In an average adult male, about 2000 mL of red blood cells will carry about 675 g of hemoglobin (based on a total blood volume of 4500 mL and a hemoglobin value of 15 g/dL). Studies

show that red cells survive in the peripheral circulation for approximately 120 ± 20 days, so that about 1% of the red cell mass is replaced daily in a normal male adult. This normal physiological state of turnover, in the absence of blood loss or increased oxygen demand, is referred to as the **basal level,** reflecting the rates of production and loss that maintain a steady state **(homeostasis)** of red blood cells in circulation. The production and maturation activity of red cell precursors that replace cells lost by normal attrition or aging (senescence) is said to represent a **production index** of 1.0; production can increase or decrease (>1 or <1, respectively) as the need to replace lost cells dictates.

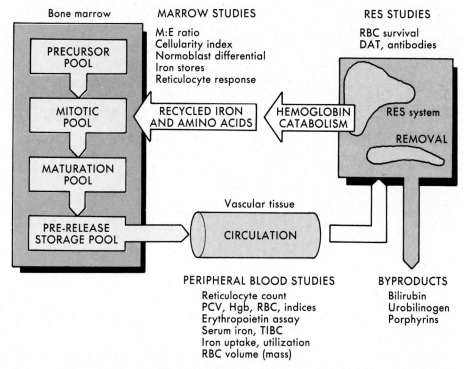

Fig. 2-2. Compartments of the erythron.
Laboratory procedures that evaluate the primary components of red cell production, circulation, and removal are listed. *PCV,* Packed cell volume; *TIBC,* total iron-binding capacity; *RES,* reticuloendothelial system; *DAT,* direct antiglobulin test, used to detect the presence of immunoglobulins coating the red cell surface.

Increased demand for oxygen-carrying capacity stimulates the erythroid precursors to increase production. This occurs during hypoxia that results from a sustained increase in muscle activity, metabolism at higher altitudes, or red cell loss. In some cases of chronic destructive anemias, the production index can increase to levels that are seven to eight times that of basal levels. Failure to compensate for blood loss can result in anemia, a deficiency in the blood's oxygen-carrying capacity. Note that increased oxygen demand, as induced by vigorous exercise or low environmental oxygen levels, can result in a similar oxygen debt despite the presence of a red cell mass that would be adequate in normal or basal conditions. Thus, anemia must be considered a *relative* condition, one that must be evaluated for the individual's needs.

Erythrocyte production can be evaluated by examining the bone marrow and the peripheral blood for the following:

1. Ratio of cellular to noncellular material in aspirated marrow (**percent cellularity**)
2. Ratio of nonerythroid cells to erythroid cells (myeloid-erythroid or **M:E ratio**)
3. Number (percent) of erythroid precursors present in a **marrow differential count**
4. Response time for production after the onset of stress or hypoxia, as measured by the appearance of large, dark **polychromatic erythrocytes** ("shift reticulocytes")
5. Total **reticulocyte count** and corrected reticulocyte count (corrected for packed cell volume): Reticulocytes are immature red cells that are released from the bone marrow to the peripheral blood, indicative of a positive hematopoietic response.

Production can also be assessed by utilizing radioactive isotopes, such as labeled iron, to determine the rate of hemoglobin synthesis, hemoglobin incorporation into red cells, and release of red cells from the bone marrow over a specified interval. The circulating red cell mass can also be labeled with radioactive chromium. The removal or destruction of red cells can be monitored by sequential sampling of the peripheral blood for iron- and chromium-labeled RBCs, resulting in calculations of survival time and turnover rate. Detection of the isotopes in the spleen or other extravascular sites permits an assessment of removal or destruction. These techniques provide data for studies of **erythrokinetics,** the dynamics of the red cell life span (Chapter 3), and **ferrokinetics,** the dynamics of iron metabolism (Chapter 4).

SUMMARY

- The erythron is defined as a dispersed tissue consisting of the immature erythrocyte precursors in the bone marrow and the mature red blood cells circulating in organs, tissues, and blood vessels.
- The primary function of erythrocytes is to transport respiratory gases to and from tissue sites of metabolism. Red cells contain hemoglobin, a protein that binds oxygen and carbon dioxide.
- Oxygen-transporting capability can be assessed by determining various red cell values: red blood cell count, hematocrit, hemoglobin concentration, and red cell indices of corpuscular volume and hemoglobin content.
- The erythron consists of distinct functional compartments: production, circulation, and extravascular components. The integrity of each component can be assessed by laboratory procedures.

3

Red Blood Cell Production and Removal

SITES OF PRODUCTION

Erythropoiesis can be first observed in the mesenchymal tissues of the embyronic yolk sac at about 3 weeks of gestational age, with the appearance of small islands of cells that form the blood vessels and earliest blood cell precursors or **hemocytoblasts.** Mesodermal blood cell production begins to decline at about week 6 of gestation, and it is completely inactive by the end of the first trimester. Erythropoiesis commences in the liver at about week 5 or 6 of gestation, and the liver remains the predominant site of blood production until the end of the second trimester, continuing to produce until about 2 weeks after birth (Fig. 3-1). Although most textbooks state that the spleen is also an important site of fetal blood formation, recent studies indicate that blood cells found in the fetal spleen may originate at other sites (Wolf et al., 1983).

The medullary cavities of the fetal bones begin producing blood cells at approximately 5 months of gestational age, and they become the dominant site of erythropoiesis by 6 to 7 months. The marrow also produces the myeloid blood cells, whereas mesodermal and hepatic production is restricted to erythrocytes. In the fetus and the young infant, all of the bones contain hematopoietic marrow, but much of this is replaced by fatty tissue as the child matures. Following birth, fatty replacement occurs rapidly in the long bones. As a result, adults maintain hematopoietic tissue primarily in the axial skeleton (vertebrae, pelvic bones, ribs, and flat bones of the skull) and the proximal ends of the femur and humerus. Even in these areas, the marrow normally consists of about 50% fatty material.

REGULATION OF PRODUCTION

Since the major function of red blood cells is to supply the tissues of the body with oxygen, it is not surprising that red cell numbers are related to oxygen delivery (Fig. 3-2). Although conflicting evidence has been presented on the specific mechanisms involved, a number of observations and experiments indicate that oxygen tension in the tissues is the critical factor for the regulation of red cell production. Oxygen delivery to the tissues is a function of the following:

1. Availability of oxygen to the organism (atmospheric partial pressure)
2. Pulmonary function, respiratory gas exchange
3. Circulatory dynamics, including cardiac output, blood viscosity, and blood vessel integrity
4. Hemoglobin concentration and total volume of red cells (quantitative sufficiency)
5. Oxygen-binding capacity of hemoglobin (qualitative sufficiency)

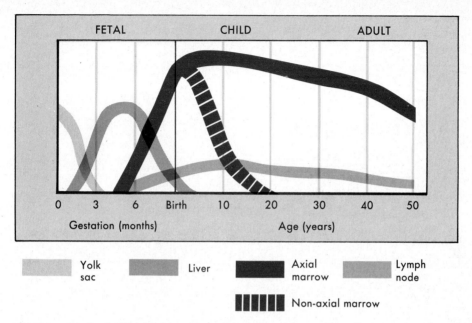

Fig. 3-1.   Sites of RBC production at different ages.
Erythropoietic sites differ as mesodermal tissues develop. Total production is highest during the rapid growth years of childhood and young adulthood. In later adult life, total production declines and most of it is confined to the marrow of the axial skeleton.

When a person relocates from sea level to a high-altitude environment (e.g, Denver or Mexico City), the difference in oxygen availability is often noticed during physical exertion. Running or climbing stairs may leave the individual feeling faint or short of breath. Although increases in respiratory rate and cardiac output compensate for the short-term deficit, a stable physiological adjustment (**acclimation**) requires a higher concentration of erythrocytes in order to maximize oxygen exchange. After 2 to 3 weeks in the new environment, the blood of a normal person will have higher hematocrit and hemoglobin values and a higher RBC count. Studies of Peruvians living near sea level (Lima) and at 14,900 feet in the Andes (Morococha) by Hurtado (1964) yielded the following comparisons, based on mean values for healthy adults:

	Sea level	15,000 feet
Atmospheric oxygen (mm Hg)	147	83
Arterial oxygen (mm Hg)	87	45
Capillary oxygen (mm Hg)	57	38
Hemoglobin (g/dL)	15	20
Total blood volume (mL)	5600	7000
Red cell volume (mL)	2600	4200
Hematocrit (%)	46	60

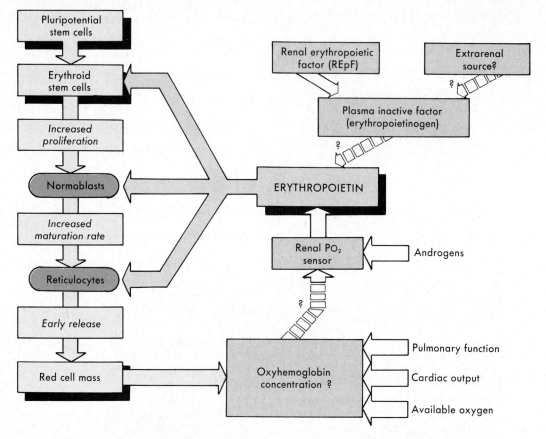

Fig. 3-2. Physiological regulation of erythropoiesis.
Erythropoietin influences the circulating red cell mass by stimulating division of committed erythroid stem cells, accelerating the maturation rate of developing normoblasts, and releasing reticulocytes before full maturity. Oxygen delivery to the tissues supposedly regulates erythropoietin production or activation, but the mechanisms are still poorly understood.

Permanent human settlements occur in the Andes at altitudes up to 17,500 feet, but this is probably the upper limit for sustained activity without the use of supplemental oxygen. Above 20,000 feet, red cell production is actually impaired and sustained hypoxia produces acute illness. Other physiological changes that facilitate acclimation include increased capillary vascularization to the tissues (this may be more important than the increase in hemoglobin content), increased pulmonary venti-

lation, and metabolic adaptation of the tissues.

Changes in **blood viscosity,** or flow properties, occur as the packed cell volume changes. A highly viscous blood moves through the blood vessels slowly (the normal circulation time of 60 seconds can be doubled!). Therefore, oxygen delivery from the lungs to the tissues can be delayed, counteracting the effects of the increased oxygen carrying capacity. This occurs in the disorder polcythemia vera, as a result of increased red cell production and release (see Chapter 17).

The first sign of an erythropoietic response to high-altitude hypoxia is reticulocytosis, the appearance of immature but non-nucleated red cells in the peripheral blood at 2 to 3 days after the onset of symptoms. Days later, the bone marrow exhibits an increased production rate. The red cell values increase slowly, until a new "normal" red cell mass and hemoglobin concentration are achieved. The reticulocyte count then returns to normal. Although many authors refer to this response as "secondary" or "relative polycythemia," a better term is **erythrocytosis.** A return to lower altitudes is accompanied by a gradual decline in red cell values to the previous "normal range." Similar changes are seen when an otherwise healthy person loses a liter or more of blood (acute hemorrhage) or is transfused with excess whole blood or packed red cells. Red cell production changes accordingly.

ERYTHROPOIETIN

The intermediary in the erythropoietic response is **erythropoietin,** a glycoprotein hormone with a terminal sialic acid residue. Depending on the assay and recovery methods used, erythropoietin appears to have a molecular weight in the range of 20,000 to 30,000 daltons and to consist of 34% carbohydrate. The exact site of manufacture is still not known for certain, but much of the evidence implicates the vascularized tissue of the kidney, probably the juxtaglomerular apparatus. Experimental animals deprived of both kidneys lack an erythropoietic response to hypoxia. Chronic renal diseases are frequently associated with a hypoproliferative anemia. Other sites of erythropoietin synthesis, including the liver, brain, lungs, and bone marrow, have also been proposed, but much of the supporting data for these extrarenal sources have been derived from studies of pathological states.

Regardless of source, erythropoietin is known to stimulate red cell production and release at several levels (Fig. 3-2):

1. Commited erythroid stem cells proliferate, resulting in an increased population of maturing normoblastic precursors. The hormone appears to act at the cell membrane, triggering a cytoplasmic protein that stimulates RNA transcription in the nucleus.
2. Normoblastic maturation time decreases.
3. Immature reticulocytes, normally stored in the marrow for three days, are released early. On Wright-stained smears these "shift" (type I) reticulocytes are identified as polychromatophilic macroocytes with irregular margins. These cells may also exhibit irregular movements in fresh (wet) preparations.
4. The walls of the marrow sinusoids, which normally retain immature red cells, are modified to facilitate reticulocyte release.

Prostaglandins may enhance erythropoietin activity, either directly (PGE_1) or via renal cyclic AMP (PGE_2). Androgen hormones stimulate erythropoietin activity, either by increasing its production or facilitating its action on the erythroid stem cells. Conversely, estrogens inhibit erythropoietin effects. This may be one of several reasons for the differences in red cell values between males and females. Inhibitory effects can be attributed also to a lipid fraction found in the kidney, and to extracts variously prepared from liver, stomach, and other tissues.

Controversy exists as to the sensing mechanism involved in the erythropoietic response. Red cell values are maintained at a relatively constant steady state, and it is difficult to visualize a mechanism that regulates a slow cellular production response based on sensitivity to rapid but minor changes in tissue oxygen pressure. Although the response to hypoxia is well documented in a variety of species under diverse physiological conditions, the decisive red cell determinants remain elusive; they may include oxyhemoglobin concentration, a hemoglobin degradation product, or some tissue respiratory metabolite (see Chapter 4).

NUTRITIONAL COMPONENTS

Several other chemical constituents play a role in normal red cell production. Iron is required for hemoglobin synthesis: both erythrocyte proliferation and erythrocyte maturation are adversely affected by a low plasma iron concentration. The role of iron is discussed in Chapter 4.

During mitosis, DNA replication occurs as a prelude to cell division. A key step in DNA synthesis requires the presence of metabolites of **folate.** These metabolites result from interactions between dietary folate (methyltetrahydrofolate) and **vitamin B$_{12}$,** an essential nutrient that is also supplied by dietary intake. Without adequate amounts of folate and vitamin B$_{12}$, DNA synthesis and cell maturation are arrested, affecting red blood cell, white blood cell, and platelet production. Cells that are released from the marrow are often large (megaloblastic) and appear to have abnormal nuclei (see Chapter 17, under Megaloblastic Anemias). Vitamin B$_{12}$ also plays a role in carbohydrate and lipid metabolism

(formation of succinyl coenzyme A) and protein synthesis (formation of the amino acid methionine).

ERYTHROKINETICS

The production of red blood cells can be qualitatively assessed by examination of the bone marrow to determine its relative cellularity and the ratio of myeloid to erythroid (M:E) cell precursors (Table 3-1). Normal marrows of adults contain about 50% cells and 50% adipose material and have an M:E ratio in the range of 2.5:1 to 4:1. However, marrow cellularity varies from bone to bone; it is almost 100% in young infants, and it increases in pregnant women during the last trimester. These values are measures of **total erythropoiesis,** the capacity of the marrow to simply produce erythrocytes. Red blood cell turnover is most conveniently measured by the reticulocyte count and expressed as a reticulocyte production index. This value, a measure of **effective erythropoiesis,** represents the red blood cells delivered to the circulating compartment that are viable and that can servein their functional capacity. Other measures of effective production include the peripheral RBC count and the RBC life span.

Measurement of the total circulating red cell mass or volume has been accomplished

Table 3-1. Erythrokinetic data (normal, 70-kg adult)

Measurement	Method	Reference values
Myeloid-erythroid ratio	Marrow count	2.5:1 to 4:1
Mitotic index*	Marrow count	44.8/1000 (4.5%)
Marrow red cell mass	Isotope scan, estimate	100 g
Periperhal blood red cell mass	Isotope label, dilution	2500 g
Reticulocyte count (relative)	Supravital stain, count	0.5% to 1.5%
Reticulocyte count (absolute)	Calculate; direct count	40 to 60 × 10^3/μL
Red cell turnover	Isotope label; calculate	0.9%/day

*Number of cells containing mitotic figures per 1000 marrow normoblasts.

by injecting dyes, such as Evans blue, allowing the dye to circulate, and determining the extent of dye dilution by colorimetric means. Dilution is directly proportional to the red cell volume. Another technique utilized the injection of compatible red cells that contained different antigens. These were then isolated with specific antisera in samples taken at later intervals, and the dilution of the heterogenous cells was used to calculate the total circulating volume. These methods were time consuming and contained large sources of error.

Progress in quantitative measurement of the erythron was accelerated with the introduction of radioisotope tracers during the 1950s. Radioactive isotopes are chemically identical to the naturally occurring stable isotopes, but they possess two properties of importance for application to clinical studies. First, radioisotopes emit gamma waves and/or beta particles with characteristic energies that are detectable at low molecular concentrations. Gamma waves can be located in deep tissues and organs by radiation detectors placed over the body. Although beta emitters are too weak to permit in vivo detection, they can be used to label blood cells and body fluids for in vitro analysis. Second, radioisotopes have characteristic physical decay rates, so that a fixed proportion of the radioactivity is lost in a given time interval. This is conveniently expressed as the "half-life" of the isotope,

or the time interval required for a given level of activity to decrease by 50%. Isotopes with half-lives of days to months can be injected into human subjects to monitor events with durations of days to months. The rapid decay of an isotope makes it possible to administer a tracer more than once without imposing a larger or lasting radiation exposure on the subject. Different isotopes, with different emission energies and decay rates, can also be given simultaneously in order to monitor physiologically interdependent but distinct events.

Two isotopes have been pivotal in defining red cell dynamics: (1) radioactive iron to monitor iron transport, storage, and incorporation into hemoglobin (Chapter 4) and (2) radioactive chromium to directly label the red cell, determine RBC volume and indicate life span. Other useful isotopes include those listed in Table 3-2.

Chromium 51 is added to blood samples in vitro. The labeled chromium enters the RBCs and binds to the beta chain of hemoglobin. After a short incubation period, the labeled blood is returned to the subject and allowed to circulate. Dilution of the radioactivity is directly related to the circulating red cell volume or mass. The radiation intensity of the injected (undiluted) blood sample is compared with counts of a sample drawn after circulation and dilution, resulting in a good estimate of the total red cell volume in milliliters. In order to com-

Table 3-2. Useful isotopes other than iron or chromium

Measurement	Isotope	Half-life	Emission	Form
Red cell volume, red cell survival	Chromium 51	27.8 days	gamma	sodium chromate
Ferrokinetics	Iron 59	45.0 days	gamma	ferric chloride
Red cell survival	Phosphorus 32	14.3 days	beta	difluorophosphate
Spleen scan: RES	Technetium 99m	6 hr	gamma	technetium sulfate

pare blood volumes of subjects at different ages, results are expressed in milliters per kilogram. Although there are problems with chromium elution from the red cells over time (see Chapter 27), the circulating cells can also be sampled over a longer interval to determine mean survival time. As the cells mature and are eventually removed from the circulation, the labeled survivors decline in number, making it possible to calculate the half-life of their survival or presence in the peripheral circulation.

NORMOBLASTIC MATURATION

Hematopoiesis is transferred from the fetal liver to the marrow during the gestational interval of 5 to 7 months. The marrow is organized architecturally into a fine reticular network of connective tissue, which serves as a supporting framework for "islands" of dividing blood cells. Circulating blood enters the marrow cavities via the nutrient arteries of the bones. These arteries branch into a fine capillary system that penetrates the bone's Haversian system, forming a vascular sinusoid within the reticulin. The sinusoids are lined with endothelial cells and a basement membrane, forming a barrier to the release of immature blood cells (erythroblasts or normoblasts, nucleated red blood cells) but providing narrow passageways for the escape of the more flexible mature cells. The capillaries collect into a venous sinus, forming an exit into the general venous circulation.

The focal centers of hematopoietic activity are termed **erythroblastic islands,** each of which consists of a macrophage surrounded by several developing red blood cells (Fig. 3-3). The macrophage (or histiocyte) is believed to accomplish a number of functions: (1) supply the developing ring of erythroblasts with nutrients, including iron; (2) phagocytize the extruded nuclei of these normoblasts as they mature to reticulocytes; and (3) phagocytize senescent red

blood cells that circulate throughout the vascular sinusoids. Each concentric ring of red cell precursors consists of several normoblasts of the same developmental stage. When the marrow is stimulated to produce red cells rapidly **(erythroplasia),** several rings of cells at different maturation stages may be seen around the central macrophage. It should be emphasized that these cellular islands are disrupted during the process of marrow aspiration and smear preparation, so that visualization of the spatial relationship between histiocyte and erythroblasts is best obtained by tissue biopsy. In preparations of living tissue observed by phase microscopy, the star-shaped macrophage is in continuous motion, contacting the surrounding normoblasts with its projecting pseudopods. Electron micrograph studies confirm the intimacy of membrane-to-membrane contact between red cell and macrophage (Bessis, 1977).

The earliest red cell stage that can be positively identified with routine morphological methods is the **pronormoblast** or **rubriblast** (Plate 1, *A*). These cells are derived from committed erythroid progenitors (erythroid stem cells, Fig. 3-2) that respond to the hormone erythropoietin. Erythrocyte stages are defined and characterized in Table 3-3. A summary of morphological features, as seen by light microscopy, is presented as a review aid in the box on page 26 and in Fig. 3-4.

Although they are too small to be seen by light microscopy, from 500 to 1000 **ferritin** molecules can be seen with the electron microscope in the cytoplasm of a rubriblast. These iron granules, to be incorporated into the hemoglobin molecule as the cell matures, positively distinguish the rubriblast from other blood cell blasts. Unfortunately, the granules are not visualized with routine iron stains, as is the ferritin content of more mature normoblasts. The nucleoli are relatively small, and they may be obscured

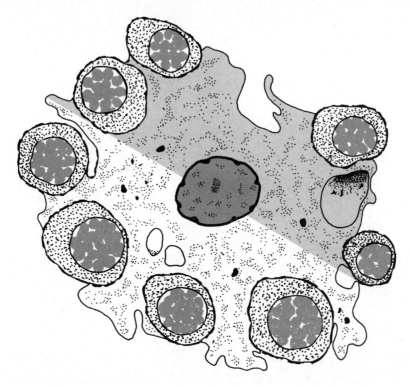

Fig. 3-3.   Erythroblastic island.
Developing normoblasts surround a marrow histiocyte. Marrow aspiration disrupts this structural relationship, but intercellular contact can be observed in living tissue preparations. (Adapted from descriptions and illustrations in Bessis, M: Blood smears reinterpreted, Berlin, 1977, Springer-Verlag).

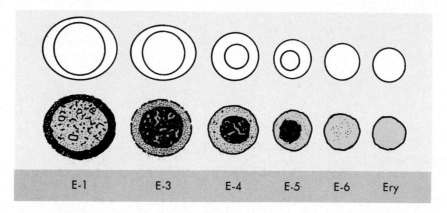

Fig. 3-4.   Normoblastic maturation.
Major changes in cell size, nucleus-to-cytoplasm ratio, and chromatin density occur as normoblasts mature. The changes are gradual, except for nuclear expulsion, which occurs at the end of stage E-5. (See Table 3-3.)

ERYTHROCYTE STAGES: MORPHOLOGICAL CHARACTERISTICS

E_1 rubriblast (pronormoblast; proerythroblast)
Size: 20-25 μm diameter
Shape: irregular, round to oval
Nucleus: comprises 80% of cell; fine reticular appearance, light staining; distinct clumps and linear strands of chromatin; 1 or 2 nucleoli, often bluish on reddish-blue chromatin
Cytoplasm: light blue in earliest cells, becomes a darker royal blue with maturation; characteristic perinuclear halo

E_2-E_3 prorubricyte (basophilic normoblast; early erythroblast)
Size: 12-16 μm diameter
Shape: irregular, round to oval
Nucleus: comprises 75% of cell; chromatin clumped as "chromocenters" of dark stain (basichromatin) against a light red-violet background (oxychromatin); typical cartwheel appearance
Cytoplasm: uniform dark blue, occasionally with a reddish tinge resulting from the early production of hemoglobin

E_4 rubricyte (polychromatophilic normoblast; intermediate erythroblast)
Size: 12-15 μm diameter
Shape: irregular to regular, round
Nucleus: comprises 25% to 50% of cell; very coarse, dark chromatin; retains cartwheel appearance; eccentric location is typical; no nucleoli; nuclear shape is even and round
Cytoplasm: blue-gray to pink-gray; smaller but distinct perinuclear halo; wide variation in color because of rapid production of hemoglobin.

E_5 metarubricyte (orthochromatic or acidophilic normoblast; late erythroblast)
Size: 10-15 μm diameter
Shape: round to slightly oval
Nucleus: comprises about 25% of cell; eccentric location is typical; very dense, pyknotic nucleus with little or no chromatin structure visible; usually round but may be cloverleaf or lobulated; nucleus extruded from cell at end of this stage
Cytoplasm: light pink to slightly blue-gray; perinuclear area may or may not be present

Reticulocyte
Size: 8-10 μm diameter
Shape: round to slightly oval; may be slightly irregular on supravitally stained smears, but very irregular on wet preparations
Cytoplasm: slightly darker than mature erythrocyte, depending on age; progressive loss of organelles (mitochondria and precipitated ribosomes) as visualized by supravital stain

Type 1 reticulocytes
Present in bone marrow and released into peripheral blood as "shift" reticulocytes during accelerated erythropoiesis; these cells have irregular shapes and may exhibit movement in fresh preparations

Type II reticulocytes

Normal peripheral blood reticulocytes with regular cell outlines; do not exhibit
movement in fresh preparations

Stress reticulocytes

Very large cells (macroreticulocytes) with increased hemoglobin content; these
appear during times of high RBC turnover, as in hemolytic anemia

Erythrocyte (mature red blood cell)

Size: 7.4-8.2 μL

Shape: deformable, round biconcave disk

Cytoplasm: pink, with a central area of pallor corresponding to the thinnest area of
the disk; extent of pallor varies with hemoglobin content of cell; transition from
center to edge is gradual

Table 3-3. Stages of erythrocyte maturation

Stage	Name	Hemoglobin (pg)	Interval (hr)	Terminal event	Percent in marrow
E-1	Rubriblast	0.0-14.4	20	Mitosis	0.1-3.5
E-2	Prorubricyte	7.2-21.6	20	Mitosis	1.7-5.5
E-3	Prorubricyte	10.8-25.2	20	Mitosis	
E-4	Rubricyte	12.6-27.0	24	Mitosis	5.0-20.0
E-5	Metarubricyte	13.5-24.5	30	Nuclear expulsion	5.0-23.8
E-6	Reticulocyte	24.5-29.5	70-75	Release from marrow	
Ery	Erythrocyte	29.5-30.5	120 days	Destroyed by RES	

Hemoglobin values from Bessis, M: Blood smears reinterpreted. Berlin, 1977, Springer-Verlag p 26;
intervals from Harris, JW, and Kellermeyer, RW: The red cell, Cambridge, Mass, 1970, Harvard
University Press; terminal events and percent in marrow from Custer, RP: An atlas of the blood
and bone marrow, ed 2, Philadelphia, 1974, WB Saunders Co.

by the blocky patches of nuclear chromatin.
In addition to a perinuclear halo of clear cytoplasm where the Golgi apparatus lies, the
otherwise blue cytoplasm may contain light
staining areas corresponding to the presence
of the centromere and mitochondria. Although barely detectable at this stage, rubriblasts contain up to 14 pg of hemoglobin,
but the intense cytoplasmic basophilia resulting from ribosomal RNA obscures the
acidophilic reaction.

Basophilic normoblasts (prorubricytes)
undergo two mitotic divisions, producing
cells that are smaller in diameter and less
basophilic in cytoplasmic staining (Plate 1,
B). As cellular hemoglobin content increases, the bluish cytoplasm becomes
slightly reddish purple. Also, the nucleus-
to-cytoplasm ratio (N:C) decreases with
each succeeding cell division, and the nuclear chromatin becomes progressively
denser. The patches of chromatin form dark
blocks (chromocenters) that take on a characteristic "cartwheel appearance," making
it easy to distinguish normoblasts from
lymphocytes. Bessis (1977) states that the

number of chromocenters always exceeds 10 (typically between 15 and 20) in normoblasts, whereas plasma cells rarely have more than 9 such clumps. Some of the ferritin molecules may aggregate in cells of this and later stages; these aggregates are visualized with iron stains (Perls' reaction or Prussion blue) with the light microscope as **siderosomes** or siderotic granules. Cells containing visible evidence of these granules are termed **siderocytes.**

Polychromatophilic normoblasts (rubricytes) are characterized by a progressively acidophilic cytoplasm that varies from grayish blue to grayish pink on Wright-stained smears (Plate 1, *C*). The N:C ratio decreases to about 1:3, and the nucleus is often eccentrically located. This is the last red cell stage that is capable of division. Although the nuclear chromatin is dark and coarse, the cartwheel appearance is still evident. Bessis (1977) lists two stages of polychromatophilic normoblasts, I and II, the latter being synonymous with the orthochromatic stage (metarubricyte). Since the latter terms are widely used in the United States, they are retained in this book. As Bessis notes, however, "orthochromatic" is a misnomer, since it implies (incorrectly) that the color and hemoglobin content of a cell at this stage are equivalent to those of the mature erythrocyte.

Orthochromatic normoblasts (metarubricytes) represent the last stage before nuclear expulsion (Plate 1, *D*). The nucleus has become **pyknotic,** with very dark and condensed chromatin, usually obscuring the typical rotary pattern. Cytoplasmic color is gray-pink to pink, reflecting the high hemoglobin content. On stained smears (and especially in wet preparations), the cell outline may be irregular and the shape somewhat distorted. Living cells undergo rapid movements, related to ejection of the nucleus (Fig. 3-5). Cells of this stage usually constitute the "nucleated red blood cells" seen in peripheral blood smears of newborn

infants and during responses to hemolytic crises.

After nuclear expulsion, the red cell membrane rapidly seals and the newly formed **reticulocyte** is retained for about 2 days in the marrow (Plate 1, *E*). As a consequence of normoblast proliferation (amplification) and the maturation interval of this cell stage, the marrow contains approximately equal numbers of reticulocytes and normoblastic precursors. Hemoglobin synthesis proceeds at the ribosomes, despite the loss of the nucleus, and continues throughout the first days of the mature erythrocyte stage. Early reticulocytes will be irregular in shape and larger in size than the more mature forms that are released into the peripheral blood. Under conditions of accelerated red cell production and release, early reticulocytes may appear in the peripheral blood ("shift" reticulocytes). These cells must mature in the peripheral circulation; thus they retain their ribosomal networks for 2 to 3 days. On stained smears, these cells will appear larger and darker **(polychromasia or polychromatophilia)** than most red cells; in wet preparations the cells may exhibit jerky movements. Macroreticulocytes ("stress" reticulocytes) may accompany metarubricytes in the peripheral blood when erythroplasia is marked and the marrow is severely stressed.

The term "reticulocyte" is another misnomer, since the cell does not contain a reticulum. The name is based on the appearance of fine blue granules and threads in cells that have been stained with supravital dyes, such as new methylene blue or brilliant cresyl blue. These dyes precipitate the ribosomes and mitochondria as they kill the cell (hardly supravital, but the designation is widely used), forming the "reticulation." The granules are not seen on Wright-Giemsa stained smears, unless they are first stained with the supravital dye. Although the alcohol in the Wright stain will decolor-

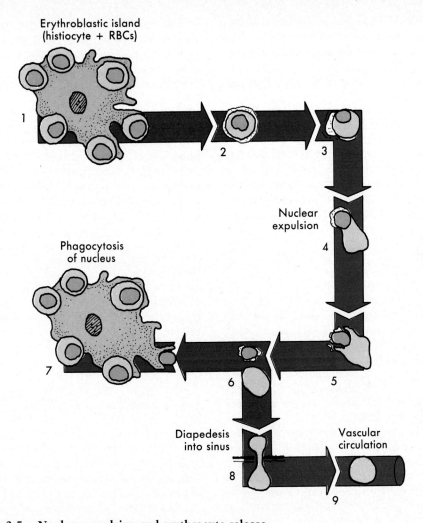

Fig. 3-5. Nuclear expulsion and erythrocyte release.
1, Normoblasts mature at the periphery of a marrow histiocyte. *2,* Orthochromic normoblasts break free from the erythroblastic island, retaining a "coat" of cytoplasm from the histiocyte. *3,* Convulsions signal the onset of nuclear expulsion *(4 and 5)* and the birth of the anucleate reticulocyte *(6)*. *7,* Marrow histiocytes (macrophages) may engulf the nucleus. *8,* After 2 to 3 days' maturation, the reticulocyte passes through the marrow sinusoidal wall (diapedesis) into the vascular circulation, where it matures to an erythrocyte *(9)*.

ize the ribosomes, the methylene blue will restain and render the reticulocytes visible for easy enumeration (Plate 1, *F*).

Reticulocytes cross from the marrow tissue into the vascular sinusoids by **diapedesis,** an amoeboid-like movement by pseudopod extension through the small gaps of the capillary wall. Although newly-formed reticulocytes are capable of considerable distension and movement, they do not locomote in the manner of white blood cells, which also cross vessel walls by the process of diapedesis. Normally, the structure of the sinusoidal barrier retains the rigid, nucleated normoblasts, whereas the deformable reticulocyte "slips" through. Thus, passage into the peripheral circulation is a function of cellular maturity as determined by membrane properties.

When the remaining organelles of the reticulocyte have disappeared and the red cell assumes its discoid shape and full hemoglobin content, the mature erythrocyte results. This anucleate, highly deformable cell will transport oxygen and other respiratory gases through some 300 miles of blood vessels during its estimated lifespan of 120 days.

EXTRAMEDULLARY HEMATOPOIESIS

Once the bone marrow assumes its role as the only site for blood cell production (excluding lymphocytes), hematopoiesis is restricted to medullary areas of the axial skeleton and proximal ends of the long bones. In certain disease states, however, increased demand for red blood cells results in conversion of the fatty marrow into red marrow. If the red marrow is not sufficient to meet the demand for new blood cells, as in cases of severe hemolytic anemias, the liver may also revert to its fetal hematopoietic function. This organ retains poorly differentiated mesenchymal cells that are apparently able to develop into selectively specialized blood cell lines (e.g., granulocyte, normoblast) when appropriately stimulated. The spleen has also been implicated as an "extramedullary" site, but recent evidence suggests that the erythrocyte precursors seen in sections of spleen may have originated elsewhere (Wolf et al., 1983). Miale (1982) lists 27 different sites apart from the marrow in which blood cell production can occur. These are mainly foci of "ectopic" hematopoiesis, sites different from those of normal fetal activity.

The potential for extramedullary hematopoiesis declines with age. Infants revert readily to hepatic blood cell production, because very little fatty tissue occupies the marrow and the marrow is already producing blood cells at full capacity. A response to erythrocyte destruction (hemolytic anemia) in adults will be met by the nonproductive marrow space first. Hepatic production becomes less likely in older adults. Conditions that result in a displacement of marrow hematopoietic tissue by fibrous tissue (myelofibrosis and myelosclerosis) or by invading and expanding tumor tissue (myeloid leukemias, lymphomas, sarcomas, myelomas, metastatic infiltrations) may also result in compensatory blood cell production at other sites. The onset of these conditions may be accompanied by the appearance of normoblasts in the peripheral blood as the marrow stromal architecture is disrupted by the fibrotic or neoplastic changes.

SENESCENCE AND REMOVAL

Red blood cells accumulate a considerable amount of membrane damage during their functional life spans. Various chemical substances encountered in the bloodstream may attach to or alter the membrane. Byproducts of metabolism often result in intracellular inclusions that mark the erythrocyte as either abnormal or senescent. As the red cell ages, the membrane becomes less pliable and the cell is less able to deform as it passes throughout the narrow spaces of the microcirculation. Some membrane surface area is lost as phagocytes of the liver and spleen remove the accumulated molecules, attached antibodies, and other debris. As a result, cell volume decreases and hemoglobin concentration increases, adding to the loss of cell deformability. Although some red blood cells lyse spontaneously in the blood vessels (**intravascular hemolysis**), under normal conditions most cells are destroyed outside of the blood vessels (**extravascular hemolysis**) by phagocytic histiocytes (macrophages) of the reticuloendothelial system (RES), located within the spleen, liver, and bone marrow.

Red cells receive the greatest stress within the red pulp of the spleen. Erythrocytes pack together (plasma volume decreases) and pass slowly through a highly reticulated network of splenic tissue. In order to return to the venous circulation, the RBCs (7 to 8 μm in diameter) must pass through small pores (2 to 3 μm in diameter) in the sinusoidal membrane. Cells that are too rigid, either because of membrane inelasticity or because of intracellular deposits (e.g., metabolic precipitates, hemoglobin crystals) are engulfed partly or entirely by the macrophages. Depending on the nature and extent of the erythrocyte abnormality, the inclusion may be extracted ("pitting"), a small part of the membrane may be removed (resulting in a schizocyte or red fragment), or the cell may be completely destroyed.

The splenic macrophages are particularly efficient at monitoring red cells for the presence of attached immunoglobulins (antibodies). The macrophages possess receptors for the Fc portion of an IgG antibody molecule; detection results in phagocytosis of the red cell. Similarly, hepatic and splenic macrophages detect the C3b component of complement, a protein that is fixed to the red cell membrane during many antigen-antibody reactions. Thus, transfused red blood cells with major antigenic differences may be marked by the immune system as "foreign" and eliminated by the RES. Some drugs can alter the molecular structures on the membranes of erythrocytes, whether autogenous (one's own) or transfused, so that they also are detected as "foreign" by RES macrophages (see Acquired Hemolytic Anemia, in Chapter 19).

Red cell destruction by the RES macrophages results in recycling of some of the cellular components for incorporation into new normoblasts, whereas other materials are degraded and excreted (Fig. 3-6). Hemoglobin is degraded into iron, protoporphyrin, and globin. Iron is either transported to marrow RBC production sites by transferrin or stored in the macrophage in the form of ferritin and hemosiderin. The globin chain is degraded for transportation in the plasma to join the general amino acid pool. The remainder of the porphyrin structure is degraded by macrophage enzymes to the compound **bilirubin**; it is subsequently transported to the liver by plasma albumin. Hepatocytes in the liver attach glucuronide to the bilirubin to produce a conjugated (direct) form of bilirubin that is excreted in the bile. As this compound, now termed mesobilinogen, passes through the intestine, it is transformed by bacterial action into the pigmented compounds, **urobilinogen** and stercobilinogen. About 70% to 80% of these compounds are eliminated as fecal urobilin and sterocobilin, and the remainder is reabsorbed into the portal circulation, where it either recirculates through the liver (enterohepatic cycle) or is excreted through the kidneys (also as urobilin and stercobilin).

The levels of a number of these degradation products can be measured in order to assess the amount of extravascular hemolysis occurring in various disorders. Indirect bilirubin levels in the plasma are indications of the quantity of protoporphyrin degraded. As the porphyrin ring is opened, a carbon and attached oxygen (carbon monoxide) are passed into the plasma, transported to the lungs, and exhaled. The level of carbon monoxide in expired air is a sensitive indicator of red cell breakdown. Urobilinogen excretion increases when red cell destruction increases, and these pigments are easily measured in the urine.

Intravascular hemolysis usually accounts for less than 10% of red cell destruction. When red cells lyse, hemoglobin is released directly into the plasma. The molecule, a tetramer of four globin chains (see Chapter

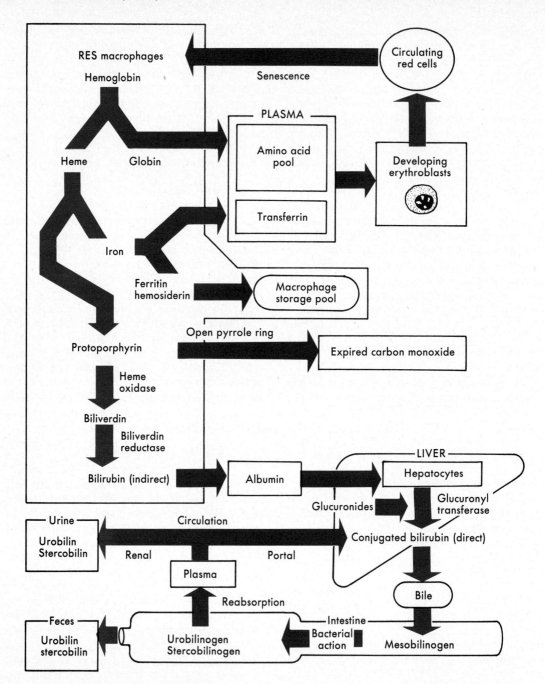

Fig. 3-6. Extravascular hemolysis.
The major pathways of red cell destruction and hemoglobin degradation involving the reticuloendothelial system. Compare this diagram with Figs. 2-2 and 3-7.

4), rapidly dissociates into two dimers (each consisting of an alpha globin and a beta globin). The dimers attach to a circulating plasma protein, **haptoglobin,** to form a large molecular complex (Fig. 3-7). Formation of the haptoglobin-hemoglobin complex prevents glomerular filtration and excretion by the kidney. RES macrophages, primarily in the liver, ingest and process hemoglobin (and haptoglobin!) in a manner similar to

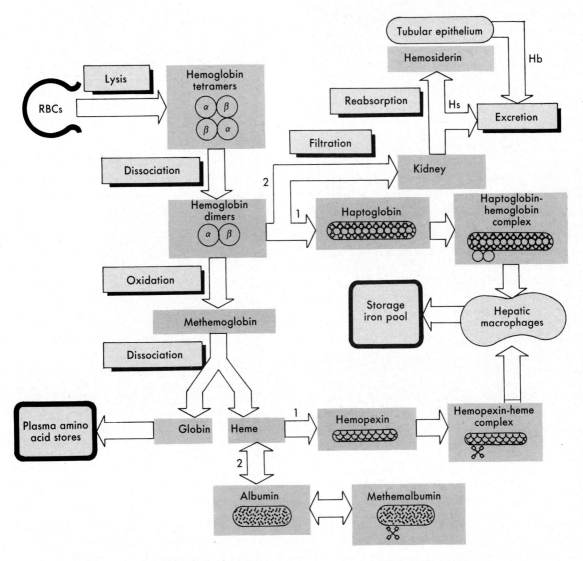

Fig. 3-7.   Intravascular hemolysis.
Pathways of hemoglobin transport resulting from red cell destruction in the blood vessels. After hemoglobin and heme arrive at the hepatic macrophages, degradation follows essentially the same pattern as that seen in extravascular hemolysis (Fig. 3-6).

what occurs during extravascular hemolysis. The concentration of haptoglobin is not sufficient to bind large amounts of hemoglobin that might be released during major hemolytic events, such as an immune reaction to incompatible blood. Some plasma hemoglobin that is not bound to haptoglobin is oxidized to **methemoglobin,** a form in which the central iron molecule is in the ferric (+3) state. Methemoglobin also dissociates, but as heme and globin. The heme attaches to a plasma protein, **hemopexin,** which is also cleared from the circulation by hepatic macrophages. If hemopexin is also depleted, because of a large concentration of free hemoglobin, heme unites with the abundant plasma protein, albumin, to form **methemalbumin.** Heme remains bound to this protein until additional hemopexin is manufactured.

Some amounts of free hemoglobin, in the dimeric form, are passed through the glomerulus. Up to 5 g/day of the filtered hemoglobin can be reabsorbed by the renal tubular cells, where the iron is released and stored as hemosiderin. Most of this iron is lost because the tubular cells are shed and excreted in the urine. Filtered hemoglobin in excess of the tubular reabsorption capacity is excreted in the urine, either as free hemoglobin or as methemoglobin.

Therefore, intravascular hemolysis can be detected by: (1) increased plasma hemoglobin, (2) decreased plasma haptoglobin, (3) the presence of plasma methemalbumin, (4) free urinary hemoglobin or methemoglobin, or (5) the presence of products processed by the RES as in extravascular hemolysis: increased bilirubin and urobilinogen.

SUMMARY

- Red cell production begins in the embryonic yolk sac at 3 weeks of gestation; production occurs predominately in the liver from 5 weeks until about 6 months of fetal age, when liver production is replaced by marrow production. Adult blood cell production is confined mainly to the axial skeleton.
- Red cell production is regulated by concentrations of oxygen in tissues. Oxygen tension is a function of environmental availability, pulmonary function, circulatory efficiency, hemoglobin concentration, and binding capacity.
- Physiological adaptations to oxygen need and availability occur: acclimation is a result of increased production (erythrocytosis), leading to increased red cell mass, hemoglobin concentration, and blood viscocity.
- Erythropoietic response is mediated by the hormone erythropoietin, which stimulates stem cell proliferation, acceleration of normoblastic maturation, and release of immature reticulocytes.
- Production of mature red cells requires iron for hemoglobin synthesis and folate and vitamin B_{12} for DNA synthesis.
- Assessment of red cell production and survival (erythrokinetics) utilizes measures of marrow cell content, reticulocyte production, and red cell mass; radioisotope techniques can trace red cell circulation patterns and establish sites and rates of destruction.
- Morphological stages of maturation can be identified with a light microscope; changes in nuclear chromatin density, nucleus-to-cytoplasm ratio, and cytoplasm color are important characteristics.
- Red blood cells are destroyed by intravascular hemolysis or by removal during passage through the spleen and the liver (extravascular hemolysis). Hemoglobin components are recycled (iron, amino acids of the globin chain) or excreted (porphyrin). Degradation by-products, such as bilirubin and urobilinogen, are indicative of red cell destruction.

4

Hemoglobin

Hemoglobin transports respiratory gases, and red blood cells transport hemoglobin. Therefore, the key to understanding the majority of red cell disorders is found in the metabolic pathways that assemble and maintain the hemoglobin molecule. Assembly involves (1) the construction of a series of tetrapyrrole ring compounds, terminating in **protoporphyrin**, (2) the formation of amino acids into polypeptide chains (**globins**), and (3) the incorporation of iron into the porphyrin rings (**heme**). Iron metabolism deserves special attention, since it is a critical process in the manufacture of hemoglobin. A disruption of the iron supply to developing erythroblasts results in a common type of anemia. Finally, this chapter examines interactions between hemoglobin and other molecules as part of the respiratory process: how hemoglobin acquires, transports, and releases oxygen at various tissue sites.

HEMOGLOBIN STRUCTURE

Hemoglobin has a molecular weight of 68,000 daltons; it comprises four chains of amino acids, each attached to a heme component (Fig. 4-1). It is the heme molecules that impart the characteristic red color to erythrocytes. The hemoglobin molecule is spatially organized, as are other proteins, at different structural levels of molecular bonding. The primary structure consists of a linear sequence of amino acids, joined by covalent bonds, composing the polypeptide chains. The peptide chains form a helix

(secondary structure), maintained by hydrogen bonds between the carbonyl (C=10) and amide (N-H) groups of certain peptides. The helix folds into a compact, roughly spherical form resembling a pretzel (tertiary structure), also maintained by hydrogen bonds, salt bridges, and van der Waals interactions. The tertiary structure is thus a monomer, consisting of a globin chain and heme group. Most of the charged (polar) amino acids face the exterior of the molecule, and most of the nonpolar amino acids are located in the interior. This electrically charged surface is an important characteristic for identifying different types of hemoglobins by electrophoretic migration. Monomers can form aggregates (quaternary structure): two chains become a dimer, and four chains form a **tetramer**. Hemoglobin in its functional form is a tetramer, consisting of two pairs of globin-heme spheres (Fig. 4-2).

Although porphyrin synthesis is constant throughout life, assembly of the globin chains differs at various stages of fetal and postnatal life. These different polypeptide structures impart varying oxygen-binding capabilities to the hemoglobin molecule, corresponding to the physiological requirements of intrauterine development. The first chains to be synthesized, between 6 and 10 weeks gestation, are designated epsilon (ϵ); a tetramer of four (ϵ_4) is named hemoglobin Gower 1. Beginning at 7 to 8 weeks of gestation, alpha (α) chains are produced; these continue to be made throughout fetal and adult life (Fig. 4-3). Initially,

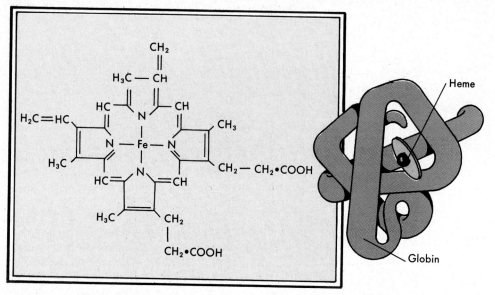

Fig. 4-1.   Structure of hemoglobin.
A, Molecular formula of heme. Each tetraporphyrin ring contains a single iron atom. **B,** Location of heme within the folded globin chain.

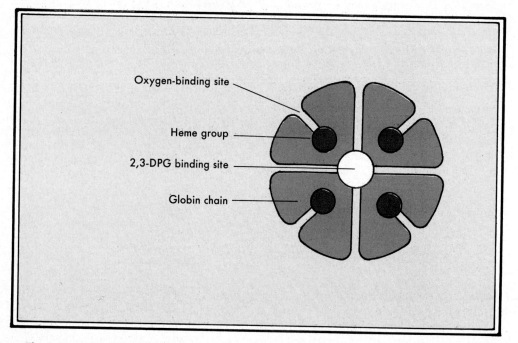

Fig. 4-2.   Hemoglobin tetramer.
Schematic model of monomer arrangement and binding sites for 2,3-DPG and oxygen.

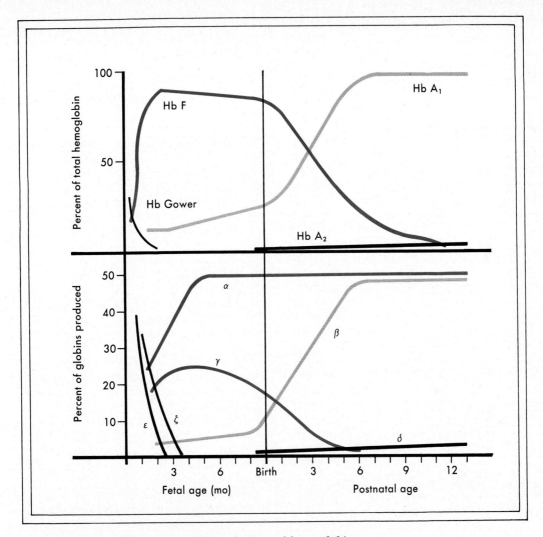

Fig. 4-3.   Development of globin chains and hemoglobins.
Sequential appearance of globin chains at different gestational and postnatal ages. Embryonic hemoglobins are produced by mesenchymal cells of the yolk sac. Production of alpha chains is required in order to produce every type of fetal and adult hemoglobin (except Portland), first in the fetal liver and subsequently in the marrow. Low beta chain production can be partially compensated for by postnatal retention of gamma chain production. Decreased alpha chain production results in a serious hemoglobin deficiency.

two alpha and two epsilon chains form a tetramer $(\alpha_2\epsilon_2)$ designated Gower 2. This is a transient hemoglobin, and it is rapidly replaced by tetramers of **hemoglobin F** (Hb F, fetal hemoglobin), consisting of two alpha and two gamma chains $(\alpha_2\gamma_2)$. Another transient hemoglobin, Portland, consists of two zeta chains and two gamma chains $(\zeta_2\gamma_2)$. Note the distinction between names of hemoglobins (tetramers) and the individual polypeptide chains (monomers) (Table 4-1). Gamma chain production declines during the third trimester of fetal life, corresponding to an increased production of beta chains. The alph-beta combination is designated Hb A (for adult) or, more specifically, **HB A$_1$,** becoming the predominant molecule within 4 to 6 weeks after birth. A fifth type of chain, delta, is also produced, beginning shortly before birth and persisting throughout adult life. Tetramers of alpha and delta chains ($\alpha_2\delta_2$) are designated **HB A$_2$.** Production of each of these chains is regulated by structural genes that are switched "on" or "off" at the appropriate developmental age by regulator and operator genes. Genes for the alpha chain are located on chromosome 16, and genes for the beta, gamma, delta, and epsilon chains are located on chromosome 11. The complete sequences of amino acids for the alpha chain (141 aa) and beta chain (146 aa) are known. Abnormalities involving structural genes result in abnormal amino acid sequences, with varying consequences for the functional properties of the resulting hemoglobin (see Chapter 18). Dysfunction of operator or regulator genes may result in the failure of a chain to appear at the expected developmental age or the persistence of a fetal type of hemoglobin during postnatal life. Other hereditary disorders affect the production rate of a particular globin chain.

HEMOGLOBIN SYNTHESIS

Each type of chain is manufactured by ribosomes in the red cell cytoplasm according to the instructions contained in the nucleotidyl sequences of structural genes **(deoxyribonucleic acid,** or **DNA)** in the nucleus. A specific gene codes for each type of polypeptide. The nuclear instructions are copied by a DNA duplicating process called **replication** before division of the cell. The assembly instructions are carried to the ribosome by **messenger ribonucleic acid (mRNA),** which is produced from the DNA by the process of **transcription.** Transcription requires an enzyme, RNA polymerase. The nucleotidyl sequence ("message") of the mRNA segment specifies the amino acid sequence for a particular type of polypeptide chain. The ribosome also consists of RNA (**rRNA,** for ribosomal) and protein; the ribosome constructs the polypeptide according to the coded message, the process of **translation.** Transfer RNAs **(tRNA)** present in the cytoplasm carry specific amino acids to the ribosomes to be attached to the growing peptide. A general, much simplified scheme of the assembly sequence is shown in Fig. 4-4.

Hemoglobin synthesis begins in the basophilic normoblast (E_2), as evidenced in electron micrographs, well before changes in color of the cytoplasm are detected on Wright-stained smears. At the time of nuclear expulsion, about two thirds of the eventual hemoglobin content of the mature cell has been realized; the remainder is synthesized by the anucleated reticulocyte. Note that polypeptide assembly occurs in the cytoplasm. Once the mRNA segment has been produced and received by the ribosome, protein synthesis occurs independent of the nucleus. Gradual loss of the remaining mitochondria and mRNA as the reticulocyte enters the peripheral circulation sig-

Table 4-1. Hemoglobin nomenclature

Peptide chains	Tetramer name	Occurrence
ϵ_4	Gower 1	yolk sac (primitive) erythroblasts
$\alpha_2\epsilon_2$	Gower 2	yolk sac (primitive) erythroblasts
$\zeta_2\gamma_2$	Portland 1	yolk sac (primitive) erythroblasts
$\alpha_2\gamma_2$	Hb F (fetal)	major fetal hemoglobin (<1 % in adults)
$\alpha_2\beta_2$	Hb A$_1$	major adult hemoglobin (98%)
$\alpha_2\delta_2$	Hb A$_2$	minor adult hemoglobin (1%-2%)

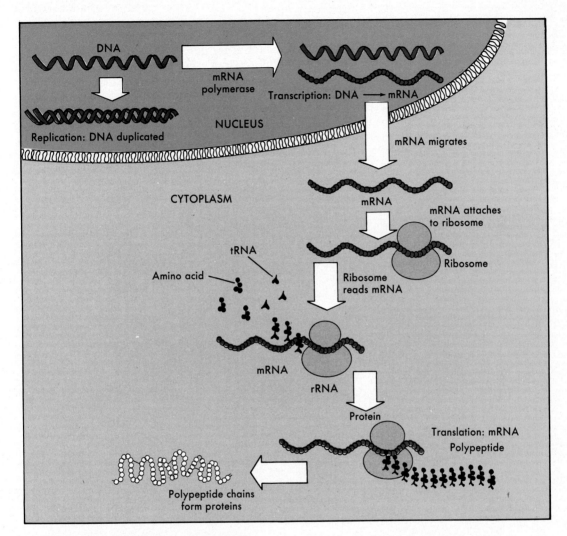

Fig. 4-4.   From DNA to polypeptide.
DNA is replicated in the nucleus during cell division. A DNA sequence contains the instructions for assembling a polypeptide chain. A complementary template of DNA, in the form of messenger RNA (mRNA), is created during transcription. The coded message passes from the nucleus to the cytoplasm to attach to a ribosome. The ribosome "reads" the mRNA sequence. Each codon of three nucleotides specifies a reaction with a species of transfer RNA (tRNA), which in turn presents a specific amino acid to the ribosome. The amino acids are attached in a linear sequence that corresponds to the nucleotidyl code of the mRNA. Translation results in polypeptide chains that are assembled with the help of specific enzymes to form complex proteins.

nals the end of hemoglobin synthesis. The average mature erythrocyte will contain approximately 640 million tetramers of hemoglobin.

Assembly of the heme structure occurs within the mitochondria and in the cytoplasm (Fig. 4-5). The major steps include (1) the formation of a porphyrin precursor from products of the Krebs (tricarboxylic acid) cycle in the mitochondrion; (2) transfer of the precursor to the cytoplasm and formation of the porphyrin ring; (3) assembly of porphyrin rings into a sequential series of four-ringed structures; (4) return of the four-ringed structure to the mitochondrion for transformation to protoporphyin; and (5) insertion of the iron molecule into protoporphyrin to form heme. Each step of heme synthesis involves a specific enzyme, and only trace amounts of excess porphyrin compounds are produced at various steps of the pathway. Excess por-

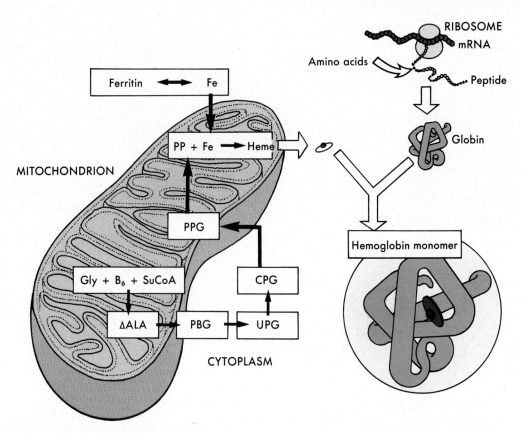

Fig. 4-5. Synthesis of hemoglobin.
Products of the Krebs cycle, glycine *(Gly)* and succinyl coenzyme A *(SuCoA)*, with pyridoxyl phosphate (vitamin B_6) form δ-aminolevulinic acid *(ALA)* in the mitochondrion. ALA passes into the cytoplasm, where enzymes convert it to porphobilinogen *(PBG)*, uroporphrinogen *(UPG)*, and coproporphrinogen *(CPG)*. CPG returns to the mitochondrion for conversion to protoporphrinogen *(PPG)* and protoporphyrin *(PP)*. Iron, derived from intracellular ferritin stores, is inserted into the protoporphyrin ring, resulting in heme. Globins manufactured by ribosomes combine with heme to form the hemoglobin monomer.

phyrin is complexed to zinc and can be measured as **free erythrocyte protoporphyrin (FEP)**. Regulation of protoporphyrin production is precisely controlled to correlate with globin production and available iron supply. Several disorders of hemoglobin synthesis can be detected when porphyrin compounds are produced and excreted in increased quantities or as altered forms of porphyrin.

Formation of the porphyrin precursor occurs within the mitochrondrion: (1) **pyridoxal phosphate (vitamin B$_6$)** forms a base derivative with glycine, and this combines with succinylcoenzyme A (produced by the tricarboxylic acid cycle) to form δ-aminoketoadipic acid; (b) this latter compound is decarboxylated by δ-**aminolevulinic acid synthase** to form δ-**aminolevulinate (ALA)**, which then passes from the mitochondrion to the cytoplasm. This is an important rate-limiting step in heme synthesis. ALA synthase is an inducible enzyme, in that its activity is affected by a large number of compound (e.g., inhibition by carbohydrates and stimulation by steroids and barbiturates). Levels of this enzyme are increased in various disorders of porphyria (Chapter 18). The action of pyridoxal phosphate is stimulated by erythropoietin, and it is inhibited by the accumulation of heme (when globin production is insufficient).

Two molecules of δ-aminolevulinate combine to form one molecule of **porphobilinogen (PBG)**, a porphyrin precursor with a single pyrrole ring. This reaction is mediated by porphobilinogen synthase, a cytoplasmic enzyme that requires zinc as a cofactor. A pair of enzymes work in concert to produce deamination and condensation of four molecules of PBG into a complex structure, **uroporphyrinogen III (UPG)**, containing four pyrrole rings. Uroporphyrinogen I synthase produces a transient molecule (uroporphyrinogen I), which is probably converted to UPG III by uroporphyrinogen III cosynthase. Only the type III compounds are precursors to heme. The type I isomers

may accumulate if enzymes of the normal pathway are destroyed by heavy metals or toxins. UPG III is converted to **coproporphyrinogen III (CPG)** by coproporphyrinogen decarboxylase.

CPG III enters the mitochondrion to be converted to **protoporphyrinogen IX (PPG)** by the action of coproporphyrinogen oxidase. Protoporphyrinogen oxidase converts PPG to the immediate precursor to heme, **protoporphyrin.** Finally, a single ferrous (+2) iron molecule is inserted into the ring structure, by the chelating action of **heme synthase** (ferrochelatase), to form **heme.** Heme leaves the mitochondrion to combine with a globin chain, forming a hemoglobin monomer.

Reticulocyte mitochondria decrease in number as the cell matures, resulting in a loss of the enzymes forming the first and last products of the heme synthesis pathway. The cytoplasmic enzymes are retained, however. Because protoporphyrin is a fluorescent molecule and much of it has not been converted to heme in the reticulocyte, these cells will fluoresce when exposed to ultraviolet light. This provides a means of automated reticulocyte counting to assess red cell production.

IRON METABOLISM

The final step in heme production requires delivery of ferrous iron to the normoblastic mitochondria. Iron is initially supplied by dietary intake, but as indicated in Chapter 3, iron is released from old red blood cells as they are destroyed by RES macrophages. Iron is thus retained, stored, and recycled for new hemoglobin synthesis in developing normoblasts. Ferrokinetics is the quantitative study of iron transport, storage, and utilization in the body. As was the case for erythrokinetics, radioisotopic tracers have been important tools for determining the pathways of iron movement. The major steps include (1) ingestion and ionic conversion of dietary iron; (2) absorption and storage in cells of the intestinal mucosa; (3) transport by plasma proteins to sites of utilization; (4) assimilation into developing normoblasts and other cellular sites of iron-containing molecules; and (5) incorporation into target molecules, such as hemoglobin, myoglobin, and cytochrome enzymes.

Iron intake and utilization can be conveniently modeled as compartments (Table 4-2), which also facilitates a discussion of approaches and methods to evaluate the iron status of an individual. The values presented in Table 4-2 are idealized averages, based on several sources. An overview of ferrokinetics (Fig. 4-6) also utilizes idealized values to demonstrate the input and output relationships between various iron compartments. The route by which iron travels to enter the red blood cell is diagrammed in Fig. 4-7 and detailed in the text below.

Ingestion. A balanced Western diet contains about 6 mg of iron for each 1000 calories of foodstuff. Based on typical caloric intakes of 2000 to 3000 calories per day, about 12 to 18 mg of iron are ingested each day. Specific foods vary greatly in iron content, and the amount of iron available is further complicated by the presence of other compounds that may facilitate or inhibit iron absorption. For example, meats rich in heme protein, such as liver (6.5 mg of iron per 100 g wet weight), contain iron that is readily absorbed, whereas bran cereals (16 mg/100 g) also contain phytates, which inhibit iron absorption. Fruits may not have high iron contents (grapefruit has 0.04 mg/100g), but high ascorbic acid (vitamin C) content enhances the absorption of what iron is present. Iron is present in food materials chiefly as ferric-protein complexes, heme-protein compounds, and ferric and ferrous hydroxides. The stomach provides an acid environment that simplifies the protein complexes and helps reduce ferric iron (Fe^{+3}) to the ferrous (Fe^{+2}) state. However, gastric hydrochloric acid, once thought to play a major part in converting iron to the absorbable ferrous state, is now thought to play only a supplementary role. The type of iron in foods ingested and the presence of enhancers and inhibitors are thought to be of more importance. There may also be some other substance, present in gastric fluid, that enhances the reduction of iron.

Absorption. Reduced iron is passed into the small intestine; absorption occurs mainly in the duodenum and to a lesser extent in the jejenum, where alkaline conditions favor the formation of ferrous hydrox-

Table 4-2. Ferrokinetic data

Compartment	Male	Female
Input-output		
Dietary ingestion	15 mg/day	15 mg/day
Absorption	1 mg/day (7%)	2 mg/day (13%)
Loss (mucosal + hemorrhage)	1 mg/day (7%)	2mg/ day (13%)
Pools		
Transport (transferrin)	5 mg (<1%)	4 mg (<1%)
Storage (ferritin + hemosiderin)	1000 mg (27%)	300 mg (14%)
Hemoglobin	2400 mg (66%)	1700 mg (77%)
Myoglobin	150 mg (4%)	120 mg (5%)
Enzymes (tissue iron)	20 mg (<1%)	15 mg (<1%)
Labile (see text)	75 mg (2%)	60 mg (3%)
TOTAL IRON	3650 mg	2200 mg

ide, the inorganic form of iron that can be transported across the intestinal cell membranes. Except for heme-protein, other forms of iron are excreted in the feces. The amount of available iron absorbed is dependent on several factors, some of which are still subjects of controversy among investigators. Generally, persons with normal body stores of iron, as reflected in plasma and tissue iron content, absorb about 5% to 10% of the iron presented to the mucosal cells. Women who are actively menstruating and children who are growing rapidly have greater demands, and they normally absorb 10% to 15% of the available iron. Since the caloric intake and the total amount of available iron per day is usually

less for women and children, the higher percentage of absorption only partially compensates for the amount of iron needed. Approximately 1.0 mg of iron per day is absorbed by a normal adult male and about 1.5 mg per day by a normal adult female. Persons with depleted iron stores, such as postpartum women and those suffering from chronic iron deficiency, can absorb up to 25% of the available iron. Increased absorption rates also occur in individuals with elevated erythropoietic activity, because of mechanisms that appear to be independent of iron stores. Increased ingestion of iron will result in an increase in *total* iron absorption, even though the *percent* of available iron that is absorbed decreases.

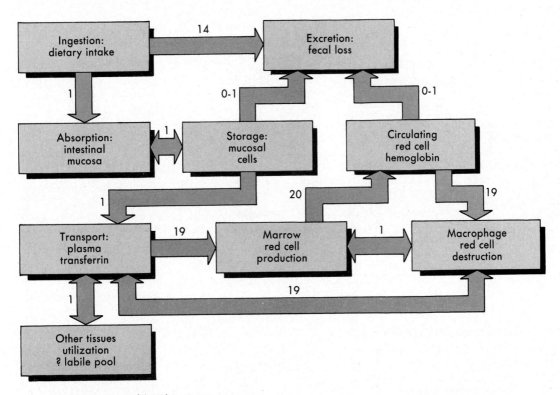

Fig. 4-6. Ferrokinetic compartments.
Numbers indicate amounts of iron (milligrams per day) that are transported between body compartments. These values do not reflect age and sex differences or account for variability in dietary habits.

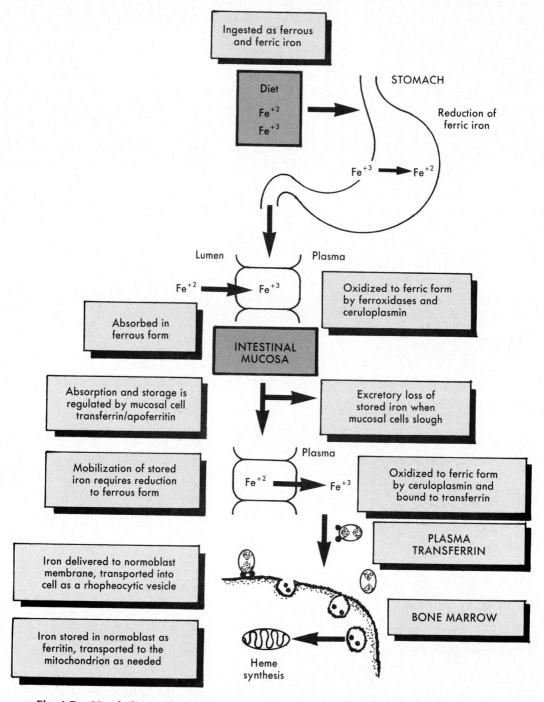

Fig. 4-7.   Metabolic pathways of iron.
Iron undergoes numerous ionic conversions during digestion, transport, and utilization.

Absorption appears to be regulated, in part, by the concentration of apoferritin and transferrin in the mucosal cell cytoplasm. **Apoferritin** is a water-soluble protein that can bind with Fe^{+2} to form **ferritin,** the primary storage form of iron. Each molecule of apoferritin can combine with up to 4000 atoms of iron (2000 or less is a more common ratio), so that the combined molecular weight of 465,000 daltons for ferritin is about 20% iron by weight. The iron is bound as a ferric oxyhydroxide core ($FeOOH$). Mobilization to or from the surrounding apoferritin shell occurs in the Fe^{+2} state, a transition in which ascorbic acid is a cofactor. Thus, absorbed Fe^{+2} is oxidized to Fe^{+3} as it is bound as ferritin, and then the Fe^{+3} is reduced to Fe^{+2} for release from the mucosal cells into the plasma of the portal circulation.

Increased iron concentration may stimulate apoferritin synthesis, assuring the availability of a storage site. Increased concentrations of the iron-transport protein transferrin may also play a role in increasing mucosal-cell iron absorption from the intestinal lumen. Previously, evidence appeared to indicate that the mucosal cells controlled iron uptake directly ("mucosal block"), but regulation of absorption is probably a complex interaction of erythropoietic activities, iron stores, and availability of transport proteins. The mucosal cells do represent a site of iron loss from the body, since these cells are shed into the intestinal lumen with their iron stores. Intestinal loss and incidental bleeding average about 1 mg per day.

Transport. Fe^{+2}, after release from the mucosal cell, is oxidized to Fe^{+3} by a copper-containing enzyme, **ceruloplasmin (CER).** Ceruloplasmin is an alpha$_2$-glycoprotein of about 120,000 to 160,000 daltons. Adult serum levels are 18 to 45 mg/dL, by nephelometric assay. Ferric iron is rapidly bound to **apotransferrin,** a beta$_1$ globulin weighing 75,000 daltons. Each molecule can bind two atoms of Fe^{+3} plus two molecules of bicarbonate (HCO_3^-), forming the iron-transporting complex, **transferrin (TRF).** Transferrin is synthesized mainly in the liver, with smaller amounts produced by the reticuloendothelial system and testes or ovaries. Adult serum concentrations are 220 to 400 mg/dL, as measured by nephelometry. Each milligram of TRF can bind 1.25 μg of iron. A widely used method to assay transferrin is to fully saturate the protein with iron and measure the resulting iron concentration, resulting in the **total iron-binding capacity (TIBC).** Actually, the TIBC overestimates transferrin by about 10% to 15%, because iron in higher concentrations also binds to albumin and other plasma proteins. The normal range for TIBC is 300 to 360 μg/dL. When serum iron concentrations are normal (70 to 180 μg/dL), about 30% to 35% of the TRF is saturated with iron. Serum iron concentrations, TIBC, and percent saturation are determinations in wide use to screen for disorders involving iron metabolism and chronic anemias (Chapter 18).

Transferrin transports iron from mucosal cells and from RES phagocytes in the liver, spleen, and bone marrow to cellular sites of iron utilization. Most of the iron goes to developing normoblasts, but some is delivered to the "tissue iron" pool for incorporation into myoglobin and various enzymes, such as cytochromes, catalase, peroxidases, and the flavoproteins.

More than 30 genetic variants of transferrin are known, based on patterns of migration on starch gel electrophoresis, but no differences in iron-binding or transport properties are apparent. Transferrin type C is present in 99% of American whites and 90% of American blacks; other transferrin types have been identified in association with specific ethnic groups.

Transmembrane transport. Transferrin delivers its two iron molecules directly to the normoblast membrane, where it binds with a specific receptor. The cell membrane invaginates, and the transferrin enters the cytoplasm as a vacuole (the process is called rhopheocytosis and the resulting vacuoles are rhopheocytic vesicles). By mechanisms not yet fully understood, the transferrin releases the iron atoms and returns to the plasma as apotransferrin to begin a new cycle of transport. Transferrin, or a molecule closely related to it, may be a component of the cytoplasm of various cells in which iron processing occurs.

Iron storage. Iron that is not incorporated into hemoglobin or other molecules is stored primarily as ferritin, by the same process described above for mucosal cells. Ferritin aggregates can be observed in tissues by electron microscopy, but not with the light microscope. Because ferritin is water soluble and forms relatively small aggregates, mobilization for transport or use is rapid; all normoblasts contain some ferritin deposits. A second form of storage is also present in the majority of normoblasts: **hemosiderin,** a larger aggregate that is not water soluble and releases iron at a much slower rate. This complex is about 37% iron by weight, and it is large enough to be seen in the light microscope, appearing as golden-brown refractile granules. The granules react with potassium ferrocyanide (**Prussian blue** or Perls' reaction) to stain light blue-green. This provides a convenient means of estimating iron stores in bone marrow, liver, and other tissues (Chapter 26). About 40% to 60% of the nucleated red blood cells will stain positively for iron; these are referred to as **sideroblasts** (Fig. 4-8, *A* and *B*). Stained granules in reticulocytes and mature erythrocytes are called **Pappen-**

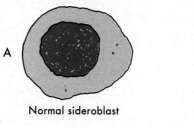
Normal sideroblast

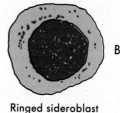
Ringed sideroblast

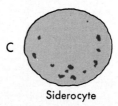
Siderocyte

Fig. 4-8. Iron deposits in red blood cells.
A, Contains none to a few siderosomes (ferritin aggregations), visualized with Prussian blue iron stain. **B,** Contains many iron granules, as hemosiderin deposits and Pappenheimer bodies. **C,** Large iron deposits in mature red cells occur as Pappenheimer bodies, seen in various red cell disorders.

heimer bodies, and the cells are often referred to as **siderocytes** (Fig. 4-8, *C*). An absence or an excess of demonstrable hemosiderin (siderotic granules) in marrow tissue is seen in a number of erythropoietic and inflammatory disorders.

A quantitative value for iron stores can be obtained by determining **serum ferritin,** which is proportional to tissue ferritin and hemosiderin. One microgram of serum ferritin corresponds to about 120 μg of iron per kilogram of body weight. As would be expected from considerations of iron use and loss, serum ferritin levels in females average less than half those of males (Table 4-3). Ferrokinetic studies indicate that an additional iron compartment of about 80 mg exists. This "labile pool" may represent a storage source other than ferritin and hemosiderin, either a diffuse cytoplasmic pool or iron associated with the lymphatic circulation.

Iron loss. Mucosal cell turnover and incidental bleeding account for about 1 mg/day of iron loss in men and women, an amount easily replaced by dietary intake. Menstruating women, however, typically lose 40 to 80 ml of blood per cycle, containing 20 to 40 mg of iron. This averages an additional 1 mg/day of iron loss during a month interval. During pregnancy, about 600 to 900 mg of iron are transferred from maternal to fetal tissues, resulting in a large depletion of iron stores in the mother. It is little wonder that unless a well-balanced diet is maintained (the exception rather than the rule in modern Western society) or supplemental iron is provided, iron-deficiency anemia is commonplace.

OXYGEN TRANSPORT

We have discussed the process for hemoglobin manufacture, and we have examined the requirements for raw materials, such as iron, that are needed to assemble the product. Next, our attention turns to hemoglobin function: how the molecule interacts with oxygen in diverse tissue environments.

Hemoglobin binds oxygen in the lungs and releases it at tissue sites of metabolism

Table 4-3. Laboratory evaluation of iron status

Determinant	Units	Male	Female
Serum Iron (fasting, morning)	μg/dl	70-180	60-180
	μmol/L	12.5-32.2	10.7-32.2
Serum iron-binding capacity (IBC)	μg/dl	250-450	250-450
	μmol/L	44.8-80.6	44.8-80.6
Serum transferrin (nephelometry)	μg/dl	220-400	220-400
Transferrin saturation	%	20-50	15-50
Serum ferritin (IRMA)	μg/L	20-300	10-120
Marrow sideroblasts (ratio to nRBCs)	%	40-60	40-60
Protoporphyrin (FEP)	μg/dl RBCs	17-77	17-77

IRMA; immunoradiometric assay.
(Data from Hillman, RS, and Finch, CA: Red cell manual, ed 5, Philadelphia, 1985, FA, Davis & Co; and Tietz, N, ed: Textbook of clinical chemistry, Philadelphia, 1986, WB Saunders Co.)

in exchange for carbon dioxide, which it returns to the lungs for expiration. Simple diffusion along a gradient of partial pressures from high to low concentration accounts for gas exchange between the alveoli and pulmonary capillary blood. However, the high oxygen demands of mammalian metabolism requires a rapid, efficient system for oxygen exchange at tissue sites. The problem is twofold: how to bind oxygen firmly at the site of uptake, yet be able to release it at the tissue site where it is needed. Once released, a mechanism must exist to prevent it from being rebound to hemoglobin. The chemical properties of hemoglobin provide such a system.

When oxygen binds to hemoglobin, the tertiary and quaternary molecular structure of the protein changes in conformation, forming **oxyhemoglobin (HbO$_2$)**. The reduced form is referred to as **deoxyhemoglobin (Hb)**. The following is the sequence of changes that occur in the transition from the deoxygenated to the oxygenated state (Fig. 4-9):

1. A single oxygen molecule attaches to the Fe^{+2} of an alpha chain heme.
2. The Fe^{+2} is displaced slightly, into the plane of the porphyrin ring.
3. The displacement results in compensatory adjustments of the alpha globin chain and the adjacent beta chain (across the α_1-β_2 interface).
4. Several salt bridges between globin chains of the tetramer are broken.
5. A molecule of **2,3-diphosphoglycerate (2,3-DPG)** is expelled from a cleft between the beta chains. Molecules of carbon dioxide, attached to the globin chains as carbaminohemoglobin (HHbCO$_2$), are also released because they have less affinity for oxyhemoglobin.
6. The other heme groups are exposed

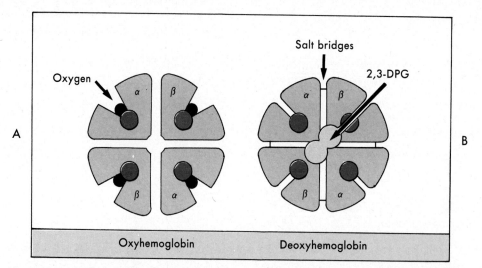

Fig. 4-9.   Interaction of hemoglobin with oxygen and 2,3-DPG.
A, Oxygen binds to hemoglobin when the iron-containing sites of the heme modules are exposed. The tetramer can bind up to four oxygen molecules (oxyhemoglobin). **B,** In the presence of 2,3-DPG and low pH, oxygen affinity decreases, salt bridges form, and 2,3-DPG interacts with the beta chains. The resulting change in hemoglobin shape prevents oxygen uptake (deoxyhemoglobin) until the red cell returns to conditions of higher pH and low 2,3-DPG concentration.

and bind oxygen molecules. This occurs more readily than with the first heme-O_2 binding, a phenomenon referred to as heme-heme interaction.

An excellent summary of the molecular events can be found in Tietz (1986, pp. 1518-1520). This sequence of events is reversed at the sites of oxygen exchange with the tissues, where a high concentration of 2,3-DPG is present. The acidic conditions (high H^+ concentration) associated with active metabolism and generation of carbon dioxide promote the formation of salt bridges between globin chains and the insertion of 2,3-DPG between the beta chains. Oxygen is released from the heme groups to diffuse through the plasma and enter cells, again following a diffusion gradient.

In summary, the uptake of oxygen by hemoglobin is favored by:

1. Increased local concentration of oxygen (pulmonary capillary and arterial blood)
2. Decreased concentration of hydrogen ions (high pH), which form salt bridges and restrict heme interaction with oxygen
3. Decreased concentration of 2,3-DPG, resulting in an oxygen-receptive hemoglobin

Conversely, oxygen release by hemoglobin is favored by:

1. Decreased local concentration of oxygen (tissue sites where oxygen is consumed)
2. Increased concentration of hydrogen ions (low pH), which form salt bridges, inhibiting oxygen binding by heme
3. Increased concentrations of 2,3-DPG available for insertion between the beta chains to inhibit oxygen uptake

Molecular rearrangements are responsible for changes in the **affinity** of hemoglobin for oxygen, and this determines the proportion of available oxygen (partial pressure, P_{O_2}) that will be bound (**percent saturation**). When partial pressure is plotted against percent saturation, a sigmoid curve results (Fig. 4-10, *A*). The slow uptake at low P_{O_2} reflects the high threshold for oxygen binding with the first heme group. Facilitated uptake of oxygen with the remaining hemes after 2,3-DPG displacement results in the rapid increase (steep slope) in saturation with a modest increase in P_{O_2}. Physiologically, oxygen binding occurs at a P_{O_2} of 95 mm Hg (mean arterial tension), when hemoglobin is 95% saturated, and oxygen is released at a P_{O_2} of 40 mm Hg (mean venous tension), when hemoglobin is 70% saturated.

The P_{O_2} at which hemoglobin is 50% saturated (**P_{50}**) is utilized to evaluate oxygen transport; normally this yields a value of 26.6 mm Hg. Various conditions can affect hemoglobin affinity for oxygen and produce a different P_{50} value, resulting in 50% saturation at a higher or lower partial pressure. Some types of hemoglobin, such as Hb F, do not interact with 2,3-DPG. These hemoglobins bind oxygen readily and release it reluctantly; therefore the partial pressure required in order to achieve any level of saturation would be less than that for normal adult hemoglobin. Thus, a curve plotted for fetal hemoglobin oxygen affinity would lie to the left of a curve for adult hemoglobin (Fig. 4-10, *B*). Any condition, such as high pH (low H^+ concentration), that results in increased oxygen saturation for a given partial pressure is said to produce a *shift to the left* in the **oxygen dissociation curve.** Conversely, low pH, high 2,3-DPG levels, and abnormal hemoglobins with low oxygen affinity will result in a *shift to the right.* Physiologically, this change in oxygen affinity (often referred to as the Bohr effect) serves a homeostatic purpose. When tissue metabolites increase, producing a state of acidosis (low pH), hemoglobin releases oxygen more readily, just what is needed to counteract the increased carbon dioxide levels. Additional 2,3-DPG is also generated under such conditions, reinforcing the shift

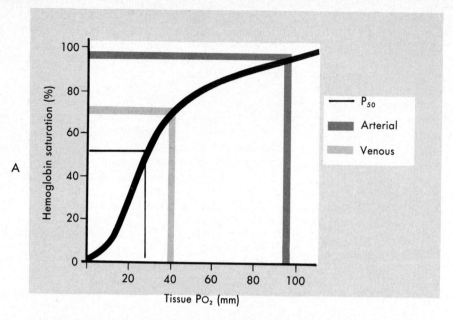

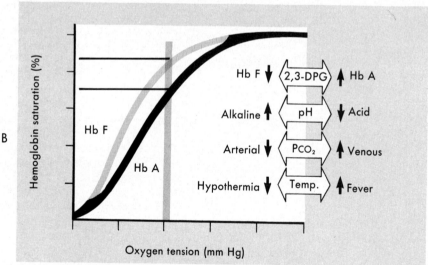

Fig. 4-10. Oxygen dissociation curves.
A, Hemoglobin saturation as a function of oxygen tension. The changes in hemoglobin's molecular shape and corresponding oxygen affinity result in a sigmoidal curve when oxygen availability (tension or partial pressure) is plotted against hemoglobin saturation (percent). The corresponding values for arterial and venous blood are shown. **B,** Shifts in oxygen dissociation curves. Differences in the affinity for oxygen between Hb F and Hb A are indicated for a given value of oxygen pressure. Because the dissociation curve of Hb F lies to the left of Hb A, a higher saturation level of oxygen occurs. The gamma chains of Hb F do not interact with 2,3-DPG as well as the beta chains in Hb A, and oxygen is bound firmly. All hemoglobins alter their oxygen affinities in response to environmental variables. The resulting shifts in oxygen dissociation are indicated for increases and decreases of 2,3-DPG, pH, P_{CO_2}, and temperature. Note that arterial blood will be high in pH (alkaline), low in P_{CO_2} and 2,3-DPG and slightly lower in temperature. The dissociation curve for hemoglobin in arterial blood will lie to the left of that for venous blood, resulting in maximum saturation. Conditions in venous blood favor maximum oxygen release.

to the right in dissociation. In the pulmonary capillaries, oxygen tension is high, blood pH is more alkaline, and the dissociation curve shifts to the left, resulting in increased efficiency of oxygen uptake.

Hemoglobin also plays a role as a buffer in maintaining blood pH, exchanging bicarbonate and chloride with tissue fluids, and various other metabolic activities. Most of these topics are beyond the intended scope of this book, but further information can be found in textbooks of biochemistry or clinical chemistry. However, one aspect of metabolism must be given further attention. In order to bind oxygen, the iron atom must be in the reduced, or Fe^{+2}, state. The next chapter discusses red cell metabolism, including the mechanisms for maintaining hemoglobin in the reduced form.

SUMMARY

- Hemoglobin is a tetrameric protein, consisting of four globin chains, each attached to a tetrapyrrole porphyrin that contains iron.
- Fetal hemoglobin, consisting of alpha and gamma chains of globin, predominates during prenatal life; adult hemoglobin, made up of alpha and beta chains of globin, predominates after birth.
- Hemoglobin is manufactured from instructions encoded in DNA that are passed by mRNA to the ribosomes, where amino acids are assembled into polypeptide chains to form the globin components.
- Heme is made in the mitochondria and cytoplasm by assembly of porphyrin rings. Excess porphyrin byproducts are excreted. ALA synthase is an important rate-limiting enzyme and vitamin B_6 is an important cofactor during early steps of heme synthesis.
- Hemoglobin synthesis requires adequate iron supplies. Dietary iron replaces most of that lost in excreted intestinal mucosa cells and through incidental bleeding. Iron deficiency is common in individuals with poor nutrition and in women during child-bearing years.
- Iron is stored as ferritin and hemosiderin, and it is transported by a protein, transferrin. Iron absorption is regulated by erythropoietic activity, mucosal cell iron stores, and transferrin availability.
- Changes occur in the tertiary and quaternary structures of hemoglobin during oxygen uptake and release. Insertion of 2,3-DPG into hemoglobin prevents oxygen binding at tissue sites. Affinity-dissociation is affected by oxygen tension, pH, and 2,3-DPG concentration. Iron must be reduced, (Fe^{+2}) for oxygen transport to occur.

5

Erythrocyte Metabolism

Intracellular metabolism is probably better defined in erythrocytes than in any other cell type. Lacking a nucleus and devoid of mitochondria, mature red blood cells are readily available in large numbers; they have proved to be an ideal tissue for measuring mechanisms of transmembrane ion exchange, glycolysis, and other enzymatic activities. Knowledge of red cell biochemistry has advanced steadily over the past five decades, providing us with a relatively clear picture of physiological processes at the molecular level. Hemoglobin function in oxygen transport was discussed in Chapter 4. Now we turn our attention to events that (1) help maintain hemoglobin in an oxygen-binding state, (2) provide the red cell with chemical energy (ATP) to maintain ionic and osmotic equilibrium, (3) generate 2,3-DPG to regulate oxygen release from hemoglobin, and (4) support the integrity of the cell membrane. Indeed, the relationship between metabolism and membrane structure is an intimate one, as can be documented in patients suffering from hereditary disorders of metabolism that result in weakened red cell membranes. The resulting hemolytic anemias are understandable as specific deficiencies of the metabolic pathways.

ENERGY METABOLISM IN THE ERYTHROCYTE
Embden-Meyerhof pathway and ATP generation

All living cells, erythrocytes included, require energy to maintain their structural in-tegrity and to participate in the diverse physiological activities that characterize complex biological processes. Shortly after reticulocytes are released from the marrow, the last remnants of mitochondrial and ribosomal structures degenerate. Oxidative metabolism is very limited, so that glucose, rather than fatty acids and amino acids, must provide most of the cell's energy needs. This is largely accomplished by the anaerobic catabolism of glucose (anaerobic glycolysis) to lactate via the **Embden-Meyerhof pathway (EMP)** (Fig. 5-1). This pathway accounts for about 90% of the glucose utilized by the red cell. Specific enzymes regulate each step in the EMP and ancillary pathways; deficiencies in these enzymes are related directly to several types of hereditary red cell disorders (Chapter 18).

Glycolysis results in a net formation of two molecules of adenosine triphosphate (ATP) for each molecule of glucose entering the pathway. Actually, two molecules of ATP are *used* during the initial hexose (6-carbon sugar) phase of the EMP. The ATP is converted to adenosine diphosphate (ADP) and the phosphates are added to hexoses to form glucose 6-phosphate and fructose, 1,6-diphosphate. Each hexose is split into two trioses (three carbon sugars), with subsequent conversion of dihydroxyacetone phosphate to glyceraldehyde 3-phosphate (Fig. 5-1). Each triose phase produces ATP at two steps; thus four ATPs are generated, while two ATPs are used, for a net gain of two ATPs. Although the efficiency of anaerobic energy production is low (about 29%,

52

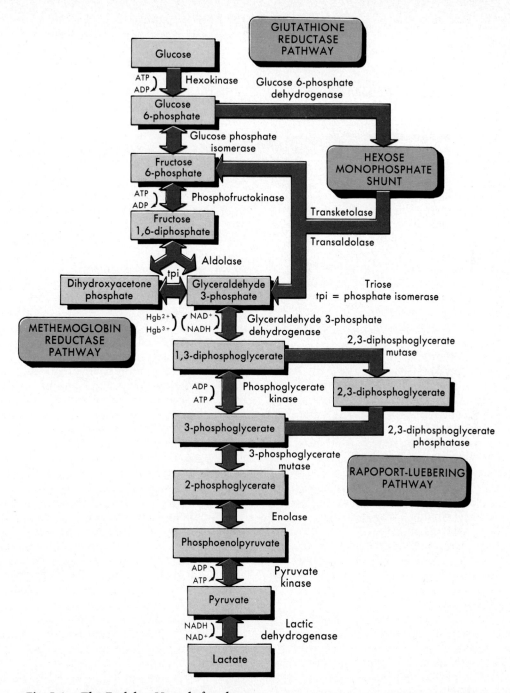

Fig. 5-1. The Embden-Meyerhof pathway.
Enzymatic catabolism of glucose to lactate generates ATP for cellular energy, produces 2.3-DPG
via the Rapaport-Luebering pathway, and reduces hemoglobin by way of glutathione and methemoglobin reductase pathways.

with the rest released as heat), it is sufficient to meet the energy needs, barely, of the circulating erythrocyte. Specifically, ATP is needed to:

1. *Activate the ATPase-based sodium pump of the cell membrane.* The membrane is leaky, allowing sodium ions from the plasma to enter the cell and potassium ions to leave the cell, each diffusing in response to a concentration gradient. One mole of ATP is required in order to pump three moles of sodium out of the cell and, by exchange, two moles of potassium into the cell. One molecule of chloride also leaves the cell, maintaining ionic balance. Lack of ATP or failure of the pump would permit ionic poisoning of critical cell functions and eventual cell death. In fact, ATP depletion is one of the major problems in blood bank donor units, limiting the survival time of stored red cells.

2. *Maintain membrane resilience and the biconcave shape of the RBC.* During its travels through the microcirculation, the erythrocyte must flex, twist, and squeeze through vessel diameters that are half, or less than half, of the cell's diameter. ATP provides energy for the phosphorylation of the cytoskeletal protein (spectrin), one of the major structural components responsible for the flexibility of the red cell membrane.

3. *Maintain membrane lipid composition.* The membrane and surrounding plasma exchange lipid compounds. Some of these reactions are regulated by enzymes that require ATP as an energy source.

Some of the enzymes of the EMP are of special interest because deficiencies in them are associated with specific hemolytic disorders. Although far from common, deficiencies of **pyruvate kinase (PK)** and **glucosephosphate isomerase (GPI)** are the most frequently encountered enzymopathies of the EMP (Chapter 18); others are quite rare, known from one or a few cases.

Hexose monophosphate shunt and glutathione reduction

About 10% of the glucose is oxidized by way of the **hexose monophosphate shunt (HMS),** also known as the pentose phosphate shunt or the phosphogluconate pathway. Although ATP is not generated by this ancillary route, the HMS does serve a critically important function. Pyridine nucleotide (nicotinamide-adenine dinucleotide phosphate, or **NADP**) is reduced (NADPH), and this maintains the reduction of a metabolically linked compound, **glutathione** (Fig. 5-2). Glutathione, in turn, prevents the oxidation and denaturation of hemoglobin and other critical RBC proteins by inhibiting the accumulation of peroxide compounds (H_2O_2). In fact, when oxidation of glutathione increases, as a result of metabolic products or the presence of oxidant drugs, HMS activity increases, resulting in a greater percentage of carbohydrate shunting and nucleotide reduction. Erythrocyte catalase also converts peroxide to water, and either enzyme system is sufficient to counteract oxidative stresses.

The key enzyme of the HMS is **glucose 6-phosphate dehydrogenase (G-6-PD)**. This enzyme occurs in numerous variant forms, differing in amino acid sequence, electrophoretic mobility, and enzymatic activity. The most common or normal variant is designated as B. The various abnormal types are listed in Chapter 18. Several forms of G-6-PD deficiency occur, and each type can compromise the linked cycle of nucleotide-glutathione-hemoglobin reduction. In addition, G-6-PD defects are relatively common, so that laboratory procedures to detect abnormalities of this enzyme are important in establishing the cause for a hemolytic anemia.

Carbohydrates entering the HMS, as glucose phosphate, are transformed into pentoses, trioses, and other sugar phosphates;

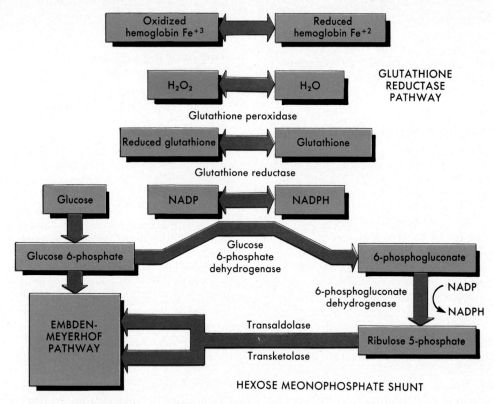

Fig. 5-2.   The glutathione reductase pathway.
The pathway is driven by activity of the hexose monophosphate shunt. Oxidants are removed,
helping to maintain hemoglobin in a reduced state.

many of these re-enter the EMP at two steps, as show in Fig. 5-1. GPI is the key enzyme for regulating activity of the HMS. Since GPI controls a bidirectional reaction, products of the HMS can be recycled through glucose 6-phosphate. Other enzymes involved in these reactions are not clinically important. Deficiencies of enzymes of the glutathion-linked reactions are associated with hemolytic anemia, although such cases are usually rare and mild.

Rapoport-Luebering pathway

The principal product of the Rapoport-Luebering pathway is **2,3-diphosphoglycer-** ate **(2,3-DPG),** the molecule that regulates hemoglobin interactions with oxygen (Chapter 4). The concentration of 2,3-DPG is equivalent to the combined concentrations of all other intermediate products of glycolysis. DPG synthesis depends on the rate of glycolytic catabolism and phosphate input, a function of phosphofructokinase activity in the hexose portion of the EMB. Regulation of 2,3-DPG synthesis occurs in response to the affinity of oxygen for hemoglobin. An increase in blood pH influences glycolytic rate and production of 2,3-DPG (both increase), which in turn influences oxygen binding to hemoglobin (decreases). Tissue demand for oxygen produces deoxygenated hemoglobin, which necessitates additional supplies of 2,3-DPG. Enzymes of this pathway are rarely associated with blood disorders, but phosphate deficiencies can result in decreased production rates of 2,3-DPG and associated problems in oxygen release.

Methemoglobin reductase pathway

An additional ancillary pathway of nucleotide reduction serves to reduce hemoglobin. The conversion of glyceraldehyde 3-phosphate to 1,3-diphosphoglycerate reduces NAD to NADH, which then drives the reduction of methemoglobin (Fe^{+3}) to hemoglobin (Fe^{+2}). The enzyme mediating this reaction is simply designated **methemoglobin reductase (MR)** (formerly, diaphorase). Since the trivalent state of iron in methemoglobin cannot combine reversibly with oxygen, the combined EMP and MR pathways are essential to counteract the various types of oxidant stress acting on hemoglobin. In normal circumstances, about 3% of the RBC's hemoglobin content is oxidized each day to methemoglobin. Methemoglobin reductase maintains the oxidized hemoglobin levels at less than 0.1% of saturation. In the absence of MR, 20% to 40% of the oxidized hemoglobin persists, not enough to be fatal but enough to compromise oxygen delivery and produce an ongoing cyanosis, or blue color of the skin (Chapter 18).

THE ERYTHROCYTE MEMBRANE

The cell membrane is much more than a passive envelope to retain cellular contents. It is a selective barrier, permitting the free passage of some materials, completely excluding many larger molecules, and quantitatively regulating the transport of others. Some materials, such as water, cross the membrane by passive diffusion in response to concentration gradients; others require active transport via specific molecular mechanisms (e.g., sodium transport by ATPase-dependent pumps). Maintenance of membrane structure is intergrally coupled to energy metabolism.

Structure of the membrane

The membrane, as currently visualized, is believed to consist of two sheets of lipid material, each of which is one molecule thick. Within this bilayer are imposed various proteins that communicate between the external and internal surfaces (Fig. 5-3). A protein skeleton is attached to the internal lipid surface, forming a reticular pattern or lattice. In addition, the external surface is coated with a diverse array of glycoproteins, complex carbohydrates, and lipoproteins, imparting antigenic structure to the membrane.

Lipids. The lipids are arranged so that the polar (charged) ends are exposed at both the external and internal surfaces of the cell. This results in a net negative charge on the outer surface of the membrane and a net positive charge on the inner surface. Analysis of the membrane reveals there are about 75 to 90 lipid molecules for each protein molecule. Most of the lipids exist in a 1:1 molar ratio of **phospholipids** and **cholesterol.** The major phospholipid components are distributed as follows:

External membrane surface	Internal membrane surface
Phosphatidylcholine	Phosphatidylserine
Sphingomyelin	Phosphatidylethanolamine
Glycolipid	Phosphatidylinositol

Cholesterol is present in an esterified form, in equilibrium with nonesterified plasma cholesterol. The ratio is maintained by lecithin-cholesterol acyltransferase (LCAT), a plasma enzyme that transfers an acyl group from lecithin to cholesterol. Deficiencies in this enzyme are known to produce membrane abnormalities. Some of the glycolipid content forms serological determinants associated with blood group antigens.

Proteins. Proteins composing the internal or peripheral cytoskeleton are organized as

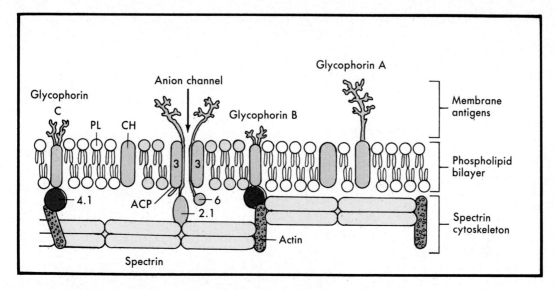

Fig. 5-3. Schematic model of the red cell membrane.
The components are not drawn to scale, nor are all of the interactions between components shown. *ACP*, Anion channel protein; *CH*, cholesterol; *PL*, phospholipid.

a lattice. This arrangement provides a flexible support system for the membrane, which is necessary for the high degree of deformability associated with passage through the microcirculation (see Hemodynamics, below). Protein analysis of red cell membranes is traditionally done by preparing the red cells in a solution of sodium dodecyl sulfate (SDS) to denature the proteins, followed by separation with polyacrylamide gel electrophoresis (PAGE) (Fig. 5-4). The bands of proteins are stained with Coomassie blue and periodic acid–Schiff (PAS) base. By means of this procedure, membrane-associated proteins have been designated by their migration positions (bands), reflecting their respective molecular weights. Several of these bands have been correlated with specific proteins and functions (Table 5-1). Since some of these proteins have not been named, they are usually referred to by band positions (e.g., "band 4.1").

The major structural component of the

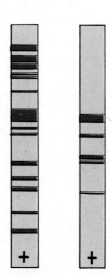

Fig. 5-4. Polyacrylamide gel electrophoresis of membrane protein components.
Bands are stained by Coomassie blue *(CB)* and periodic acid–Schiff *(PAS)*.

Table 5-1. Membrane protein components

	Name	Molecular weight*	Function
PAGE band			
1,2	Spectrin	220-240	Cytoskeleton structure
2.1	Ankyrin	210	Attach spectrin to band 3
3	Anion channel	95-97	Transport anions and glucose across membrane
4.1		72	Cytoskeleton support
4.2		79	
5	Actin	43	Bridge between spectrin units; attach spectrin to membrane
6	G-6-PD	35	Enzymatic activity
7		29	
8		21	
PAS band			
1	Glycophorin A†	83	Attach cytoskeleton to membrane; carries blood group antigens
2	Glycophorin C	45	Attach cytoskeleton to membrane
3	Glycophorin B	25	Carries some blood group antigens

*In kilodaltons, based on Kurantsin-Mills, J, and Lessin, LS: The red cell membrane. In Lichtman, MA, ed: Hematology and oncology, vol. 6, New York, 1980, Grune & Stratton, pp 75-78.
†Glycophorin identities conform to Mueller, TJ: The red-cell membrane skeleton and the hereditary anemias, Lab Management 24:37-41, 1986.

cytoskeleton is **spectrin,** which comprises bands 1 and 2 of the SDS-PAGE system. Spectrin is organized as tetramers and oligomers of alpha and beta subunits. The beta spectrin units of the peripheral lattice are attached to the integral proteins of the phospholipid bilayer by **ankyrin,** a protein that migrates with beta spectrin and must be separated by an additional procedure (it is assigned band 2.1 for clarification). Ankyrin appears to attach the cytoskeleton to one of the transmembrane proteins, **band 3,** which serves as a polarized anion chan-nel. Band 3 protein is arranged within the lipid layer so that its polar groups (negative charge) face the lumen of the transmembrane channel, permitting chloride and bicarbonate ions to pass. Glucose is also transported across the membrane by way of the anion channel protein (ACP). Cations, such as potassium and sodium, are mostly excluded. Two other proteins, **actin** and **band 4.1,** link spectrin oligomers with each other and with two transmembrane sialoglycoproteins, **glycophorin A** and **glycophorin C.** Actin is a protein with contractile properties: as a bridge element, it may permit rearrangement of the spectrin network and thus contribute to the pliability of thered cell. Glycophorins are embedded in the phospholipid bilayer. They provide attachment points for the underlying cytoskeleton, they may serve as sites of membrane enzymatic activities, and some support the complex glycolipids and glycoproteins that serve as red cell antigens.

The functions of many of the membrane components are not known at this time. The difficulties in preparing membranes for protein analysis has led to some disparities between investigators in assigning components to PAGE bands. For instance, extracted glycophorins form dimers (including heterodimers of A and B), resulting in two or more bands with the same protein component. The information in Table 5-1 is a composite of data from sources that utilize different criteria for band identification, but revision and standardization of membrane component nomenclature can be expected in the near future.

Membrane function

Spectrin is also associated with ATPase activity, utilizing ATP generated from glycolysis. Leakage of cations across the semipermeable membrane occurs by passive diffusion, but active transport is required to counteract the process. About 70% of active cation transport is provided by an ATP-dependent pumping mechanism, in which sodium ions are transported out of the cell and potassium ions are brought into the cell (Fig. 5-5). Export of a chloride ion compensates for the outward movement of surplus positive charge. The other 30% of active transport is ATP independent. The relationship between energy metabolism (glycolysis), ATPase activity, and cytoskeletal structure is not clear, much less the mechanisms by which changes in cell shape occur. Much of what is known has been derived from studies of RBC membrane structure and metabolism in patients with

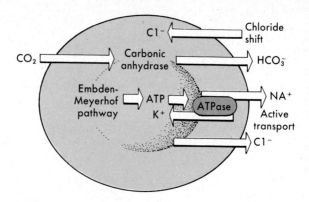

Fig. 5-5.   Ion transport across the red cell membrane.

An ATPase-activated sodium-potassium pump compensates for ion leakage across the membrane. Some chloride is pumped out with sodium. Chloride enters as an isohydric exchange for bicarbonate (chloride shift) during carbon dioxide transport.

hemolytic disorders associated with specific deficiencies in membrane components (Chapter 19).

HEMODYNAMICS: THE RED BLOOD CELL IN VIVO

At rest, the erythrocyte forms a biconcave disk. This is the form traditionally illustrated in books and represented by the dried cell corpses of peripheral blood smears. Yet for most of its life span an erythrocyte of 7 to 8 μm in diameter must pass through capillary vessels of 2 to 3 μm in internal diameter. During its time in the microcirculation, the red cell loses much of the accompanying plasma, resulting in increasing frictional forces and potential membrane damage. Tests for membrane deformability are beyond the capabilities of most clinical laboratories, but scientists involved in experimental cell research utilize animal models to obtain a picture of the changes that occur in erythrocytes (Fig. 5-6). Studies of blood cell flow in vessels constitute an investigational subdiscipline called cytorheology. Such studies reveal that RBCs can be stretched to 3 or 4 times

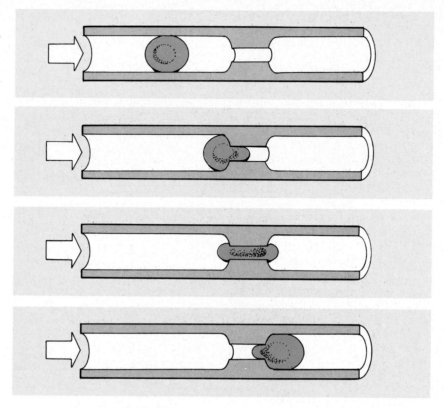

Fig. 5-6. Erythrocyte deformability.
Red cells elongate as they pass through small vessels, as demonstrated in vitro in capillary tubes. Diapedesis from marrow hematopoietic sites to a blood vessel lumen requires still greater deformation.

their diameter, assume a variety of shapes under different flow velocities, and pass through pores in the vascular endothelium that are less than 1 μm in diameter.

Young red cells are more pliable than older cells, when cells of equal size are compared. Larger cells (macrocytes), however, tend to be more fragile than normocytes, and red blood cells of newborn infants are more fragile and less pliable than those of adults (RBC life spans are typically 60 to 80 days in neonates). As red cells circulate, accumulating damage to the membrane, coupled with a gradual decrease in the efficiency of metabolic pathways, re-

sults in membrane aging. Inability to conform to the narrow passages of the capillaries eventually leads to cell lysis or removal by RES macrophages. Cells with abnormal membranes, such as spherocytes, are considerably less pliable than normal cells, and their survival times are proportionately shorter.

ANTIGENIC STRUCTURE OF THE MEMBRANE: IMMUNOHEMATOLOGY

The erythrocyte surface is coated with hundreds of different types of complex molecules. Some of these are glycolipids, identified with the lipid bilayer, but others are glycoproteins and complex carbohydrates, associated with the integral glycophorins. Most of these complex molecules terminate in **sialic acids,** residues that possess a strong negative charge, with the result that erythrocytes repel each other. These complex molecules are capable of stimulating immune responses in animals that lack the same configuration of molecular determinants or antigenic specificity. Thus, red blood cells bearing specific surface antigens can cause the production of antibodies in recipients whose cells lack the antigens. To date, over 300 red cell antigens have been described; most of these are organized into about 15 genetic systems of blood groups. Studies of red cell antigens and their corresponding antibodies form the subject matter of **immunohematology;** application of this knowledge is the basis for transfusion therapy or blood banking. A lengthy discussion of red cell immunogenicity is beyond the scope of this textbook (see Additional Reading at the end of this section), but it is necessary to comprehend some basic principles in order to understand some of the hemolytic anemias that can occur.

Most red cell antigens are believed to be integral components of the membrane. Antigen molecular structure is determined by genes that specify enzymes involved in their construction. For example, construction of the ABO blood group antigens involves genes located on chromosome number 9 (Fig. 5-7). The terminal portions of the ABO antigens are oligosaccharides that are attached to a glycolipid component. Genes of the ABH blood group system code for enzymes, **glycosyltransferases,** that add sugars to the glycolipid, The first product in this system is produced when the *H* gene codes for an enzyme, L-fucosyltransferase, that attaches the sugar L-fucose to a mucopolysaccharide precursor. Inheritance of an *A* gene results in construction of an enzyme that attaches the sugar *N*-acetylgalactoseamine to the "H substance" formed by action of the *H* gene. Note that gene designations are written in italics, whereas their products, the antigens, are written as roman letters. Similarly, the *B* gene codes for the enzyme D-galactosyltransferase. Inheritance of the *0* gene, however, apparently does not produce a detectable enzyme. This gene is recessive to both the *A* and *B* genes, and it is silent or amorphic in expression. Individuals that inherit an *0* gene from each parent (they are homozygous) produce H substance, but no other sugars are added. Antigens of other blood group systems are constructed from precursor components in a similar manner. Some systems, such as ABO, P, Ii, and Lewis, share common precursors; the chemical natures of others are different or still unknown. The proteinaceous Rh antigens, for example, are integral components of the red cell membrane. Deletion of the genes responsible for construction of the Rh antigens results in a weekened membrane and shortened erythrocyte survival. Other antigens, attached to peripheral or nonessential membrane components, can be eliminated without apparent effects on red cell survival.

SUMMARY

- Erythrocytes obtain energy, in the form of ATP, from the anaerobic metabolism of glucose via the Embden-Meyerhof pathway.
- ATP functions to (1) drive the sodium-potassium pump to actively transport cations across the RBC membrane; (2) maintain membrane integrity and regulate cell shape, and (3) maintain membrane lipid composition.
- The hexose monophosphate shunt drives a series of reduction reactions that help maintain hemoglobin in a reduced, oxygen-binding state. G-6-PD is a key enzyme for activation of this pathway.
- The Rapoport-Leubering pathway generates 2,3-DPG for interaction with hemoglobin.
- Additional hemoglobin reduction is provided by the methemoglobin reductase pathway.

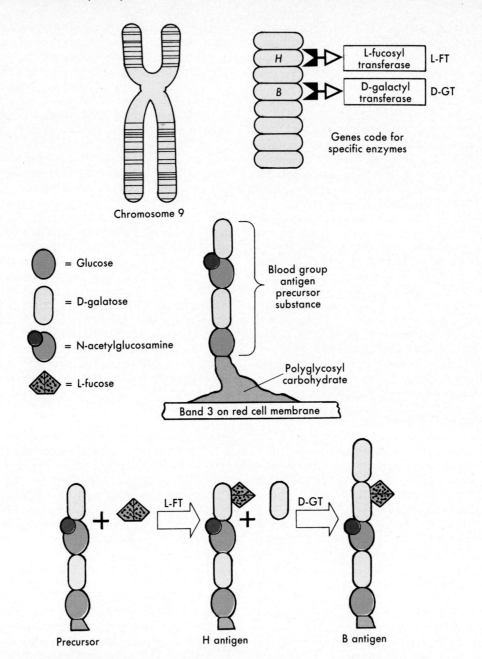

Fig. 5-7. Formation of B blood group antigen.
The gene, *H*, codes for an enzyme, L-fucosyltransferase. The enzyme attaches L-fucose to a carbohydrate precursor substance associated with membrane glycophorin, producing H substance. Another gene, *B*, produces D-galactosyltransferase, which attaches D-galactose to H substance, resulting in the B antigen.

- Erythrocyte membranes consist of a phospholipid bilayer, cholesterols and other lipids, and specialized proteins. Proteins can be identified as stained bands on gel electrophoresis. Spectrin and actin form a flexible cytoskeleton underlying the membrane. Glycophorins serve as connecting points between membrane and spectrin and as foundations for some of the blood group antigens.
- Red cells are capable of considerable deformation in shape as they pass through the microcirculation. The cytoskeleton and ATP play major roles in cell shape change.
- Genes code for enzymes that assemble the blood group antigens on the outer surface of the red cell membrane. ABO antigen determinants consist of carbohydrates added sequentially to a mucopolysaccharide precursor substance.

SUGGESTED READINGS—SECTION II

Benesche, RE, Benesch, R, and Yu, CI: The oxygenation of hemoglobin in the presence of 2,3-diphosphoglycerate: effect of temperature, pH, ionic strength, and hemoglobin concentration, Biochemistry 8:2567-2571, 1969.

Bessis, M: Corpuscles: atlas of red blood cell shapes, Berlin, 1974, Springer-Verlag.

Bessis, M: Blood smears reinterpreted, Berlin, 1977, Springer-Verlag.

Brånemark, PI: Intravascular anatomy of blood cells in man, Basal, 1971, S Karger.

Bunn, HF, and Forget, BG: Hemoglobin: molecular, genetic and clinical aspects, Philadelphia, 1986, WB Saunders Co.

Custer, RP: An atlas of the blood and bone marrow, ed 2, Philadelphia, 1974, WB Saunders Co.

Diggs, LW, Sturm, D, and Bell, A: The morphology of human blood cells, ed 5, North Chicago, Ill, 1985, Abbott Laboratories.

Finch, CA: Erythropoiesis, erythropoietin, and iron, Blood 60:1241-1246, 1982.

Finch, CA, and Huebers, H: Perspectives in iron metabolism, N Engl J Med 306:1520-1528, 1982.

Harris, JW, and Kellermeyer, RW: The red cell, Cambridge, Mass, 1970, Harvard University Press.

Hillman, RS, and Finch, CA: Red cell manual, Philadelphia, ed 5, FA Davis & Co.

Hurtado, A: Acclimatization to high altitudes. In Weihe, WH, ed: Physiological effects of high altitude, New York, 1964, Macmillan, Inc.

Kurantsin-Mills, J, and Lessin, LS: The red cell membrane. In Lichtman, MA, ed: Hematology and oncology, vol 6, New York, 1980. Grune & Stratton, pp 75-78.

LaBounty, LA: Iron metabolism and the identification of iron deficiency and anemia, J Med Technol 3:81-84, 1986.

LaCelle, PL, Evans, EA, and Hochmuth, RM: Erythrocyte membrane elasticity, fragmentation and lysis, Blood cells 3:335-350, 1977.

Lichtman, MA, ed: Hematology and oncology vol 6, New York, 1980, Grune & Stratton.

Lichtman, MA: The ultrastructure of the hemopoietic environment of the marrow: a review, Exper Hematol 9:391-410, 1981.

Lux, SE: Dissecting the red cell membrane skeleton, Nature 281:426-429, 1979.

Lux, SE: Spectrin-actin membrane skeleton of normal and abnormal red blood cells, Semin Hematol 16:21-51, 1979.

Marchesi, VT: The red cell membrane skeleton: recent progress, Blood 61:1-11, 1983.

Marcus, D, ed: Blood group immunochemistry and genetics, Semin Hematol 18:1-77, 1981.

Miale, JB: Laboratory medicine: hematology, ed 6, St Louis, 1982, The CV Mosby Co.

Mueller, TJ: The red-cell membrane skeleton and the hereditary anemias, Lab Management 24:37-41, 1986.

Perutz, MF: The hemoglobin molecule, Sci Am 211:644-679, 1964.

Perutz, MF: Hemoglobin structure and respiratory transport, Sci Am 293:92-133, 1978.

Pfafferott, C, Wenby, R, and Meiselman, HJ: Morphologic and internal viscosity aspects of RBC rheologic behavior, Blood Cells 8:65-78, 1982.

Rapoport, SM: The reticulocyte, Boca Raton, Fla, 1986, CRC Press.

Tietz, N, ed: Textbook of clinical chemistry, Philadelphia, 1986, WB Saunders Co.

Tippett, P: Chromosomal mapping of the blood group genes, Semin Hematol 18:4-12, 1981.

Williams, WJ, Beutler, E, Ersler, AJ, and Lichtman, MA, eds: Hematology, ed 3, New York, 1983, McGraw-Hill Book Co.

Wolf, BC, Luevano, E., and Neiman, RS: Evidence to suggest that the human fetal spleen is not a hematopoietic organ, Am J Clin Pathol 80:140-144, 1983.

SECTION III
The Normal Leukocyte

6

Introduction to White Blood Cells

DISCOVERY OF WHITE BLOOD CELLS

Although white blood cells were probably observed by various microscopists during examinations of blood, Hewson is usually given credit for the first descriptions, contained in a paper published in 1774. He also described the human lymphatic system and the lymphocytes associated with it. Unlike the pigmented red cells, the translucent and less numerous leukocytes were difficult to observe and descriptions were vague. In the 1840s, William Addison described granulocytes and made the association between the presence of white cells and the formation of pus as a result of infection. This association is not as straightforward as it might seem today. Earlier observations indicated that the capillaries, along with larger blood vessels, formed a "closed circulatory system." Since the blood cells were contained within the vessels and pus was observed to occur extravascularly in tissues, support for a hemic origin of pus formation was not convincing. Addison reported several experiments to show that white cells were attracted to sites of induced irritation, but his observations were generally ignored until Waller observed white cells in the process of crossing the vessel walls of a frog tongue. In fact, numerous investigations would later demonstrate that leukocytes use the bloodstream only as a transport medium; their functional lives occur almost entirely in the extravascular tissues!

The first white cell counts were reported by Vierordt in 1851, but it was the advent of triacid staining techniques by Ehrlich in 1877 that permitted rapid progress in the characterization of white blood cells. These stains made it possible to distinguish nuclear details and cytoplasmic contents and to classify leukocytes as distinct morphological types. The association of certain granulocytes with sites of infection and pus formation was clearly established, setting the stage for Metchnikov's observations in the 1880s on phagocytosis and those of many others on changes of white cell numbers and types in association with disease states. Because lymphocytes did not display obvious amoeboid movement and because of their association with the lymphatic system, their function remained a mystery for several decades. Indeed, many hematologists considered these small mononuclear cells, present in most of the tissues examined, to be precursors for the other blood cells. Advances in staining methodology shifted the focus of white cells studies from living material to fixed blood smears for many years, but the primary role of the leukocyte as an essential part of host defense was well established.

TYPES OF WHITE BLOOD CELLS

Leukocytes can be classified in a number of different ways. The simplest morphological distinction considers white blood cells as either **mononuclear,** those that contain a single nuclear lobe, or as **polymorphonuclear (PMN),** those that contain more than one nuclear lobe. This distinction is often used to characterize the cell contents of body fluids, such as spinal fluid, as to the nature of an infectious process. Polymorphonuclear cells are the granular leukocytes (**granulocytes**) associated with bacterial infections and pus formation, whereas mononuclear cells are characteristic of viral and fungal infections, tumor infiltrates, and other pathological processes.

Each distinct cell type can also be assigned to one of several stages of maturation, starting with an immature **blast** form that divides and differentiates into one or more intermediate forms. Blast cells are usually confined to the tissue sites of white blood cell production (**leukopoiesis**). Intermediate stages may or may not undergo mitosis; some are found in the bloodstream, while others remain at production sites. Mature forms are fully committed to perform one or more host defense functions. These cells travel the bloodstream to tissue sites for further differentiation, specialization, or activation. Thus, a sample of blood in a normal individual reveals white cells in transition. The numbers and degree of maturation of each cell type are relatively constant for individuals of a given chronological age (see Table 7-3). Changes in the relative numbers of each cell type or in the degree of maturation of circulating cells can be indications of a pathological process.

Mononuclear blood cells can be further divided into **lymphocytes,** cells associated with the lymphatic system that are produced at various organ and tissue sites, and **monocytes,** cells produced in the bone marrow that migrate to body tissues to serve as phagocytic macrophages. There are several types of lymphocytes, characterized by immunological techniques that detect specific molecules on the cell's outer membrane. Some types of lymphocytes interact with tissue macrophages to identify "foreign" molecules and cells; other lymphocytes produce globulin proteins as **antibodies** that help neutralize or further identify the for-

eign materials (Chapter 9). Monocytes are the migratory or intermediate forms of **macrophages,** tissue cells that recognize, process, and engulf invading foreign materials or **antigens** (Chapter 10).

The polymorphonuclear cells are so named because the most mature stages contain a nucleus that has segmented into two or more lobes (Fig 6-1). These cells also contain a variety of granules, and the term "granulocyte" is commonly used. Both of these terms can be misleading, however, since one type of granulocyte usually retains a single, nonsegmented nucleus, and the earliest stages (blasts) of the granulocytes may not contain demonstrable granules.

The triacid stain of Ehrlich was based on the chemistry of aniline dyes: some components of the stain reacted with hydrogen ions in the cellular components (acidophilic), others reacted with hydroxyl ions (basophilic) and others reacted with both (neutrophilic). The nucleus of the cell, containing large amounts of basic chromatin, attracts acidic and neutral dyes, resulting in a complex stain of blue and purple-red shades of color with the dyes typically employed. The cytoplasmic granules, however, contain specific enzymes that attract certain basic dye components preferentially. Some granulocytes contain acidophilic granules that react with eosin, a common basic stain component. These granules are stained bright orange to orange-red; the cell is called an **eosinophil.** Other cells, **basophils,** contain granules that attract the dark blue to purple acidic dye component. **Neutrophils** contain granules that combine with both components, usually staining a lilac to faint pink color. The cytoplasmic background also reacts with these dyes, depending on the relative RNA content, to produce cytoplasmic color varying from a deep basophilic blue to an acidophilic pink. Other cellular components, such as the mitochrondria, centrioles, and centromere, are

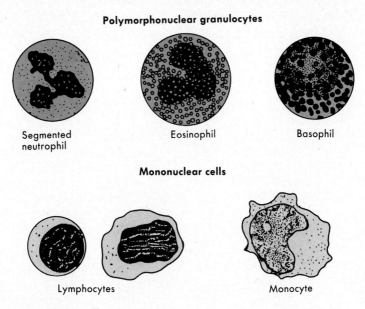

Fig. 6-1.   White blood cell types.
Representations of mature leukocytes found in peripheral blood, based on nuclear segmentation and granule content. Basophils often contain only a single nuclear lobe. The granulation of leukocytes may vary greatly in density and contrast, particularly in basophils.

not stained, and these may appear as colorless areas in some types of cells.

Maturation of granulocytes is characterized by progressive segmentation of the nucleus Early cell stages, normally present only in the bone marrow, are large cells with a single, round or oval nucleus. The nuclei of neutrophils and eosinophils indent to form a band before or during release from the marrow. The nuclei of circulating neutrophils rapidly condense and lobulate to form three to five segments connected by thin strands of chromatin. Mature eosinophils rarely form more than two or three nuclear lobes, and basophils may contain a single or bilobed nucleus (Fig. 6-1).

The peripheral blood contains lymphocytes of different sizes, monocytes, neutrophils in the band and segmented stages, eosinophils, and basophils. Recognition of each cell type, including normal variant forms and numerous pathological manifestations, is the basis for the **differential white cell count** (Chapter 26). Each type of white blood cell has several unique physiological roles in host defense, topics that are discussed in Chapters 8 to 10. A brief introduction to leukocyte cell function is included in this chapter to facilitate the learning of morphological characteristics (Table 6-1).

LEUKOCYTE FUNCTION: AN OVERVIEW

If one can imagine an organism as a nation, then the white blood cells are the armed forces and the "immune system" is the Department of Defense. Leukocyte defenses against invading microorganisms and other substances foreign to the body involve activities of two types. The first line of protection consists of cells that can recognize, locate, engulf, and kill microbes. The process of ingestion is **phagocytosis,** and the primary phagocytes are neutrophils and monocytes. Eosinophils and some lymphocytes are also capable of limited phagocytic activity. Organisms apparently acquired phagocytosis as a defense mechanism early in the evolutionary pagent, since the simplest invertebrates possess wandering ameboid-like cells that engulf microbes and remove cellular waste materials. The second major defense element, involving soluble proteins distributed in the plasma and extracellular fluids, evolved much later and is present only among the vertebrates.

A phagocyte, such as a mature neutrophil in the peripheral blood, has molecular receptors located on its outer membrane that react with (detect) substances that indicate an infection or inflammatory process has begun. These substances include molecules present in the cell walls of some bacteria, products resulting from tissue destruction at the site of invasion, chemicals released by other phagocytes responding to the microbes, and proteins manufactured by lymphocytes (antibodies) in response to the invasion. Phagocytes respond much like the familiar amoebae of pond water: they orient toward a gradient of increasing concentration of the stimulatory chemicals and then migrate to the source of the molecules, a process called **chemotaxis.** Migration occurs through the bloodstream and across the blood vessel walls (diapedesis) and through the tissues to reach the site of infection. Engulfment of the bacteria is also similar to that of free-living ameboid cells: the cell membrane of the phagocyte extends and surrounds the microbe to form a vacuole (Fig. 6-2). The vacuole encloses the microbe and is then referred to as a **phagosome.** Organelles, appearing as granules in the cytoplasm of the phagocyte, contain lysozymes and acid hydrolases. The granules move to the vacuole and fuse with the membrane, forming a **phagolysosome.** The granular contents enter the vacuole to help digest the microbe, which is also being attacked by other chemical processes generated during phagocytosis (see Chapter 8, under Oxidative Metabolism). The capacity for ingesting and killing microorganisms varies with type of phagocytic cell and type of microbe. Generally, neutrophils respond more rapidly and in greater numbers than do monocytes, but monocytes ingest and kill more cells than do the neutrophils, which are destroyed by their own secretory products. Some types of microorganisms generate a diminished phagocytic response, others may actually inhibit chemotaxis, and still others are capable of surviving and reproducing inside the phagocytic vacuoles!

Eosinophils respond to foreign materials by different mechanisms. Eosinophils ap-

Table 6-1. Major activities of white blood cells

(50%-75% of peripheral leukocytes)	
Granulocytes	
Neutrophils	Phagocytize bacteria
Eosinophils	Destroy parasites, participate in mucosal immune responses
Basophils	Transport and release substances involved in immune and inflammatory responses
(3%-11% of peripheral leukocytes)	
Macrophages	
Monocytes	Phagocytize bacteria, fungi, degenerating blood cells, and products of tissue damage
	Processing and presenting antigens
(20%-45% of peripheral leukocytes)	
Lymphocytes	
T lymphocytes	Regulate activities of other lymphocytes
B lymphocytes	Plasma cells that produce antibodies
Natural killer cells	Destroy tumor cells and cells infected with viruses

pear to be specialized for protecting mucous tissues, such as the nasal and oral membranes, lining of the gut, and respiratory surfaces. These cells respond to allergens, such as those causing hay fever and other types of hypersensitivity, and to invasion by some types of parasites. The parasite may be a worm larva or metazoic cell many times larger than the eosinophil, so that engulfment is not a practical course of action. Eosinophils surround the parasite and extrude the lysozyme granules, by a process called **exocytosis,** directly onto the parasite's cell membrane. Attack by the eosinophils is mediated by antibodies produced by lymphocytes, interactions with the tissue phase of monocytes (macrophages), and in concert with neutrophils. They are also involved in removing fibrin deposits that are formed during the inflammatory response.

Basophils are involved in certain types of immune responses. These cells carry numerous large granules containing, among other products, histamine and heparin. Histamine is released by the basophil when the immune system is stimulated by certain types of foreign proteins or antigens, such as those associated with many allergic conditions. Histamine in the bloodstream and tissues produces dilation of peripheral blood vessels, causing local redness, swelling and pooling of blood, and constriction of respiratory smooth muscle, such as during attacks of asthma. Heparin is an anticoagulant, helping to inhibit blood clotting during some types of tissue injury.

Although monocytes are considered to be an immature, transient phase of tissue macrophages, they are fully capable of vigorous phagocytosis when they encounter microorganisms. In fact, one might think of monocytes as "blood macrophages." Originating in the bone marrow from cells that also give rise to the granulocytes, monocytes spend a short time in the bloodstream, then enter the body tissues, ready to respond to

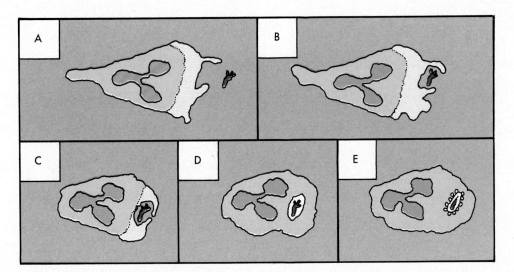

Fig. 6-2. Phagocytosis of a microbe.
A segmented neutrophil approaches (**A**) and makes contact with a microorganism (**B**). Extension of the cell membrane around the microbe (**C**) results in the formation of a phagosome or ingestion vacuole (**D**) so that the microbe is inside the PMN. Only two dimensions are illustrated here, but the PMN completely encloses the vacuole. Lysosomes and other granular contents fuse with the membrane (**E**) to enter the vacuole and aid in digestion of the microbe.

chemical signals sent by other blood cells. Often this involves signals sent by neutrophils during bacterial ingestion. First to arrive at the site of infection, the neutrophils rapidly digest the microbes, also destroying some of the surrounding tissue and themselves, producing one of the common signs of inflammation: pus and tissue necrosis. It is the macrophages that clean up this residue of surviving microbes, tissue fragments, and dying neutrophils. Macrophages are also more adept at ingesting fungal cells and viruses than are the neutrophils. The differences in these phagocytic capabilities can be seen in patients suffering from deficiencies in one type of cell or the other and the corresponding lack of control of particular infectious agents. Some macrophages function at fixed tissue sites, such as the alveolar macrophages of the lungs, Kupffer cells in the liver, reticuloendothelial cells of the spleen, microglial cells of the brain. Others such as the Langerhan's cells of the skin, migrate with antigens they encounter to the lymphoid tissues. Some of these macrophages recognize and remove antibodies produced by lymphocytes attached to foreign cells; others present invading antigens to other cells of the immune system.

Lymphocytes are produced both in the bone marrow and in the lymphatic tissues. They form part of the **humoral** defense system, since they primarily produce products that interact with antigens in the plasma and tissue fluids. These products, the antibodies, are manufactured and released into the bloodstream by specialized lymphocytes called **plasma cells,** a differentiated type of **B lymphocyte.** Antibody production is regulated by other types of lymphocytes, **T lymphocytes,** which can recognize antigens and either suppress or induce B lymphocyte activities. Still other types of lymphocytes are specialized to destroy viruses and to monitor developing tumor cells (neoplasms). The interactions between various lymphocytes, macrophages, and granulocytes are described in Chapter 9. Additional humoral defense factors include the **complement** system, a sequence of protein fragments that helps recruit phagocytes to target microbes, various acute-phase proteins associated with inflammation, and components of the hemostatic and coagulation mechanisms (Chapter 11).

In addition to the leukocytes commonly encountered in the peripheral blood, a number of other cells of myeloid origin are found in the bone marrow and at other tissue sites. The marrow contains **megakaryocytes,** large multinucleated cells that give rise to the blood platelets, small cellular fragments that help initiate hemostasis and blood clotting (Chapter 12). Reticulum cells (macrophages), osteoblasts and osteoclasts, and lipid storage cells are also present in the marrow as structural and functional elements. The connective tissue and mucosal epithelium contains **mast cells** (a tissue cell that is morphologically similar to circulating basophils) and **tissue eosinophils.** These cells play roles in immune reactions in concert with lymphocytes and macrophages.

SUMMARY

- The functional roles of some types of white cells (granulocytes) were established when the relationship between pus formation, infection, and phagocytosis was discovered during the nineteenth century.
- Morphologically distinct leukocytes include mononuclear cells (lymphocytes and monocytes) and polymorphonuclear (PMN) cells (the granulocytes: neutrophils, eosinophils, and basophils).
- White blood cells reproduce and differentiate in the marrow or in the lymphatic organs (lymphocytes), utilize the bloodstream as a transport medium, and fulfill their functional destinies as mediators of host defense in the peripheral tissues and other organs of the body.

- Specific granulocytes are named on the basis of their cytochemical reactions with triacid stains: eosinophilic (red-dye attracting), basophilic (dark-dye attracting), and neutrophilic (attracts both dyes).
- Leukocytes conduct host defense activities by phagocytosis and digestion of microbes and by secreting soluble antibodies that combine with and neutralize foreign materials. Many of these activities are shared and coordinated by different white cell types, in concert with a complement protein system and other elements of the inflammatory response.

7

Leukopoiesis

STEM CELLS AND COLONY FORMING UNITS

Morphologically, stem cells are small, mobile, mononuclear cells that can differentiate into one or more cell lines. Identification of these cells in the marrow has been difficult because the cells resemble lymphocytes and lack distinguishing features. Much of the evidence for their existence is based on studies in which marrow cells are removed from a laboratory animal and grown in tissue culture. The donor animal is either irradiated or treated with chemical agents that destroy the remaining blood forming tissues of the marrow and spleen. Cells believed to be undifferentiated precursors are infused into the treated donor in an attempt to reestablish hematopoietic tissue. In mice, these cells appear as small colonies in the spleen; therefore the stem cells are defined as **colony forming units (CFU),** or more specifically, CFU-S, designating spleen. Analysis of chromosomes from these cells indicate that each microscopic colony of dividing cells was started by a single injected stem cell.

These cells replicate to establish clones of blood forming tissue, a characteristic referred to as "self-renewal." Furthermore, each CFU-S has the potential to differentiate into one or more of the various lines of leukocytes. This should not be surprising, since every diploid cell of an organism contains all of the genetic information needed to form every type of specialized, mature cell at various stages of life. Which genes operate and which genes remain inactive is determined by complex developmental mechanisms interacting with specific environmental triggers and regulators. Ultimately, the precursor of every cell is a fertilized egg! What is not clear is to what degree some of the different types of CFU represent the forerunners of various blood cells.

Developmentally, embryonic blood cells are derived from undifferentiated mesenchymal cells. These have been difficult to identify in the marrow, and different experimental approaches have resulted in a bewildering assortment of overlapping terms to describe the various stem cell stages. Until such time as an assay or technique can provide definitive identification, the earliest blood-forming unit can be simply termed the **primitive stem cell.** This cell probably also gives rise to other mesenchymal derivatives, such as osteoclasts and osteoblasts, fibroblasts, marrow histiocytes, and lipocytes (fat cells). Slightly more differentiation would produce a cell that could form any blood cell, equivalent to the "hematopoietic stem cell" of some authors (Fig. 7-1). This is designated the CFU-LM on the basis of culture and transplantation experiments, but it is more widely known as the **pluripotential stem cell (PSC).** Depending on the actions of physiological feedback mechanisms, many of which are still hypothetical, the PSC can become "committed" to a lymphoid or myeloid line, in the form of **multipotential stem cells (MSC),** which may also be referred to as "lymphoid stem cells" and "myeloid

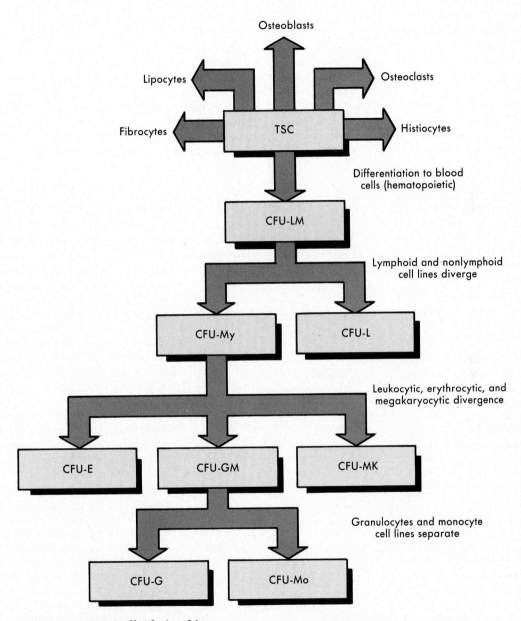

Fig. 7-1.   Stem cell relationships.
One model for hematopoietic cell lineage. The number of stem cell stages is not known nor is the degree to which in vitro experiments (cell cultures) represent in vivo relationships.

stem cells," respectively. Unfortunately, these terms are used somewhat informally and interchangeably, whereas names derived from the capacity to form a clone of an identifiable cell type is based on experimental results that are reproduceable. The problem with a stem cell nomenclature based on colony forming units is that most of the work is done on non-human tissues and there is no guarantee that the maturation and repopulation kinetics of cell transplantation experiments represent normal blood cell origins.

Lymphoid precursors migrate from the bone marrow to the lymphoid tissues (thymus, spleen, lymph nodes, etc.) to mature into functionally specialized lymphocytes (Chapter 9). The CFU-S probably represents the myeloid MSC, which can differentiate further into separate stem cell pools or colony forming units of the erythroid

---

STEM CELL DESIGNATIONS AND SYNONYMS

Totipotent stem cell (TSC)
Primitive stem cell
Undifferentiated Reticulum Cell

Pluripotent stem cell (PSC)
Hemohistoblast
Colony forming unit, lymphoid/myeloid (CFU-LM)
Hematopoietic stem cell

Multipotent stem cells (MSC)
Colony forming unit-spleen (CFU-S)
Lymphoid stem cell (CFU-L)
Myeloid stem cell (CFU-My)

Committed stem cells
Colony forming unit-Granulocyte/Monocyte (CFU-GM)
Colony forming unit-Erythrocyte (CFU-E)
Colony forming unit-Megakaryocyte (CFU-MK)
Colony forming unit-Granulocyte (CFU-G)
Colony forming unit-Monocyte (CFU-Mo)

(CFU-E), megakaryocytic (CFU-MEG), and granulocyte-monocyte (CFU-GM) types. Additional restriction of phenotypic expression in the CFU-GM produces separate granulocytic and monocytic stem cells. These may or may not be the marrow cells that are identifiable as myeloblasts and monoblasts. Again, the number of cell intermediates and their respective characteristics remain to be identified. The relationship between marrow precursors, blood cells, and tissue components is diagrammed in Fig. 7-2.

MARROW STRUCTURE

Blood cell differentiation and maturation occurs in an environment that is structurally well organized and complex. The cellular material observed in tissue cultures and in marrow aspirations obtained from patients provides a misleading picture of the in vivo relationships between marrow elements. Human bones consist of a relatively dense outer layer (cortex) and a central, "spongy" area of trabecular bone. The trabecular system contains fat cells ("yellow marrow") and an extensive capillary network supported by fibrous connective tissue ("red marrow"). The capillaries form a complex network, the **marrow sinus,** which returns blood to the venous system leaving the bone. It is in the spaces between branches of the sinus that blood cell proliferation and maturation occur (Fig. 7-3). The luminal surface of the sinusoidal capillaries consists primarily of a single layer of endothelial cells; the outer or abluminal surface is partly covered by adventitial **reticulum cells.** The reticulum cells also extend cytoplasmic projections into the adjacent hematopoietic tissue, producing a fibrous network to which the hematopoietic elements attach. Reticulum cells were once believed to be hematopoietic, possibly a type of early stem cell, but more recent evidence indicates that they serve as a structural support.

Mature blood cells must migrate across the sinusoidal endothelia to enter the circu-

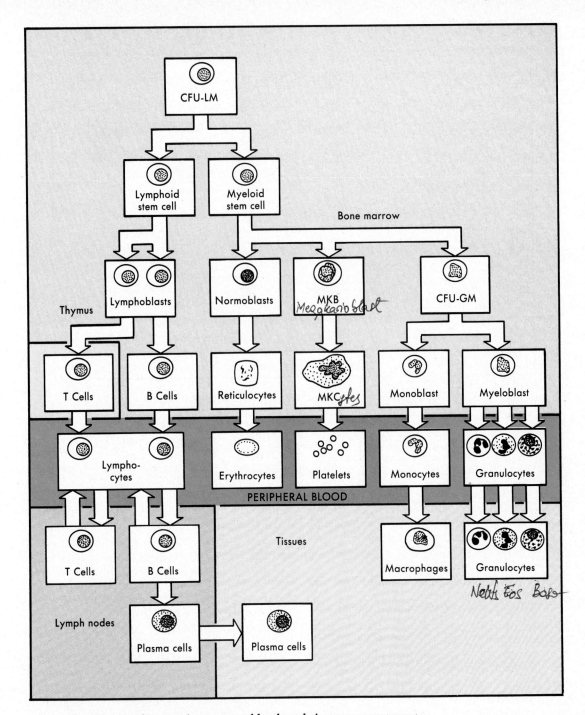

Fig. 7-2.   Leukocytes in marrow, blood, and tissue compartments.
Not all tissue-blood cell relationships are depicted. Lymphocytes, for example, recirculate between various organs, lymphatic vessels, and the bloodsteam.

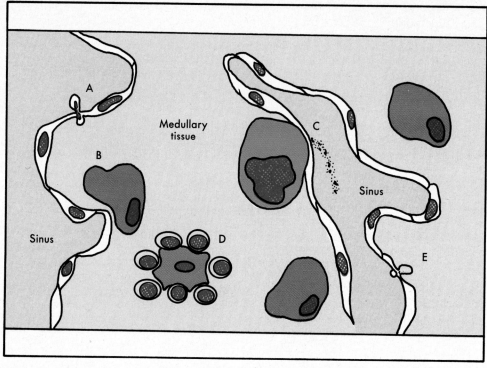

Fig. 7-3. Structure of the hematopoietic marrow and sinuses.
Depiction of relationships between the hematopoietic tissue of the marrow (medullary tissue) and the capillary sinuses. *A*, Passage of a neutrophil through the endothelial lining of the sinus; *B*, large lipocytes (fat cells) that comprise a large portion of the marrow space; *C*, release of a platelet strand from a megakaryocyte adjacent to a sius; *D*, erythroblastic island; *E*, passage of a reticulocyte through the endothelial lining.

lation (Fig. 7-4). Endothelial cell membranes contain small pores or fenestrations that permit the passage of mature cells that are relatively more deformable and retain the more rigid and less motile precursors. Indeed, the sinusoidal passage of reticulocytes after nuclear expulsion (Chapter 3) may be analogous to the release of neutrophils as a result of nuclear segmentation. In either case, pathological processes can facilitate the release of immature cells by affecting the cellular composition of the sinusoidal lining.

Marrow leukocyte precursors form clusters of maturing cells, similar to the erythroblastic islands of maturing normoblasts. These aggregates are usually disrupted during marrow aspiration, but they are sometimes preserved in biopsy sections. Groups of granulocytes and lymphocytes are usually found at some distance from the sinus walls, whereas megakaryocytes are often adjacent to the endothelium.

The total **cellularity** of the marrow in a normal, stable adult is about 50%, with the rest of the space occupied by lipid deposits. This figure is much higher in newborns, where hematopoietic activity is maximal, and it may be slightly lower in persons over 60 years of age. During times of hematopoi-

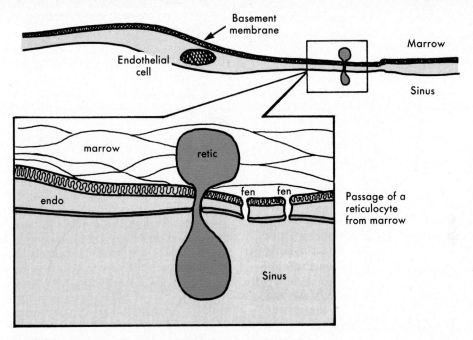

Fig. 7-4. Passage of a blood cell from the marrow.
Reticulocytes pass through fenestral openings *(fen)* or pores at specialized areas of the endothelial cells *(endo)* lining the sinuses.

etic demand, such as a response to infection or hemorrhage, cellularity can increase to almost 80% or more. **Hypercellular** or **hyperplastic** marrows are also seen in myeloproliferative diseases in which cell reproduction is uncontrolled (Chapter 20). Failure of blood cell proliferation, due to nutritional deficiencies or because of exposure to toxic agents, results in a **hypocellular** or **hypoplastic** marrow. The proportion of myeloid cells (granulocyte and monocyte precursors) to erythroid cells (normoblasts), called the **myeloid to erythroid ratio (M:E),** is approximately 2:1 to about 5:1 in an adult.

PHYSIOLOGICAL REGULATION OF LEUKOPOIESIS

Proliferation of committed stem cells of the erythroid line (CFU-E) are, in part, regulated by erythropoietin (Chapter 3). A number of similar mechanisms have been pro-

posed to explain leukopoietic responses to microbial invasions and other demans for white blood cells (Fig. 7-5). The clearest evidence to date has been derived from studies of CFU-GM cells in tissue culture. In vitro proliferation of these bipotential stem cells requires the presence of a colony-stimulating factor (CSF) which has been isolated in several forms of **colony stimulating activity (CSA):** substances that stimulate neutrophil, monocyte, neutrophil + monocyte, or eosinophil production (Burgess, 1980). Varieties of CSA are released by marrow macrophages, circulating monocytes, endothelial cells, T cell blasts in culture, and activated lymphocytes, but their production and regulation is still unclear. CSF has also been referred to as "leukopoietin" or "granulopoietin," but the number of different agents and their actions in vivo are still under investigation.

Release of granulocytes from the marrow storage pool may be regulated by another agent, **neutrophil releasing activity (NRA),** which may account for the immediate response of neutrophils to bacterial sepsis. Additional substances have been tentatively identified as products or lymphocytes that may regulate production or release of CSAs by other cells. At least one product, **lactoferrin,** is found in neutrophilic granules that appears to inhibit the release of CSA by monocytes and macrophages. This may provide a negative feedback control for neutrophil proliferation and release. The role of lactoferrin in neutrophil microbicidal function is discussed in Chapter 8.

LEUKOCYTE KINETICS AND ENUMERATION

The differential white blood cell count, a classification and enumeration of peripheral or marrow leukocytes, is one of the fundamental analyses of hematology. The **absolute concentration** of each cell type is expressed as number/µL or number/L and the **relative concentration** is expressed as a percent of the total differential count. Traditionally, the total white blood cell count (WBC) and differential were done manually, using a hemacytometer and stained blood smear, respectively. Specific leukocyte types were rarely counted directly, an exception being eosinophils, which can be diluted with a stain and visualized in a hemacy-

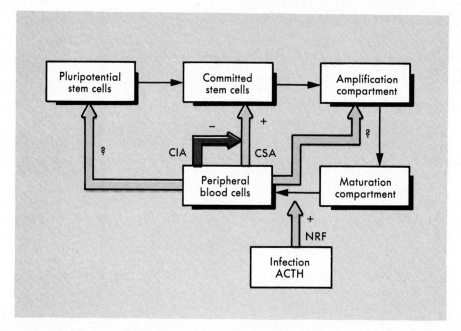

Fig. 7-5.   Regulation of leukopoiesis.
Differentiation, maturation, and release of granulocytes from the marrow are separate processes that are regulated by substances released from mature neutrophils, monocytes, and lymphocytes. Some mediators stimulate cell proliferation (colony stimulating activity, *CSA*) and others inhibit the stimulatory mediators (colony inhibitory activity, *CIA*). Bacterial sepsis and steroid compounds can stimulate the release of granulocytes from the marrow storage compartment (neutrophil releasing factor, *NRF*). A variety of potential mediators have been identified in tissue culture, but the nature of their physiological activities in vivo is still unclear.

tometer (Chapter 27). Therefore it was common practice to obtain the absolute leukocyte count and then classify and tabulate 100 white cells by percent. Multiplying each percentage by the total white count resulted in an indirect measure of the absolute concentration of neutrophils, lymphocytes, and other leukocytes:

Lymphocytes/μL = Lymphocytes, decimal fraction × leukocytes/μL

Most complete blood counts now are done by automated instruments, including differential counts based on many hundreds to thousands of cell identifications. The increased precision of these methods permits a much finer discrimination of sequential differences in leukocyte values so that a patient's disease course or response to therapy can be followed. As a result, it is becoming more common and useful to report both the relative and absolute values of each leukocyte type.

The relative amounts of white cells present in marrow and peripheral blood samples are determined by their rates of production, maturation times, circulation intervals, and turnover rates. Studies of leukocyte kinetics, like those of erythrocytes, have employed radioisotopic markers to document production rates and survival times. Unfortunately, data for some types of white cells are difficult to interpret, either because of the relatively fewer cells involved or because of their migrations and transformations after release from the marrow. Other data is derived from in vitro studies, usually cell cultures, or from manipulations of hematopoietic tissue in other animals, such as mice. Even the data obtained in humans, but as a result of pathological processes, must be interpreted and applied to normal human physiology with some caution.

The reproductive potentials of white blood cell stages increase with differentiation from earliest stem cell through the morphologically recognizable marrow precursors. At each stage, some cells differentiate to provide a source of cells for the next maturation compartment and other cells provide a pool for self-replication (Fig. 7-6). Expansion of a cell clone is most rapid after the unipotential stem cell differentiates to the next most mature form, either a blast or early identifiable stage of a cell line. Mitotic doubling results in a committed stem cell producing several differentiated offspring, a process called **amplification.** Thus, a single erythroblast or myeloblast produces 16 erythrocytes or myelocytes, respectively.

The maturation and circulation times of different types of white cells vary considerably (Table 7-1). Total lifespans also vary; some types of lymphocytes, in the form of immunological memory cells, may persist for several years. Monocytes enter the tissues and may become fixed macrophages with similar lifespans. On the other hand, neutrophils probably survive for only a few days after leaving the marrow. Blood con-

TABLE 7-1. Leukocyte kinetics

Type of leukocyte	Time in compartment (hrs)		Cell numbers (blood:tissue)	Recirculate in blood
	Marrow	Blood		
Neutrophil	240	8-12	1:20	No
Lymphocyte	72		1:20	Yes
Monocyte	60	8-14	1:400	Yes
Eosinophil		1-20	1:400	Yes

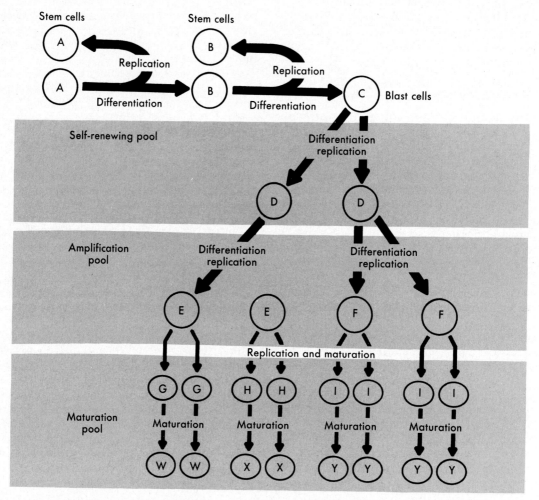

Fig. 7-6. Model of cell replication and differentiation.
Stem cells divide to provide progeny for maturation and to maintain a relatively constant marrow population. Sequential differentiation results in identifiable, committed blast cells that are not self-renewing. They undergo several sucessive divisions, amplifying the number of cell progeny. Note the difference in maturation sequences between stages derived from E cells and F cells. All F cells become Y cells, but E cells can undergo further differentiation at later stages of maturation.

centrations of each cell type depend on both the numbers of cells moving into and out of the circulation and on the amount of time spent in the circulation (Fig. 7-7). Leukocyte values, expressed as percents of resident cells, are given for the bone marrows of normal adults in Table 7-2.

There exists considerable variation in absolute and relative white cell concentrations in the peripheral blood as a function of age (Table 7-3 and Fig. 7-8). The most dramatic changes take place within hours after birth as the total leukocyte and neutrophil densities first rise then slowly decrease during infancy and early childhood. High blood neutrophil concentrations are replaced by a predominance of lymphocytes, which also reverses at about 4 years of age. Phagocytic cells are thus numerically more evident during the first few days

TABLE 7-2. Normal values for marrow cell differential counts

Cell	Mean percent	Range percent
Red cell series		
Rubriblasts	0.6	0.2-1.4
Prorubricytes	1.4	0.4-2.4
Rubricytes	21.0	17.8-29.2
Metarubricytes	5.0	1.0-12.0
Granulocytic series		
Myeloblasts	1.0	0.2-3.6
Promyelocytes	3.0	1.0-6.0
Neutrophilic Myelocytes	10.0	6.0-18.0
Neutrophilic Metamyelocytes	12.0	6.0-18.0
Band neutrophils	14.0	9.0-20.0
Segmented neutrophils	12.0	5.0-20.0
Eosinophilic myelocytes	1.2	0.2-3.0
Eosinophilic metamyelocytes	1.4	0.4-3.2
Band eosinophils	1.2	0.2-2.2
Segmented eosinophils	2.0	0.4-3.0
Basophils (all stages)	0.2	0.1-1.0
Other myelogenous cells		
Monocytes	2.0	0.4-3.0
Megakaryocytes	0.2	0.1-1.0
Lymphoid cells		
Lymphocytes	10.0	3.0-24.0
Plasma cells	0.8	0.2-2.8
Miscellaneous		
Reticulum cells	0.6	0.2-2.0
Mitotic cells	0.4	0.2-2.0
MYELOID:ERYTHROID RATIO		2:1-5:1

Considerable variation exists between published sources for marrow cell values (Custer, 1974; Diggs et al, 1985; Dittmer, 1961; Miale, 1982; Wintrobe et al, 1981). The counts presented here are compilations that are intended to represent typical reference values.

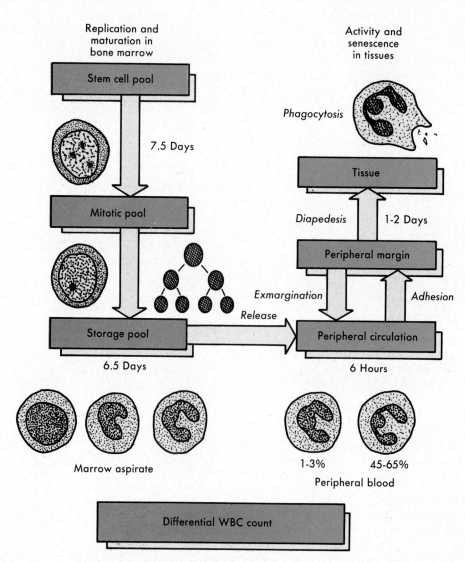

Fig. 7-7. Leukocyte transit in the peripheral blood.
The neutrophils seen on a peripheral blood smear are transients, subject to the kinetic variables of release from the marrow, demand in the tissues, and interchange between blood vessel margin and lumen.

TABLE 7-3. Mean leukocyte values in peripheral blood ($\times 10^3/\mu L$)

Age	WBC	SEG	BAND	LYM	MONO	EOS	BASO
Birth	18.2	9.4	1.7	5.5	1.1	0.4	0.1
12 Hours	22.8	13.2	2.3	5.5	1.2	0.5	0.1
24 Hours	19.1	9.8	1.8	5.8	1.1	0.5	0.1
1 Week	12.1	4.7	0.8	5.0	1.1	0.5	0.05
2 Weeks	11.4	3.9	0.6	5.5	1.0	0.4	0.05
1 Month	10.8	3.3	0.5	6.0	0.7	0.3	0.05
6 Months	12.0	3.3	0.5	7.3	0.6	0.3	0.05
1 Year	11.5	3.2	0.4	7.0	0.6	0.3	0.05
2 Years	10.6	3.2	0.3	6.3	0.5	0.3	0.05
4 Years	9.1	3.5	0.3	4.5	0.5	0.3	0.05
8 Years	8.3	4.1	0.3	3.3	0.4	0.2	0.05
12 Years	8.0	4.2	0.2	3.0	0.4	0.2	0.05
18 Years	7.7	4.2	0.2	2.7	0.4	0.2	0.05
21 Years	7.0	4.0	0.1	2.2	0.5	0.2	0.05

Mean leukocyte values are presented, rather than ranges, to facilitate comparisons of cell ratios by age.

of life, followed by the development of the immune system and the presence of circulating lymphocytes during early childhood, then finally a gradual shift to the adult pattern that once again favors phagocytic cells.

LEUKOCYTE MATURATION

The stages of white blood cell differentiation and maturation have been well known since the advent of trichrome staining at the turn of the century. Generally, the morphological changes with maturation follow the same patterns as those of the erythroid series: (1) subsequent divisions result in smaller cell size, (2) nucleus to cytoplasm ratio (N/C) decreases as cytoplasmic functions become active and specialized, (3) nuclear chromatin becomes progressively more clumped and coarser and nucleoli become less prominent or absent with the loss of replicative ability, (4) specific cytoplasmic products and granules appear, and (5) cytoplasmic basophilia gives way to other colors in conjunction with a reduction of RNA, except in some types of lymphocytes. Two excellent sources for detailed morphological descriptions and illustrations are a widely circulated atlas (Diggs, Sturm, and Bell, 1985) and a monographic discussion of morphological interpretation (Bessis, 1977).

Although there is still considerable debate as to the maturational relationships between different blood and tissue leukocytes, a general scheme can be presented for the purposes of organizing discussions of white cell differentiation (Fig. 7-9). The specific evidence for these lineages and descriptions of each cell stage are presented in the relevant sections of Chapters 8, 9, and 10. The relationship between eosinophils and other granulocytes has been unclear for some time. Earlier schemes showed a myeloblast or committed myeloid stem cell giving rise to three equal lines of granulocytes: neutrophilic, eosinophilic, and basophilic (Fig. 7-10, A). Work with precursors in tissue culture indicate that an earlier stem cell, committed to the eosinophil series (CFU-EOS), may coexist. The same problem exists with regard to basophils: are they derived from the CFU-GM, a committed myeloid stem cell, or a separate line of

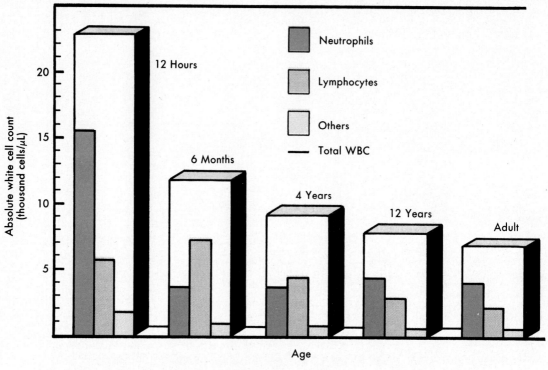

Fig. 7-8. Relative peripheral WBC components change with age.
Neutrophils comprise the majority of circulating white blood cells shortly after birth. Lymphocytes dominate during early childhood, coinciding with increased immunological activity. Lym-
phocyte/granulocyte ratios reverse before puberty and remain relatively constant throughout life.
The total leukocyte count declines slowly after infancy.

an earlier precursor (Fig. 7-10, *B*)? Tissue basophils and eosinophils were once thought
to be variants of blood basophils and eosinophils; then they were believed to be funda-
mentally different but morphologically convergent. Now biochemical evidence suggests that their morphological similarities
may indeed be reflections of shared ancestry.

The early separation of the lymphocytic
cells from all other blood cells is now well
established, as is the relationship of the
megakaryocytic and erythroid lines to the
myeloid series. The continuity of the
monocyte-macrophage line and its late separation from the neutrophil precursors is
also supported by biochemical, immunological, and tissue culture studies. These relationships are meaningful in attempting to
understand the development and manifestations of myeloproliferative diseases. More
than one cell line is often abnormal in
these neoplastic processes, showing identical chromosome abnormalities or other genetic markers that indicate a defect arising
in a particular stem cell clone.

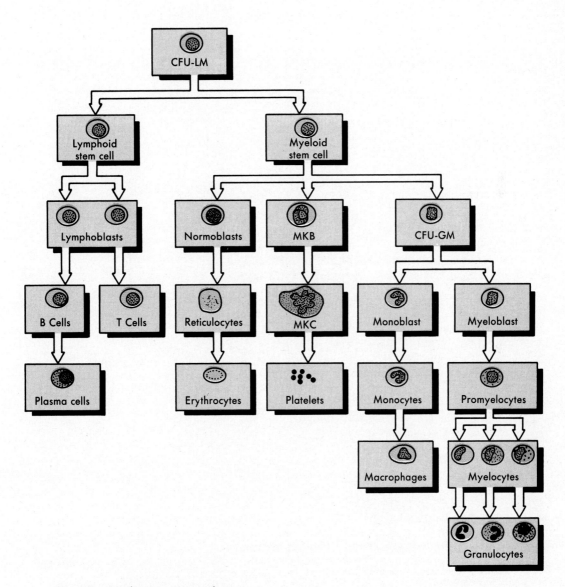

Fig. 7-9.   Leukocyte maturation.
A general model of leukocyte differentiation and maturation shows the relationships of the mature cell lines and stem cells. Intermediate stages are not shown for all cells.

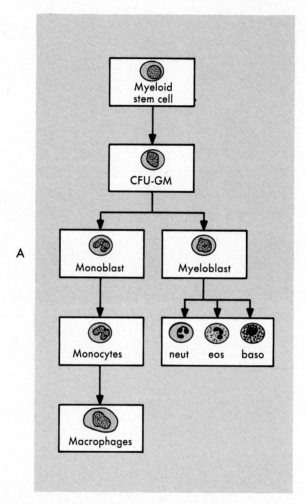

Fig. 7-10.   Alternate schemes of leukocyte maturation.
Granulocyte precursors may be represented by a myeloblast that is common to all three cell types (A) or each granulocyte cell line may derive from a separate stem cell line (B). Tissue granulocytes, including mast cells, may differentiate from peripheral granulocytes or from other stem cells.

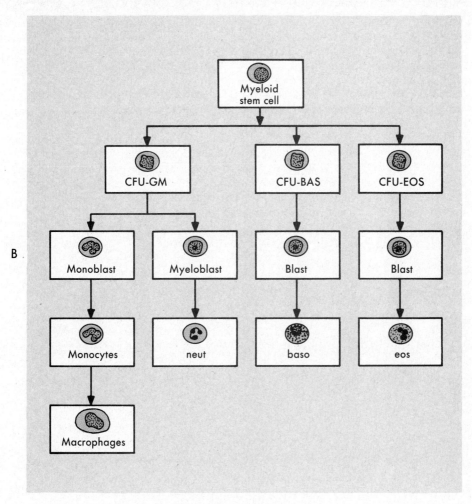

Fig. 7-10, cont'd.
See legend on facing page.

SUMMARY

- Colony-forming units (CFUs) are hemo-topoietic precursors or stem cells that reproduce to establish a line of identifiable blood cells. Early stem cells can differentiate to establish several lines.
- Pluripotential stem cells can "commit" to either a myeloid or lymphoid cell line by giving rise to the appropriate multipotential stem cell. These in turn differentiate into specific cell lines represented by unipotential stem cells.
- Lymphoid stem cells migrate to the lymphoid tissues to mature and differentiate into specialized lymphocytes; myeloid stem cells remain in the marrow to form colonies of erythrocytes, megakaryocytes, granulocytes, and monocytes.

- Blood cells are released from the marrow hematopoetic tissue into a complex capillary sinus. Normal cells attain mature characteristics that permit them to cross the sinusoidal endothelial cell barrier.
- The normal adult marrow is about 50% cellular and 50% lipid stores and connective tissue. The cellular component consists of about 2 to 5 times as many non-erythroid elements as it does erythroid cells.
- Proliferation, maturation, and release of leukocytes is regulated by a number of specific agents, some of which are elaborated by circulating white blood cells.
- Absolute densities of peripheral blood white cells are expressed in number/μL, and relative densities are stated as a percent of the total leukocyte count.
- Leukocyte maturation is accompanied by a decrease in cell size, a decrease in nucleus to cytoplasm ratio, increased coarseness of nuclear chromatin, decrease and disappearance of nucleoli, appearance of cytoplasmic granules and products, and a decrease in cytoplasmic basophilia.

8

The Granulocytes

THE NEUTROPHIL

Neutrophils are the most numerous white cells of the peripheral blood in both newborn infants and in adults (during early childhood the majority cells are lymphocytes, corresponding with development of the immunological defense system). Examination of the bone marrow reveals that neutrophils and their immediate precursors make up the predominant cell in this tissue also, a function of the high peripheral cell density and the rapid turnover (short lifespan).

Neutrophil concentration in the blood is a function of three processes: (1) input from the marrow storage compartment (2) ratio of freely circulating cells to those adhering onto the endothelial cell lining of the blood vessels (marginal pool), and (3) the rate of emigration from blood to tissues by diapedesis (see Fig. 7-7). The capability of the marrow storage pool to respond to peripheral demands for replacement neutrophils depends on the number of replicating precursors and the rate of maturation. Normally, when neutrophil turnover is in a steady state, the marrow releases cells with segmented or band-shaped nuclei. These stages possess the requisite organelles and enzymes for host defense, and the cell is able to deform and pass through tissues more readily. Earlier stages are retained in the marrow unless physiological responses to a pathological stimulus deplete the peripheral blood. Under these conditions, maturation time may be reduced, and the pool of self-replicating granulocyte precursors may expand to compensate for the deficit (see Chapter 21 for a discussion of benign responses to acute infections).

Neutrophil maturation

Maturation from a myeloblast to a segmented neutrophil involves several obvious morphological changes and many less obvious but equally important biochemical alterations. As with the red cells, neutrophil differentiation is associated with a loss of mitotic activity and the appearance of specialized organelles (Table 8-1). The nuclear chromatin becomes coarser and more basophilic, the nucleus to cytoplasm ratio decreases, and the number of visible nucleoli decreases from several to none by the myelocyte stage. The shape of the nucleus undergoes a dramatic metamorphosis, from an irregular sphere to an indented form, finally fragmenting into several lobes connected by thin strands of chromatin (Fig. 8-1). The cytoplasm exhibits maturational changes similar to those of the rubricytes: a progressive loss of basophilia associated with a decrease in RNA content.

The myeloblast (see plate 2A). The **myeloblast** is the first stage (M_1) of the granulocytic series that is identifiable by light microscopic morphology. It may be difficult to distinguish myeloblasts from other blasts in the peripheral blood unless one uses special stains or infers their identity from the presence of other immature cells of the same line. A myeloblast can be distinguished

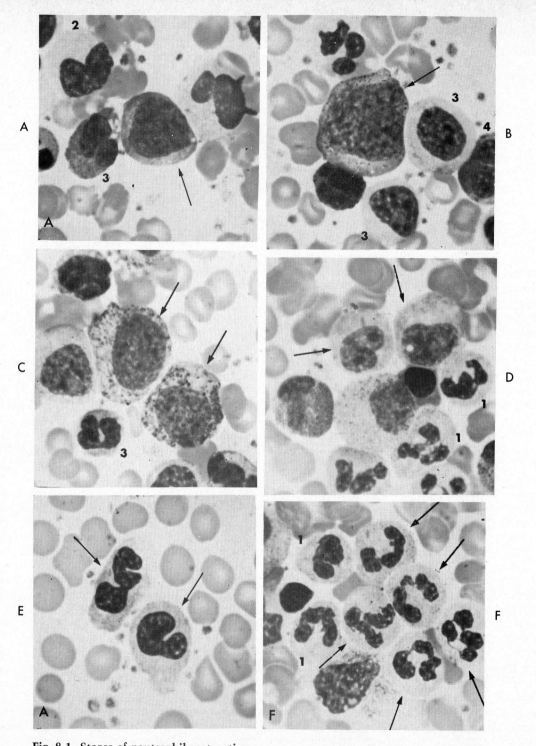

Fig. 8-1. Stages of neutrophil maturation.
The nucleus undergoes the most dramatic changes as a myeloblast matures to a segmented neutrophil. Accompanying changes in the cytoplasm occur with the appearance of primary and secondary granules. **A,** Myeloblast; **B,** promyelocyte; **C,** myelocyte. **D,** metamyelocyte, **E,** band neutrophil; **F,** segmented neutrophil.

Table 8-1. Neutrophil changes associated with maturation

	Cell stage	Mitosis	Primary granules	Secondary granules
M_1	Myeloblast	Yes-1	None or few	None
M_2	Promyelocyte	Yes-1	Many, prominent	None visible
M_{3-4}	Myelocyte	Yes-2	Moderate, distinct	Many, prominent
M_5	Metamyelocyte	No	Few, indistinct	Many, light
M_6	Band form	No	Few, indistinct	Many, faint
M_7	Segmented form	No	Few, indistinct	Many, faint

from a promyelocyte by its lack of cytoplasmic granulation, although some workers reserve the use of myeloblast for cells that contain a few fine azurophilic granules. Peroxidase stains can distinguish myeloblasts from lymphocytic and erythroblastic precursors, although the reaction can be quite variable. The nucleus is composed of very fine nonaggregated chromatin that stains light blue to reddish-purple with Wright's stain. From 2 to 5 distinct nucleoli are usually present. The nucleus is often bordered at one side by a distinct perinuclear zone. A 4:1 nucleus to cytoplasm ratio leaves a small rim of cytoplasm surrounding the roughly round to oval nucleus, which frequently has an irregular or pentagonal periphery. The cytoplasm is typically basophilic because of the high density of ribosomes and increased RNA content. Myeloblasts are about 12 to 20 μm in diameter. They exist at the M_1 stage for about 1 day and then undergo a single mitotic division.

The presence of many large, reddish-purple granules characterizes **promyelocytes,** the second granulocytic stage. These azurophilic granules are nonspecific in that they are shared by the other granulocytes (eosinophils and basophils). They are also referred to as the **primary granules** since they are the first to appear during cell maturation. They are synthesized only during the promyelocyte (M_2) stage, which lasts about 2 days and terminates in one mitotic division. The number of granules varies from cell to cell, and some authors have

proposed the terms "early" and "late" promyelocytes to distinguish morphological varieties. These granules are peroxidase positive, and a lipid component reacts with Sudan black stain, providing a second cytochemical reaction for the identification of large mononuclear cells in blood and marrow smears. The cell size, 12 to 20 μm, is the same as that of a myeloblast, but the nucleus to cytoplasm ratio is less, usually from 3:1 to 2:1. The chromatin is still fine, but some aggregation is evident. One to three nucleoli are also visible, although these can be obscured by heavy granulation. The nucleus is more regular in outline, round or oval, and it may be eccentrically located. The cytoplasm is less basophilic than that of neighboring myeloblasts, although some variability in staining reaction should be expected at either stage. Because granule synthesis is very active at this stage, the large Golgi complex may be represented by a distinctly clear juxtanuclear region. Although promyelocytes of different mature granulocyte types cannot be distinguished on the basis of routine blood stains, electron microscopy and specialized cytochemical stains can identify eosinophilic precursors from those of neutrophils.

The myelocyte (see plate 2C). The **myelocyte** undergoes two mitotic divisions (stages M_3 and M_4), accounting for an interval of 4 days. These are the last replications of the granulocytic maturation and amplification sequence, in which one myeloblast has produced up to 16 myelocytes. This theoretical multiple is probably not realized under normal conditions of reduced granulopoiesis, in which marrow macrophages consume some mitotic products and recycle the cell contents. Myelocyte cell diameter varies greatly, from 10 to 18 μm; larger cells are generally premitotic and smaller cells are postmitotic. The nucleus to cytoplasm ratio decreases from about 2:2 to 1:1, and the oval or round nucleus is often eccentrically located. Chromatin is finely granulated in early myelocytes and more aggregated in later cells. The nucleolus is no longer visible on routine-stained smears. A prominent perinuclear area is characteristic.

This stage is defined by the appearance of **secondary granules** that contain products specific for a particular type of granulocyte. Thus a myelocytic stage can be identified for neutrophils, eosinophils, and basophils by specific granules that are characteristic for each cell type. Primary granules are also present, but they are not as numerous because the original content, synthesized only at the promyelocytic stage, has been apportioned among several cells during mitosis. Neutrophilic secondary granules stain a faint reddish-purple to bluish color with Wright's stain. Their biochemical contents are listed in Table 8-2 and described below. Some of these granules may be actually synthesized during the late promyelocytic stage, but they are difficult to detect because of the density of azurophilic granules. The cytoplasm of neutrophils stain a light gray-blue to polychromatic pink-gray, depending on the degree of granule synthesis. One should remember that cell maturation is a continuous process and that a population of myelocytes in a marrow smear will display the variable characteristics of cells of heterogeneous age and biochemical activity.

The metamyelocyte (see plate 2D). Metamyelocytes are characterized by further aggregation of nuclear chromatin, the appearance of basiphilic and oxyphilic chromatin patchiness, and a progressive decrease in cytoplasmic basophilia. Cell diam-

Table 8-2. Chemical contents of neutrophils

Product and location	Function
Primary granules (nonspecific lysosomes)	
Acid hydrolases	?Digest microbes in phagosomal vacuole
Neutral proteases	Break down proteins of ingested microbes
Myeloperoxidase	Potentiates HOCl killing of microbes
Acid phosphatase	?Digest microbes during phagocytosis
Cationic bacteriocidal protein	Alters microbial membrane permeability
Lysozyme arginase	Hydrolyzes microbial mucopeptide cell wall
Secondary granules (specific)	
Lactoferrin	Iron binding protein, inhibits bacteria
Lysozyme (muramidase)	Hydrolase, attacks microbial cell walls
Vitamin B12 binding R-protein	Similar to plasma transcobalamin III
Collagenase	Dissolve tissue basement membranes
Cytoplasmic membrane	
Alkaline phosphatase	Microbial digestion?
NADPH oxidase	Generation of superoxide anion
Cytoplasm	
Catalase	Destroys cytoplasmic hydrogen peroxide
Superoxide dismutase	Converts superoxide to hydrogen peroxide

eter ranges from 10 to 18 μm, but the nucleus-to-cytoplasm ratio has stabilized at approximately 1:1. Indentation of the nucleus begins at this stage, forming an outline that varies from slightly reniform (kidney-shaped) to that of a broad V shape. This stage (M_5) lasts for about 2 days, occurring as a component of the marrow storage compartment. Living cells are motile whereas myelocytes and earlier stages exhibit little or no movement. Furthermore, metamyelocytes appear to be effective in responding to and eliminating microbial invaders. When severe bacterial infection exhausts the circulating and marginal neutrophil compartments, metamyelocytes and bands from the marrow storage pool represent a "ready reserve" of phagocytes.

The band neutrophil (see plate 2E). Further indentation of the nucleus results in the formation of a **band neutrophil.** The nuclear chromatin stains deep blue to purple and it is aggregated as coarse granules. The major morphological change involves nuclear shape, and considerable debate exists as to the criteria for assigning neutrophils to stages M_5 (metamyelocyte), M_6 (band), and M_7 (segmented neutrophil). The controversy exists because of granulocytic responses to infection (see further discussion in Chapter 21). When the marrow storage pool is activated, resulting in an increase in circulating bands, a more severe and possibly progressive infection is indicated. The appearance of less mature forms **(shift to the left)** is often more significant than mere changes in total leukocyte or neutrophil count. Therefore, it is important to define the reference limits for the number of band forms that are present normally. If different laboratories or hematology workers use different criteria for inclusion or exclusion of a band, misinterpretation of changes in the blood picture of a patient can result.

Band forms normally account for about 0 to 3% of the total leukocyte count or 0 to 5% of the neutrophil count. A band can be defined as a cell whose nucleus has indented to a point between uniform thickness and one half of the thickness of the arms of the U (Fig. 8-2). The indentation must have proceeded to at least the center of the nucleus or the cell would be classified as a metamyelocyte. Other hematologists may be more conservative in defining bands, excluding cells that show any constriction beyond uniform thickness. On the other hand, other workers define a segmented form as a cell with distinct nuclear lobes connected only by a fine chromatin strand or filament (0.5 μm or less). A filament is not wide enough to have distinctly visible chromatin material present. The arms of the band may show concentrated areas or poles of chromatin. By these criteria, band forms include a greater number of cells with relatively marked constrictions; thus the normal differential leukocyte percentages will be higher.

Band forms function as mature neutrophils; they are highly motile and they are biochemically active in destroying phagocytized microbes. They have a 2-day life span, lasting about one day in the marrow and one day in the peripheral blood.

The segmented neutrophil (see plate 2F). Polymorphonuclear (PMN) or **segmented neutrophils** ("segs") are the mature phagocytes that migrate through tissues to destroy microbes and respond to inflammatory stimuli. This stage (M_7) has a total lifespan of about 5 days. Progressive constriction of the nucleus results in lobulation and a condensed chromatin that stains very dark blue or purple. Segs are from 9 to 16 μm in diameter and appear approximately spherical on a blood smear. The nuclear lobes may be spread out so that the connecting filaments are clearly visible, or the lobes may overlap or twist (Fig. 8-3). Extensions and appendages of the nucleus may also be present, including the condensed, lyonized x chromosome of females. Routine differential white cell counts consider segmented forms as a single catagory,

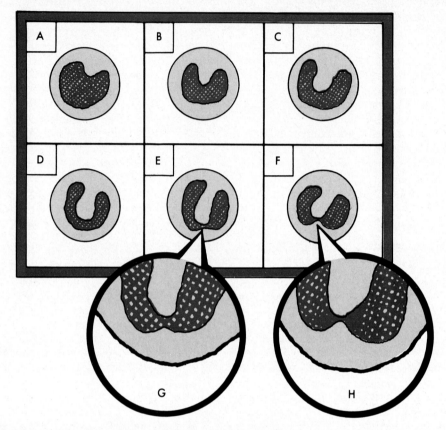

Fig. 8-2. Nuclear morphology of the band neutrophil.
Criteria for inclusion or exclusion of a cell as a band neutrophil varies among workers. Slight indentation of the reniform metamyelocyte (**A**) progresses to 50% of the nuclear diameter (**B**). Both of these cells may be considered metamyelocytes. As the indentation crosses the center of the cell (**C**) and the band becomes equally thick (**D**), inclusion as a band is widely accepted. Further constriction of the connecting portion (**E and G**) results in a cell accepted as a band by some and as an early segmented form by others. The constricted portion is half or less the width of the lobes and chromatin can be seen between the nuclear edges (**G**). Complete constriction to a thin filament excludes chromatin (**F and H**), resulting in a cell that is classified universally as a segmented form.

but their relative maturation in the peripheral blood can be recognized by classifying the cells on the basis of the number of distinct, visible lobes (Fig. 8-4). The cytoplasm stains a light beige to pink color, and the granules are fine and evenly dispersed. Primary granules may not be distinct because the azurophilic reaction is diminished in mature cells.

Neutrophil function

The primary (possibly only) role of neutrophils is to resist invasion of the host by microorganisms, mostly bacteria. After release from the bone marrow, band and segmented forms circulate in the peripheral blood for several hours. About 40% to 60% of the blood neutrophils, at any time, are adherent to the endothelial cells of the

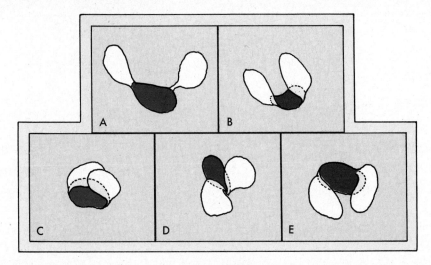

Fig. 8-3. Nuclear lobes of segmented neutrophils.
The apparent configuration of a three-lobed nucleus (**A**) can be misleading because of folding and twisting of the lobes (**B** to **E**). The center lobe is in color so that the three-dimensional relationship can be appreciated.

blood vessels (Fig. 8-5), comprising the **marginal pool** or compartment. Leukocytes marginate prior to crossing the vessel lining to enter the tissues, but they also adhere in response to diverse stimuli: some anesthetics, the onset of hemodialysis, the presence of malaria parasites, and some viruses. Increased margination can produce a pseudoneutropenia, but this condition is usually reversible. Demargination or release from the endothelium occurs in response to severe exercise, stress, and the administration of epinepherine. These "fight or flight" responses produce a pseudoneutrophilia. Thus the total leukocyte and absolute neutrophil counts do not include the actual number of cells present in the blood vessels, but only those that are freely circulating (nonadherent). Passage into the tissues by diapedesis occurs in response to inflammatory stimuli and other factors associated with infection.

Chemotaxis. Phagocytic cells respond to specific molecules by orienting and migrating toward the source of the stimulus. Ori-

Segmentation		Percent
	1 Lobes (band)	0-5
	2 Lobes	10-30
	3 Lobes	40-50
	4 Lobes	10-20
	5 Lobes	0-5
	> 5 Lobes	Rare

Fig. 8-4. Classification and frequency of occurrence of normal segmented forms.

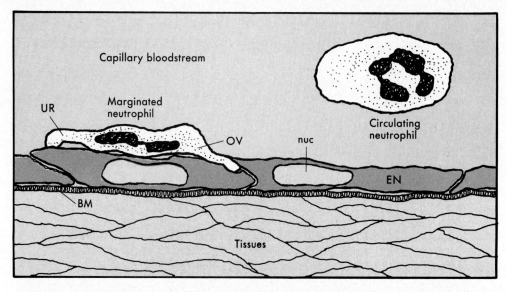

Fig. 8-5. Margination of neutrophils to the vascular endothelium.
The circulating neutrophil is amorphous in form; the marginated neutrophil is commencing diapedesis by extending a pseudopod between endothelial cells. *BM,* basement membrane; *EN,* endothelial cell; *nuc,* nucleus of endothelial cell; *OV,* oral veil; *UR,* adhesive uropod.

entation and movement toward the source is termed **chemotaxis**; increased activity without directional movement is termed **chemokinesis.** Neutrophils possess membrane receptors for specific chemicals, including the C5a fraction of complement, formylated terminal peptides (N-formyl-met-leu, N-formyl-met-leu-phe), and metabolic products of the arachidonic acid pathway (hydroxyeicosetetraenoic acid, or HETE, and leukotriene B_4). Other chemotaxins include lymphokines, secretions of activated mast cells, products of macrophages, monocytes, and other neutrophils, molecules associated with microbial cell walls and metabolism, and proteins of the kinin pathway. The synthetic peptides have provided clues to the chemotactic behavior of neutrophils. For example, there are about 50,000 membrane receptors for f-met-leu-phe. After the chemotaxin binds to the receptor, a polarized contraction spreads across the membrane, reorganizing the cy-

toskeleton. Increased quantities of calcium and other ions move across the membrane, activating the cyclic AMP and GMP pathways. Phospholipase is also activated, resulting in the release of arachidonic acid and generation of prostaglandins and leukotrienes (compare these activities with those of platelets, Chapter 12). Note that neutrophils provide some of the stimulatory products to activate or recruit additional neutrophils. This cascading or amplifying action assures that sufficient cells are attracted to an inflammatory site to combat the infection. When inflammatory stimuli decrease, the release of cellular products also decreases and phagocyte recruitment ceases.

Locomotion. Neutrophil movement is somewhat ameboid but only occurs when the cell is in contact with a surface. Cells removed from the blood stream are spherical and they die and dry on a glass slide before appreciable shape change has occurred.

When the cells are placed in a chamber or under a sealed coverslip, their movements are easily observed with a phase microscope (Fig. 8-6). The transition from a floating spherical form to an activated amoeboid or bipolar form can be accelerated by stimulating the cell with a chemotaxin (e.g., f-met-leu), fresh serum containing complement, or an extract of a microbial agent (yeast, gram-positive cocci, or lipopolysaccharides from gram-negative bacilli are often used). The leading edge forms a veil-like canopy or protopod that extends and retracts agranular pseudopods. These are difficult to see without either a phase microscope or reduced light, and they are barely discernible on stained smears. The posterior or trailing edge often forms a blunt adhesive structure, the uropod. This structure attaches the neutrophil to the substrate with several cytoplasmic filaments, so that the cell creeps across surfaces in the fashion of an inchworm, alternately extending the protopod while holding with the uropod, then attach-

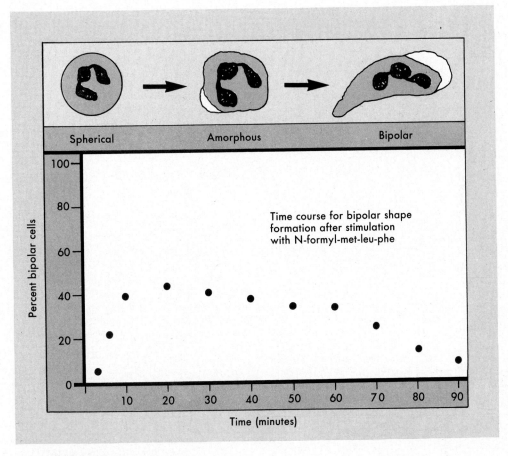

Fig. 8-6. Bipolar shape formation.
Change of neutrophil shape from resting spherical form to actively motile bipolar form in response to an artificial oligopeptide. Response curve is typical for whole blood, collected in EDTA, from a normal individual.

ing with the pseudopods while releasing the uropod. Movement through the endothelial lining occurs by extending the pseudopod between endothelial cells, dissolving the basement membrane with a protease or collagenase, then pulling the elongated cell through the opening. Bessis (1977) reports rates of movement at 19 to 40 μm per minute. Neutrophils move toward the chemical stimulus by orientation along the molecular gradient similar to the chemotactic behavior of many free-living protozoans. Circulating cells may marginate in capillaries near inflammatory sites by responding to local concentrations of chemotaxins. Young or old cells can leave the circulation, so that migration is not necessarily age dependent. Migration also occurs across linings of the gastrointestinal tract, genitourinary tract, and lungs and many of these cells are excreted.

Phagocytosis. Ingestion of a microorganism at a site of infection involves several specific steps (see Chapter 7). When the neutrophil arrives at the source of chemotactic signals, recognition of the microbe requires stimulation of other membrane receptors. If the microbe has been coated with antibodies, the phagocyte can detect the F_c portion of the immunoglobulin. Opsonization of the microbe with C3b, a complement fragment, can also be detected by neutrophil membrane receptors. Recognition is followed by attachment of the phagocyte membrane to the microbe; the microbe is surrounded, and an internal vacuole, the **phagosome,** is created by a process called "endocytosis." With the onset of endocytotic ingestion, various biochemical processes are activated, including a sharp uptake of oxygen by the cell (the **respiratory burst**).

Lysosomal granules move toward, contact, and fuse with the phagosome, forming a **phagolysosome.** The lysosomes may also fuse with the cytoplasmic membrane and with each other. Fusion with the cytoplasmic membrane may result in exocytosis, or release of the granule contents outside of the cell to attack microbes too large to be ingested. External release of acid hydrolases and other reactive enzymes can also result in destruction of normal tissues and produce a state of pathological inflammation (Chapter 21). Degranulation of the cytoplasm occurs as the granule contents are expelled either into the phagolysosome or extracellularly. After digestion of the microbe is completed, the vacuole contents are expelled by exocytosis.

The ingested microbes are killed by a combination of events. Nonoxidative events are those involving the granule contents: various enzymes that attack cell wall and membrane components of the microbe. The low pH inside the phagolysosome is also a factor, but most nonoxidative factors are probably digestive rather than lethal. The real killing power of a neutrophil comes from the generation of powerful oxidants that result from the respiratory burst.

Oxidative metabolism

The increased uptake of oxygen by activated phagocytes can be documented in a cellular respiration chamber (Fig. 8-7). The oxygen is converted to superoxide (O_2^-) by a membrane-bound enzyme, **NADPH oxidase** (NADH oxidase may also be involved). The generation of suitable quantities of NADPH is a function of the cellular hexose monophosphate shunt and **glucose-6-phosphate dehydrogenase.** Deficiencies of this latter enzyme can result in decreased levels of NADPH and inability to generate oxidants. Production of superoxide can be evaluated with a simple assay, the **nitroblue tetrazolium (NBT)** test. Neutrophils are incubated in the NBT and they incorporate it intracellularly. Formation of superoxide changes NBT, a clear substrate, to formazon, a blue material visualized as deposits in the cytoplasm. Lack of the colored deposits indicates a deficiency in superoxide generation (the procedure is presented in Chapter 27).

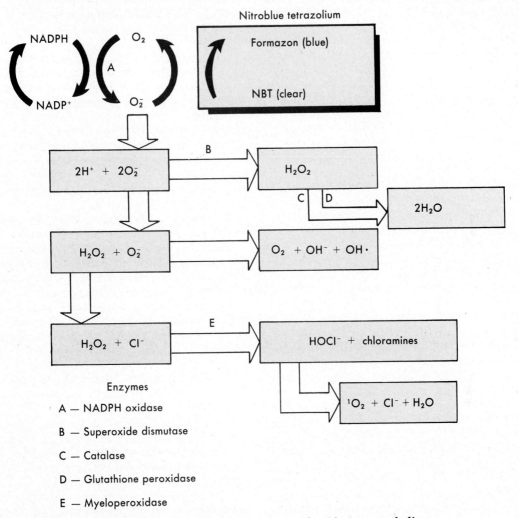

Fig. 8-7. Pathways for generating lethal products of oxidative metabolism.
Constituents released into the phagolysosome that may kill certain microbes are shown in color.

Superoxide is probably not a lethal product for most microbes, but it does act as intermediary for the generation of other agents that are effective. Superoxide, in an acid environment, is converted to hydrogen peroxide and oxygen (Fig. 8-7). Hydrogen peroxide combines with additional superoxide to produce hydroxyl ions (OH^-) and radicals ($OH^\bullet$) and with chloride ions to produce hypochlorite ($HOCl^-$), the major ingredient of household bleach, and chlorinated amines. This reaction is catalyzed by **myeloperoxidase (MPO)**, the major enzyme of the primary granules. MPO is also present in monocytes in smaller amounts, but it is lacking in the more mature macrophages. The neutrophilic MPO content in some people may be markedly decreased without an associated increase in bacterial infections, indicating the number of different mechanisms that are utilized in antimicrobial defense. One product that does appear to be highly effective is generated from hypochlorite. Singlet oxygen ($^1O_2$) exists for only a few microseconds, yet it may be one of the most lethal agents generated in the oxidative process.

Hydrogen peroxide formation also interacts as a positive feedback for the generation of additional NADP and stimulation of the HMP shunt. Glutathione peroxidase converts reduced glutathione (GSH) and H_2O_2 to glutathione (SG) and water. Glutathione reductase reduces the glutathione and NADPH to NADP (see Fig. 5-2).

Death of the microbes can be demonstrated with fluorescent stains, such as auramine O. Incubation of a microbe culture, such as *Escherichia coli,* with the dye results in the bacterial cells staining a bright green under ultraviolet illumination. As the bacteria are ingested and killed, the microbes change color from green to yellow to orange-red. This technique permits a determination of the maximum number of microbial cells ingested, the time required to kill them, and the consequences of specifically determined defects and disorders. For example, a typical neutrophil can ingest more than 30 cells of a *Pseudomonas sp.* but only kill about 20 of them (Boggs and Winkelstein, 1983). The destructive effects of the phagolysosomal activities are cumulative, and a neutrophil eventually incurs autolysis, literally digesting itself with its own enzymes.

Other cellular products

Lactoferrin is an iron-binding glycoprotein associated with lysosomes. Extracellular release of this chemical may inhibit bacterial growth by removing their source of iron. Curiously, this same molecule has been identified as a possible inhibitor or blocking agent of colony stimulating activity (CSA) for granulopoiesis.

Leukocyte alkaline phosphatase (LAP) was once believed to be a component of the secondary granules, but current evidence associates LAP primarily with the cell membrane. LAP content increases when neutrophils are activated. This can be demonstrated by a histochemical technique that provides a substrate for the enzyme. Increased neutrophil LAP content is seen in patients with reactive leukocytosis (especially in those with severe bacterial infections), during the third trimester of pregnancy, and in patients with myeloproliferative disorders (Chapter 20).

Muramidase or lysozyme is a hydrolase found in the lysosomes. Levels are increased in the abnormal cells associated with granulocytic leukemia. **Cathepsins,** along with other proteases, help break down fibrin clots. Neutrophils also contain **plasminogen,** the precursor of plasmin, that acts to remove fibrin deposits and promote the healing of inflamed areas. **Lysozyme arginase** is a product of the primary granules. It hydrolyzes the cell walls of certain types of bacteria.

THE EOSINOPHIL

Eosinophils are formed from committed stem cells (CFU-GM) that probably give rise to the neutrophil-monocyte line and to eosinophils and basophils. Although the existence of a true eosinophilic blast is still debatable, distinctly eosinophilic cells can be recognized at the promyelocytic stage by ultrastructural features and differences in myeloperoxidase. In addition, the humoral regulatory factors for eosinophil production and maturation appear to be distinct from those for neutrophils. Distinct eosinophils are recognized on Wright-stained smears at the myelocyte stage by the appearance of the large, bright orange granules (eosin-attracting) for which they are named.

Maturation

Eosinophilic myelocytes are about 10 to 18 μm in diameter with an irregular round to oval outline (Plate 3A). The nucleus is oval to round and may be slightly indented; it is often eccentrically located, occupying one half to two thirds of the cell (N/C ratio = 2:1 to 1:1). Like that of neutrophilic myelocytes, the chromatin pattern is slightly aggregated with a fine granulation, but this may be obscured by the large specific granules. A single nucleolus may be visible. The cytoplasm may be more basophilic than that of the corresponding neutrophilic stage. The granules are considerably larger (0.5 to 1.5 μm diameter) than those of neutrophilic myelocytes and they often stain bluish-purple in early stages. The granules of late myelocytes take on the typical red-orange color, but this difference led to misinterpretations of the bluish granules as evidence of a shared basophilic and eosinophilic lineage.

Eosinophil kinetics is still a poorly understood subject, but the maturation time in the bone marrow is believed to require 3 to 6 days, including an **eosinophilic metamyelocyte** stage. This cell has most of the same properties of the myelocyte, except that the chromatin is more condensed and patchy and the N/C ratio is more typically 1:1. The cytoplasm is less basophilic, usually a pink to pink-gray color.

Release of **band eosinophils** and mature **eosinophils** (Plate 3B) from the marrow is followed by a transit time of about 8 to 12 hours through the peripheral blood. Most of the cells accumulate in the tissues, especially in the gut and lungs, so that a distribution ratio of about 300:1:200 (marrow: blood:tissues) results. The mature cells are about 10 to 16 μm in diameter and represent about 1% to 3% (50-300 per μL) of the peripheral blood leukocyte count. Actually, band neutrophils are seldom encountered in the peripheral blood, they comprise only about 1% of the cells in the marrow (see Table 7-2). Most of the circulating eosinophils are bilobed though few attain three or four lobes. The lobes are usually very regular and ovoid, in contrast to the lobes of

neutrophils, which tend to be stringy and irregular (Fig. 8-8).

Function

Eosinophils provide a line of defense against parasitic infections and they also inactivate some of the products released from mast cells during anaphylactic reactions. They are particularly active during infections of helminths and they attack the schistosomula larvae of *Schistosoma mansoni* by releasing granule contents onto the surface of the parasite. Eosinophils respond chemotactically to immune complexes, granular products of mast cells, complexes of complement (C5a and C5-6-7), histamine

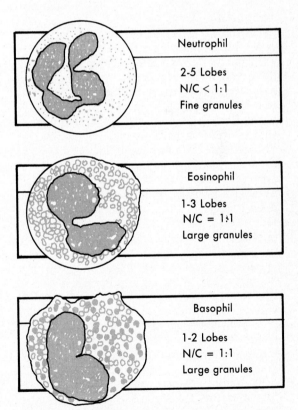

Fig. 8-8. Morphological features of neutrophils, eosinophils, and basophils, comparing the shape and size of nucleus and granules of mature granulocytes.

(a basophil product), soluble factors released from lymphocytes, and an eosinophilic chemotactic factor (ECF) released from neutrophils. The cells respond to stimulation by increasing NADPH oxidase activity 3 to 6 times that of resting levels. They are capable of limited phagocytosis and exhibit a marked uptake of oxygen after ingestion, but their major activity involves exocytosis of the granule contents.

The granules contain an arginine rich protein of 10,800 daltons, **major basic protein (MBP),** which is toxic to both parasitic and host tissue. MBP accounts for about 50% of the total granular protein content, and a crystalloid fraction of MBP is the substance of **Charcot-Leyden crystals,** found in exudates, secretions, bronchial washings, and stool specimens in association with parasitic infestations. Other granular molecules include acid hydrolases, histaminase (neutralizes histamine), aryl-sulphatase B (inactivates the slow-reacting substance of mast cells that mediates the anaphylactic reaction), phospholipase D (inactivates platelet-activating factors), a peroxidase that is different from myeloperoxidase, acid phosphatase, ribonuclease, cathepsins, and cationic proteins. Alkaline phosphatase is present, but it is closely associated with the nuclear and mitochondrial membranes and does not stain with routine histochemical techniques. Glycogen particles and mitochondria are especially numerous. The functional roles of some of these products are still not well understood. For example, a benign absence of eosinophilic peroxidase, due to an autosomal recessive trait, is associated with a decrease in specific granules and phospholipids and an increased tendency toward nuclear segmentation, but without apparent pathological consequences.

Eosinophil densities in the peripheral blood vary diurnally; they peak near midnight and are at the lowest levels just before noon. Adrenocorticotropic hormone (ACTH) produces a transient decrease in circulating eosinophil levels, and steroid compounds generally inhibit their release from the bone marrow and stimulate their passage into the tissues. Patients with Cushing's syndrome secrete large amounts of ACTH, and the peripheral blood may show little or no signs of eosinophils, but tissue and marrow examination demonstrates that these patients are not truly eosinopenic. Eosinopenia does accompany stress reactions and most bacterial infections because of the stress-steroid reaction and the recruitment of eosinophils to inflammatory areas. Unlike neutrophils, eosinophils can reenter the peripheral circulation from the tissues. However, the extent to which they marginate and emarginate is not as well documented as that for neutrophils.

The destruction of metazoan parasites by eosinophils has received considerable attention. Coating of the parasite by IgG, IgE, or activated complement results in close adherence of the eosinophil to the invader's cell wall. Exocytosis of the granular contents produces lesions on the cell wall surface, which opens the parasite to further invasion by eosinophils, neutrophils, and macrophages. The extent to which eosinophilic attacks merely limit parasitic spread, rather than dispose of the worms, is debatable. As is the case with the inflammatory reaction of neutrophils, eosinophils can damage host tissue, sometimes producing a more adverse condition than that caused by the parasites. For example, the formation of a granuloma around schistosome eggs in hepatic tissue produces much of the liver damage associated with this type of infection. Other effects and conditions associated with eosinophils are presented in Chapter 21.

THE BASOPHIL

Basophils are the least common of the normal leukocytes seen in the peripheral blood, accounting for less than 1% of the total white cell count. The relationship to

similar-appearing **mast cells** or tissue basophils is uncertain. Earlier evidence suggested that the morphological similarities
may have been convergent and that they
were derived from different cell lineages,
but more recent biochemical and ultrastructural observations indicate that the
circulating blood basophils and the semi-
fixed tissue cells share common precursors
and functional roles.

Basophil precursors can be identified biochemically at the promyelocyte stage on
the basis of specific granule contents, but
routine morphological recognition begins
with the **basophilic myelocyte.** Basophils
mature in the same manner as other granulocytes, forming metamyelocytes and
band forms, but these are not seen often in
marrow smears and they are usually not
categorized; most differential counts
merely report the total basophil percent or
absolute count. The specific granules of the
basophilic myelocyte and later stages are at
first truly basophilic, then metachromatic,
in reacting with routine stains. The granules normally range in size from 0.2 to 1.0
µm, but some may be as large as 2.0 µm.
They are also water soluble, due to the
presence of acid mucopolysaccharides, so
that improper fixation prior to staining
may result in cells that have poorly stained
granules or the appearance of cytoplasmic
vacuoles.

Basophils are the smallest circulating
granulocytes, averaging 10 to 15 µm in diameter (see Plate 2C). The nucleus to cytoplasm ratio is about 1:1, and the nucleus is

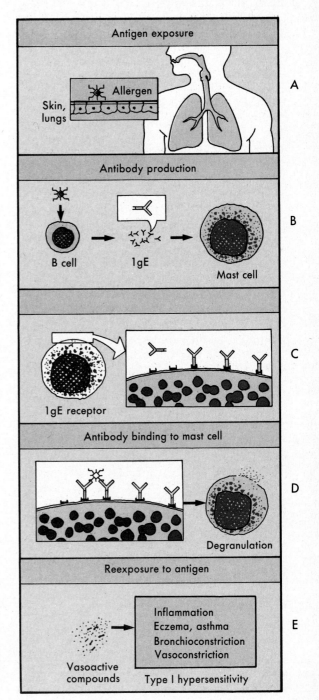

**Fig. 8-9. Allergens, mast cells, IgE, and degranula-
tion.** An antigen (**A**) enters the body through the skin
or a mucosal surface and invokes the formation of IgE
antibodies (**B**) by B lymphocytes. The antigen-specific
IgE attaches to the outer surface of mast cells (**C**). Representation of the antigen and reaction with the bound
IgE (**D**) results in a degranulation reaction by the mast
cells. The vasoactive products (**E**) produce allergic responses that range from simple inflammation to anaphylactic shock.

most often unsegmented or bilobed, rarely with three or four lobes. The chromatin is usually coarse and patchy, staining a deep blue to reddish-purple. The cytoplasm is a homogenous pale blue, but this is often obscured by the large dark granules. Because the average basophil density is only 0.5% of the total leukocyte count, a finding of zero basophils in a routine differential count is not significant. Buffy coat or other concentration techniques are needed to evaluate a true basopenia. Increases are also not common; most cases of basophilia are associated with chronic myelogenous leukemia and some myeloproliferative disorders (Chapter 20).

Basophils contain large amounts of **heparin,** an anticoagulant (this is one of the acid mucopolysaccharides). They also contain significant amounts of the amino acid, histidine, which is converted by basophilic histidine carboxylase into **histamine,** a powerful vasoactive compound. Other cellular contents include various dehydrogenases, serotonin, and diaphorases. No lysozymes have been detected. Basophils display very limited amoeboid movement and they are less active as phagocytes than are eosinophils. The cytoplasm exhibits a diffuse positive PAS reaction and very weak reactions for peroxidase, alkaline phosphatase, and Sudan black. An increase in blood basophils may be associated with a bleeding disorder due to the increased levels of heparin. Degranulation of basophils and the release of histamine results in vasoconstriction and bronchioconstriction, components of the anaphylactic reaction that are seen in mast cell degranulation. Basophils may also be participants in delayed hypersensitivity (cell mediated immunity) and they may help deposit immune complexes in tissues.

TISSUE GRANULOCYTES

Mast cells or tissue basophils participate in immune reactions involving IgE. Lymphocytes produce IgE antibodies to specific allergens, such as pollen, dust mite feces,

proteins in animal fur, etc. The antibodies attach to the outer membrane of the tissue basophils (Fig. 8-9). Reintroduction of the specific antigen results in two adjacent IgE molecules on the mast cell being "bridged." A sequence of membrane and intracellular reactions occur, leading to degranulation of the cell and release of the vasoactive compounds into the tissues and peripheral blood. These products produce the devastating reactions **(anaphylactic shock)** associated with hyperimmune responses to hymenopteran insects (wasps, bees, and ants). Eosinophils are attracted to the sites of granule release and they can neutralize some of the compounds. Mast cells are believed to be long-lived and, unlike neutrophils, they can synthesize new products and granules.

Other tissue granulocytes (eosinophilic and neutrophilic) are also observed in tissue sections, including bone marrow, but the significance of these cells remains obscure. Many hematologists, in fact, consider tissue neutrophils or "Ferrata cells" to be artifacts of tissue preparation. Illustrations and a discussion of these cells can be found in the atlas of blood morphology by Diggs et al. (1985).

SUMMARY

- Neutrophils are the most common cells in the peripheral blood of adults. Blood concentrations reflect input from the marrow storage pool, the ratio of marginated to freely circulating cells, and the rate of diapedesis into the tissues.
- Neutrophils mature from a granulocytic-specific myeloblast to a promyelocyte that produces primary granules to a myelocyte that produces secondary or cell type-specific granules. Each of these stages is accompanied by mitosis and amplification of cell numbers.
- Later stages of neutrophil maturation do not include mitotic division: metamyelocytes, band forms, and segmented neutrophils are accompanied by changes in nuclear shape. Band and segmented forms circulate in the blood and tissues as phagocytes.
- Neutrophils respond to chemical stimuli that are indicative of inflammation and the presence of microorganisms. Chemotaxis directs

the neutrophil to the site of infection, where recognition and ingestion (phagocytosis) of the microbe occurs.

- Formation of a phagocytic vacuole also stimulates the production of reactive oxygen forms, hydrogen peroxide, hypochlorites, and hydroxyl molecules. These oxidative products kill most of the microbes ingested. Generation of these molecules depends on enzymes of the hexose monophosphate shunt and myeloperoxidase.

- Eosinophils are active against metazoan parasites, which they attack by exocytosis of granular contents, such as major basic protein (MBP) and acid hydrolases. They also participate in immune responses involving basophils and mast cells.

- Eosinophils decrease in response to stress and ACTH; diurnal variations occur as peaks of peripheral blood concentration at night and low levels during the day.

- Basophils contain heparin (an anticoagulant) and histamine (a vasoactive compound). They are the least common normal cell of the peripheral blood.

- Mast cells are similar in morphology and biochemistry to basophils. They mediate responses to allergens that involve IgE antibodies. Rapid degranulation by mast cells results in hyperimmune responses to certain toxins, such as bee and wasp stings, producing life-threatening anaphylactic reactions of vasoconstriction and bronchioconstriction.

9

Lymphocytes

Lymphocytes interact with molecules and cell surfaces, determine whether the chemical structures are foreign (non-self) or part of the host (self), and produce a neutralizing immune response, if necessary. Lymphocytes are found throughout the tissues, with concentrations in the spleen, lymph nodes, and thymus. Less than 5% of the total lymphocyte mass ciculates in the blood at any time and most of these are intermitotic or "resting" forms. The total body mass of lymphocytes for an average adult is about 10^{12} cells, and the daily production rate is about 10^9 cells. Lymphocytes are produced in the bone marrow from lymphoid stem cell precursors, but they mature in various lymph tissues to specialize in manufacturing immunoglobulins (antibodies) or to interact with and direct the activities of other cells of the immune system. Because antibodies are protein components of the plasma, this phase of host defense is often referred to as **humoral immunity;** the phase involving cellular interactions between different types of lymphocytes and between lymphocytes and other leukocytes is termed **cell-mediated immunity.** Some of the diverse functional activities of lymphocytes (sometimes referred to as "immunocytes") are listed on page 109.

Terms associated with lymphocyte maturation and differentiation have been used in different ways by immunologists and hematologists so that a considerable amount of confusion arises when one consults various textbooks. The lymphoid organs and tissues are often divided into a "primary" or "central" system and a "secondary" or "peripheral" system. Although there is general agreement that the bone marrow is a primary source of lymphoid stem cells (derived from the hematopoietic stem cell, Chapter 7), other sites of lymphocyte development may be classified differently. The thymus and spleen may be viewed either as primary tissues of lymphoid origin or as secondary tissues of differentiation and function, depending on fetal, neonatal, or adult status of the individual. Various patches of lymphoid tissue (lymph nodes, Peyer's patches, and other concentrations associated with mucosal surfaces) are generally considered as secondary. In the following discussion, the bone marrow and thymus will be regarded as the **primary lymphoid organs,** and all other tissues are **secondary lymphoid organs.**

An additional distinction must be emphasized in presenting lymphocyte maturation. Morphological changes do not correlate well with functional/immunological changes. This fact is responsible for much of the earlier confusion about the appearance of lymphocytes in patients with viral infections or inflammations. Immature-appearing cells, in these cases, are mature cells exhibiting an immune response. We begin with morphology.

LYMPHOPOIESIS
Morphological cell stages

The lymphoid stem cells in the bone marrow are small to medium-sized mono-

MAJOR ACTIVITIES OF THE IMMUNE RESPONSE SYSTEM

Antibody mediated (humoral) immunity

Inhibition of viral reproduction

Neutralization of toxic substances

Destruction of encapsulated bacteria (e.g., pneumococcus)

Rejection of foreign tissues and cells (e.g., transfusion reaction of incompatible blood; hyperacute rejection of incompatible organ and skin transplants)

Recognition and destruction of some neoplastic growths

Formation of immune complexes, involvement in autoimmune diseases

Response to allergens; initial events associated with anaphylactic shock

Cell mediated immunity

Elimination of some intracellular microbes (e.g., *Legionella*, *Mycobacterium*, some viruses, fungi, and protozoa)

Surveillance and destruction of some types of neoplasms

Rejection of foreign tissues by infiltration (acute and chronic reactions)

Graft versus host disease (GVHD) (e.g., bone marrow transplants)

Contact dermatitis (localized skin response to some metals, chemicals, or plant toxins)

---

nuclear cells that are indistinguishable from other undifferentiated blasts. Like other early progenitors, these cells are capable of self renewal and of giving rise to a maturing line of lymphocytes. These cells are generally referred to as **lymphoblasts** by hematologists, based on morphological appearances (see Plate 3D). The cells are 12 to 20 μm in diameter with a round to oval nucleus, sometimes eccentric in location. The nucleus to cytoplasm ratio is about 4:1 and the periphery of both the nucleus and the cell may be irregular in outline. The fine, highly dispersed nuclear chromatin stains a light reddish-purple, and one or two pale blue or colorless large nucleoli are visible. The cytoplasm is usually agranular and deeply to moderately basophilic, with marginal (peripheral) intensity a common characteristic.

Prolymphocyte is a term that has been applied to lymphocytic cells that appear to be less morphologically mature than the typical, circulating cells, but most references now identify this stage as simply a prelymphocyte or an immature lympho-cyte. When immunological studies are performed, these cells can be identified as belonging to specific subsets of lymphocytes; unfortunately, simple morphological criteria do not permit identification. Mature cells undergoing blast transformation for mitotic amplification may also be included in this stage. Cell size ranges from 10 to 18 μm, the N/C ratio ranges from 4:1 to 3:1, and nuclear chromatin may appear more condensed and patchy than in the blast. Nucleoli are less distinct and usually only one is visible. The cytoplasm is less basophilic than that of the blast, but it remains agranular.

Mature **lymphocytes** (see Plate 3E) actually include a number of highly specialized lymphocyte subsets and phases of differentiation. Morphologically, lymphocytes in the peripheral blood have been described on the basis of size and cytoplasmic granularity (Fig. 9-1). **Small lymphocytes** are the most common, ranging in size from 6 to 10 μm (diameters vary widely from reference to reference). The nucleus is usually round or slightly oval, occasionally showing a

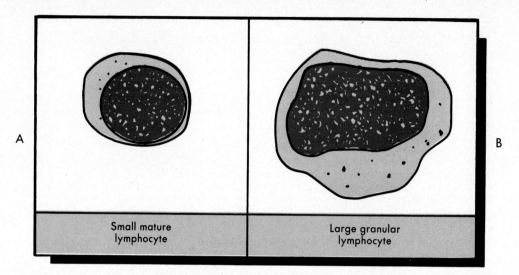

Fig. 9-1.   Variations in lymphocyte size and granularity.
A, Small mature lymphocyte; **B**, large granular lymphocyte.

small indentation due to the adjacent centrosome. Except in the smallest cells, the nucleus is about 7 μm in diameter, a size that has been convenient for estimating the size of surrounding erythrocytes (Chapter 15). Nuclear chromatin stains a dark reddish-purple to blue with large dark patches of condensed chromatin. The nuclear structure often appears blurred or indistinct, in comparison to that of granulocytes. The N/C ratio is high (5:1 to 3:1), and the cytoplasm is often seen only as a peripheral ring around part of the nucleus. Either it is agranular or it contains a few distinct azurophilic granules. Cytoplasmic color can vary greatly, from a typical sky blue to a very deep dark blue. Cells with basophilic cytoplasms represent activated lymphocytes that are synthesizing protein.

Large granular lymphocytes (LGL) are also regarded as mature cells that contain additional cytoplasm, usually associated with immunological activation and increased protein synthesis. Cell size ranges from about 10 μm to about 18 μm, but these are arbitrary values. Some authors provide

size ranges that distinguish small, medium, and large cells, but the usefulness of sizing in most clinical applications remains to be demonstrated. From one to six large (0.3 to 0.6 μm) azurophilic granules, identifiable as lysosomes by electron microscopy, are visible. Like that of the small lymphocytes, the cytoplasm of LGLs is typically sky blue but it can be deeply basophilic. The cell outline may be very irregular or amorphous. LGLs may include cells that appear to be intermediates transforming to plasma cells; these may be described as **plasmacytoid** or preplasma cells (see below). Other large granular lymphocytes have been correlated functionally with natural killer (NK) and cytotoxic T cells, but the correspondence is not predictive or useful for identification and enumeration.

Lymphoid organs and tissues

All hematopoietic tissues arise first in the yolk sac of the embryo. During the fetal stage of development, the liver and spleen serve as centers of blood cell development, to be replaced by the bone marrow shortly after birth. Committed (unipotential) stem cell of the lymphoid line produce two lines of lymphoblasts that yield the pre-B and pre-T cells mentioned above. It is not certain as to the number of precursor stages that exist from the lymphoid stem cell to the first identifiable B and T cells. **B lymphocytes (B cells)** are defined as the antibody producing line of cells associated with humoral immunity. They were originally named after their sites of maturation, first discovered in chickens, the bursa (B) of Fabricius. The equivalent structure in humans is believed to be the bone marrow, but the aggregation of lymphoid patches located along the intestines (**GALT, gut-associated lymphoid tissue**) is also a possible site. Functional maturation of the B lymphocyte occurs either in unidentified areas of the bone marrow or in the GALT.

T lymphocytes (T cells) mature in the **thymus,** a bilobed organ found in the lower neck and upper chest (Fig. 9-2). This structure develops from the third and fourth branchial pouches, along with the parathyroid glands, and becomes fully functional during fetal life. It reaches maximum size and mass (about 40 g) by puberty, after which the organ slowly atrophies to a remnant of tissue in the young adult. Interestingly, failure of the thymus to develop results in a severe immunodeficiency (Di George's syndrome, Chapter 21) due to a lack of T lymphocytes, but removal of the thymus at or after birth produces only minimally adverse effects.

Maturation of lymphocytes in the bursal equivalent and thymus results in cells that are **immunocompetent,** that is, able to respond to antigenic challenges by directing the immune responses of host defense. These cells, prior to antigen exposure, have been named "virgin" lymphocytes. They migrate, via the blood stream and lymphatic system, to the lymph nodes, spleen, and assorted GALTs (e.g., the appendix, tonsils, and adenoid glands) to await antigen presentation and activation. In contrast to most other blood cells, lymphocytes traverse the body (**recirculation**), reentering the blood and lymphatics, migrating through the spleen and lymph nodes to communicate with other lymphocytes and macrophages (Fig. 9-3). Because of the functional specialization and complex patterns of recirculation involving different lymphocyte subsets, it is difficult to determine the life span of these cells. Estimates of survival range from 10 to 20 days for some antibody-producing B cells to over 25 years for some T cells.

Structure of the lymph node

The lymphatic system is a set of channels that drains extravascular fluid (lymph) from the tissues of the body, especially at the joints of the appendicular and axial skeletons. Located at intervals along the channels are **lymph nodes,** roughly spherical structures composed of a structural reticulum and a series of interconnecting sinuses. The lymph fluid, carrying white blood cells and environmental antigens, enters the node through an afferent channel, passes through the sinuses, and exits by way of an efferent channel. The sinuses are lined with macrophages that can detect and remove antigenic molecules from the lymph. In addition, the node serves as a mechanical filter to remove cellular debris, dead microbes, and fibrin clots. Each node consists of an outer cortex, partitioned into discrete follicles, and an inner medulla that is more or less continuous with the lymphatic capillaries (Fig. 9-4). B lymphocytes predominate in the cortex and T cells dominate the medulla. The cortex expands and contracts due to increases and decreases in B cell density, a function of immunological response. The center of each follicle, referred to as a germinal center, contains the youngest B cells. The medulla also contains germinal centers, composed of T cells, that respond to antigenic stimulation. The thymus, spleen, and most lymphatic tissues are organized in this manner.

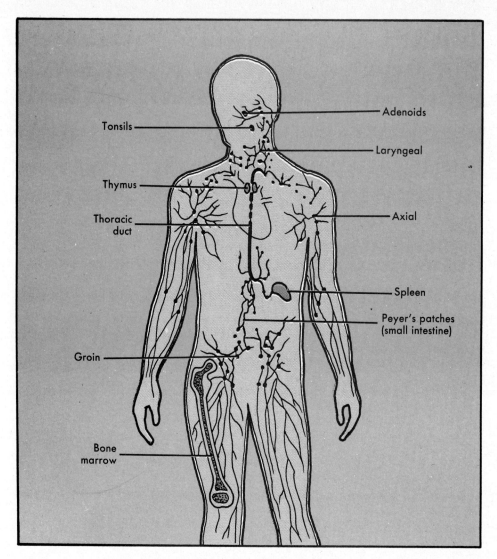

Fig. 9-2.   Location of major lymphoid tissues.
The bone marrow also contains lymphoid cells.

T lymphocytes continually migrate through the nodes, exiting via the efferent capillaries, passing through a progressively larger series of channels to enter the thoracic duct and into the venous blood circulation. The T cells thus recirculate, passing through arterial and capillary vessels to reenter the tissues by crossing the endothelial linings of venules. B cells also recirculate (they comprise about 20 to 30% of the peripheral blood lymphocytes), but they are shorter-lived and tend to be more localized in the spleen and lymph tissue. Very little is known about the movements of other lymphocyte types.

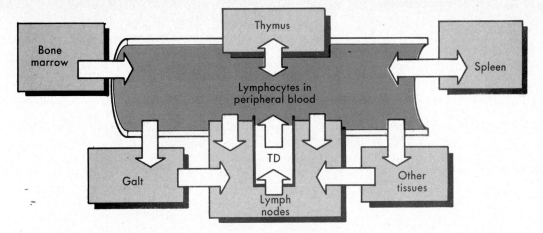

Fig. 9-3. Lymphocyte recirculation compartments.
Lymphocytes originate in the primary tissue (bone marrow) and circulate through the blood-stream to the thymus (also a primary tissue) and to the secondary sites. Recirculation occurs as the lymphathic vessels collect lymphocytes from various tissues. After passage through the major thoracic nodes, lymphocytes enter the major lymphatic ducts, including the thoracic duct (TD), and return to the venous circulation.

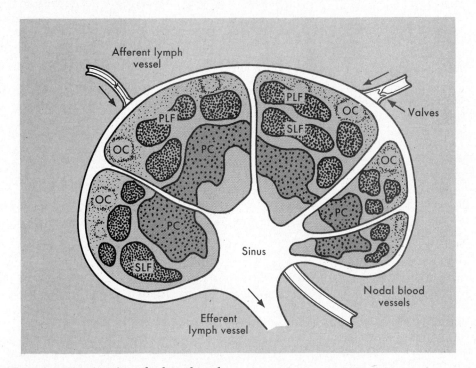

Fig. 9-4. Cross-section of a lymph node.
Lymphocytes enter the node through an afferent vessel (valves prevent backflow). B cells prolif-erate in the outer cortex (OC). Primary and secondary lymphoid follicles (PLF and SLF) contain B cells surrounded by macrophages (antigen-presenting cells) and T lymphocytes. The number of follicles is an indication of immunological activity. The paracortical area (PC) consists of T lym-phocytes. Plasma cells, producing antibodies, lie in the medulla between the PC and sinus. The latter collects antibodies and recirculating cells for discharge through the efferent vessel.

The spleen

The **spleen** was introduced in Chapter 3 as an organ of erythrocyte removal. It represents the largest reservoir in the body for both lymphocytes and macrophages. Gross inspection of a cross-sectioned spleen reveals areas of red pulp, containing a fine capillary network lined by macrophages, and a white pulp that consists of lymphocytic follicles, similar in organization to lymph nodes. Blood enters the spleen by arteries to terminate in either type of pulp or in a reticular network, the marginal zone. A portion of the blood passes rapidly through the spleen by entering the sinuses directly and out through the splenic veins. Most of the blood supply, however, passes through the tortuous capillary network of the white and red pulps, subject to inspection and phagocytosis by the RES system macrophages.

The immunological role of the spleen is similar to that of other secondary lymphoid tissue, serving as a reservoir for lymphocytes, especially B cells. Antigens transported in the blood are introduced to macrophages and T cells in the white pulp, which subsequently initiate and coordinate antibody production from adjacent B cells. Microbes that are not removed by circulating phagocytes (primarily, neutrophils) or the fixed macrophages of the liver are passed through the red pulp and phagocytosed along with other cellular debris and abnormal red blood cells.

FUNCTIONAL MATURATION OF LYMPHOCYTES

Although lymphocytes have been described and characterized as morphological entities for over 100 years, it is only during the last 25 years that detailed information on their function has become available. Most of these advances have resulted from developments in immunological methodology, in particular the use of monoclonal antibodies to identify cell surface antigens. Lymphocytes act as the directors and the effectors of the immune response. Most of these activities involve the reception of molecular messages via specific glycoproteins located on the external surface of the cytoplasmic membrane. As lymphocytes mature, their identities and functions are specified by these antigenic structures. Unfortunately, progress in this field of technology is so recent and has developed so rapidly that terminology and interpretation of the data has resulted in some confusion and the necessity to qualify most statements with a caution that "the following information is subject to revision at any time." Fortunately, this minor inconvenience is amply compensated by the excitement of witnessing an entire field of science develop in only a few brief years.

The development of B and T lymphocytes is traditionally separated into sequential phases of **antigen-independent** and **antigen-dependent** maturation. Differentiation from the lymphoid stem cell to the "virgin" lymphocyte proceeds from genetic instructions (DNA and RNA) coupled with hormonal influences of the maturation environment (thymus or bone marrow). Antigen-dependent maturation involves exposure of the B or T cell to a specific antigen resulting in the expression of surface receptor molecules that can recognize the foreign antigen upon representation.

Maturation of T lymphocytes

Lymphoid stem cells produce committed T cell precursors in the bone marrow (Fig. 9-5), but the number of maturation stages at this point is difficult to determine. They are recognized as members of the T lineage because of the presence of the antigenic markers T9 and T10. These antigen designations correspond to a set of monoclonal antibodies utilized by Coulter Electronics, Inc. Equivalent names for antibodies produced by Ortho Diagnostics and Becton Dickinson are compared with the cluster differentiation (CD) nomenclature recommended by the World Health Organization (Table 9-1). In addition, stem cells and early B and T cells share an enzyme, **terminal de-**

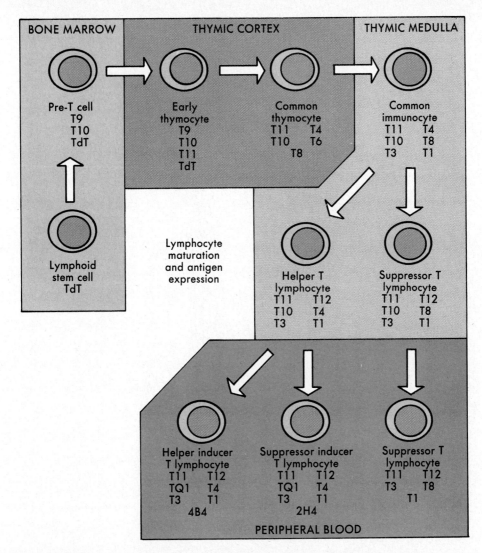

Fig. 9-5. Maturation and surface marker differentiation of T lymphocytes.
As the T lymphocyte matures, various membrane proteins and cytoplasmic enzymes appear and
disappear. These are useful in identifying cell stages seen in lymphoid malignancies.

oxynucleotidyl transferase (TdT), that is lost
during early maturation. This enzyme is a
convenient marker for identifying the lineage of immature cells seen in acute leukemia (Chapter 20).

Committed pre T cells migrate to the cortex of the thymus to become **early thymo-**

cytes. These cells express T11, an antigen
that was first identified with T cell specificity as a receptor for sheep red blood cells
(SRBC). When mixed in vitro, the sheep
cells formed rosettes around T cells containing the "E" (for erythrocyte) receptor
but not other lymphocytes. Further differ-

Table 9-1. Lymphocyte surface markers

Antigen	Mol. wt.	Positive cells	Monoclonal antibodies		
			Ortho	B-D	Coulter
CD1	49 KD	Thymocytes	OKT6	Leu 6	T6
CD2	45;55 KD	T, NK cells; (E rosette)	OKT11	Leu 5B	T11
CD3	20; 30 KD	T cells	OKT3	Leu 4	T3
CD4	55 KD	T_H cells, MHC-2	OKT4	Leu 3	T4
CD5	67 KD	T cells, some B cells; CLL	OKT1	Leu 1	T1
CD6		T cells			T12
CD7	40 KD	T, NK cells; ALL		Leu 9	
CD8	32; 43 KD	T_S, T_C cells, some NK cells	OKT8	Leu 2a	T8
CD9		Leukemic cells			BA-2
CD10	40; 100 KD	Pre-B; ALL cells	OKT10	CALLA	J5
CD11		NK, some T cells; (C_3b)	OKM1	Leu 15	MO1
CD15		Activated T cells		Leu M1	
CD16		NK cells, Fc		Leu 11	NK15
CD19	40; 80 KD	B cells; CLL, pre-B ALL cells		Leu 12	B4
CD20	35 KD	B cells		Leu 16	B1
CD21	140 KD	B cells; (C_3d)		CR2	B2
CD22		B cells; CLL, HCL cells		Leu 14	
CD23		Lymphoblasts			
CD24		B cells; CLL, pre-B ALL cells			BA-1
CD25		Activated and infected T cells		IL-2	

ALL, Acute lymphocytic leukemia; *CLL,* chronic lymphocytic leukemia; *HCL,* hairy cell leukemia. Based on data compiled by the World Health Organization and leukocyte typing procedures established by Ortho Diagnostics, Inc. (Raritan, NJ), Becton Dickinson Immunocytometry Systems (Moutain View, CA), and Coulter Electronics, Inc. (Hialeah, FL).

entiation in the cortex results in **common thymocytes** that display T4, T6 and T8. Antigens T4 and T8 will become the characteristic markers for two functional subsets of T cells. Therefore, the term "common" indicates a prcursor that shares these functional specificities. Antigen T6 appears to be unique to the common thymocyte, since it is lost when the cell migrates to the medulla. It is here that the thymocyte, a "virgin" lymphocyte, is exposed to the dirty world of foreign proteins and microbes. Macrophages play a role, discussed in Chapter 10, in presenting antigens to the thymocyte. A hormone produced in the thymus, **thymosin,** also functions in the maturation process. The thymocyte attains a unique identity, producing a receptor molecule on its cell surface that allows it to react to its particular antigen when they meet once again. Also, two new markers characterize this immunocompetent T cell, T1 and T3.

This cell still shares T4 and T8 and is termed a **common immunocyte** in Figure 9-5.

Further differentiation in the medulla, accompanied by mitotic division, produces a subset of cells expressing T4 (the **helper T cell, T_H**) and a separate subset expressing T8 (the **suppressor T cell, T_S**). Both populations also display a new marker, T12. These cells are ready to leave the maturation nest and migrate through the bloodstream, enter tissues, lymphatics, and visit lymph nodes and spleen. Many of the cells probably localize in particular nodes or splenic follicles, whereas other continually recirculate. During its peripheral travels, further differentiation of the helper cell occurs, forming a helper inducer and suppressor inducer cell, identifiable by the appearance of new surface markers. Normally, a $2:1$ ratio of helper to suppressor T cells is present in the peripheral blood, usually measured by reaction with monoclonal antibodies to T4 and T8, respectively. Reversal of this ratio is characteristic of some immunodeficiency disorders, including acquired immunodeficiency syndrome (AIDS). Loss of suppressor activity, the "brakes" of the immune system, can result in a hyperactive immune response, as seen in some autoimmune disorders.

B cell maturation

Despite determined efforts, the bursal equivalent in humans has not been positively identified. Committed B cells either stay in the bone marrow or they migrate to GALTs to undergo maturation. The antigen-independent phase takes place in the bursa equivalent, producing immunocompetent B cells that migrate to spleen and lymph nodes to await antigen-dependent stimulation. The first unique feature that identifies B cells is the appearance of immunoglobulin chains in the cytoplasm (Fig. 9-6). Immunoglobulins consist of light and heavy molecular weight chains. The heavy chain (μ) of IgM is synthesized first, characterizing the **pre-B cell.** Other markers appearing at this stage or earlier include Ia, B1, B4, BA-1, and CALLA, a marker used to identify blast cells in acute leukemias. The next stage of maturation, the **early** or **immature B cell,** has cytoplasmic (cIg) and surface immunoglobulin (sIg) in the form of complete heavy and light chain molecules of IgM. CALLA is no longer present, but the other B markers persist. The surface-bound IgM is structurally different from the IgM molecules that normally circulate in the plasma. Receptors for complement proteins (C3b and C3d) and the Fc portion of an immunoglobulin (IgG) also appear. All of this occurs while the cells reside in the marrow, prior to antigen stimulation.

The **mature B cell** produces two types of surface immunoglobulin: IgM and IgD. The amount of IgD appears to be related to the degree of B cell maturation, and it must be expressed before the cell is able to respond to antigenic stimulation. Exposure to foreign antigen occurs in the marrow or bursal equivalent and the virgin B cell becomes immunocompetent. A decrease in surface IgD follows stimulation, although a small subset of B cells may maintain IgM + IgD. Specialization of the immunocompetent B cell results in the production of a particular class of sIg: either IgM, IgG, IgA, or IgE, which can recognize (bind to) a specific antigen. Except for cells that produce only IgM, most B cells produce IgM plus one of the other immunoglobulin classes. Mature B cells migrate to the secondary lymphoid tissues (lymph nodes and spleen, etc.) to reside as resting or intermitotic cells until reexposure to their specific antigens. Some of these cells are long-lived, serving as **memory B cells.** The number of cell copies for each type of antigen is unknown; it may depend on the nature of the antigen and how often it is encountered.

When reexposure to the antigen occurs, the memory cell or a committed mature B cell with the corresponding antibody re-

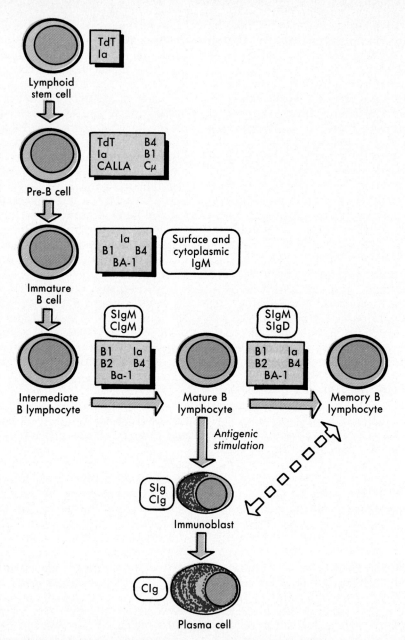

Fig. 9-6.   Maturation and differentiation of B lymphocytes.
CIg, Cytoplasmic immunoglobulin; *SIg,* surface immunoglobulin. The number of stages is not well defined, nor is the relationship between memory cells and antibody-producing cells.

sponds by transforming into a clone of effector cells, the plasma cells or plasmocytes. These cells rarely appear in the peripheral blood, but they are morphologically distinct and they are common in lymph node aspirates and tissue sections of the spleen. They are the antibody factories, secreting up to 2000 immunoglobulin molecules per second for several days.

During transformation, an immature intermediate cell stage can be identified, variously referred to as a proplasmocyte, plasmacytoid lymphocyte, Turk cell, and lymphocytoid plasma cell. Some texts also described a cell stage with a morphologically less mature appearance as a plasmoblast, but immunological evidence indicates that this is probably a mature B cell that has undergone **blast transformation.** B cells in tissue culture respond to mitogenic substances (materials that induce mitosis) by increasing DNA synthesis and proliferating as a clone of cells. These cells have the fine nuclear chromatin and basophilic cytoplasm of typical immature cells, but these cells are immunocompetent and they express the antigenic markers and enzymes of fully differentiated cells. Since most of these cells are localized in the lymphoid organs at the time of stimulation, they are found only occasionally in the peripheral blood, usually during acute viral infections and as signs of inflammatory responses. Indeed, the association between plasmacytoid lymphocytes and viral infections led earlier hematologists to designate these cells as "virocytes."

Plasmacytoid lymphocytes are about 15 to 20 μm in diameter with irregular cell outlines. The N/C ratio varies greatly, from 3:1 to 1:1. The nucleoli (usually 1 or 2) may be distinct or partially obscured by the moderately granular chromatin. The nucleus is either central or slightly eccentric. Color of the cytoplasm also varies from sky blue to moderately basophilic. A perinuclear clear zone, due to a prominent centrosome, is usually evident. Development of the endoplasmic reticulum and Golgi complex imparts a marbled appearance to the stained cytoplasm that increases with maturation of the cell. The cytoplasm is agranular, but colorless vacuoles are often seen.

Mature **plasma cells** (see Plate 3F) are often oval or fan shaped, measuring 12 to 20 μm in length and 8 to 15 μm in width. The nucleus is characteristically eccentric and oval in shape. A 2:1 to 1:2 N/C ratio is typical. The nucleus may be bilobed or multilobed, especially in patients with lymphoid blood dyscrasias. The perinuclear zone is very distinct, appearing white in the deeply basophilic cytoplasm. Nuclear chromatin is condensed and very patchy, appearing as dark blocks on a reddish-purple background. The cytoplasm stains deep blue to gray blue, depending on the stain and the ribosomal content of the individual cell. The increased RNA content can be readily demonstrated by staining the cell with pyronine, producing a bright red color. Granules are not present, but vacuoles may be numerous. Although these cells are not normally present in the peripheral blood, they comprise from 0.2% to 2.8% of the marrow white cell count.

Other lymphocytes

An additional type of T effector cell can be identified by its ability to lyse abnormal host cells, particularly those infected by viruses and those arising as neoplastic clones (tumor cells). These **cytotoxic T cells (T_C)** are not morphologically distinguishable from most other lymphocytes, but they do express the T8 antigenic marker and they recognize class 1 MHC (major histocompatability complex) antigens that are present on all nucleated cells. The cytotoxic T cell recognizes and binds to the membrane of the abnormal target cell. Changes in target cell permeability are followed by swelling and lysis; the T_c cell survives to attack additional targets.

In addition to cells that are identifiable as

T and B lymphocytes, a third population exists. These cells were previously named "null" cells because of negative reactions with antibodies that were used during early investigations for T and B cell antigens. Morphologically, these cells appear as large granular lymphocytes and they comprise about 3% of the peripheral blood lymphocytes. Some of them are able to destroy abnormal cells, such as those infected by viruses and tumor cells, without interacting with antibodies or T cells; they have been designated as **natural killers (NK).** Their identity is unclear in that they display heterogeneous reactions for other surface markers, and their responses to interferon and various lymphokines varies. Most NK cells express T3, T4, T8, and M01, a myeloid cell marker. Another subset of lymphocytes (K cells) lyse target cells, but by the mechanism of antibody-dependent cell cytotoxicity (ADCC). They have surface receptors for IgG, but they appear to be distinct from mature B cells.

LYMPHOCYTE FUNCTION

Lymphocytes conduct host defense by producing immunoglobulins (antibodies), lysing cells, and interacting with other leukocytes to neutralize microbes and foreign substances that enter the body. Foreign substances include blood and tissues that are transplanted from a donor to a genetically nonidentical recipient, an unfortunate complication for modern mankind that was not anticipated by the evolutionary forces of natural selection.

Immunoglobulin production

Antibodies are produced by B lymphocytes and plasma cells to react with antigens. Most antigens are proteins or glycoproteins with complex molecular structures. The antibody may be confined to the cytoplasm of the B cell (clg), expressed as a molecule bound to the cell surface (slg), or secreted into the plasma to circulate as a component of the globulin fraction of protein. The area of the antigenic molecule that an antibody binds to is called a **determinant.** Although an infinite number of these binding sites is *theoretically* possible, only a few actually stimulate an antibody response by the effector cells. A particular cell clone only recognizes a single specific determinant. This specificity is what makes it possible for the immune system to discriminate between the host's own molecules (self) and those external to the host (non-self).

Antibodies are composed of one of five major classes of immunoglobulin (Table 9-2). Each antibody is composed of peptide chains that are classified by molecular weight as light (lambda and kappa) or heavy (mu, gamma, alpha, delta, and epsilon). The basic structure of lg is a dimer of two light chains (either kappa or lambda but not

Table 9-2. Properties of immunoglobulins

Class	Mol wt	Plasma concentration	Percentage of plasma immunoglobulin	Binds complement	Crosses placenta
IgM	950 KD	80-170 mg/dL	5-10	Yes	No
IgG	150 KD	750-1750 mg/dL	75-85	Yes	Yes
IgA	160 KD	170-280 mg/dL	5-15	Yes*	No
IgD	180 KD	2-4 mg/dL	< 1	No	No
IgE	190 KD	0.1-1.0 mg/dL	< 1	No	No

*By the alternate pathway

both) and two heavy chains (Fig. 9-7, *A*). For example, IgG is composed of two kappa or lambda chains plus two gamma chains and IgA is composed of two kappa or lambda chains and two heavy alpha chains. IgM is pentameric, consisting of 10 light chains (5 pairs) and 10 heavy mu chains (5 pairs) (Fig. 9-7, *B*). Note that both the light and heavy chains consist of a variable region and a constant region. The variable region is a sequence of amino acids that is specifically directed at the antigen that the antibody will bind to; therefore it is unique. The constant region is an amino acid sequence that is shared by other immunoglobulins of the same class or subclass. The terminal fragment (Fc) of Ig can be recognized by receptors on lymphocytes, macrophages, and granulocytes.

The sequence of Ig production is an important indicator of cell maturation stage, useful for identification and characterizing B cell neoplasms (Chapter 20). As stated earlier, IgM is the first to be synthesized, appearing first as a single heavy chain (mu) in the cytoplasm of early B cells. The complete molecule is produced and assembled in later B cell stages. When the cell is immunocompetent and able to respond to antigenic stimulation, IgM is the first anti-

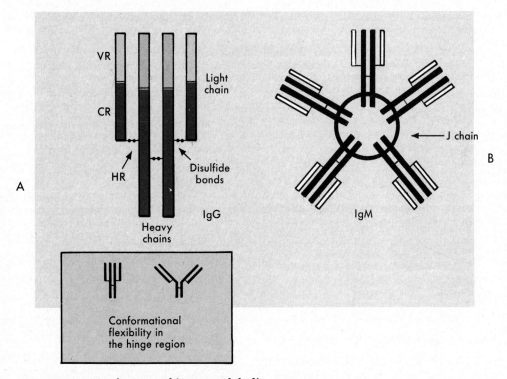

Fig. 9-7.   Major features of immunoglobulin structure.
The variable region (VR) contains the amino acid sequences that recognize a particular antigen determinant (idiotype). The constant region (CR) contains a portion that is recognized by macrophages and neutrophils. Conformational changes occur in the hinge region (HR), permitting the antibody to bind to determinants of variable spatial arrangement. Disulfide bonds are indicated by blackened dots. IgM is a pentamer of IgG-like molecules connected by a J chain. **A,** IgG, **B,** IgM.

body to be secreted (the primary response). Restimulation of mature B cells or plasma cells by the same antigen results in production and release of IgM plus the additional immunoglobulin synthesized by that cell. Most cells synthesize IgG, but many of the lymphocytes associated with mucosal tissues, sometimes referred to as the mucosal-associated lymphoid tissue, or MALT (essentially synonymous with GALT), synthesize IgA or IgE. This secondary, or **anamnestic response,** is more rapid and produces more antibody than the initial reaction. Thus a typical immune response to a viral infection produces an initial release of IgM to first antigen exposure and a release of IgG after re-exposure (Fig. 9-8). Each antigen exposure and cycle of antibody production is accompanied by a clonal expansion

of the responding B cells, but most of these are retained in the lymph nodes or spleen. Swollen lymph nodes, tonsils, and adenoids are evidence of B cell stimulation, but changes in the numbers and appearance of peripheral blood lymphocytes are usually subtle.

Intercellular communications

A detailed discussion of the interactions between lymphocytes and other cells involved in immune responses is beyond the scope of this book, but the interested reader is referred to any of the introductory texts of immunology cited in the Section III bibliography. Host response to an infection involves a number of physiological systems that act both independently and in concert (Fig. 9-9). In addition to the direct phago-

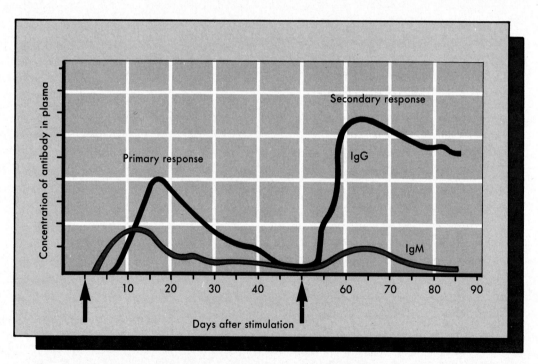

Fig. 9-8.   Antibody production responses to sequential exposures of an antigen.
The secondary response is more rapid and results in greater immunoglobulin production than the primary response. IgM occurs first after initial presentation of an antigen (arrow), but IgG is dominant after restimulation (second arrow).

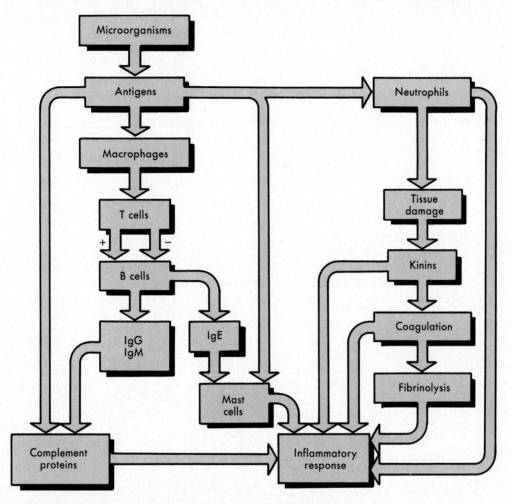

Fig. 9-9. Interaction of physiological systems in host defense.
Some of the relationships between phagocytosis, antibody production, the coagulation cascade,
fibrinolysis, kinin-bradykinin pathway, and the complement system. Many more interactions
and feedback loops occur during a host's response to infection.

cytic activities of granulocytes (Chapters 7
and 8) and monocyte-macrophages (Chapter
10), plasma proteins enhance the detection
and destruction of microbes by coating
them with molecules (the process is called
opsonization) that are recognized by lymphocytes and phagocytes. **Complement** is
an additional class of proteins that helps
mediate the antibody-dependent lysis of tar-

get cells. During infection, the inflammatory response is triggered by these mediators and by activation of the coagulation
and plasminogen pathways (Chapters 13
and 14). Deficiencies involving any of these
pathways can impair the host's ability to respond to infection.

Lymphocytes and macrophages cooperate
in directing cellular responses to infection

by synthesizing and secreting substances called **lymphokines** and **monokines,** respectively (Table 9-3). Microbial antigens are usually recognized by macrophages and monocytes, either at the tissue site of entry, in the spleen, or in the bloodstream (Figure 9-10). If the antigen is T cell dependent, the macrophage presents identifying information of its molecular determinants to T helper cells located in the medullary areas of the lymph nodes. T-independent antigen determinants are presented directly to B cells to stimulate antibody production. The T helper cell binds to the antigenic determinant and to class II MHC antigens on the macrophage. This activates the macrophage, and it secretes the monokine, **interleukin-1 (IL-1),** which stimulates the T_H cell to proliferate and secrete a lymphokine **interleukin-2 (IL-2).** IL-1 is also known as lymphocyte activating factor (LAF), and IL-2 is called T cell growth factor (TCGF). Bioassays for these substances utilize cell responses in tissue culture to measure the integrity of lymphokine production and reception. T suppressor cells also develop receptors for IL-2 and they may be stimulated to suppress activities of the T helper and B cells, acting as a negative feedback control for the immune response. Activated T helper cells also secrete groups of substances, collectively known as B cell growth factor (BCGF) and T cell replacing factor (TCRF), that stimulate B cells to differentiate and proliferate. The sequences of molecular events in these interactions are very complex but current investigations promise to reveal a great deal about the manner in which immunological protection occurs.

Metabolism and chemical constituents

Glycogen deposits are usually small and appear as localized aggregates when stains are used. The PAS reaction in normal lymphocytes is usually negative or very faintly positive, although a stronger reaction may be seen in the abnormal lymphocytes of leukemia patients. Peroxidase reactions are negative, but lymphocytes are strongly positive for acid phosphatase (associated with lysosomes) and beta glucuronidase. Specific esterase (napthol AS-D chloroacetate esterase) is also absent in lymphocytes, but weekly positive reactions to nonspecific esterases (alpha-napthyl acetate and butyrate

Table 9-3. Mediators of lymphocyte function

Mediator	Mol wt	Origin	Target	Function
IL-1 (LAF)	15 KD	Macrophages	T_H and B cells	Activate T and B cells
IL-2 (TSF)	14.5 KD	activated T_H cells	activated TH and NK	T cell proliferation; stimulate NK
BCGF (BSF)	12; 19 KD	activated T_H cells	B cells	stimulate B cells
TCRF	various	activated T_H cells	B cells	B cell proliferation and differentiation
Thymosin	3; 5 KD	Thymic epithelial cell	Thymocytes	T cell differentiation
Thymopoietin	5.5 KD	Thymic epithelial cell	Thymocytes	thymocyte differentiation
Suppression	2 KD	Thymic epithelial cell	T_S cells	stimulate T_S cells

BCGF, B cell growth factor; *BSF,* B cell stimulating factor; *IL,* interleukin; *LAF,* lymphocyte activating factor; *TCRF,* T cell replacing factor; *TSF,* T cell stimulating factor.

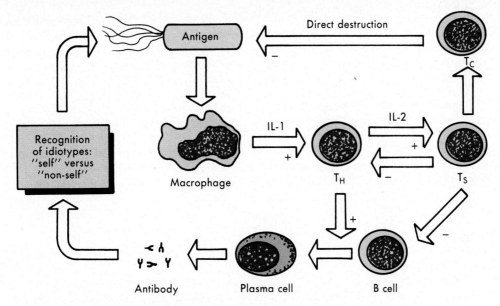

Fig. 9-10.   Interactions between lymphocytes and macrophages.
IL-1, interleukin 1 (LAF); *IL-2*, interleukin 2 (TSF); T_C, cytotoxic T cell; T_H, T helper cell; T_S, T suppressor cell. Cytotoxic T cells may destroy cells infected with viruses, some types of tumorous cells, or cells with membranes modified by drugs.

esterases) occur under some conditions (see Chapter 27 for procedures and interpretations). A circular organelle in the cytoplasm, the gall body, contains alpha napthyl acid esterase (ANAE).

The other major participants in the immune response, the monocyte-macrophages, are discussed in the next chapter.

SUMMARY

- Lymphocytes are the major mediators of the immune response: soluble antibodies are secreted into the plasma to neutralize foreign antigens (humoral immunity), and other cells act as effectors to lyse target cells (microbes, virally infected cells, tumor cells) or to direct the attack of phagocytes (cell-mediated immunity).
- Lymphocytes arise and mature in primary lymphoid tissues, the marrow for B lymphocytes that produce antibodies, and the marrow and thymus for T lymphocytes

that serve as regulators of humoral and cell mediated immunity. Mature lymphocytes reside in the secondary lymphoid organs, the spleen, lymph nodes, and mucosal-associated tissues; they recirculate through the body by way of the blood and lymphatic systems.

- Morphological stages include the lymphoblast, prolymphocyte, mature lymphocyte, and plasma cell. Variations of these stages are seen in activated cells that are responding to infection or inflammation. Functional stages are identified by the appearance of antigenic markers on the cell surface and the synthesis of immunoglobulins.
- Monoclonal antibodies against the surface proteins indicate that maturation, differentiation, and interaction with other cells occurs in specified areas of the spleen, thymus, and lymph nodes. T cells specialize as inducers or suppressors of the im-

mune response or as effectors that directly lyse target cells. B cells become antibody-producing specialists, plasms cells, after stimulation by a specific antigen during maturation.

- Mature B and T cells can serve as memory cells, retaining the ability to recognize antigens and mount a rapid response of blast transformation and proliferation following re-exposure.
- Plasma cells produce immunoglobulins of the IgM class; most produce an additional class (IgA, IgG, IgD, or IgE) as a result of stimulation and maturation. Each B cell or plasma cell produces a single antibody specificity that binds to a particular antigenic determinant.
- Lymphocytes communicate with each other and with macrophages and other white cells by secreting lymphokines. These substances regulate the activation, inhibition, and growth responses of their target cells.

10

Monocytes and Macrophages

Phagocytic cells have been recognized as important components of host defense for quite some time. Early anatomists and physiologists devised the term "reticuloendothelial system (RES)" as a collective term for the aggregations of phagocytes that existed in virtually every tissue and organ of the body. However, even they recognized that these cells did not form a "system" as much as the fact that they simply shared some functional attributes. The organs in which they are found have other, primary functions, there is no apparent connection between reticulum and endothelium, and the relationship between the different types of phagocytic cells themselves was not well established. Furthermore, granulocytes are also phagocytic, but these were not usually included as components of the RES. This term has now been replaced by **mononuclear phagocytic system (MPS)**, or monohistiocytic series, to denote a cell lineage derived from bone marrow precursors that gives rise to wandering (motile) and fixed (nonmotile) macrophages throughout the body. The terms **macrophage** and **histiocyte** are used somewhat interchangeably by hematologists, but some workers prefer to restrict use of the former to cells that are actively phagocytic and known to be derived from marrow monocytes. The latter term is used for cells that are not phagocytic, cells that are nonmotile (fixed in place), or whose origins are not yet determined. By this definition, the fixed dendritic cells of the thymus and spleen would be regarded as histiocytes.

MONOCYTE PRODUCTION AND MATURATION

Monocytes are produced by differentiation from the bipotential stem cell, CFU-GM, which gives rise to committed stem cells of the granulocytic and monocytic lines (see Chapter 7). The factors that help determine the number of cells passing through each line are still unknown, but a colony-stimulating factor (CSF) with a monopoietic hormone-like effect is secreted by macrophages in tissue culture. Bacterial endotoxins and secretions from T cells stimulate the release of CSF. About 3% to 11% of the circulating white cells are monocytes, increasing in some infections involving intracellular bacteria (i.e., tuberculosis, *Legionella*, and *Salmonella*).

The **monoblast** is the first stage of monocyte-macrophage maturation (Plate 4 A). It is about 12 to 20 μm in diameter, has an N/C ratio of 4:1 to 3:1, and, like most myeloid blasts, has a round to oval nucleus with fine, lightly dispersed chromatin. From one to four nucleoli may be visible. The nucleus may be either central or eccentric and it may show evidence of indentation or folding. The cytoplasm is agranular, stains moderately to lightly basophilic, and often has an intensely stained periphery and a prominent perinuclear clear zone. Monoblasts never appear in the normal peripheral blood and they are rarely identifiable in the marrow without using special stains. In monocytic leukemias, they can be identified as the most immature forms in clusters of cells with obvious monocytic features.

Myeloblasts and monoblasts are so similar in light microscopc morphology that identification of *individual* cells should not be attempted without other lines of evidence.

Myeloblasts contain large amounts of peroxidase, show a strong positive reaction to Sudan black, and possess nonspecific and specific esterases (alpha-naphthyl chloroacetate esterase), whereas monoblasts have relatively little peroxidase, display a weak or negative reaction to Sudan black, and contain only the nonspecific esterases (alpha-naphthyl butyrate esterase). These reactions are fairly consistent for normal cells, but they do not necessarily apply to leukemic cells, in which abnormalities of cytoplasmic constituents can produce ambiguous staining results (Chapters 20 and 27).

Promonocytes are generally regarded as the first stage to be recognized solely by morphological criteria (see Plate 4-B). They are slightly larger, 14 to 22 μm in diameter, and they show the typical signs of maturity: an N/C ratio of 3:1 or 2:1, chromatin that is slightly more condensed than that of the blast, fewer nucleoli, and better evidence of nuclear folding and indentation. Many cells have a nucleus that displays a prominent central crease, or "peaked cap." Promonocytes are also not seen in the normal peripheral blood, but they may be recognized occasionally in a smear of the bone marrow. The chromatin may have an open, lacy appearance, with distinct individual fibers forming a reticulum. The cytoplasm is bluish gray, evenly stained, and it may contain extremely fine reddish purple granules. The cell outline is usually irregular, forming blunt pseudopods. Promonocytes probably pass through 2 to 3 mitotic divisions in the marrow, requiring about 60 hours. The Golgi apparatus and endoplasmic reticulum are prominent in electron microscopic studies.

Mature **monocytes** are released from the marrow shortly after transition from the promonocytic stage. Unlike neutrophils, there does not appear to be a storage pool in the marrow. Monocytes are quite variable in size, from 10 to 30 μm in diameter, making them the largest cells normally seen in the peripheral blood (see Plate 4C). They have an N/C of 2:1 to 1:1, and the nucleus is often band-shaped (horseshoe) or reniform (lima bean). The chromatin is arranged in a fine reticular pattern but it stains darker than that of preceding stages. A nucleolus may be present but it is usually obscured by the chromatin. The cytoplasm is a lighter blue-gray to sky blue. Fine granules, much smaller than the azurophilic granules of lymphocytes, are evenly dispersed through the cytoplasm. These granules are bound by membranes, creating the appearance of tiny vacuoles. This gives the cytoplasm a "ground glass" appearance, the classical term used to describe monocytes and distinguish them from large lymphocytes and myelocytes. Vacuoles are often present and they may be numerous in cells that are responding to infections. The cell outline is often very irregular and forms pseudopods, a consequence of ready adherence to glass surfaces and active motility.

As the monocyte matures, lysosomal contents consisting primarily of acid hydrolases (acid phosphatase and acrylsulfatase) increase while peroxidase decreases. Transit time in the peripheral blood is debatable: references cite times from 8 hours to 100 hours. About three times as many monocytes compose the marginal pool, adhering to vessel endothelia, as compose the freely circulating pool. Like neutrophils, chemotactic stimuli result in margination and emargination responses as the cells migrate to the site of inflammation. They diapedese into the tissues, but unlike neutrophils, they survive for weeks or months and they can phagocytize numerous particles without self-destruction.

The monocyte metamorphoses into a **macrophage,** its final mature form, during its travels through the tissues (see Plate 4D). The cell expands as a result of increased cytoplasmic content and the nucleus becomes round or slightly ovoid. Nucleoli again become prominent and the cytoplasm assumes a sky blue color in stained smears. These cells are not normally found in the blood, but some may enter by way of recirculation through the lymphatic system and they can be demonstrated in buffy coat concentration techniques. Macrophages evidently retain the ability to proliferate, which they may do in response to inflammations. This is most commonly seen in granulomas, lesions that result from accumulations of mononuclear cells around a site of infection that cannot be resolved directly by phagocytosis. More than one macrophage may attempt to ingest the same cell or particle, resulting in a merger of cytoplasms and forming a multinucleated giant cell.

MACROPHAGE FUNCTION

As macrophages mature, they may become specialized morphologically and functionally as a component of a particular organ or tissue (Table 10-1). It is not clear whether all of these cells are derived in the same manner from marrow precursors. For example, the dendritic cells are not phagocytic, but they possess many of the immunological properties of other macrophages.

In general, the roles of macrophages can be separated into two fundamental activities: phagocytosis and antigen presentation.

The biochemistry and physiology of phagocytosis in monocytes and macrophages is very similar to that of neutrophils. The generation of toxic oxygen molecules relies on an activated hexose monophosphate shunt. Myeloperoxidase is not present, but additional acid hydrolases may provide compensatory digestive and killing power. Chemotactically, neutrophils are more motile and they are the first to arrive at a site of inflammation, where their initial activities attract the monocytes. Slower but more efficient, these larger phagocytes ingest more bacteria and clean up the cellular debris of autolysed neutrophils, damaged normal tissue, and fibrin clots. This sequence of arrival can be demonstrated by using a Rebuck skin window (Fig. 10-1). A small abrasion is made on a shaven and cleaned forearm. A coverslip is taped over the site and replaced by a clean coverslip every few hours. When the coverslips are fixed and stained, they show that neutrophils arrive within the first few hours to be replaced by monocytes at 12 to 16 hours. By 24 to 48 hours, many of the monocytes have been transformed into macrophages. This proce-

Table 10-1. Specialized macrophages and histiocytes

Macrophage type	Location	Function
Monocytes (immature macrophages)	Blood	Phagocytosis
Macrophages	Tissues	Phagocytosis; antigen presentation to T and B cells
Histiocytes	Bone marrow	Phagocytosis
Kupffer cells	Liver	Phagocytosis
Langerhans cells	Skin	Antigen presentation to T cells in lymph nodes
Marginal zone macrophages	Spleen	Phagocytosis; antigen presentation to B cells
Follicular dendritic cells	Lymph nodes	Antigen presentation to B cells
Interdigitating cells	Thymus	Antigen presentation to T cells
Alveolar macrophages	Lung	Phagocytosis
Microglial cells	Brain	Phagocytosis
Intraglomerular mesangium	Kidney	Phagocytosis

dure can be used as a crude assay for the chemotactic integrity and mobility of neutrophils and monocytes in immunodeficiency disorders (Chapter 21).

Antigen presentation is a derivative of phagocytosis. A wandering macrophage encounters a foreign particle or microbe that is recognized as non-self. The antigen is ingested but the specific determinants that are "foreign" are preserved and combined with an RNA component. The antigenic determinant is expressed on the macrophage cell surface and carried to a lymph node for presentation to T helper cells, or in some cases, directly to B cells. Presentation target depends on whether the antigen is T cell dependent or not (see Chapter 9). The macrophage secretes a monokine, IL-1, which activates the target lymphocyte. Three forms of this protein are known: alpha IL-1 activates B cells, beta IL-1 activates T helper cells, and gamma IL-1 stimulates cytotoxic T cells. Binding to the target lymphocyte is possible because the lymphocyte recognizes the specific antigenic determinant and because the macrophage expresses an immune-associated antigin (Ia) that mediates cooperative interactions between these cells. The lymphocyte also stimulates the macrophage, enhancing its metabolism and lysosome synthesis. Activated macrophages are sometimes referred to as "angry" because they are then capable of nonspecific target cell destruction at increased rates.

Macrophages have surface receptors forthe Fc fragment of IgG, IgM, and, in a few cells, for IgE. Microbes that have been

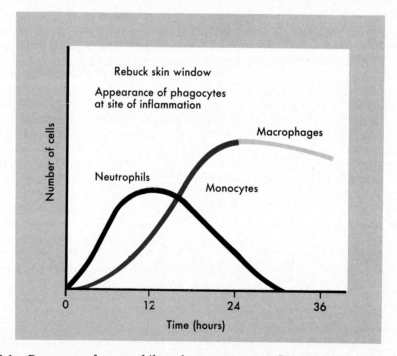

Fig. 10-1.   Responses of neutrophils and monocytes to inflammation.
A Rebuck skin window is used as an assay for chemotactic and motility responses of phagocytes. Neutrophils appear first, to be replaced by monocytes. Many of these transform into macrophages.

coated with these antibodies or with complement (C3b) are readily attacked by the phagocyte. They also respond to alpha-interferon, a substance released from virally infected cells. Lymphocytes can release a protein that inhibits macrophage motility (migratory inhibition factor, MIF), resulting in localization of macrophages with the MIF receptor.

In addition to phagocytosis and antigen presentation, macrophages secrete (1) a pyrogen that induces the fever response; (2) complement components; (3) a type of interferon; (4) capillary growth factors to help maintain blood vessels; (5) chemotactic factors to attract neutrophils to sites of inflammation; and (6) a stimulatory factor for hepatocytes to secrete fibrinogen, a major protein of the coagulation cascade. Macrophages possess enzymes of the arachidonic pathway, which produce prostaglandins. Some of these inhibit activated T cells, providing an additional negative control over the immune response.

SUMMARY

- The mononuclear phagocytic system consists of cells derived from marrow precursors (CFU-GM) that differentiate as the monocytic line. Monoblasts and promonocytes mature in the bone marrow and transform to peripheral blood monocytes.
- Immature cells of the monocytic line require cytochemical staining or immunological methods of positive identification, since they share many of the morphological features of the granulocytic precursors. Nonspecific esterase is positive and specific esterase is negative in normal monocytes.
- Monocytes can enter the tissues by diapedesis and perform phagocytic functions similar to those of neutrophils. They are longer-lived than PMNs and usually transform into tissue macrophages.
- Macrophages function as phagocytes and/or antigen presenting cells. They interact with lymphocytes by carrying the anti-

genic determinant of a foreign particle to the lymph nodes for binding with specific antigenic markers on B, T, or T_C cells. Interaction is mediated by secretion of a monokine, interleukin-1.
- Specialized macrophages reside in various tissues to monitor blood, lymph, alveolar membranes, and serous membranes for microbes and foreign particles. Some of these cell types are fixed (histiocytes) and other remain mobile.

SUGGESTED READINGS—SECTION III

Babior, BM: The respiratory burst of phagocytes, J Clin Invest 73:599, 1984.

Barrett, JT: Textbook of immunology: an introduction to immunochemistry and immunobiology, ed 5, St. Louis, 1988, the CV Mosby Co.

Bessis, M: Blood smears reinterpreted, Springer-Verlag: Berlin, 1977, Springer-Verlag.

Bessis, M, and de Boisfleury, A: A catalogue of white cell movements (normal and pathologic), Blood Cells 2:365, 1976.

Boggs, DR, and Winkelstein, A: White cell manual, ed 4, Philadelphia, 1983, FA Davis Co.

Borregaard, N, and Tauber, AI: Subcellular localization of the human neutrophil NADPH oxidase, J Biol Chem 259:47, 1984.

Burgess, AW, and Metcalf, D: The nature and action of granulocyte-macrophage colony stimulating factors, Blood 56:947, 1980.

Calvert, JE, Maruyana, S, Tedder, TF, et al: Cellular events in the differentiation of antibody-secreting cells, Semin Hematol 21:226, 1984.

Clark, P, Normansell, DAE, Innes, DJ, and Hess, CE: Lymphocyte subsets in normal bone marrow, Blood 67:1600, 1986.

Cline, MJ: The white cell, Cambridge, Mass, 1975, Harvard University Press.

Diggs, LW, Sturm, D, and Bell, A: The morphology of human blood cells, ed 5, Chicago, 1985, Abbott Laboratories.

Dinarello, C, and Mier, JW: Interleukins, Ann Rev Med 37:173, 1986.

Dittmer, DS, editor: Blood and other body fluids, Washington, DC, 1961, Federation of American Societies for Experimental Biology.

Dutcher, T: Bands, polys, and atypical lymphs—one more time! Lab Med 6:19, 1975.

Gleich, GJ, and Loegering, DA: Immunobiology of eosinophils, Ann Rev Immunol 2:429, 1984.

Krensky, AM: Lymphocyte subsets and surface molecules in man, Clin Immunol Rev 4:95, 1985.

Miale, JB: Laboratory medicine: hematology. ed 6, St. Louis, 1982, The CV Mosby Co.

Ogawa, M, Porter, PN, and Nakahata, T: Renewal and commitment to differentiation of hemopoietic stem cells (an interpretive review), Blood 61:828, 1983.

Presentery, B: Cytochemical characterization of eosinophils with respect to a newly discovered anomaly, Am J Clin Pathol 51:451, 1969.

Reinherz, EL, and Schlossman, SF: The differentiation and function of human T lymphocytes, Cell 19:821, 1980.

Roitt, IM, Brostoff, J, and Male, DK: Immunology, St. Louis, 1985, The CV Mosby Co.

Rose, N, Frieman, H, and Fahey, J, editors: Manual of clinical immunology, ed 3, Washington, DC, 1986, American Society of Microbiology.

Schiffman, E: Leukocyte chemotaxis, Ann Rev Physiol 44:553, 1982.

Snyderman, R, and Goetzl, EJ: Molecular and cellular mechanisms of leukocyte chemotaxis, Science 213:830, 1981.

Stutman, O: Ontogeny of T cells, Clin Immunol Allergy 5:191, 1985.

Sullivan, TJ: The role of eosinophils in inflammatory reactions, Prog Hematol 11:65.

Thorup, OA Jr: Leavell and Thorup's fundamentals of clinical hematology, ed 5, Philadelphia, 1987, WB Saunders Co.

Unanue, ER: Antigen-presenting function of the macrophage, Ann Rev Immunol 2:395, 1984.

Weller, PF, and Goetzl, EJ: The human eosinophil: roles in host defense and tissue injury, Am J Pathol 100:793, 1980.

Wilkinson, PC: Chemotaxis and inflammation, ed 2, Edinburgh, 1982, Churchill-Livingstone.

Williams, WJ, Beutler, E, Ersler, AJ, and Lichtman, MA, editors: Hematology, ed 3, New York, 1983, McGraw-Hill Book Co.

Zucker-Franklin, D: Ultrastructural evidence for the common origin of human mast cells and basophils, Blood 56:534, 1980.

SECTION IV
Hemostasis and Coagulation

11

Introduction to Hemostasis and Coagulation

MECHANISMS TO PREVENT BLOOD LOSS

Hemostasis is the component of host defense that functions to stop and prevent blood loss (exsanguination). Although this process is most often presented as a mechanism that responds to trauma, the system also operates continuously, forming and removing microscopic-sized clots, repairing minor damage in the vasculature, and participating in the inflammatory response. Physiological mechanisms to control fluid loss appeared early in the evolution of multicellular organisms (Ratnoff, 1987). Although these processes are probably analogous rather than homologous, the solutions to the problem of fluid loss involve similar components in lower animals (invertebrates) and in mammals: tissue contraction to restrict fluid flow, aggregation of a cellular component to form a plug or solid barrier, and solidification (gelation) of fluid proteins to stabilize the cellular plug and provide an adherent material. All of these factors operate in a sequential and interactive fashion to effect hemostasis in humans (Table 11-1).

Injury to tissue and disruption of circulatory system integrity activates hemostatic and inflammatory responses simultaneously (Fig. 11-1). Activation of the so-called contact factors of the plasma results in stimulation of the coagulation cascade by an intrinsic pathway in addition to the extrinsic mechanism due to tissue factors.

Inflammatory responses are initiated by way of **kallikrein** and **bradykinin** responses. These plasma proteins also help activate the **plasminogen system,** producing a proteolytic product that enzymatically digests the fibrin clots (**fibrinolysis**) produced by the coagulation cascade. Plasmin and inflammatory mediators stimulate the **complement cascade,** which results in additional inflammatory responses, including mast cell activation and the release of vasoactive amines. Complement and antibodies attract phagocytic leukocytes to the injury site to remove microorganisms; recruitment of phagocytes requires increased rates of diapedesis across the vascular endothelium and a higher rate of blood delivery to the inflamed tissues. Stimulation of mast cells during injury results in the release of chemical mediators that increase vascular permeability and produce vasodilation. The blood **platelets** contain additional products that are released upon activation of the coagulation process. There are many processes and interactions between the components of response to tissue injury and infection that are not included here, but the interested reader can refer to a textbook of immunology or one of the review papers listed at the end of this section.

TISSUE AND VASCULAR FACTORS

The importance of the **vascular endothelium** has been appreciated only in recent

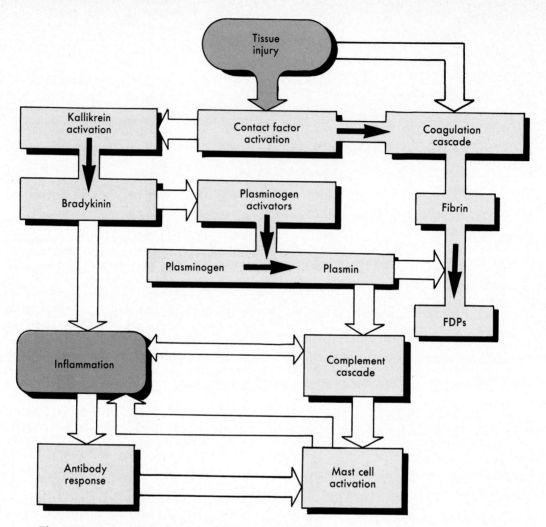

Fig. 11-1.   Interacting systems of host defense following tissue injury.
The relationships between hemostatic processes and inflammatory responses are complex and involve every cellular component of the hematopoietic tissue as well as numerous constituents of the plasma and tissues.

years. These cells form a relatively continuous monolayer on the inner, or *luminal*, surface of the blood vessels (Fig. 11-2), and the cells can be sometimes seen on peripheral smears as a contaminant of blood collection. Disruption of this monolayer, due to trauma or to nutritional deficiencies, exposes the underlying basement membrane of collagenous material. When circulating platelets contact the collagen, biochemical and structural changes occur that lead to the formation of platelet aggregates and fibrin clots. Gaps in the endothelial lining can be plugged by adhering platelets, preventing further stimulation by the collagen layer.

Table 11-1. Events in hemostasis and coagulation

Component	Action	Result
Vascular	Vessel/tissue injury	Collagen exposure
Platelet	Collagen reacts with platelet membrane receptor	Platelet activation
Coagulation	Contact factors of intrinsic pathway of factor VII of extrinsic pathway activated	Cascade of coagulation products Lead to formation of fibrin from fibrinogen
Platelet	Shape change, from disc to sticky sphere	Platelets adhere to vessel walls
Platelet	Biochemical activation and release of granule contents	Activation and recruitment of other platelets to aggregate
Thrombus	Platelets trapped in fibrin mesh with lytic proteins	Clot formed and hemostasis is achieved
Fibrinolysis	Plasminogen activated	Plasmin begins clot lysis for eventual dissolution

Endothelial cells in different vessels may be ultrastructurally specialized for the transport of materials from blood to tissues. Openings through the endothelial layer permit the passage of phagocytic cells. Openings can occur as small pores or fenestrations through individual cells or as very small gaps between adjacent cells (tight junctions). In some tissues, the endothelium may not form a continuous barrier. The vascular lining is **thromboresistant,** or nonreactive to platelets and coagulation protein, because of a proteoglycan secreted by the endothelial cells. This material, **heparan sulfate,** is deposited on the luminal surface and interacts with and potentiates antithrombin III, a natural circulating anticoagulant, to prevent the formation of clots (thrombi).

The vascular endothelium is not merely a passive boundary, however. Endothelial cells *actively* prevent the formation of platelet plugs and fibrin clots by secreting **prostaglandins.** One such substance, **prostacyclin,** inhibits aggregation of platelets to each other at a lower concentration than is necessary to prevent adherence of platelet to exposed collagen surfaces. Thus platelets can seal the exposed vessel wall without forming a large plug that would block circulation. Prostacyclin is especially important in the vasculature of the lungs, where platelets are present in large numbers. It stimulates the cyclic AMP cycle of the platelets, making them less reactive to aggregating stimuli. The endothelial cells secrete plasminogen activators which lead to the production of plasmin and the degradation of any thrombi that do form. Thrombomodulin, a receptor complex of 74,000 daltons, is secreted onto the endothelial cell membrane, where it activates protein C and degrades coagulation factors V and VIII. Endothelial cells also possess a membrane-

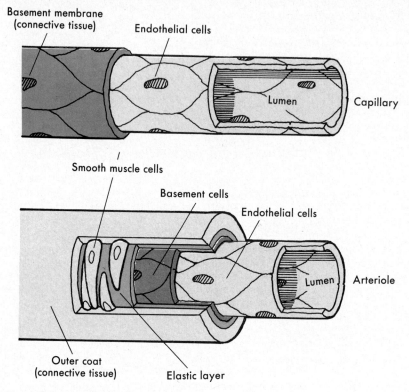

Fig. 11-2.   Structure of blood vessel boundaries.
Comparison of capillary (top) and arteriole (bottom) cross section. Arterioles and veins are surrounded by a layer of contractile cells, as well as elastic fibers.

bound enzyme that destroys ADP and other amines that stimulate platelet aggregation. In addition, endothelial cells participate in antigen processing as part of the immune response and they synthesize the von Willebrand's factor (vWF) component of coagulation factor VIII, fibronectin, and collagen. Considering the many interactions between endothelium and blood components, it is easy to understand how damage to the vessel tissue can lead to both bleeding manifestation and thrombogenesis.

The vessel response to trauma and hemorrhaging is critical to achieving hemostasis. Capillaries usually seal directly and immediately, without involvement of plate-

lets and clotting mechanisms. Arterioles and venules have larger lumens, and the formation of a platelet plug is required to repair breaks and stop blood flow. Larger arteries and veins contain contractile fibers and elastic materials. Trauma to these vessels stimulates mast cells that release vasocontrictors, resulting in a smaller luminal cross section and a larger surface area–to–volume relationship. Extensive coagulation and plug formation may be required to contain blood loss from larger damaged vessels. With continuing blood loss, lowered blood pressure and circulatory shunting (shock) helps reduce the rate of local hemorrhaging, although not without systemic risk.

PLATELET COMPONENTS

Platelets provide the physical mass to form hemostatic plugs, especially in damage involving arterioles and venules. The biochemical and structural events involved in adherence and aggregation responses are described in Chapter 12. Platelets also provide important cofactors and reaction surfaces for some of the reactions of the coagulation process. These are detailed in Chapter 13. Mentioned above is the observation that platelets are able to seal gaps in the endothelial lining, covering the collagenous subendothelial surface. More controversial studies indicate that platelets may actually contribute membrane material to help repair and extend the endothelial lining. When circulating platelet numbers are low, repair activities are limited, and "leaky" blood vessels result in localized bleeding into surrounding tissues (Chapter 22). In vitro studies with tissue cultures indicate that platelets produce growth factors that stimulate mitosis in endothelial cells, fibroblasts, and smooth muscle cells.

THE COAGULATION CASCADE

Plasma gelation is an effective means of preventing body fluid loss for any animal. Moreover, the fibrin mesh can entrap blood cells and platelet plugs, adding mass and rigidity to form an effective barrier at breaks in blood vessels (Fig. 11-3). Activation of contractile proteins in the platelets causes the entire clot to shrink (**clot retraction**), expelling the serum and forming a smaller but more stable hemostatic seal. This also permits partial blood flow through the injured vessel.

The major problem with any physiological response system is one of control: (1) how to turn it on when it is needed, (2) how to keep it turned off when it is not needed, and (3) how to limit the response to what is needed. The first problem is one of activation. A series of reactions are connected in a cascading fashion, in that the product of one reaction is the activator for a subsequent reaction. The inactive form of each coagulation protein is an enzyme precursor called a **zymogen.** Coagulation factors have been assigned roman numerals, although names are often retained for some, such as fibrinogen (I) and prothrombin (II). Activation occurs when a specific protease either cleaves a peptide bond or causes a conformational rearrangement in the zymogen molecule (Fig. 11-4). Activated proteins are designated by the letter a (e.g., XIIa, Va). For some reactions, cofactors are needed to aid in conformational rearrangement (e.g., calcium) or provide a reaction surface (e.g., phospholipid on the platelet surface). The activated molecule is a serine protease that acts on the next zymogen in the series. As a result, the final product of the coagulation cascade (fibrin) is separated from the initial reactants by several events. Therefore every molecule that participates in the cascade must be normal and present in sufficient quantity to permit the process to continue.

Equally important are the mechanisms that prevent inappropriate activation of the cascade. Natural or innate inhibitors and anticoagulants circulate in the plasma, limiting the initiation and extent of fibrin formation (Table 11-2). **Antithrombin III (AT-III)** is a potent neutralizer of thrombin, one of the key activated proteins of the cascade. It slowly forms a 1:1 complex with thrombin, but this process is greatly accelerated by the addition of **heparin,** a sulfated mucopolysaccharide that is released from basophils and mast cells. Platelets and endothelial cell surfaces contain heparan sulfate, a closely related molecule. Heparin reversibly binds to lysine residues on the AT-III molecule, producing conformational changes at a second site with arginine residues. This change enhances the reaction between serine residues on thrombin and arginine residues on AT-III, and a stable complex between enzyme and inhibitor forms. Heparin serves as a catalytic enzyme: it is

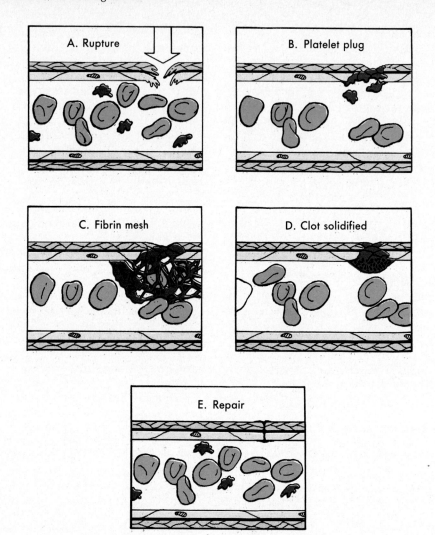

Fig. 11-3.   Formation and retraction of a fibrin clot.
A, Traumatic rupture of a small blood vessel exposes basement membrane. **B,** Platelets adhere to the exposed collagen and aggregate to form a plug. **C,** Localized plasma gelation produces a fibrin mesh that entraps red cells around the platelet plug. **D,** Platelet contraction produces clot retraction, solidifying the clot and allowing partial circulation through the vessel. **E,** Plasmin produces dissolution of the clot coincident with adjacent tissue repair.

released to enhance additional AT-III molecules. Heparin is obtained commercially from various animal tissues and employed as a medical anticoagulant to inhibit thrombosis during the acute phase of treat-

ment for pulmonary and cardiac disorders (Chapter 24).

Protein C is an additional protease inhibitor that inactivates coagulation factors V and VIII during their interactions with

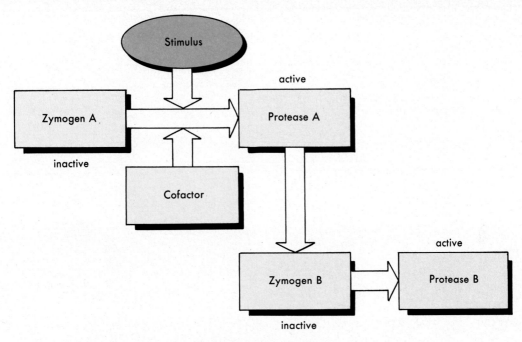

Fig. 11-4. Activation of zymogen precursors into active proteases.
The general form of reactions within the coagulation and fibrinolytic systems.

platelets. Although it is present in very small amounts, it is rapidly activated to its enzymatic form by thrombin in association with endothelial thrombomodulin and calcium ions (Fig. 11-5). Protein C activity on the phospholipid surface of platelets is enhanced by the presence of protein S. There is also a circulating inhibitor that inactivates protein C. Both protein C and S are vitamin K–dependent factors (along with coagulation factors II, VII, IX, and X) synthesized by the liver. Disruption of vitamin K synthesis by administration of the oral anticoagulant, warfarin sodium (Coumadin), results in deficiencies of these proteins. Protein C is also a participant in the fibrinolytic process (Chapter 14).

Other natural coagulation inhibitors are

Table 11-2. Coagulation inhibitors and anticoagulants

Component	Function	Molecular weight (Daltons)
Antithrombin-III	Neutralize thrombin, XIIa, XIa, IXa, Xa, and kallikrein. Cofactor for heparin effects.	56,000
alpha$_2$-macroglobulin	Inhibit XIIa, XIa, kallikrein	360,000
alpha$_1$-antitrypsin	Inhibit XIa, thrombin, kallikrein	55,000
C1 inactivator	Inhibit XIIa, XIa, kallikrein	40,000
Protein C	Degrade Va and VIIIa; inhibit Xa on platelets	62,000
Protein S	Cofactor for protein C	

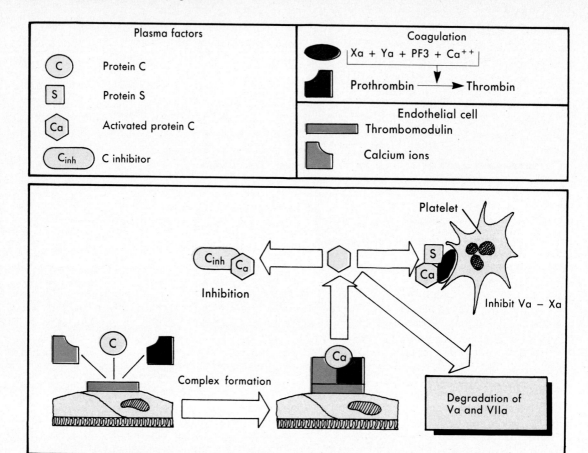

Fig. 11-5.   Interactions of protein C with the coagulation and fibrinolytic systems.
Protein C is activated (C_a) by thrombin and thrombomodulin on the surface of endothelial cells in the presence of calcium ions. Excess protein C can be bound by a circulating inhibitor (C_{inh}). C_a degrades the activated forms of factors V and VIII and interferes with the formation of the Va-Xa complex on the phospholipid surface of platelets. Protein S is a cofactor in the latter action.

known, but their in vivo activity is not fully understood. **Alpha-2-macroglobulin** can bind with and neutralize thrombin, kallikrein, trypsin, collagenase, and plasmin, but the bound enzymes are not completely inactivated. Instead, the inhibitor-protease complex may be a means of sequestering enzymes from complete inactivation by other inhibitors while providing a slow, controlled clearance of the proteases from

circulation by macrophages of the liver and spleen. Other inhibitors include alpha$_1$-antitrypsin and C1 inactivator, but these probably play minor or secondary roles in the coagulation process.

FIBRINOLYSIS

Dissolution of the clot is necessary for tissue repair to proceed and for normal blood circulation to resume. Again, a fine balance between clot formation and removal must exist if hemostasis is to be effective. Fibrinolysis is initiated by incorporating components of the plasminogen-plasmin system into the formation of the fibrin clot. **Plasmin** is yet another serine protease, in this case, one that enzymatically attacks the fibrin molecule, producing a series of degradation products (FDPs) that are cleared from the circulation by macrophages (Chapter 14).

SUMMARY

- Hemostasis and the inflammatory response are closely linked as components of host defense. Injury to tissue involves responses of the blood platelets to produce a hemostatic plug, the plasma coagulation system to produce a fibin clot, the fibrinolytic system to dissolve the clot, the bradykinin system to mediate tissue reactions and stimulate phagocytic recruitment, the complement cascade to facilitate phagocytosis, and the immune system to neutralize and remove foreign particles.

- The vascular endothelium provides both a passive and active boundary for transport of materials and cells between blood and tissues. Endothelial cells secrete a number of products that interact with platelets (von Willebrand's factor, prostacyclin, ADPase), with coagulation factors (thrombomodulin, antithrombin III, heparan sulfate), and with the fibrinolytic system (plasminogen activators).

- Hemostasis consists of vessel responses to trauma (vasocontriction), the formation of a cellular plug by adherence and aggregation of circulating platelets, and the gelation of plasma to form a mesh composed of red blood cells, platelets, and fibrin.

- Homeostatic control is maintained by a series of activators and inhibitors at various steps in the hemostatic process. Inactive coagulation proteins, zymogens, are converted to active proteases in a sequence or cascade of reactions. Other molecules inhibit the formation or activity of these enzymes.

12

The Normal Platelet

Platelets are small, disc-shaped cellular fragments that provide an early response to blood vessel damage and bleeding. Platelets (or "thrombocytes," the equivalent term used in most animals) are anucleate, but the cytoplasm contains a variety of organelles and chemical substances that function to maintain blood vessel integrity, initiate hemostasis, and promote coagulation. Tissue damage results in the release and exposure of materials that promote platelet stickiness and clumping; the accumulated mass serves as a barrier to blood loss. The platelet surface also facilitates activities of the coagulation cascade, resulting in the formation of a fibrin clot that strengthens and stabilizes the initial platelet plug.

THROMBOPOIESIS: PLATELET PRODUCTION
Maturation from megakaryoblast to megakaryocyte

Platelets are fragments of the cytoplasm of megakaryocytes. These large granular cells of the bone marrow are derived from pluripotential hematopoietic stem cells (Chapter 7) that also give rise to granulocyte and erythrocyte precursors. The stem cells replicate from time to time, maintaining a steady level of the self-renewing clone. An unknown stimulus results in some of the stem cells "committing" to the thrombocytic or megakaryocytic lineage, forming CFU-MK cells (Fig. 12-1). Some evidence suggests that the formation and subsequent expansion of CFU-MK numbers is in response to a proliferation hormone,

thrombopoietin, analogous to erythropoietin. Other investigators believe that thrombopoietin may regulate platelet production by controlling later stages of megakaryocyte maturation and platelet release. Much of the evidence for the existence and physiological effects of thrombopoietin are derived from studies of patients who have been infused with excess platelets or in patients with a low circulating platelet mass.

Subsequent cell stages of the megakaryocytic series are unique among blood cells. Whereas mature cells of the red cell and white cell lines are smaller than their respective precursors (due to mitotic division of cell contents), mature megakaryocytes are larger than the earlier forms. Committed stem cells (CFU-MK) mature to **megakaryoblasts** (MKB), the first designated megakaryocytic precursor. From this point on, DNA replicaton in the MKB occurs without concurrent division of the cytoplasm. As a result, the cell changes from the normal diploid (2N) state to a polyploid state. Each doubling of the nuclear contents, a process called **endomitosis,** or endoreduplication, increases the ploidy, from 4N to 8N to 16N and so forth. The cytoplasmic contents also increase, by accumulation and synthesis, resulting in large polyploid **promegakaryocytes.** Endomitosis is the analogue of amplification seen in early stages of granulocyte and normoblast production. Maturation of promegakaryocytes into **megakaryocytes** (MKC) can occur at various states of ploidy, although most of the cells in a normal marrow are either 8N

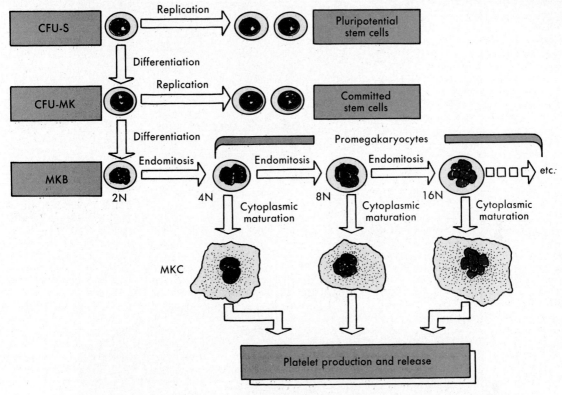

Fig. 12-1.   Thrombopoiesis: derivaton of megakaryocytes.
Cell lineage and megakaryocytes, a composite representation. *CFU-S*, Colony forming unit, spleen; *CFU-MK*, colony forming unit, megakaryocyte; *MKB*, megakaryoblast; *MKC*, megakaryocyte. The CFU-MK and MKB may be identical or cells differing slightly in maturation and commitment; neither stage has been identified morphologically. Continued endomitosis can result in promegakarocytes with higher ploidys (32N, 64N, etc), each giving rise to platelet forming megakaryocytes.

or 16N. Maturation consists of structural rearrangements and synthetic activities in the cytoplasm: (1) synthesis of extensive endoplasmic reticulum, (2) formation of demarcation membranes that isolate the cytoplasm into small zones, (3) the formation of storage granules containing a variety of chemicals, (4) synthesis of filaments, microtubules, and small canals within the zones, and (5) creation of energy-generating systems. The cytoplasm becomes highly granular and the demarcation membranes become increasingly distinct. After about five days of maturation the MKC cytoplasm fragments into hundred to thousands of individual **platelets,** which pass from the bone marrow into the blood circulation (Fig. 12-2).

Considerable disagreement exists among investigators as to the number of early stages and their characteristics. As a result, maturation stages have been assigned various names and numbers by different authors (Table 12-1). Recent studies employ immunological and histochemical techniques to positively identify the megakary-

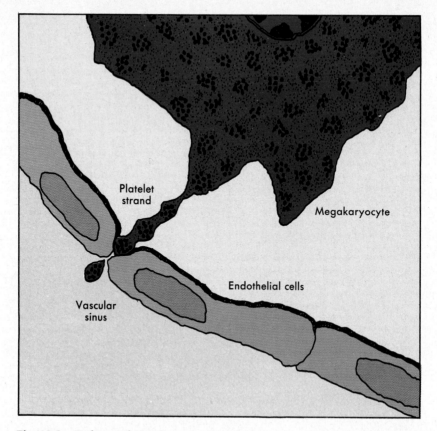

Fig. 12-2.   Release of platelet strand from bone marrow into venous sinus.

oblast, a stage questioned by Bessis (1977) but designated by Williams and Levine (1982). Assignment of cell size and nuclear ploidy to some early stages is also not definitive at this time, but a tentative scheme is indicated in Fig. 12-1. The CFU-MK and MKB may be synonymous or distinct stages with differences in DNA synthetic activity and ploidy. T.C. Bithell, in Thorup (1987) states that the CFU-MK may be 4N, whereas most other authors indicate that amplification by endomitosis begins later, in the promegakaryocytic, or MK_2 stage (Bessis, 1977).

Platelet production

Several points regarding platelet production are relatively well documented, however. The degree of endomitosis is a function of platelet demand, as indicated in thrombocytopenic patients that exhibit increased marrow productivity. MKCs with higher ploidy numbers (16N to 32N) are associated with increased amounts of cytoplasm and with greater platelet numbers released per cell. Thus an MKC of 8N may produce 500 to 1000 platelets, whereas an occasional MKC of 64N may produce up to 4000 platelets. An average MKC releases 1000 to 1500 platelets. Thrombopoietin or a related factor apparently communicates the peripheral platelet deficit to the marrow, resulting in the production of MKCs of higher ploidy, up to 128N in some pathological conditions (Chapter 23). In addition, thrombopoietin may speed up the process of cyto-

Table 12-1. Stages of megakaryocyte maturation

| Cell name | Designation | | Cell size | Nuclear Ploidy |
	Bessis	Levine		
Megakaryoblast	—	I	15-40 μm	2N
Promegakaryocyte (basophilic MKC)	MK_1	II	20-60 μm	4N-32N
Granular megakaryocyte	MK_2	III	30-90 μm	8N-32N
Mature megakaryocyte	MK_3	IV	40-120 μm	8N-32N

plasmic maturation and fragmentation. Other evidence indicates that the size of MKCs (ploidy) and the number of MKCs formed may be regulated by independent processes.

Although earlier investigators had reported that nuclear lobulation was a direct indicator of ploidy, later studies have refuted this. Chromosome and DNA studies indicate that 76% of the marrow MKCs are 16N, about 16% are 32N, and 8% are 8N; 4N and 64N cells are rare (Bessis, 1977). Altogether, MK_1 cells comprise 10% to 15% of marrow MKCs, MK_2 cells are 60% to 70% and MK_3 cells are 10% to 20% of the total. One estimate of the MKC mass gives values of 5.4 to 6.8×10^6/kg body weight. Platelet release from a single MKC is probably simultaneous or of short duration, rather than by a slow "budding" process, as indicated by earlier studies of stained marrow sections. Beck (1985) reports an estimate of 50 platelets released per day per N of ploidy (i.e., 800/day from a 16N MKC).

Morphological characteristics of MKC stages

Four stages are listed with data compiled from a number of sources (Table 12-1). The first stage, the **megakaryoblast** (Levine stage I), is identifiable in marrow sections stained for specific peroxidases and by immunological methods for MKC antigens. The nucleus is usually round or oval with a regular outline. Two to six distinct nucleoli are present in a nuclear background of fine chromatin. Nucleus to cytoplasm ratio is about 10:1. The cytoplasm is basophilic and agranular; there may be blunt projections at the periphery. Size estimates vary from 10 μm or less to more than 50μm in diameter.

The **promegakaryocyte** (MK_1 or Levine stage II) is much more obvious in marrow sections and smears. The nucleus is usually irregular and lobulated. A more condensed chromatin may contain 0 to 2 indistinct nucleoli. Nucleus to cytoplasm ratio has decreased to 4:1 to 7:1, depending on ploidy. The more abundant cytoplasm may contain a few azurophilic granules; background color is orthochromic or lightly basophilic. Cell diameter ranges from 25 μm to 80 μm.

Granular megakaryoctes (MK_2 or Levine stage III) have condensed, multilobulated nuclei. Nucleoli may be absent or present as many small, indistinct light areas that can be best seen in well-spread cells on thin areas of the marrow smear. Nucleus to cytoplasm ratio is 2:1 to 1:1, and the cytoplasm is very finely and diffusely granular. No evidence is seen of the coarse granules that will become individual platelets.

Mature or **platelet-forming megakaryocytes** (MK_3 or Levine stage IV) have N/C ratios of less than 1:1. The cytoplasm contains coarse clumps of granules, especially at the cell periphery. Evidence of fragmentation or "budding" may be present, although the latter may be an artifact of preparation. Diggs, Sturm and Bell (1985) use the term **metamegakaryocyte** for this stage.

Platelet (thrombocyte) is the individual cytoplasmic fragment released into the blood. Some authors restrict the term "thrombocyte" to the equivalent cells of birds and lower vertebrates, whereas other hematologists use the two names interchangeably. The prefixes *mega-* and *micro-* can be affixed to thrombocyte to indicate abnormal size. Micromegakaryocytes (8 to 15 μm diameter) are sometimes seen in marrows undergoing blast crisis in chronic myeloid leukemia (Chapter 20).

Post-thrombocytic megakaryocytes consist of a condensed nucleus with little or scant amounts of cytoplasm remaining. The nucleus is phagocytosized by marrow macrophages and the nucleotides and amino acids are recycled within the hematopoietic environment.

Platelet formation

Organization of the megakaryocytic cytoplasm into distinct zones begins at the MK$_1$ stage with the formation of **demarcation membranes** (Fig. 12-3). The membranes are actually tubules that communicate throughout the cell and to the extracellular environment. As the cytoplasm matures

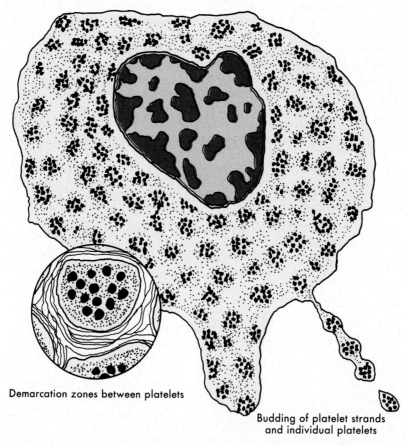

Demarcation zones between platelets

Budding of platelet strands and individual platelets

Fig. 12-3.   Formation of platelets by fragmentation of cytoplasm.

(MK$_2$ stage), glycoproteins form on the membrane's luminal surface, eventually to become the external coat of the platelets after they are released. Additional tubules form from the endoplasmic reticulum to become the canaliculi of the mature platelet. A centrosome, located near the periphery of the nucleus, contains a Golgi complex that produces various granules and lysosomes. The azurophilic granulation disperses evenly throughout the cytoplasm to give the granular megakaryocte its distinct appearance.

Further maturation results in aggregation of the granules into groups of 10 to 12 granules, separated from adjacent groups by channels of clear cytoplasm, constituting "platelet territories." Electron microscopy reveals that these territories or zones contain organelles (small mitochondria, ribosomes, and azurophilic granules, some glycogen deposits, and lysosomes). Studies of platelet release with time-lapse cinematography by Bessis revealed that the megakaryocyte deforms and extends cytoplasmic processes consisting of an elongated strand of several platelet zones. The extensions undergo periodic contractions so that the individual or small groups of platelets are fragmented from the cell. The process of extension and fragmentation probably requires from 3 to 12 hours, but there also is evidence that peripheral fragmentation may occur simultaneously, with release of most or all of the platelets within minutes. The platelet strands diapedese from the marrow into the venous sinuses and thus to the peripheral circulation. Most of the strands are further fragmented during diapedesis so that individual platelets are released into the bloodstream, but occasional strings of platelets can be seen in some platelet disorders (see Chapter 23).

Platelet distribution

After release, platelets are circulated to the spleen, where they remain for 2 to 4 days, before distribution throughout the body. The **splenic platelet pool** is an important consideration in diseases in which splenomegaly occurs and in evaluating thrombocytopenia on the basis of peripheral blood platelet counts. At any time, about 20% to 35% of the platelet mass is present in the spleen and, as is the case with red blood cells, this proportion can increase dramatically in individuals with splenomegaly and drop to zero following splenectomy. Platelets and some megakaryocytes are found in the lungs, kidneys, and liver. When suitable concentration techniques are used, one can also demonstrate a low concentration of MKCs in peripheral blood (about 12 MKC/ml). About 65% to 80% of the platelets released from the marrow are present in the peripheral blood, surviving about 8 to 12 days.

Reference values for platelet concentration in the blood vary from one investigator to another. Lower limits have been cited from 130,000 to 200,000/μL, and upper limits from 350,000 to 450,000/μL. Radioisotopic methods have been used to estimate both the survival time and life span of circulating platelets and the rate of release from the bone marrow. Harker and Finch (1969) determined that about 31,000 to 39,000 platelets/μL of blood were released from the marrow each day. Platelet size distribution can also vary widely, as reported in different studies. Diameter ranges from 2 to 5 μm and volume from 5 to 10 fL (Bessis, 1977). Bithell in Thorup (1987) cites values of 2.9 to 4.3 μm diameter, 0.7 to 1.1 μm thickness and 5.2 to 7.7 fL volume. About 5% to 10% of the platelets seen on a smear from a normal individual may be slightly larger (macrothrombocytes). These larger forms have often been regarded as younger, that is, freshly released from the marrow, because they are more prevalent in patients with accelerated platelet production and this correlates with a decrease in MKC ploidy *(shift to left)*.

The fate of platelets is controversial. They are removed from the circulation by splenic macrophages, as are other blood cells. However, the basis for their demise is uncertain. Do platelets have finite lifespans of several days, after which they undergo degenerative processes, becoming vulnerable to phagocytosis? Or is it a random process by which a determinable proportion is removed, based on physiological need and production kinetics?

PLATELET STRUCTURE

Platelets are discoid cytoplasmic fragments, containing a variety of chemicals and organelles of a highly specialized nature. However, this is not apparent in routine stained smears in which only a small clump of azurophilic granules are visible. Electron microscopy reveals several types of granules, mitochondria, tubules, microfilaments, and a multilayered covering (Fig. 12-4).

The periphery

The platelet surface interacts with the blood vessel surface and with the plasma coagulation proteins and is therefore the sender and receiver of biochemical messages that initiates hemostasis. The outermost **external coat** (glycocalyx) is a layer of sialoglycoproteins, 10 to 50 nm thick. Onto this surface are adsorbed some of the plasma coagulation proteins and factors that promote adhesion of the platelet to vascular endothelial cells. Beneath the external coat lies a trilaminar **plasma membrane** (protein-lipid bilayer), about 7 to 8 nm thick, which communicates directly with the system of tubules (canalicular system) into the interior of the cell. A **cytoskeleton** of microtubules lies under the plasma membrane, serving to maintain and change the shape of the platelet during aggregation and hemostatic plug formation.

The **canalicular system** provides access for cellular contents to the exterior surface. It is continuous with the plasma membrane, forming an invagination so that the canalicular lumen is exterior to the cell. Platelet products that are stored in and released from various granules pass across the

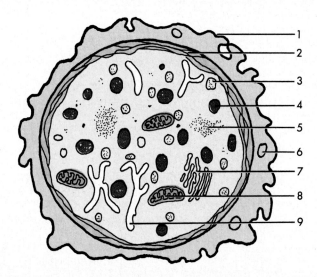

Fig. 12-4. Platelet ultrastructure, based on electron micrography.
1, Outer coat or glycocalyx; *2*, plasma membrane and cytoskeleton of microtubules; *3*, alpha granule; *4*, dense body; *5*, glycogen granules; *6*, pinocytotic vesicle; *7*, Golgi apparatus; *8*, mitochondrium; *9*, section of open canalicular system.

canalicular membrane to the extracellular environment, usually to attach to the platelet surface.

Cytoplasm

The cytoplasm contains small **mitochondria** and glycogen deposits. Glycogen synthetase is also present to provide an energy releasing mechanism for biochemical synthesis, secretion, and contractile activities via anaerobic glycolysis. Nucleotides (mainly AMP, ADP, and ATP) are distributed in the cytosol, membranes, and mitochondria for metabolic needs. Contractile proteins are dispersed throughout the cell, composed mainly of **thrombosthenin** (platelet actomyosin) in the form of microfilaments, with much of it concentrated as a peripheral band of microtubules beneath the plasma membrane.

Granules are classified into two basic types, based on appearance on transmission electron micrography (TEM) thin sections. **Alpha granules** correspond to the azurophilic granules of Wright-stained smears and have thin walls on TEM preparations. Alpha granules consist of two types: **lysosomes** containing acid hydrolases and alpha granules proper that contain a diversity of products (Table 12-2). Thick-walled, relatively opaque organelles, the **dense bodies**, contain fewer but no less important products.

PLATELET FUNCTION

Platelets have three primary functions: (1) react to vessel injury by forming an aggregative plug or platelet mass that can slow or stop blood loss, (2) help activate and participate in plasma coagulation as a more effective means of forming a barrier to extensive blood loss, and (3) maintain the endothelial lining of blood vessels.

Hemostatic plug formation (Fig. 12-5)

Adherence. Injury to a blood vessel disrupts the architecture of the luminal surface. When endothelial cells are damaged or

Table 12-2. Contents of platelet granules

Constituent	Function
Alpha granules	
Albumin	May inhibit fibrinolysis
α_2-antiplasmin	Inhibits activity of plasmin, prevents clot lysis
β-thrombo-globulin (BTG)	Weak antiheparin activity
Factor V	Component of coagulation complex on platelet surface
Factor VIII:vWF	Attach platelet to endothelium (adherence)
Fibrinogen	Provides fibrin matrix for platelet aggregation and plug formation
Fibronectin	Connecting molecule between platelets (aggregation) and from platelet to endothelium
Platelet-derived growth factor (PDGF)	Mitogen, promotes migration and proliferation of endothelial and smooth muscle cells in vessel walls
Platelet factor 4 (PF-4)	Antiheparin activity
Thrombospondin (TSP)	Connecting molecule, platelet aggregation
Dense bodies	
Adenine nucleotides	ADP activates and recruits platelets (aggregation)
Calcium	Cofactor in platelet-mediated coagulation reactions
Epinephrine	Aggregating agent; vasoconstrictor
Serotonin (5-HT)	Vasoconstrictor

displaced or when they degenerate, platelets in the blood stream are exposed to the underlying substrate of collagen and subendothelial factor VIII:vWF (see Chapter 11). Collagen stimulates changes in platelet function and morphology that result in adherence of the platelet to the damaged area of the blood vessel. The platelet transforms from a compact disc into a slightly broader, platelike form with increased surface area

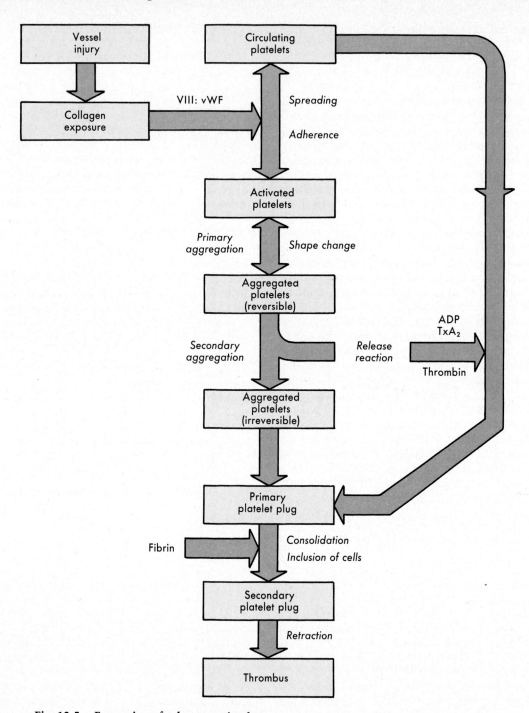

Fig. 12-5. Formation of a hemostatic plug.
Major processes of plug and thrombus formation following traumatic damage to a blood vessel.

for contact. Adherence may involve a number of different biochemical mechanisms, but the process is poorly understood. Endothelial cells secrete **fibronectin,** a 450,000 Dalton protein, that is stored in the alpha granules of platelets and is released when platelets are activated. Fibronectin has been shown to bond platelets to collagen, a process that may also require the activation of coagulation factor XIII. In fact, fibronectin is present in tissues throughout the body and may be an essential component of the "glue" that binds cells together. The basement membrane and elastic fibers may also serve as sites of adherence in vivo. Platelets will also bind to a number of artificial substrates, especially glass, and this can be used as a basis for in vitro testing, but the biochemical mechanisms for adherence may not be the same.

An additional protein is necessary for optimal platelet-collagen binding. The largest component of coagulation factor VIII, variously known as VIII:ag, VIII:vWF, or **von Willebrand's factor,** is secreted by platelets and by vascular endothelial cells. Deposits of this protein enhance platelet-collagen interactions; deficiencies in VIII:vWF result in the bleeding disorder, von Willebrand's disease (see Chapter 24). Adherence is the first step in formation of a hemostatic barrier and it is the stimulus that activates the next phase, aggregation of platelets to each other.

Shape change. Attachment to a surface brings about reversible changes in the platelet, collectively referred to as **activation.** Morphologically, the platelets undergo a dramatic change in shape, from the flattened disc of the adherent form to a sphere with long, irregular arms (Fig. 12-6). As a result, surface area increases greatly to facilitate interaction with other platelets and proteins of the coagulation cascade.

Shape change involves movements of the microtubules and other elements of the platelet cytoskeletal system. Actin and myosin-like proteins, similar to that found in

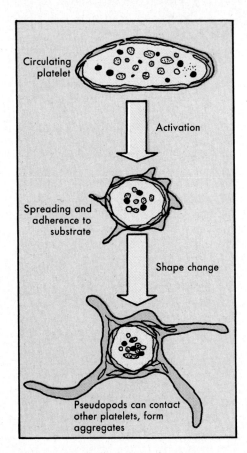

Fig. 12-6. Adherence and shape change. Diagrammatic representation of platelet shape change following collagen exposure and activation.

muscle tissue, provide the molecular apparatus for contractility of the central portion of the platelet and extension of the pseudopodial arms. At the same time, many of the granules and other organelles become "centered" so that they lie adjacent to openings of the canalicular system. Up to this point, change of shape is reversible; lack of additional stimuli will eventually result in a return to the discoid, nonadherent form of circulating platelet. The release of granule contents usually commits the platelet to aggregation and the formation of a hemostatic plug.

Release reaction. Centering of organelles is required before the secretion or release of substances from the platelet However, release of granule contents is not simple. Which granules and which contents are involved depends on the substance and the level of concentration that stimulates the platelet. This process requires energy, supplied by nucleotide metabolism and intracellular calcium. Weak stimulation, such as that provided by ADP, results in the release of dense body contents. Dense bodies contain ADP, and this is secreted into the accumulating mass of platelets to stimulate ADP release by the dense bodies of other platelets (an example of physiological *amplification*, in which a cell product or activity produces an increasing level of similar activity in other cells of the same population). Strong stimulation, e.g, as provided by collagen from damaged vessels or by thrombin from coagulation processes, results in the release of substances from dense bodies and alpha granules. Thorup (1987) lists more than 30 products that can be released from stimulated platelets. Once release is initiated, additional stimulation and release proceeds until the process is disrupted, either by inhibitory mechanisms or by diminishment of the original activating conditions. A graded response allows the amount of platelet recruitment to be limited in the presence of minor vessel trauma, but it can result in amplification when substantial injury requires formation of a large plug in a short time interval.

Aggregation. Platelets attach to other platelets because of changes that occur on their outer coats and as a result of the formation of molecular complexes that join them. Aggregation can occur without releasing ADP **(primary aggregation)**, a reversible process, or as a permanent change that results in release of ADP and activation of a platelet thromboxane-prostaglandin pathway **(secondary aggregation)**. Natural primary aggregating agents include ADP, epinepherine, vasopressin (antidiuretic hormone), and platelet activating factor (PAF). Secondary agents include thrombin, collagen, and ADP in high concentrations.

Deposits of materials secreted by the platelet transform the outer coat into a "sticky" substrate. A number of different molecular receptors have been identified on the platelet surface, and glycoproteins appear to be important in establishing platelet-platelet connections. Hereditary disorders of specific glycoproteins have been identified in association with bleeding disorders that are characterized by defective platelet aggregation (Table 12-3).

The growing mass of platelets forms the primary hemostatic plug in vivo. This plug, unless stabilized by fibrin strands contributed by plasma protein coagulation, is only a temporary structure. Aggregation and attachment of a functional plug occurs within 15 to 30 seconds after vessel injury, but stabilizaton may take several minutes. A bleeding time determination provides an overall assessment of platelet plug formation, dependent on platelet concentration (count), qualitative function, and vessel integrity. Platelet aggregation can be tested in vitro by photometrically measuring change in platelet shape and rate of clumping as a response to any of several physiological agents (Fig. 12-7). The clot retraction test assesses consolidation of the platelet plug into a thrombus or clot (see Chapter 28 for details and interpretations of procedures).

Procoagulant activities

Platelets play several roles in the coagulation mechanism: (1) they secrete proteins that serve as cofactors in two key steps of the coagulation cascade; (2) the outer coat is a template or reacting surface for some coagulation steps; and (3) they participate directly in initiating coagulation at the contact phase. Most of these processes occur concurrently or in sequence with hemostatic function.

Coagulation cofactor. Platelet factor 3 (PF-3) is a phospholipoprotein contained on or

Table 12-3. Platelet surface glycoproteins

Glycoprotein	MW (kilodaltons)	Notes
Ia	165	Binds thrombin and ristocetin; interacts with factor VIII; high content of sialic acid
Ib	177	Binds plasma-derived vWF; F_c receptor; absence seen in Bernard-Soulier syndrome (BSS)
IIa	155	
IIb	160	Binds platelet-derived vWF; deficient in thrombasthenia
IIb/IIIa		Calcium-dependent binding site for fibrinogen and fibronectin, exposed by action of thrombin
IIIa/IV	95	IIIa is decreased in thrombasthenia
V	65	Cleaved by thrombin; decreased in BSS
IX	22	Complexed with Ib, about 25,000 sites; decreased in BSS
150/135	198	Fibronectin receptor

within the plasma membrane. PF-3 participates in the formation of factor Xa on the platelet surface by complexing with IXa, VIII, and CA^{++} (see Chapter 13 for details). The next reaction in the sequence also occurs on the platelet surface: PF-3 forms an enzymatic complex with Xa, V, and Ca^{++} to convert plasma prothrombin to thrombin. PF-3 secretion and spatial organization on the membrane coincides or closely follows the release reaction and other steps involved in secondary aggregation.

Surface template for hemostasis and coagulation reactions. Specific receptor molecules have been identified on the platelet membrane and/or outer coat; these glycoproteins bind to coagulation proteins and to substances that facilitate platelet-platelet and platelet-endothelium interactions (Table 12-3). Analysis of the glycoproteins is usually done with SDS-PAGE separation (the electrophoretic technique used to separate RBC membrane proteins) or by identification with monoclonal antibodies directed against determinants on the receptor molecules. Glycoprotein (GP) IIb/IIIa is present in an inactive form in nonstimulated platelets, but the site appears to be modified by thrombin during platelet activation. GP IIb/IIIa serves as a reactive site for fibrinogen and fibronectin, enhancing the aggregative stimulus of ADP. An additional fibronectin receptor is identified as GP 150/135 and it may help, in concert with fibrinogen, to stabilize platelet aggregates. Two distinct sites bind von Willebrand's factor: GP Ib is the receptor for vWF that circulates in the plasma and GP IIb interacts with vWF released from platelet granules. Other sites bind coagulation factors V, VIII, and Xa, but these have not been characterized as well.

Contact phase initiation. Platelets that have been biochemically activated are capable of proteolytically activating coagulation factors XI and XII in vitro, similar to the manner in which tissue factors initiate the contact phase of coagulation. The extent to which this occurs in vivo is not clear.

Maintenance of vascular lining

Platelets secrete products that help repair and maintain the vascular endothelium. **Platelet derived growth factor (PDGF)** is a mitogen present in alpha granules. PDGF stimulates endothelial cell migration and proliferation, especially after traumatic disruption of the vessel wall lining. Some ultrastructural and isotopic labeling experi-

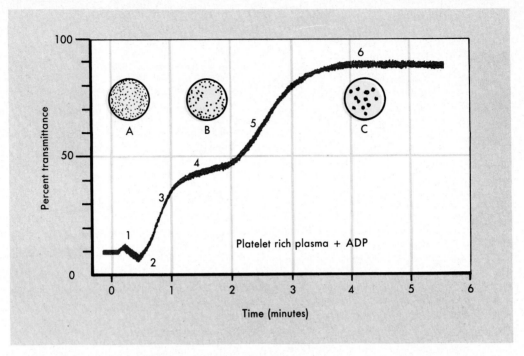

Fig. 12-7.   In vitro aggregation as a measure of platelet activation response.
Aggregation curve, plotted as change in light transmittance over time, for a platelet suspension responding to low concentrations of ADP. Insets A, B, and C represent platelet dispersion at various phases of aggregaton. 1, Shape change; 2, rebound from shape change (may not be present); 3, primary wave of aggregation (reversible); 4, plateau prior to release reaction; 5, secondary wave of aggregation (irreversible) following release reaction; 6, plateau (maximum aggregation).

ments suggest that platelets attach to the gap junctions between endothelial cells and that platelet membrane and/or cytoplasm is actually transferred to the endothelial cell. Serotinin and ADP, from the dense bodies, also promote endothelial cell integrity. Regardless of the mechanisms, individuals with chronic thrombocytopenias show evidence of deteriorating vascular linings: petechial hemorrhages and increased capillary fragility result.

Platelet biochemistry

The biochemical pathways and metabolic requirements of platelets are as complex as those of nucleated cells, and the functional nature of these cytoplasmic fragments may be more diverse than that of many complete cells. Much of the cytoplasmic content is manufactured before the platelet breaks free from the nucleated megakaryocyte, although other substances are either synthesized during activation of the circulating platelet or they are adsorbed from the plasma. In addition to the granule contents described in Table 12-2, two other biochemical systems require elaboration: nucleotidyl metabolism and the thromboxane-prostaglandin pathway.

Nucleotide metabolism (Fig. 12-8)

Three nucleotides predominate within the platelet: **cyclic adenosine monophosphate (cAMP)**, adenosine diphosphate (ADP), and

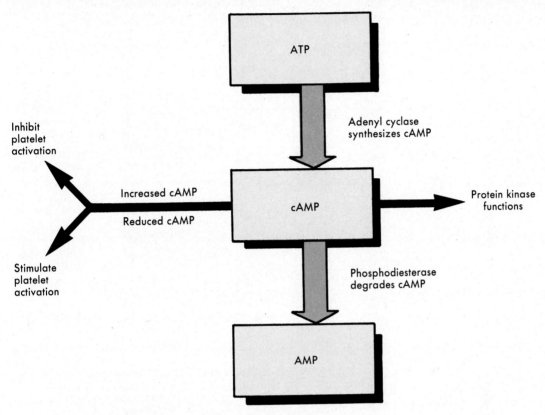

Fig. 12-8. Nucleotidyl regulation of platelet activation.
The central role of cyclic adenosine monophosphate is regulated by the enzymes adenyl cyclase and phosphodiesterase. Increases in cAMP inhibit platelet activation and decreases in cAMP enhance activation. Cyclic AMP also regulates protein kinases, cyclooxygenase, and phospholipase metabolism.

adenosine triphosphate (ATP). ATP is a major energy source for metabolic reactions, as it is in other cells. ADP is a stimulant for platelet aggregation, as described above. About 60% of platelet ADP is contained within the dense bodies, and it is this source that is expelled from the cell during the release reaction. The remaining ADP content is dispersed in the cytoplasm as part of the metabolic machinery. Cyclic AMP levels are closely regulated in resting platelets by the enzymes *adenyl cyclase* and *phosphodiesterase,* but a number of substances can inhibit or stimulate the ac-

tivity of these enzymes, producing dramatic changes in the concentration of cAMP. Thus agents that increase adenyl cyclase activity (e.g., prostacyclin, prostaglandins PGE_1 and PGD_2, and adenosine, plus a number of commonly prescribed drugs) produce higher levels of cAMP which, in turn, inhibits platelet activation and release reaction. Substances that inhibit phosphodiesterase activity and the degradation of cAMP to AMP accomplish the same result. Conversely, agents that inhibit adenyl cyclase promote low levels of platelet cAMP and increase sensitivity of the platelet for

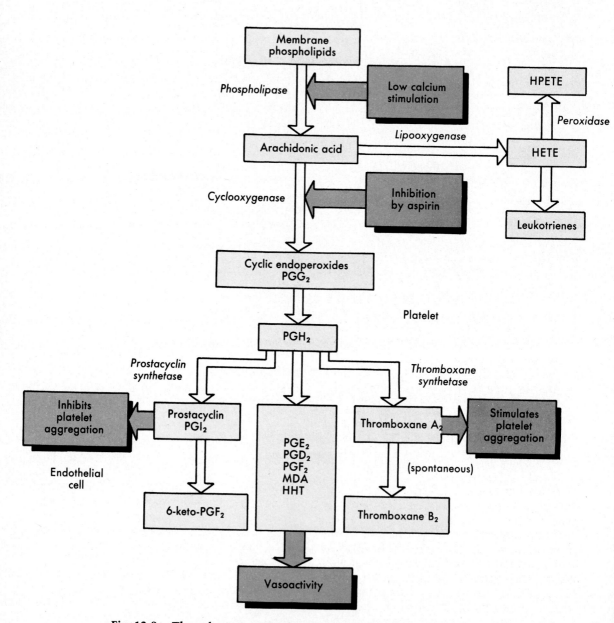

Fig. 12-9.   Thromboxane-prostaglandin metabolism.
The major pathways of arachidonic acid, thromboxane, and prostaglandin synthesis.

activation. Among adenyl cyclase inhibitors are collagen, thrombin, epinephrine, platelet activating factor (PAF), and thromboxane A_2. Cyclic AMP may also be important for calcium ion release; low levels of cAMP are correlated with the release of Ca^{++} from canalicular storage sites. Calcium release is also important in platelet-platelet binding during aggregation and as a cofactor in coagulation reactions occurring on the outer coat. Cyclic AMP also regulates the protein kinase that controls phosphorylation of the actin-myosin system, producing contractile changes in cell shape.

Thromboxane-prostaglandin pathway (Fig. 12-9)

Activation of a platelet is initiated by the binding of a suitable substance, such as thrombin or epinephrine, to its plasma membrane receptor. As a result of this membrane-associated change, hydrolysis of membrane phospholipid by *phospholipase A_2* occurs, producing **arachidonic acid** and its immediate metabolites, the cyclic endoperoxides or prostaglandins PGG_2 and PGH_2. These substances are collectively known as "labile aggregating substances (LASS)" and, in fact, arachidonic acid is often used as an aggregating agent to test platelet function. Conversion of arachidonic acid to the endoperoxides is regulated by an important rate-limiting enzyme, **cyclooxygenase.** Activity of this enzyme is inhibited by salicylic acid (aspirin), producing partial to total platelet dysfunction (Chapter 23). The endoperoxides are either released and converted to *prostacyclin* by an endothelial cell enzyme or they remain in the platelet to be converted to one of several prostaglandins or into **thromboxane A_2 (TxA_2).** This latter substance, although extremely short-lived, is believed to be the in vivo agent that activates platelets and produces release and aggregation reactions during plug formation. In addition, TxA_2 is a powerful vasoconstrictor, further abetting the hemostatic process. It should also be ap-

parent that amplification of platelet activation by thromboxane occurs in a positive feedback loop, just as it does with ADP.

The prostaglandins formed from cyclic endoperoxides either enhance thromboxane function (PGE_2) or enhance adenyl cyclase activity (PGD_2), thus providing both positive and negative feedback regulation of platelet activation. Prostacyclin (PGI_2), produced outside of the platelet by leukocytes as well as vascular endothelium, also enhances adenyl cyclase regulation of cAMP synthesis (Fig. 12-8).

SUMMARY

- Platelets function in three primary roles: to form a hemostatic plug following injury to blood vessels, to provide cofactors and a surface for reactions of the coagulation cascade, and to maintain and repair the vascular endothelium.
- Platelets are derived from polyploid megakaryocytes in the bone marrow by a process of cytoplasm fragmentation.
- Platelets are present in the peripheral circulation for 8 to 12 days; normal blood concentrations range from 130,000 to 450,000 per μL. About 20% to 35% of the peripheral platelet mass is sequestered in the spleen.
- Platelets are discs of 2 to 5 μm diameter consisting of a complex outer coat and plasma membrane, an underlying cytoskeletal region of contractile microtubules, a system of tubular canals that communicate from the interior of the platelet to the exterior, and a cytoplasm filled with numerous granules, mitochondria, glycogen deposits and various organelles.
- Granules are of two main types: alpha granules with diverse contents (e.g, factor V, vWF, fibrinogen, PF-4, PDGF, and BTG) and dense bodies (ADP, serotonin, Ca^{++}).
- Formation of a hemostatic plug results when collagen from a damaged vessel wall stimulates platelets to adhere, un-

dergo shape change, release granule contents, attract other platelets to form an aggregate, and promote fibrin formation (coagulation) to strengthen the plug.

- Adherence depends on interactions between platelets and endothelia that involve von Willebrand's factor and fibronectin; aggregation is a response to thrombin, thromboxane, and ADP produced by activated platelets.
- Platelets participate in coagulation by secreting PF-3, which complexes with coagulation factors IXa, VIII, and Ca^{++} to form Xa, then with Xa, V, and Ca^{++} to convert prothrombin to thrombin. Platelets may also serve as contact activators of XI and XII.

- Generation of thromboxane and platelet prostaglandins by way of arachidonic acid is regulated by cyclooxygenase, an enzyme that is inhibited by aspirin ingestion. These products provide positive and negative feedback regulation of platelet activation, primarily by regulating platelet cAMP levels.

13

The Coagulation Cascade

When viewed in its entirety, even in a simplified form, the coagulation cascade can appear bewildering, a formidable challenge to understand, much less memorize. For this reason, the pathways will be introduced in a simplified form first, one set of reactions at a time, before the feedback loops and most important intermediate steps are described. Although there are a number of ways to approach the study of coagulation, this text will present the reactions in reverse order, starting with the formation of fibrin, the goal and final product of the clotting process. This method has two advantages: (1) the end of the process is established and the molecular reactions are understandable as means to that end; and (2) the generation of thrombin is explained before encountering most of the other reactions. Since thrombin is involved in activating many of the enzymes of the preceding reactions, the significance of its presence is more readily appreciated.

Therefore, we begin by examining the **common pathway** of coagulation, in which a **fibrin polymer** or plasma clot is formed from a circulating protein, **fibrinogen** (Fig. 13-1). This reaction requires the presence of a protease, **thrombin,** to split peptides from the fibrinogen molecule. Thrombin must be activated from a precursor zymogen (see Chapter 11), **prothrombin.** This is accomplished on the surface of activated platelets, in which calcium, platelet phospholipid, and two plasma coagulation factors form a complex. One of these factors, the Stuart-Prower factor, or **factor X,** must be activated to **Xa** by products from one of two other pathways.

The **extrinsic pathway provides a serine protease, activated factor VII,** along with calcium and a tissue factor, to activate factor X. Reactions in this pathway are stimulated by injury to tissue and the release of substances from outside ("extrinsic") to the plasma. Factor X can also be activated by products of the **intrinsic pathway,** generated by the sequential reactions of proteins within the plasma. These reactions culminate in a complex of activated **factor IX, factor VIII,** and calcium in association with the phospholipid (PF-3) of platelets. The extrinsic pathway is able to activate factor X very rapidly, since there are fewer reaction steps involved. Although the intrinsic reactions are more complex and slower, they account for the majority of the coagulation activity in vivo. The differences and relationships between these two pathways will be more apparent in the detailed discussions below.

THE COMMON PATHWAY

The production of a fibrin clot from fibrinogen is dependent on the generation of a potent enzyme, thrombin. The structures of these molecules are the keys to understanding how they function and the nature of deficiencies that result in clotting disorders.

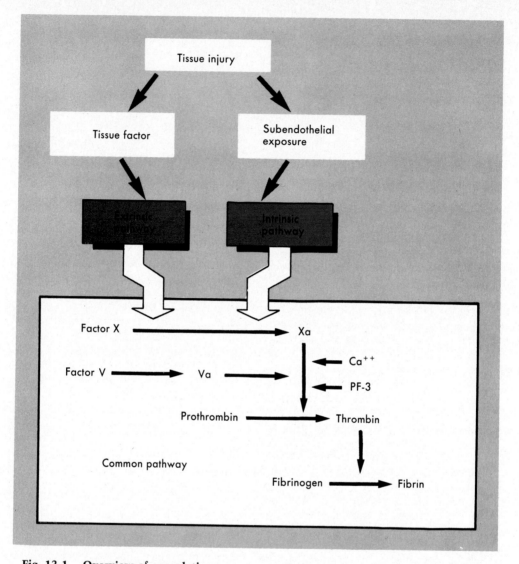

Fig. 13-1.   Overview of coagulation.
Relationship between the three pathways, emphasizing the major events of the common pathway.

Fibrinogen to fibrin polymer

Fibrinogen (factor I) is a plasma euglobulin weighing 340,000 daltons. Plasma concentrations normally range from 200 to 400 mg/dL, and about 60 to 100 mg/dL is required to attain hemostasis. The molecule is synthesized in the liver and circulates in the blood with a half-life of 80 to 120 hours. Fibrinogen migrates between the beta and gamma globulin fractions on routine protein electrophoresis. It consists of three pairs of polypeptide chains, designated Aα, Bβ, and γ that are interconnected by disulfide bonds (Fig. 13-2). The molecule is tri-

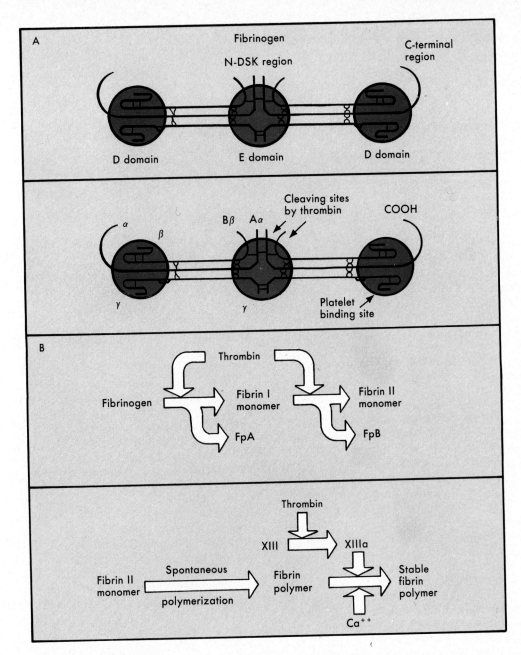

Fig. 13-2. Fibrinogen.
The major regions and domains of the fibrinogen molecule. The three pairs of polypeptide chains are coiled into nodules, forming a central E domain and two lateral D domains. The N-terminals of the polypeptides converge as a disulfide knot (N-DSK). The reaction sequence for the conversion of fibrinogen into a stabilized fibrin polymer. Thrombin is active at several steps. *Fp*, fibrinopeptide.

nodular in structure, consisting of three regions, a central E domain and two lateral D domains. In each of these domains, the polypeptide chains are intertwined, forming complex bundles. The domains are separated by relatively linear strands of the three polypeptides. The molecule is polarized, as are other proteins, displaying the carboxyl (COOH) ends from the D domains and the amine (N-terminal) ends from the E domain. The alpha and beta strands form a specialized nodule called the N-terminal disulfide knot (N-DSK). The carboxyl terminus in the D domain provides a binding site for the GP IIb/IIIa receptors on platelet membranes that must be bridged for platelet aggregation to occur (see Chapter 12). Thus fibrinogen has a functional role as an intact monomeric molecule and as a transformed polymer.

The formation of a fibrin mesh of crosslinking molecules requires polymerization. Fibrinogen is negatively charged at each of the terminal residues, preventing it from reacting in this fashion. Thrombin, however, cleaves a small peptide sequence from the Aα and Bβ chains, changing the residual charge in the N-DSK region. As a result, the E domain of one fibrinogen molecule binds to the D domains of four other molecules. Each of its own D domains bind to two other E domains, resulting in a two-dimensional lattice or mesh of molecules arranged side-by-side and end-to-end (Fig. 13-3).

Cleavage of the Aα chain occurs first, resulting in the release of **fibrinopeptide A** (1800 daltons) and the formation of **fibrin I monomer.** The Bβ chain is attacked next, releasing **fibrinopeptide B** (1500 daltons) and the formation of **fibrin monomer II.** Spontaneous polymerization then occurs as the E and D domains of adjacent molecules link by hydrogen bonds. The specific configurations of the domains also aid the assembly of the lattice, but these interactions are less well documented. The resulting **fibrin polymer** is unstable and will easily dissolve in denaturing solutions of urea or

monochloroacetic acid, providing the basis for a test to detect unstable polymers (Chapter 28). The final step in fibrin formation results in the establishment of covalent cross links between the polymers.

Fibrin stabilizing factor (FSF or **factor XIII)** is an alpha-2 globulin weighing 320,000 daltons (plasma XIII) or 143,000 daltons (platelet XIII). The plasma factor is believed to be synthesized in the liver and circulates as a tetramer of 80,000 dalton subunits with a half-life of about 100 to 175 hours. Platelet XIII is synthesized by megakaryocytes and exists as a dimer, but it exhibits the full functional capabilities of the plasma factor. Factor XIII is converted from a proenzyme to a transamidinating enzyme (XIIIa) by thrombin. The presence of calcium ions is required for the dissociation of *a* and *b* chains (subunits) and activation of plasma XIII, but platelet XIII can be activated without calcium. Both types of XIIIa stabilize the fibrin polymers by crosslinking the gamma chains of D domains with the alpha chains of adjacent D domains; the bridge is made between glutamine and lysine residues. Similar reactions of XIIIa occur in linking the endothelial cell protein, **fibronectin,** to collagen and fibrin residues, a mechanism believed to be important in cell adherence and tissue growth and repair.

The stabilized clot provides an effective hemostatic barrier that can withstand collison with blood cells, changes in pressure and fluid flow, and rapid attack by most proteolytic mechanisms. Incorporation of factor XIII into the clot is assured by the presence of platelets, and its importance is seen when this factor is absent or functionally deficient. Fortunately, only 1% of the normal plasma levels (about 100 µg/dL) or 1 µg/dL is required to maintain hemostasis.

Generation of thrombin from prothrombin

Thrombin (factor IIa) obviously plays an important role in the coagulation mechanism, serving as the activating enzyme for

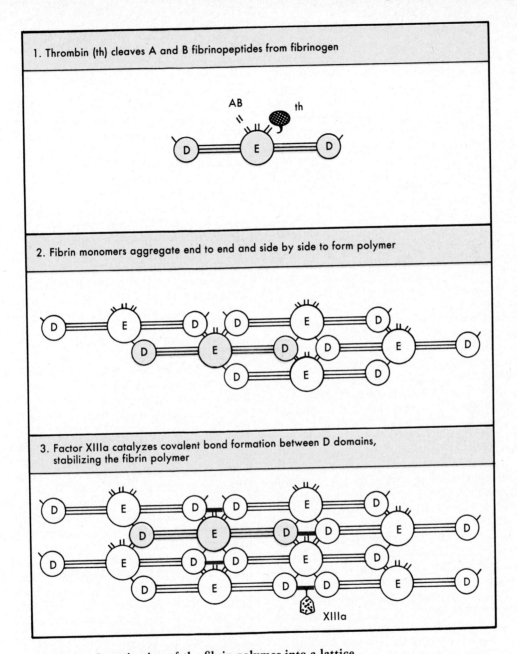

1. Thrombin (th) cleaves A and B fibrinopeptides from fibrinogen

2. Fibrin monomers aggregate end to end and side by side to form polymer

3. Factor XIIIa catalyzes covalent bond formation between D domains, stabilizing the fibrin polymer

Fig. 13-3. Organization of the fibrin polymer into a lattice.
After removal of the A and B peptide fragments from fibrinogen, connections between E and D domains of adjacent fibrin monomers produce a two-dimensional array or lattice. The polymer is subsequently stabilized by covalent bonds by the action of the transamidase, factor XIIIa.

factor XIII and the protease to cleave fibrinogen at two steps. It also acts in concert with the endothelial protein, thrombomodulin, to activate protein C (see Chapters 11 and 14). As will be described later, thrombin activates other zymogens and cofactors of the common and intrinsic pathways.

Thrombin is generated from a precursor, **prothrombin (factor II)** catalyzed by factor Xa in the presence of Factor V (a cofactor), calcium ions, and platelet phospholipid (Fig. 13-4). Prothrombin is a monomeric alpha-2 globulin weighing 69,000 daltons and is synthesized by the liver. It is one of the vitamin K−dependent coagulation factors, and it circulates in the plasma at concentrations of 8 to 15 mg/dL and a half-life of 70 to 110 hours. About 20% of the normal concentration must be present to ensure hemostasis.

Prothrombin binds to platelet phospholipid surfaces to interact with the other components of the **prothrombinase complex.** Carboxyglutamic acid residues at the N-terminal of the protein bind to the phospholipid with the help of calcium ions. Factor Xa, with the help of cofactor V, cleaves prothrombin at two points, forming first an intermediate (prethrombin 2) that is then cleaved to form the active protease, thrombin.

The synthesis of prothrombin and the other vitamin K−dependent factors (VII, IX, X and protein C) by the liver deserves special mention because of the relationship between drugs and disorders that interfere with vitamin K, resulting in clotting disorders. The monomeric (single chain) molecule possesses two nodular loops, the F_1 and F_2 regions, consisting partly of the carboxyglutamic acid residues mentioned above. These loops are synthesized by a reaction requiring vitamin K, a process that is inhibited by warfarin sodium, the coumarin drugs used as oral anticoagulants. These drugs are widely administered to outpatients for long-term therapy after heart attacks to diminish coagulation factor function and prevent thrombosis. They also provide the basis for widely used rodent poisons, but in doses high enough to produce uncontrolled hemorrhaging.

The prothrombinase complex is able to convert prothrombin into thrombin at rates of 10,000 or more faster than would occur with Xa alone. This is due to both the proximity of the reactant molecules in the complex and to conformational changes that occur in prothrombin as it binds to cofactor V and the platelet phospholipid. As thrombin is generated, it activates factor V, producing an additional increase (amplification) in thrombin generation. Thrombin can also cleave the prothrombin molecule between fragments 1 and 2 on N-terminal end, reducing the affinity of prothrombin to bind with the calcium-phospholipid-factor V complex.

Proaccelerin or **labile factor (factor V)** is a globulin weighing 330,000 daltons that is synthesized by the liver. It circulates at concentrations of about 4 to 14 μg/mL with a half-life of about 12 to 30 hours. Hemostasis is maintained with concentrations of 5% to 10% of normal. Factor V is also known as the labile factor because it deteriorates rapidly in stored blood (along with factor VIII). Although it exists as a multimeric zymogen and functions in this form as a cofactor, the most active form is probably monomeric, produced by cleavage with thrombin. It can also be inactivated by thrombin or by plasmin.

Stuart-Prower factor (factor X) is a dimeric alpha globulin weighing 59,000 daltons, synthesized by the liver in a vitamin K−dependent process, circulating at concentrations of 3 to 10 μg/mL with a half-life of 24 to 65 hours. About 5% to 10% of the normal concentration is required to maintain hemostasis.

We can now turn to the next step back in the process, which is activation of factor X from the intrinsic and extrinsic pathways.

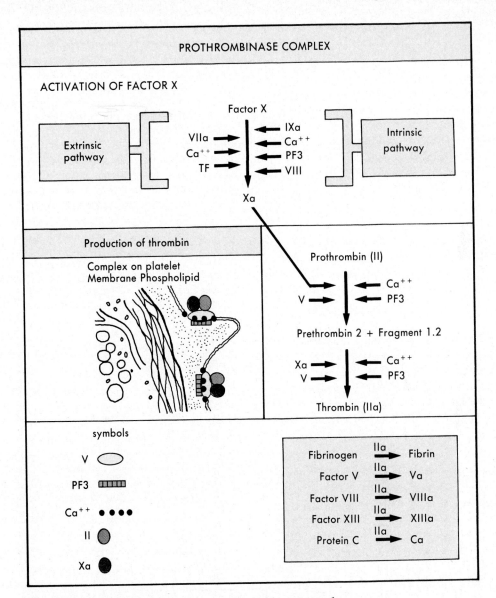

Fig. 13-4. Reactions involving the prothrombinase complex.
Reactions of the common pathways, from the activation of factor X to the generation of thrombin. The inset diagrams the proposed relationships between components of this complex, an arrangement that is probably similar to the plasma thromboplastin complex formed during the intrinsic pathway. Some of the many actions of thrombin are listed in the inset at bottom right.

THE EXTRINSIC PATHWAY

Since the extrinsic mechanism involves fewer steps, we shall dispense with it first. Factor X is activated by a complex consisting of calcium ions, phospholipid derived from tissue sources, and activated factor VII in the presence of a tissue thromboplastin cofactor (Fig. 13-5).

Proconvertin, or **stable factor (factor VII),** is monomeric and weighs about 50,000 to 63,000 daltons, although estimates as high as 100,000 have been reported. It is synthesized in the liver by a vitamin K–dependent process and circulates in the plasma at concentrations of 0.5 to 1.0 μg/mL. It has a very short biological half-life, 4 to 6 hours, so that it rapidly disappears from the blood if synthesis stops. It is therefore the first factor to respond to coumarin therapy and its presence can be monitored by the prothrombin test (Chapter 28).

The structure of factor VII is similar to that of prothrombin and the other factors with prominent carboxyglutamic acid loops. Calcium and phospholipid bind to the loops, forming a tight association with factor X and tissue thromboplastin (factor III). Like factor V, proconvertin has some activity as a zymogen but it is greatly enhanced in the activated form. Initially, factor VII is probably activated because of conformational changes associated with complex formation. The interaction between factors X and VII provides a perfect example of an amplification or positive feedback cy-

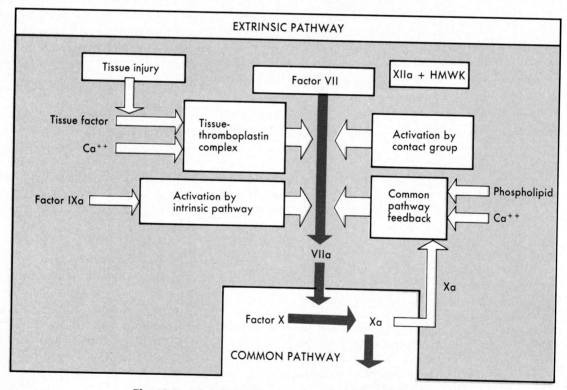

Fig. 13-5.   Major reactions of the extrinsic pathway.
Generation of factor VIIa following activation of tissue factors.

cle; factor VIIa activates factor X to Xa, and Xa accelerates the conversion of factor VII to VIIa. Contact factors (XIIa complex) and factor IXa of the intrinsic pathway also accelerate the activation of factor VII; VIIa enhances factor IX activation (see Fig. 13-8).

Tissue factor, or **tissue thromboplastin (factor III),** is a glycoprotein present on the membrane of most somatic cells of the body. It is not a single molecular entity; thus size estimates range from 45,000 to over 1,000,000 daltons, depending on the type of tissue from which it is derived. Tissue factor consists of a protein and a phospholipid component. Red cell membranes, platelets, brain tissue, placenta, and lung tissue are concentrated sources for factor III. Tissue thromboplastin does not circulate in the plasma per se, unless significant damage occurs to the tissues (intravascular hemolysis of red cells, spontaneous abortion, traumatic head injury are notable examples). Endothelial cells and monocytes also contain significant amounts of tissue factor and the endothelium can provide small amounts of cofactor to initiate factor VII activation when vessel linings are damaged.

THE INTRINSIC PATHWAY
Activation of factor X

The alternate mechanism for activating factor X is by means of a complex involving factors VIII and IX in association with (take a guess!) calcium and phospholipid. This complex is sometimes referred to as **plasma thromboplastin,** analogous to the activating role of tissue thromboplastin. The association of components is very similar to the prothrombinase complex: calcium bridges link factor IX to a phospholipid surface provided by platelets.

Plasma thromboplastin component (PTC), or **Factor IX,** is also known as Christmas factor and antihemophilic Factor B because deficiencies of this protein are associated with a specific type of hemophilia (Chapter 24). Factor IX is monomeric and

either an alpha- or beta-globulin weighing 55,000 to 62,000 daltons. It is synthesized by the liver and circulates in the plasma at concentrations of 3 to 4 µg/mL with a half-life of 12 to 24 hours. About 20% to 30% of the normal levels are required for coagulation. As with the other vitamin K–dependent factors, factor IX possesses residues of carboxyglutamic acid that are the binding sites for calcium-phospholipid. Activation is a two step process in which factor XIa cleaves factor X to form an inactive intermediate dimer, then removes a peptide sequence from one chain to produce the serine protease, factor IXa (Fig. 13-6). The protease, in association with cofactor VIII, acts on factor X to initiate the common pathway.

Antihemophilic Factor (AHF), or **Factor VIII,** circulates as a multimeric complex consisting of two different functional subunits. The coagulation cofactor is designated **VIII:C,** and the component which facilitates platelet adherence to subendothelial surfaces is termed "von Willebrand's factor," or VIII:vWF (see Chapter 12 for a discussion of its interactions with platelets). The total molecular weight for factor VIII, containing both functional attributes, is about 1,200,000 daltons. The larger part of this is VIII:vWF and it is strongly antigenic and participates in platelet aggregation induced by the antibiotic, ristocetin. Unfortunately, separate designations were applied to proteins assayed by these different techniques, but VIII:Ag and VIII:R are essentially synonymous with VIII:vWF.

Factor VIII:C has a molecular weight of about 270,000 daltons and a circulating half-life of about 10 to 16 hours. Plasma concentrations range from 5 to 10 µg/mL and about 25% to 35% of this level is required for hemostasis. Deficiencies in VIII:C result in hemophilia A, the classic "bleeder's disease," and deficiencies of VIII:Ag are seen as von Willebrand's disease (Chapter 24). The synthesis, structure, and function of factor VIII is still poorly under-

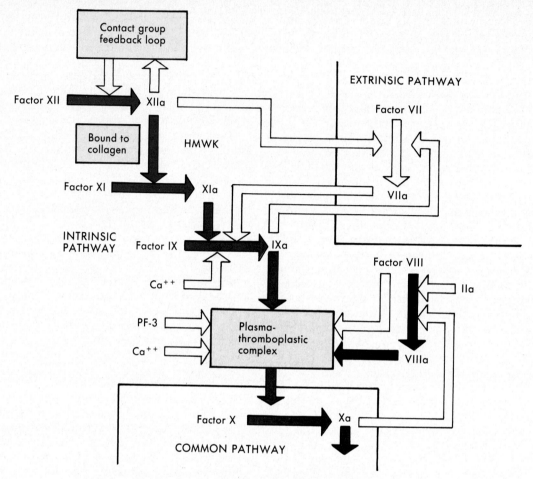

Fig. 13-6. Major reactions of the intrinsic pathway.
Generation of factor IXa and the plasma thromboplastin complex.

stood, despite intensive investigative effort. In addition to platelet functions, factor VIII:vWF may serve as a carrier molecule for VIII:C. The two subunits are not covalently bound, and they can be disassociated in the presence of calcium ions, such as occurs in the plasma thromboplastin complex on platelets. Factor VIII, like cofactors described previously, functions as a conformational link between factor IXa and factor X, but small amounts of thrombin and activated factor Xa, through positive feedback, can produce VIIIa and increase its cofactor activity significantly. Large amounts of thrombin destroy the functional properties, similar to its action on prothrombin, providing a negative feedback loop that limits the extent of coagulation and prevents depletion of the cofactors.

Sites of synthesis for factor VIII are still debatable for VIII:C, but VIII:vWF is produced in megakaryocytes and by endothelial cells lining the blood vessels. Much of the factor VIII content of the body is ex-

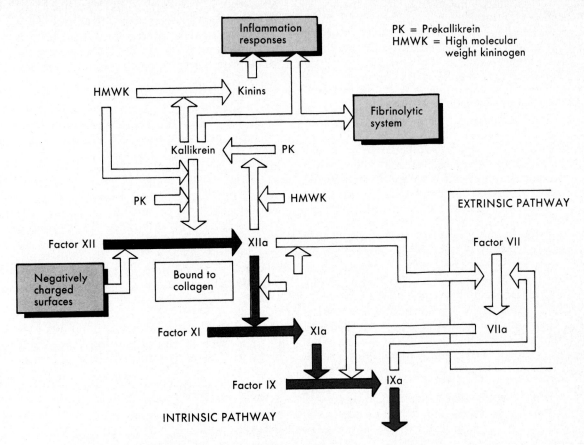

Fig. 13-7.   Major reactions of the contact factor group.
Generation of factor XIIa and the relationship between the contact phase and mediators of the inflammation response.

travascular, but the kinetics of its formation and movement are not known.

Activation of factor IX

Factor IX is converted from a zymogen to a protease by the action of factor XIa in the presence of calcium. Activated factor VII of the extrinsic pathway can also produce activation, effectively bypassing the need for input from reactions "upstream" in the intrinsic cascade.

Plasma thromboplastin antecedent (PTA), or **Factor XI,** is a beta or gamma globulin weighing 160,000 to 200,000 daltons that is synthesized by the liver. Vitamin K is not required. Circulating concentrations range from 2 to 7 μg/mL, with a half-life of 48 to 180 hours. About 20% to 30% of the normal levels are required for coagulation, and deficiencies of factor XI are described as hemophilia C.

Factor XI is dimeric, consisting of identical polypeptide chains. It circulates as a complex with another protein, **high molecular weight kininogen (HMWK),** which serves as a cofactor for its activation by Factor XIIa (Fig. 13-7). Factors XI and XII and their cofactors are often referred to as the contact factors because their activation is initiated by contact with negatively charged surfaces, such as subendothelial basement membrane, that are exposed during injury to tissues and vessels.

Activation of contact factors

The formation of factor XIIa occurs through several mechanisms associated with tissue injury and inflammation.

Hageman factor (factor XII) is a monomeric gamma globulin weighing 80,000 daltons that is synthesized by the liver and circulates freely in the plasma at concentrations of 27 to 45 μg/mL with a biological half-life of about 40 to 60 hours. Activation occurs in one of two ways: the molecule binds to exposed collagen to undergo conformational rearrangement to XIIa as an intact molecule, or the molecule is proteolytically fragmented into smaller molecules (XIIf) that are enzymatically active. Surface-bound factor XIIa activates factor XI, converts prekallikrein into kallikrein, and activates plasminogen in the fibrinolytic system.

High molecular weight kininogen (HMWK), or **Fitzgerald factor**, serves as a cofactor for reactions involving factor XIIa, which can also activate factor VII in the extrinsic pathway, an additional reminder that the two pathways are far from independent. It has a molecular weight of 120,000 to 200,000 daltons. The cofactor is synthesized in the liver and circulates in the plasma at concentrations of 70 to 100 μg/mL. HMWK is also the precursor molecule of bradykinin, which mediates inflammatory reactions involving vascular permeability and dilation, production of pain at inflammatory sites, and prostaglandin synthesis.

Prekallikrein (PK), or **Fletcher factor**, is the precursor for a serine protease, **kallikrein**, which also activates plasminogen. Kallikrein acts as a chemotactic factor to recruit phagocytes and stimulates the complement cascade. Both prekallikrein and kallikrein are involved in a feedback loop that activates factor XII to XIIa. PK is a monomer with a molecular weight of 80,000 to 85,000 daltons. It circulates in the plasma at concentrations of 30 to 50 μg/mL in association with HMWK. Cleavage by factor XIIa results in the conversion of monomeric PK into dimeric kallikrein, a reaction that again requires HMWK as a cofactor of XIIa. There also exists in the plasma a low molecular weight kininogen (LMWK), weighing 80,000 daltons, that is not involved in the coagulation cascade.

Interestingly, deficiencies of factor XII, PK and HMWK are not normally associated with bleeding disorders, although the decreases can be detected with the appropriate laboratory procedures (see Chapter 28). Only small amounts of factor XIIa are necessary to initiate the intrinsic pathway, and this can be bypassed by other mechanisms. The feedback amplification loop of kallikrein helps generate additional amounts of factor XIIa, but most of this is in the form of fragments (XIIf) that are not surface bound. These smaller molecules are principally active in initiating fibrinolysis and altering vascular permeability.

THE COAGULATION PROCESS: PUTTING IT ALL TOGETHER

Having worked backward from the final product, a stabilized fibrin clot, through the common pathway to the initiating stimuli of the extrinsic and intrinsic pathways, we can now visualize the entire coagulation cascade and comment on the role of specific components (Fig. 13-8 and Table 13-1). Each step and component must be related in order to appreciate the testing strategies employed in attempting to diagnose a bleeding disorder.

The role of **calcium (factor IV)** is critical to several steps in the process. Its removal from the blood prevents fibrin formation, and it is the basis of many of the commonly employed anticoagulants: cationic oxalates, fluorides, citrates, and ethylenediamine-

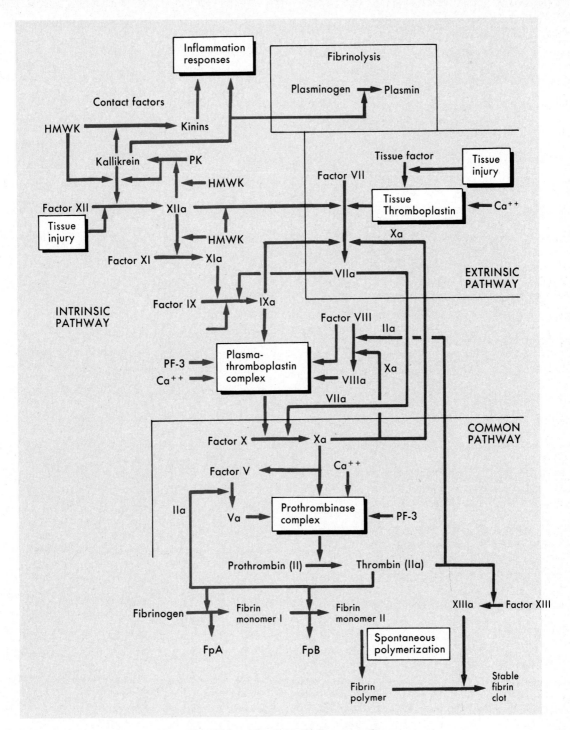

Fig. 13-8.   The coagulation cascade.

TABLE 13-1. Summary of coagulation factors

	Factor	Molecular weight (kd)	Plasma concentration	Biological half-life (hours)	Production site	Type of factor	Minimum for hemostasis	Other notes
I	Fibrinogen	340	200-400 mg/dL	120	Liver	Substrate	60-100 mg/dL	Stable in stored blood
II	Prothrombin	69	80-150 μg/mL	70-110	Liver (vitamin K)*	Protease	20-40 μg/mL	Stable in stored blood
III	Tissue thromboplastin	50-400			many tissues	Cofactor		Heterogeneous molecules
IV	Calcium ions	40 d	4.2-4.8 mg/dL			Cofactor		Values for plasma ionized calcium
V	Proaccelerin	330	4-14 μg/mL	12-30	Liver	Cofactor	20-40 μg/mL	Labile in stored blood; heat labile
VII	Proconvertin	50-63	0.5-1.0 μg/mL	4-6	Liver (vitamin K)	Protease		Stable in stored blood; heat labile
VIII	Antihemophilic factor (AHF)	1200	5-10 μg/mL	8-16	VIII:C unknown	Cofactor and protease	2-3 μg/mL	Labile in stored blood; smaller part of complex with VIII:vWF
IX	Plasma thromboplastin component	55-62	3-4 μg/mL	20-24	Liver (vitamin K)	Protease	1-2 μg/mL	Stable in stored blood; heat labile

X	Stuart-Prower factor	59	3-10 µg/mL	24-65	Liver (vitamin K)	Protease	0.3-1.0 µ/mL	Moderately stable in stored blood; heat labile
XI	Plasma Thromboplastin Antecedent	160-165	2-7 µg/mL	60-70	Liver	Protease	0.4-2.0 µg/mL	Concentration increases in stored blood; contact factor
XII	Hageman Factor	80	27-45 µg/mL	40-60	Liver	Protease	Not required	Stable in stored blood; contact factor
XIII	Fibrin stabilizing factor	320	10 µg/mL	100-175	Liver, platelets	Transamidase	0.1 µg/mL	Stable in stored blood; heat labile
PK	Prekallikrein (Fletcher factor)	80-85	30-50 µg/mL		Liver	Cofactor and protease	Not required	Contact factor complex; inflammation response mediator
HMWK	High molecular weight kininogen (Fitzgerald factor)	120-200	70-100 µ/mL		Liver	Cofactor	Not required	Contact factor complex; inflammation response mediator

*Factors dependent on vitamin K–mediated carboxylation for functional competence.

tetraacetic acid (EDTA). It is the only participant that is not a protein or lipoprotein and therefore it is not directly comparable to other coagulation factors in terms of half-life, concentration, and molecular weight. Calcium appears to serve primarily as a bridge between the phospholipid surface of platelets and the serine proteases IXa and Xa. It is also involved in the complex between tissue factor and factor VIIa, the activation of factor VII by factor Xa, and the conversion of factor IX to IXa by factor XIa. There is also indirect evidence that calcium may perform a stabilizing role, since factors V and VIII are rapidly degraded in plasmas from which calcium has been chelated.

Platelet phospholipid or **platelet factor 3 (PF 3)** is also a necessary component of the complexes involving cofactors and calcium. Platelets possess specific receptors to bind some of the coagulation proteins (V, VIII and Xa) and they probably facilitate the close association of enzyme, substrate, and cofactor in these reactions. Phospholipids can also stimulate the initial events of the contact phase.

To facilitate study of the coagulation process, the factors have been organized into functional groups (see box). The **fibrinogen group** includes the larger molecules that are consumed during fibrin formation and, as a result, are absent from serum. The **prothrombin group** of factors consists of smaller molecules synthesized by the liver, requiring vitamin K to convert the glutamic acid residues to gamma-carboxyglutamic acid residues. These are also the factors that calcium interacts with on the phospholipid surfaces of platelets. The **contact group** contains the components involved in initiation of the intrinsic pathway after exposure to negatively charged surfaces. During testing procedures to isolate a factor deficiency, some factors can be removed from the

---

COMPARATIVE LISTS OF FACTOR PROPERTIES

Related groups

Fibrinogen group	Prothombin group	Contact group
I Fibrinogen	II Prothrombin	XI PTA
V Proaccelerin	VII Proconvertin	XII Hageman factor
VIII AHF	IX PTC	Prekallikrein
XIII FSF	X Stuart-Power factor	HMWK

Factor presence in reagents

Aged serum	Aged plasma	Adsorbed plasma
II Prothrombin*	I Fibrinogen	I Fibrinogen
VII Proconvertin	II Prothrombin	V Proaccelerin
IX PTC	VII Proconvertin	VIII AHF
X Stuart-Power factor	IX PTC	XI PTA
XI PTA	X Stuart-Power factor	XII Hageman factor
XII Hageman factor	XI PTA	XIII FSF
XIII FSF*	XII Hageman factor	

---

*Usually present in decreased amounts.

plasma by **adsorption with barium sulfate** or aluminum hydroxide, leaving other factors; **aged serum** contains factors that are relatively stabile but not those that are more labile. Adding these solutions with their partial factor contents to a plasma that may be deficient in one or more coagulation factors and then testing the mixture can help determine the nature of the deficiency (see Chapter 28). Finally, the coagulation factors can be separated into functional categories as serine proteases, cofactors, substrates, or others.

Mechanisms that limit the extent of coagulation

Coagulation is a carefully controlled process, finely tuned to respond to injury while maintaining blood circulation. There are several mechanisms that limit the extent of clotting, both spatially and temporally:

1. Localization of fibrin formation to specific areas is assured by the presence and participation of platelets as a reacting surface. Injury to blood vessels attracts platelets that adhere, aggregate and then serve as the organizing structure for the coagulation complexes, plasma thromboplastin and prothrombinase. The platelet plug also forms a physical barrier that slows circulation and inhibits the dispersal of platelets that may be activated while passing through the injured area. The fibrin mesh completes the isolation of the injury site.
2. Consumption of key cofactors (factors V and VIII), the major substrate (fibrinogen), and the thrombin precursor (factor II) limit the amount of fibrin that can be formed.
3. Degradation of components occurs as thrombin levels increase and the fibrinolytic system is activated. Thrombin has a negative feedback effect at high plasma levels, especially on cofactors V and VIII. Factor VIIIa is especially sensitive to deactivation by plasmin and activated protein C.

4. Circulating inhibitors and anticoagulants, such as antithrombin III, limit the amount of thrombin formation, especially in areas outside of the injury zone. The protease inhibitors are described in Chapter 11.
5. Circulating precursors and proteases are continuously removed by hepatocytes in the liver

Failure of any or all of these mechanisms can result in an uncontrolled hemostatic response, disseminated intravascular coagulation (Chapter 24). This can occur if the initiating stimulus is abnormally potent (e.g., certain snake venoms, massive red cell destruction, the introduction of urokinase or streptokinase into the blood), if deficiencies in inhibitors or their synthetic pathways are present, or in the presence of damaged blood vessels that stimulate widespread platelet aggregation and the formation of microthrombi.

It is also apparent that the in vivo process of coagulation occurs somewhat differently than the in vitro process of mere clotting. The interactions between different components and the participation of tissue factors and cellular components, especially endothelial cells and platelets, requires that the results of laboratory procedures must be interpreted carefully. Nevertheless, the laboratory can provide confirmation and, in some cases, detect the primary defects of many coagulation disorders.

SUMMARY

- The coagulation cascade can be separated into three processes: a common pathway that culminates in the conversion of a plasma protein, fibrinogen, into stable fibrin clots; an extrinsic pathway that is mediated by tissue components, culminating in activation of factor X of the common pathway; and an intrinsic pathway that is initiated by contact with exposed subendothelial surfaces and mediated by a sequence of plasma proteins, culminating in the activation of factor X in the common pathway.

- Many of the coagulation factors exist in the plasma as inactive zymogens. Either from conformational change or, more commonly, from trypsin-like cleavage by a specific serine protease, the zymogen is activated to also become a protease.

- Thrombin is a major protease, formed from prothrombin in the common pathway. It is the enzyme that converts fibrinogen to fibrin, activates factor XIII to stabilize the fibrin polymer, activates cofactors and zymogens at earlier steps in the cascade (feedback amplification), and promotes aggregation of platelets.

- Several key factors (II, VII, IX, X and protein C) are synthesized in the liver, and vitamin K is required in a step that carboxylates critical glutamic acid residues to carboxyglutamic acid. When vitamin K is deficient or is inhibited by coumarin (warfarin) type anticoagulants, the factors are synthesized but are nonfunctional

- The contact phase of the intrinsic pathway activates factor VII, which results in feedback loops that generate kallikrein from prekallikrein. Kallikrein is an important mediator of the inflammatory response.

- Factor VIII is an important cofactor of the intrinsic pathway. It is the largest molecule of the cascade, consisting of a coagulant subunit (VIII:C) and the von Willebrand's factor (VIII:vWF) which acts as a carrier for VIII:C and is critical for platelet adherence to basement membranes and other surfaces. Deficiencies in either factor VIII component result in the most common coagulopathies, hemophilia A and von Willebrand's disease, respectively.

- Calcium and platelet phospholipid play important roles in coagulation. Calcium links cofactors to the phospholipid complexes at critical steps of the intrinsic and common pathways and serves as a cofactor in several other reactions. Calcium removal by chelating agents is an effective means of in vitro anticoagulation.

- Feedback interactions between coagulation components result in a fine control system that limits the extent of the clotting response. Other limiting mechanisms include the degradation of precursors by thrombin and plasmin at high concentrations, the presence of circulating inhibitors and anticoagulants, localization of key reactions to activated platelet surfaces at the points of injury, and the clearance of precursor molecules by the liver.

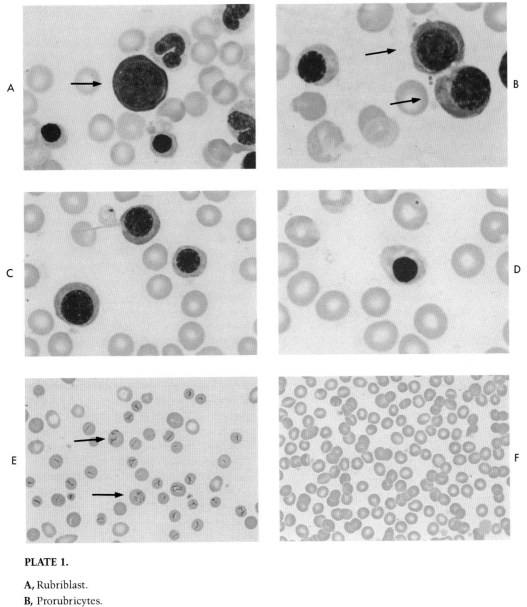

PLATE 1.

A, Rubriblast.

B, Prorubricytes.

C, Rubricytes.

D, Metarubricyte.

E, Reticulocytes. New methylene blue counterstained with Wright's.

F, Mature erythrocytes.

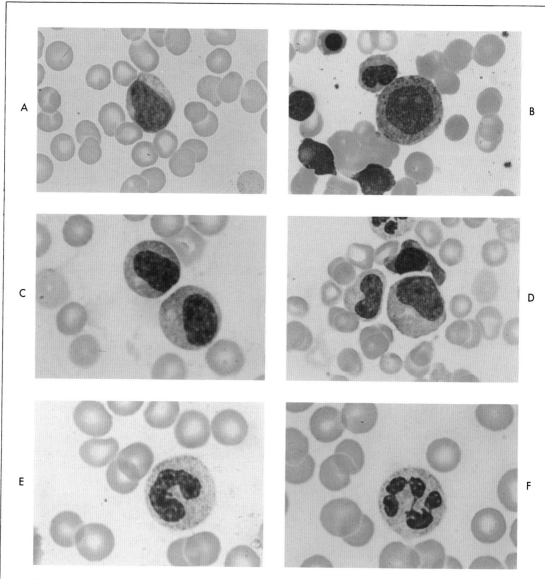

PLATE 2.

A, Myeloblast, from peripheral blood, acute myelogenous leukemia.

B, Promyelocyte.

C, Myelocytes.

D, Metamyelocyte *(left)* and late myelocyte *(right)*.

E, Band neutrophil.

F, Segmented neutrophil.

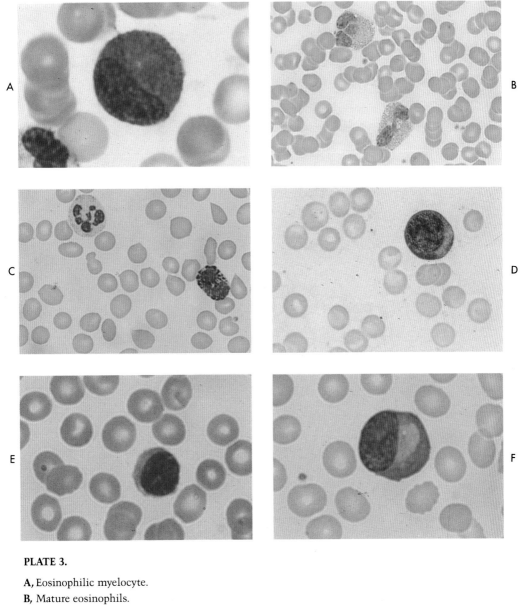

PLATE 3.

A, Eosinophilic myelocyte.

B, Mature eosinophils.

C, Basophil and segmented neutrophil.

D, Lymphoblast.

E, Small, mature lymphocyte.

F, Plasma cell.

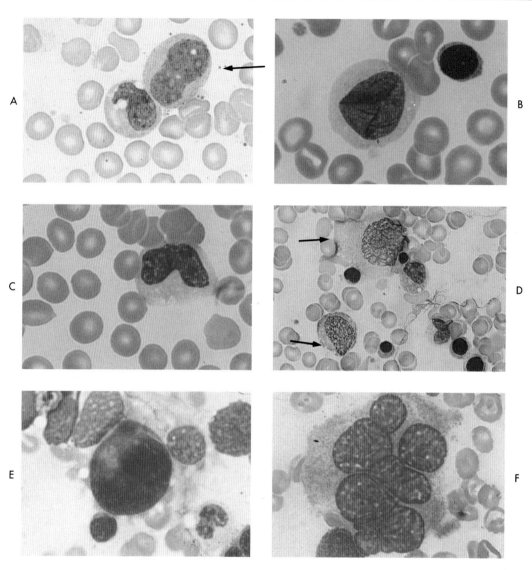

PLATE 4.

A, Monoblast *(arrow)* and immature monocyte.

B, Promonocyte, from a case of monocytic leukemia.

C, Mature monocyte.

D, Macrophages in bone marrow.

E, Megakaryoblast.

F, Megakaryocyte.

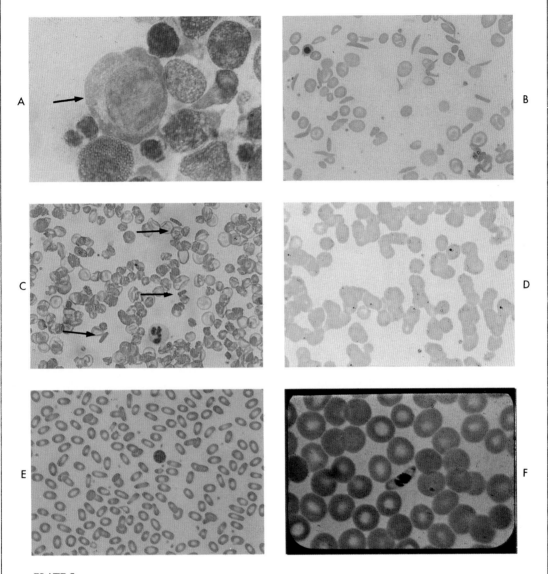

PLATE 5.

A, Megaloblast *(arrow)* in pernicious anemia.

B, Sickle cell crisis. Sickle cells and target cells predominate.

C, Hemoglobin C disease. Three crystals are evident *(arrows)*.

D, Howell-Jolly bodies. Compare erythrocyte inclusions to platelets *(lower right)*.

E, Elliptocytosis.

F, Malaria: band form of *Plasmodium falciparum*.

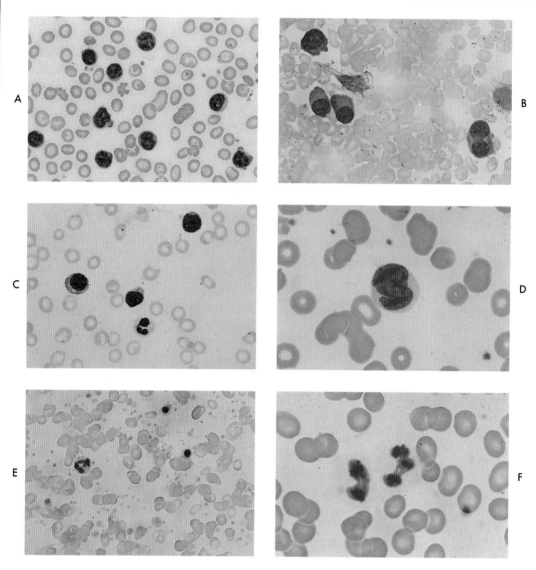

PLATE 6.

A, Chronic lymphocytic leukemia, peripheral blood.

B, Plasma cell leukemia, bone marrow. Note binucleated cell.

C, Acute myelogenous leukemia: myeloblast with Auer rod.

D, Myelomonocytic leukemia: immature monocytoid cell.

E, Myeloid metaplasia. Note platelet size and density, nucleated red blood cells.

F, Myelodysplastic syndrome: agranular neutrophils, peripheral blood.

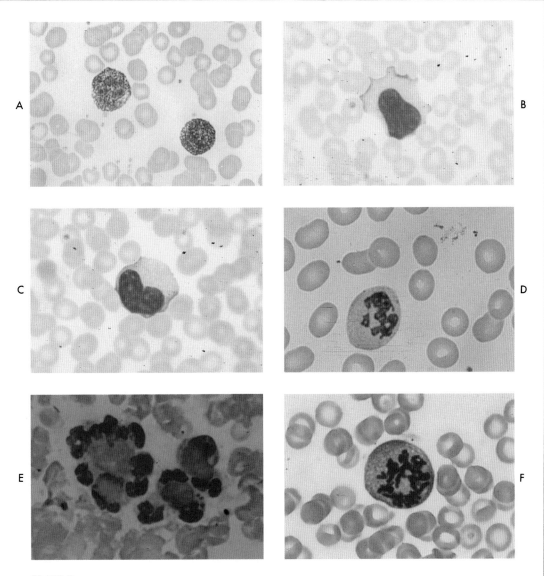

PLATE 7.

A, Alder-Reilly anomaly in a neutrophil and lymphocyte from a case of Hurler's syndrome.

B, Large reactive lymphocyte from a case of infectious mononucleosis.

C, Monocytoid lymphocyte from a case of infectious mononucleosis.

D, Hypersegmented neutrophil from a case of plasma cell leukemia.

E, LE cell phenomena, rosette formation by neutrophils.

F, Blood cell during mitosis, normal bone marrow.

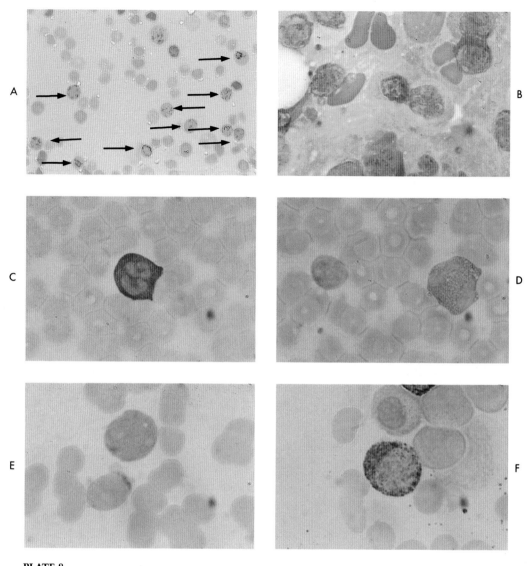

PLATE 8.

A, New methylene blue stain for reticulocytes *(arrows).*

B, Prussian blue stain for iron deposits, bone marrow: sideroblastic anemia.

C, Periodic acid—Schiff stain of neutrophil.

D, Periodic acid—Schiff stain of lymphocyte (negative) and eosinophil (weakly positive).

E, Non-specific esterase positive cells, bone marrow: monocytic leukemia.

F, Specific esterase, positive cell *(center)* and negative cells, bone marrow.

14

Fibrinolysis

Cheryl Dahl McRoyan

Fibrinolysis is the process whereby fibrin deposits are removed to restore circulation in blood vessels and to facilitate the repair process following tissue injury. The fibrinolytic system includes (1) the plasma protein, **plasminogen,** the zymogen precursor of the proteolytically active enzyme, **plasmin;** (2) various plasminogen activators (zymogens) in the plasma and in the vascular endothelium, which are activated by other hemostatic components and secreted into the circulation; and (3) protein inhibitors, primarily alpha$_2$-antiplasmin inhibitor, which bind to and inactivate plasmin (Fig. 14-1). As fibrin clots form, plasminogen adheres to the fibrin surface and is activated to plasmin. Plasmin enzymatically degrades the fibrin clot to form low molecular weight fragments that are rapidly cleared from the plasma by the liver. Circulating plasmin is rapidly inactivated by alpha$_2$-antiplasmin inhibitor, thus limiting fibrinolysis to localized sites of fibrin deposition. Pathologic defects in the fibrinolytic system can result in a thrombotic tendency due to ineffective fibrin degradation or a hemorrhagic tendency due to uncontrolled fibrin degradation.

COMPONENTS OF THE FIBRINOLYTIC SYSTEM
Plasminogen

Plasminogen, synthesized in the liver, has a bilogical half-life of about 2 days and exists in plasma as a single chain glycoprotein with a molecular weight of 81,000 daltons. The molecule contains 790 amino acid residues with 24 disulfide bonds and no free sulfhydryl groups. Two major molecular forms, differing in carbohydrate content, have been identified. Native plasminogen has an NH$_2$-terminal glutamic acid residue (Glu-plasminogen). A modified plasminogen molecule, formed by autocatalytic conversion of Glu-plasminogen into Lys-plasminogen, has an NH$_2$-terminal of lysine, valine, or methionine. Activation of plasminogen to the proteolytic enzyme occurs most efficiently on the surface of a fibrin deposit. Plasminogen contains specific lysine-binding sites for fibrin, triple-loop structures called *kringles.* Interaction of plasminogen and the fibrin mesh results in cleavage at amino acids Arg$_{560}$-Val$_{561}$ and the formation of the double chain serine protease, plasmin. Sequestration within the clot protects plasmin from inhibition by circulating antiplasmin, and degradation of the fibrin molecule proceeds. Abnormal plasminogens have been described in individuals with a history of thromboembolic disease (Chapter 24).

Plasminogen activators

An important key to understanding the complex interactions between clot formation and removal is in the way in which plasminogen, the proenzyme, is activated to become plasmin, the protease. Plasminogen activators are found in most tissues and body fluids, existing both as precursor zymogens and as active forms. Heart tissue, the renal medulla, and various endocrine organs contain lysosomes that serve as activators if tissue trauma occurs. Plasminogen can be activated by three different mechanisms.

1. Intrinsic or plasma activation of plasminogen involves activated Hageman factor (factor XIIa), prekallikrein (PK or Fletcher factor), high molecular weight kininogen (HMWK or Fitzgerald factor), factor XIa, and possibly other plasma proteins. These proteins form active enzymes during initiation of the intrinsic contact phase of fibrin formation (Chapter 13). XIIa is believed to facilitate the conversion of a *plasma proactivator* into a plasminogen activator (see Fig. 14-1). Deficiencies of the contact factors have not been associated with bleeding disorders, but various thrombotic disorders associated with deficiencies in Hageman factor and Fletcher factor have been reported. Because of these activating effects of intrinsic coagulatin factors, fibrinolytic processes are set in action concurrently with the for-

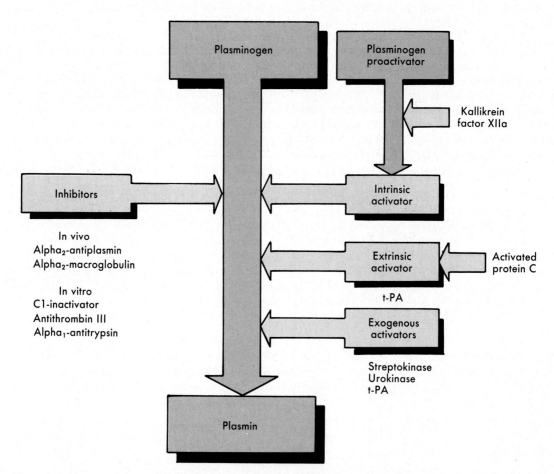

Fig. 14-1.   Activation and inhibition of the fibrinolytic system.

mation of fibrin, thus ensuring the eventual removal of the clot.

2. Extrinsic or extravascular activation of plasminogen involves **tissue plasminogen activator (t-PA),** a 70,000 dalton protein that is synthesized and released into the circulation by endothelial cells. Release of t-PA from the endothelium can be stimulated by a number of mechanisms, including venous stasis, exercise, vasoactive drugs, anoxia, hypoglycemic agents, hypotensive shock, and several factors that appear during thrombus formation, such as thrombin and activated protein C. T-PA has a high affinity for fibrin, which acts as its cofactor, and very efficiently activates plasminogen on the fibrin surface, resulting in clot degradation. Impaired release and/or diminished production production of t-PA has been reported in several families with thromboembolic diseases.

3. Exogenous activation of plasminogen can be induced by the enzymes streptokinase and urokinase, agents that are used in the treatment of thrombosis. The aim of fibrinolytic therapy employing these plasminogen activators is to deliver the enzymes into the blood stream at or near the site of the fibrin clot. Fibrin-bound plasmin-ogen in the clot is converted to plasmin, dissolving the clot. However, neither streptokinase nor urokinase has a specific affinity for fibrin (it is not required as cofactor for these agents) and they can indiscriminately activate circulating and fibrin-bound plasminogen at other sites, producing further widespread vascular complications.

Plasmin

Plasmin is the proteolytic enzyme formed from plasminogen. The primary physiologic function of plasmin is to digest fibrin clots in a thrombus. As fibrin is digested, a sequence of protein fragments, **fibrin degradation products (FDPs),** are formed. These fragments exert an anticoagulant effect due to their ability to interfere with thrombin and fibrin polymerization. Plasmin is also capable of degrading fibrinogen to form FDPs, and it can degrade factors V and VIII, resulting in additional anticoagulant effects.

Inhibitors of fibrinolysis

The inhibitors of fibrinolysis serve to limit and regulate plasmin activity (Table 14-1). The inhibitors include: antithrombin III, alpha$_2$-antiplasmin, alpha-antitrypsin,

Table 14-1. Components of the fibinolytic system

Component	Function	Molecular weight (daltons)
Plasminogen	Plasmin precursor	81,000
Tissue plasminogen activator	Extrinsic activation	70,000
alpha$_2$-antiplasmin	Plasmin inhibitor	67,000
alpha$_1$-antitrypsin	Plasmin inhibitor	55,000
alpha$_2$-macroglobulin	Plasmin inhibitor	360,000
Antithrombin III	Plasmin inhibitor	56,000
C1-inactivator	Plasmin inhibitor	40,000
Fragment X	Degradation product	270,000
Fragment Y	Degradation product	165,000
Fragment D	Degradation product	85,000
Fragment E	Degradation product	55,000
Fragment DD	Degradation product	170,000

alpha$_2$-macroglobulin, and C1-inactivator. The action of alpha$_2$-antiplasmin occurs as a rapid and irreversible inhibition of plasmin in the circulation, interference with the absorption of plasminogen to fibrin, and interaction with factor XIIIa to cross-link the alpha$_2$-antiplasmin to fibrin to inhibit plasmin within the fibrin clot. An individual with a congenital deficiency of alpha$_2$-antiplasmin exhibits a severe hemorrhagic tendency due to premature lysis of fibrin clots. Antiplasmin rapidly neutralizes plasmin in a 1:1 stoichometric ratio in the fluid phase (plasma). Enough of this inhibitor is normally present to inactivate about half of the potential blood plasmin that could be formed at any time in the circulation. Antiplasmin also slowly inactivates IXa and XIIa, thus removing one source of further plasminogen activation. The other inhibitors have a minimal role in inhibiting plasmin and generally they are involved only after alpha$_2$-antiplasmin is depleted. Alpha$_2$-macroglobulin binds plasmin slowly, but it does not prevent fibrinolytic activity during transport. The other plasma protease inhibitors, alpha$_1$-antitrypsin, antithrombin III, and C1-inactivator, have been shown to slowly inhibit plasmin in vitro, but their role as inhibitors of in vivo fibrinolysis is thought to be very minor.

FIBRIN DEGRADATION

Essentially, fibrinolysis begins when intrinsic and extrinsic fibrin formation is initiated by vascular injury. Surface activation of the contact factors (XII, XI and Fletcher factor) results in intrinsic fibrin formation and also in activation of plasminogen. Kallikrein, the activated form of Fletcher factor (prekallikrein), appears to be the most important of the contact factors to serve as a plasma activator. As fibrin formation proceeds, tissue plasminogen activator (t-PA) is released from vascular endothelial cells. Fibrin formation at the site of injury is accompanied by binding of plasminogen and t-PA to the fibrin surface, the most effective site for plasminogen activation to form plasmin.

Plasmin functions as an active serine protease to degrade its principal substrates. Fibrinogen and fibrin. Plasmin also digests factors V and VIII, further limiting fibrin formation. Degradation of fibrinogen initially yields a series of peptides and a protein fragment, **fragment X** (Fig. 14-2). Degradation of fragment X yields two products, **fragment D** and **fragment Y.** Fragment Y, a transient intermediate, is quickly split by plasmin into a second fragment D and a **fragment E.** The fragments resulting from fibrinogen degradation may have intact Aα and Bβ chains, which are lacking in fragments formed from fibrin.

Degradation of noncross-linked fibrin (fibrin monomer) is essentially identical to that of fibrinogen in both the kinetics and the structure of the derivative fragments. Cross-linked fibrin is degraded by plasmin at a slower rate and the degradation products (FDPs) are distinctive because of the covalent and noncovalent bonds that hold the fibrin domains together. Each FDP complex consists of two fragments that represent portions of linked fibrin monomers joined at their terminal domains by cross-linked bonds. The smallest unique product of cross-linked fibrin is fragment DD, which consists of two fragment D portions. The smallest complex is a combination of fragment DD and fragment E, joined by noncovalent bonds. Larger complexes are simply combinations of longer portions of each fibrin polymer chain, subject to further degradation by plasmin.

Some of the fragments, particularly fragments X and Y, possess anticoagulant properties that function principally by interference with fibrin polymerization. Fibrin degradation products also interfere with platelet aggregation, they can exaggerate the hypotensive effects of bradykinin, and inhibit some immunological responses. Once formed, FDPs have a circulating half-life of

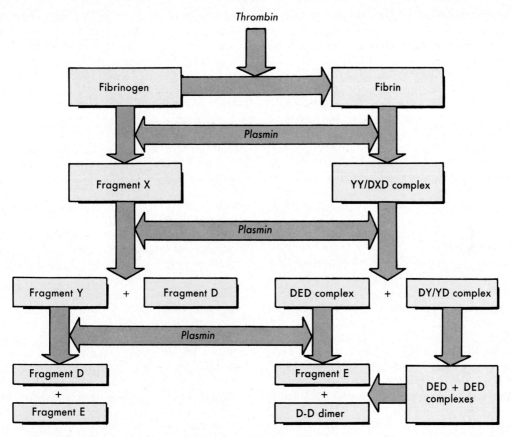

Fig. 14-2. Degradation of fibrinogen and fibrin.
Plasmin is involved at several steps in the formation of FDPs. Molecular weights of the fragments are listed in Table 14-1.

three to six hours before they are cleared from the circulation by cells of the reticuloendothelial system. Excess plasmin present in the circulation is rapidly inactivated by alpha$_2$-antiplasmin.

THROMBOLYTIC AGENTS

The aim of thrombolytic agents is to initiate fibrinolytic processes to remove pathological deposits of intravascular fibrin. These deposits cannot be left for spontaneous removal by intrinsic mechanisms; vascular patency must be restored as rapidly as possible so that tissue damages are mini-

mized. Two agents, streptokinase and urokinase, are available clinically with FDA approval. A third agent, tissue plasminogen activator, is currently employed in clinical trials.

Streptokinase

Streptokinase (SK) is the most widely used agent. SK is a bacterial protein produced by group C strains of beta hemolytic streptococci. SK forms a complex with plasminogen, activating the conversion of free plasminogen and fibrin-bound plasminogen to plasmin, which results in fibrin digestion and the formation of FDPs. Since SK is not highly selective in its activation of plasminogen, hemorrhage can be an unwanted complication. SK is also very antigenic, stimulating the production of antistreptococcal antibodies and causing patients to be resistant to further SK therapy. SK administration results in a rapid decrease in plasminogen and fibrinogen levels, as well as the appearance of high levels of FDPs, with their corresponding anticoagulant effects. A number of laboratory tests may be used to monitor the effects of SK therapy, although the thrombin clotting time is sufficient for most instances.

Urokinase (UK)

Urokinase, isolated from human urine or kidney tissue culture, is a trypsin-like enzyme. UK will convert plasminogen to plasmin directly, leading to fibrin and fibrinogen degradation and the appearance of FPDs. Unlike SK, UK is not antigenic; however, its short half-life and high cost are serious drawbacks to its general use as a thrombolytic agent. Due to the generalized conversion of plasminogen to plasmin during UK therapy, the major complication of UK use is bleeding. Laboratory monitoring of the effects of UK therapy is similar to that used with SK therapy.

Tissue plasminogen activator (t-PA)

Tissue plasminogen activator is the newest agent available for thrombolytic therapy. Therapeutic t-PA has been isolated from melanoma cell lines and has been produced by utilizing recombinant DNA technology. Since t-PA has a high affinity for fibrin, most conversion of plasminogen to plasmin occurs on the surface of fibrin, with little effect on circulating plasminogen. Thus the risk of unwanted bleeding appears to be much less with t-PA than with SK or UK therapy. However, some bleeding due to systemic fibrinogenolysis has been seen with larger doses of t-PA.

SUMMARY

- Fibrinolysis is the enzymatic degradation of fibrin clot deposits by plasmin to restore normal blood circulation and tissue integrity.
- A circulating plasma protein, plasminogen, is the precursor for plasmin. Conversion from precursor to active enzyme is stimulated intrinsically by contact factors (XII, XI, Fletcher factor, and Fitzgerald factor) and extrinsically by tissue plasminogen activator (t-PA).
- Plasminogen activation is inhibited primarily by alpha$_2$-antiplasmin.
- Degradation of fibrin and fibrinogen results in the formation of protein fragments or fibrin degradation products (FDPs). FDPs are an indication of fibrinolytic activity; plasma FDP levels are used to monitor thrombolytic disorders and therapy.
- Therapy for disorders resulting in fibrin deposits includes administering exogenous plasminogen activators, such as streptokinase and urokinase. These agents produce systemic fibrinolysis and can result in uncontrolled hemorrhage; t-PA may be more specific with less side effects.

SUGGESTED READINGS — SECTION IV

Akiyama H, Sinha D, Seaman FS, et al: Mechanism of activation of coagulation factor XI by factor XIIa studied with monoclonal antibodies, J Clin Invest 78:1631, 1986.

Aoki N: Genetic abnormalities of the fibrinolytic system, Semin Thromb Hemostasis 10:42, 1984.

Aoki N, and Harpel PC: Inhibitors of the fibrinolytic enzyme system, Semin Thromb Hemostasis 10:24, 1984.

Beck WS, editor: Hematology, ed 4 Cambridge, Mass, 1985, MIT Press.

Bessis M: Blood smears reinterpreted, Berlin, 1977, Springer International.

Bick RL: The clinical significance of fibrinogen degradation products, Semin Thromb Hemostasis 8:302, 1982.

Biggs R, and Rizza CR, editors: Human blood coagulation, Haemostasis and thrombosis, ed 3, Oxford, 1984, Blackwell Scientific Publications.

Burstein SA, and Harker LA: Control of platelet production, Clin Haematol 12:3, 1983.

Caen JP, Cronberg S, and Kubisz P: Platelets, Physiology and pathology, New York, 1977, Stratton Intercontinental Medical Book Corp.

Castellino FJ: Biochemistry of human plasminogen, Semin Thromb Hemostasis 10:18, 1984.

Clouse LH, and Comp PC: The regulation of hemostasis: the protein C system, N Engl J Med 314:1298, 1986.

Colman RW, Hirsch J, Marder VJ, and Salzman EW, editors: Hemostasis and thrombosis: basic principles and clinical practice, Philadelphia, 1982, JB Lippincott.

Comp PC, and Clause L: Plasma proteins C and S: the function and assays of two natural anticoagulants, Lab Management 23:29, 1985.

Duchett F: Thrombolytic therapy, Semin Thromb Hemostasis 10:87, 1984.

Esmon CT: Protein C and S, Semin Thromb Hemostasis 10:109, 1984.

Fedor B, and Kruithof I: Tissue plasminogen activator: chemical and physiological aspects, Semin Thromb Hemostasis 10:6, 1984.

Gerwirtz AM: Human megakaryocytopoiesis, Semin Hematol 23:27, 1986.

Haller CJ, and Radley JM: Time-lapse cinematography and scanning electron microscopy of platelet formation by megakaryocytes, Blood Cells 9:407, 1983.

Hemker HC, Van Rijn JLML, Rosing J, et al: Platelet membrane involvement in blood coagulation. Blood Cells 9:303, 1983

Hirsch J, and Brain EA: Hemostasis and thrombosis: A Conceptual Approach, ed 2, New York, 1983, Churchill Livingstone.

Holmsen H: Platelet metabolism and activation, Semin Hematol 22:219, 1985.

Holt JC, and Niewiarowski S:Biochemistry of granule proteins, Semin Hematol 22:151, 1985.

Levine RF: Isolation and characterization of normal human megakaryocytes, Br J Haematol 45:487, 1980.

McGann MA, and Triplett DA: Laboratory evaluation of the fibrinolytic system, Lab Med 14:18, 1983.

Nemerson Y, and Bach R: Tissue factor revisited, Prog Hemostasis Thromb 6:237, 1982.

Nurden AT, and Caen JP: Specific roles for platelet surface glycoproteins in platelet function, Nature 255:720, 1975.

Oates JA, Hawiger J, and Ross R, editors: Interaction of platelets with the vessel wall, Bethesda, Md, 1985, American Physiological Society.

Rao LVM, Rapaport SI, and Bajaj SP: Activation of human factor VII in the initiation of tissue factor-dependent coagulation, Blood 68:685, 1986.

Rosenberg RD, and Rosenberg JS: Natural anticoagulant mechanisms, J Clin Invest 74:1, 1984.

Santoro SA: Thrombospondin and the adhesive behavior of platelets, Semin Thromb Hemostasis 13:290, 1987.

Schick BP, and Schick PK: Megakaryocyte biochemistry, Semin Hematol 23:68, 1986.

Schumacher HR, Garvin DF, and Triplett DA: Introduction to laboratory hematology and hematopathology. New York, 1984, Alan R. Liss, Inc.

Sirridge MS, and Shannon R: Laboratory evaluation of hemostasis and thrombosis, ed 3, Philadelphia, 1983, Lea & Febiger.

Sten M: Fibrinolysis: an overview, Semin Thromb Hemostasis 10:1, 1984.

Suzuki K: Activated protein C inhibitor, Semin Thromb Hemostasis 10:154, 1984.

Thompson AR, and Harker LA: Manual of hemostasis and thrombosis, ed 3, Philadelphia, 1987, FA Davis Co.

Thorup OA Jr: Leavell and Thorup's fundamentals of clinical hematology, ed 5, Philadelphia, 1987, WB Saunders Co.

Triplett DA: Laboratory evaluation of coagulation, Chicago, 1982, American Society of Clinical Pathologists Press.

Triplett DA: Tissue plasminogen activator (t-PA) and fibrinolysis, Clotter's Corner 43, 1986. (Organon Teknika Corp, Durham, NC 27713.)

Williams N, and Levine RF: The origin, development and regulation of megakaryocytes, Br J Haematol 52:173, 1982.

SECTION V
Hematopathology

15

Introduction to Hematopathology

Understanding and attempting to alleviate problems that occur to the complex structures and functions of the tissues and cells of the body require a thorough knowledge of the *normal* homeostatic state. In the preceding chapters, an introduction to hematopoietic mechanisms and relationships has been presented so that the elements of pathological changes can be appreciated. Several points are emphasized in the following chapter with regard to the organization and description of hematological diseases. Hematopathology, in this text, includes disorders of the blood forming organs, primarily the bone marrow, diseases of the lymphoid and reticuloendothelial tissues that result in blood-borne manifestations, and bleeding and thrombotic disorders.

Distinctions will be made, when known, between diseases that have a **genetic** basis and those **acquired** from an environmental source. Acquisiton can be **prenatal** (before birth), **perinatal** (at the time of birth), or **postnatal** (anytime after birth). Some diseases, therefore, are **congenital** (a child is born with the condition, which may be genetic or acquired in the intrauterine environment), some are primarily characteristic of childhood, others affect adults, and some are most typical of geriatric populations. Also, diseases of the hematopoietic tissues will be classified as **primary,** an abnormality of the blood itself, or **secondary,** as a result of another disorder that is associated with manifestations in the blood cells or plasma coagulation and immune factors.

Defects can be structural or functional (usually they are both, but it may be easier to detect evidence of one or the other). The deficiency may be partial or complete, it may be **localized** in a specific tissue or cell lineage, or it may be **systemic,** involving several tissues and organs. Some diseases are **progressive,** becoming worse despite therapeutic intervention, whereas others are **self-limiting** in that the normal defense mechanisms of the body are able to contain it. Unfortunately, many of the diseases involving hematopoietic tissues include the cellular and/or humoral components of host defense. Finally, some diseases are **idiopathic,** arising by unknown mechanisms and undetermined cause.

GENETIC DISEASES

Hereditary diseases are due to specific abnormalities or deficiencies in the nucleotidyl codes of genes, passed on from generation to generation by definable mechanisms of gene assortment and interactions. Readers that have not had a course or biological component in genetics should review a basic biology text or one of the sources listed in the bibliography of this section. A few terms are reviewed here and in the glossary to facilitate a preliminary understanding. Characteristics of an individual (e.g., eye color, skin pigment, blood group, and amino acid sequence of enzymes) are expressed physically as traits or **phenotypes.** These traits can be seen and measured by appropriate techniques. The instructions for assembling most of these molecular constituents are contained within the **genotype,** the **deoxyribonucleic acid (DNA)** sequences inherited in the chromosomes from each parent. The conversion of DNA sequences into proteins was described in Chapter 4 for hemoglobin. Genetic changes can involve specific substitutions of one amino acid for another, resulting in alterations in the bonding interactions of polypeptides. In critical regions, a single gene mutation can render a large macromolecule such as hemoglobin ineffective at binding or releasing oxygen. Several of these abnormalities are described in Chapter 18. More substantial changes in genetic material can involve a large area of a chromosome, for instance, as a deletion, inversion, or translocation. Usually, numerous abnormalities occur in divergent organ systems. When a disorder is characterized by a consistent pattern of clinical and physical signs, the term **syndrome** is used to define the set of abnormalities. Chromosomal abnormalities are frequently associated with malignant growths of cells (tumors or neoplasms), such as the leukemias and lymphomas (Chapter 20), and confirmation of the presence of these conditions can be obtained by analyzing the chromosome set or **karyotype** for morphological abnormalities.

Changes in genes do not necessarily result in a clinical disease. A mutation can occur at a noncritical portion of a peptide, having no observable effect on the molecule's function. Many variant types of hemoglobin, for instance, are detectable only by biochemical techniques; they exist as hereditable curiosities that provide clues to the structure and function of the molecule. The basis for other inherited **anomalies** (e.g., Pelger-Huët, Chapter 21) is not clear, but there does not appear to be a functional disorder associated with the variant morphological pattern.

When a particular gene form or **allele** is inherited from only one parent and a different form from the other, the offspring is **heterozygous** for that gene (e.g, *A* gene and

B gene for blood group antigens of the ABO system). The same allele from each parent results in a **homozygous** genotype. Some alleles in a gene set are expressed in preference to others: genes can be **dominant, recessive,** or **codominant.** For the ABO blood group system, these terms can be illustrated as follows:

Maternal gene	Paternal gene	Offspring genotype/phenotype		Gene relationship
A	*B*	*AB*	AB	Codominant heterozygous
A	*O*	*AO*	A	Heterozygous, *A* dominant
O	*O*	*OO*	O	Homozygous

The appearance and severity of an inherited disease in a family depends on several factors. If the abnormal gene is dominant, then all individuals with the gene will express the disorder. Recessive genes will only be expressed as a homozygous state, provided that there is a dominant allele to supress it. This is normally the case with genes present on the **autosomes,** the set of 22 pairs of chromosomes inherited by both males and females. An additional pair of chromosomes are sex-specific, however, with XX determining female characteristics and XY determining male characteristics. The female sex chromosomes obey the same rules for allelic expression as the autosomes, but the male pair is heterologous, differing in gene content. For this reason, a male inheriting an abnormal gene on the X chromosome will express it, even though it would otherwise be recessive, because it is the only copy. Alleles on the Y chromosome or the X chromosome of the male are said to be **hemizygous,** and the resulting traits are said to be **sex-linked.** Obviously, males are much more likely to express such a genetic based disorder, since they only need to inherit a single recessive allele, whereas a female child would require two alleles, one from each parent, in order to express the disease.

Persons that have a single recessive allele

but do not express the disease phenotypically are said to be **carriers**. Carriers of some abnormal alleles may display a very mild form of the disease (e.g., sickle cell trait). Fig. 15-1 illustrates these terms in the form of a hypothetical **pedigree**, a chart of the inheritance pattern of disease "Z". Some alleles of genes are carried without expressing a phenotypic product; these are "silent", or **amorphic** (without form).

CORRELATING PHYSIOLOGY, DISEASE, AND LABORATORY RESULTS

The need to relate normal physiology with pathology has been emphasized throughout this textbook. The next step, evaluation of laboratory analyses of body fluids and tissues, is the essence of clinical laboratory science. The practices of clinical medicine and pathology are indisputably the prerogatives of physicians; the laboratory professional neither diagnoses nor institutes therapy. However, familiarization with medical practice and methods of treatment can facilitate the interpretation and validation of laboratory results as a component of patient care. Just as the physician must possess some knowledge of the laboratory and other allied health services in order to make best use of these services, the laboratory scientist must be able to communicate with the physician concerning the uses and limitations of laboratory procedures. Laboratory hematology has become increasingly specialized, and the amount and variety of information available from computer analyses has made it essential that technologists be knowledgeable about the physiological and pathological processes they are evaluating. Two types of approaches—the case history and the algorithm—are particularly useful in developing an integrated knowledge of hematological processes.

CASE HISTORIES

This is the traditional method of medical study and review, following the course of a

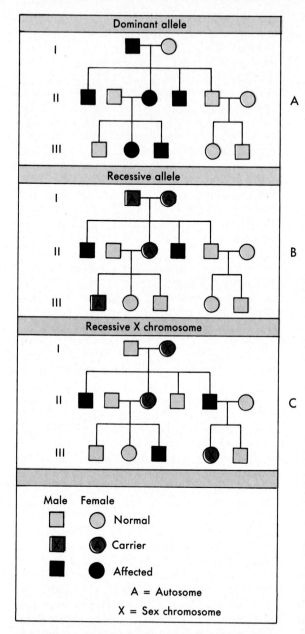

Fig. 15-1. **Sample pedigree charts to illustrate inheritance patterns.**

A, A dominant trait carried by autosomes. **B,** A recessive trait carried by autosomes. **C,** A recessive trait carried by the X sex chromosome (sex-linked).

patient from first presentation of complaints or symptoms to final or most recent disposition of the case. Several case histories are presented in the following chapters to illustrate the progress and typical laboratory findings of a disorder. These are only examples—they do not represent the diversity of presenting symptoms, complications, and therapeutic regimens that might be encountered. Blood cell patterns are manifestations of patholgoical processes, not the disease itself. Therefore, case data is an aid to understanding the correlations between laboratory results and underlying hematopathology, not an attempt to assign specific laboratory values to specific diseases. Of course, some laboratory findings are, for all practical purposes, definitive for the recognition of a particular condition (e.g., the presence of hemoglobin S in sickle cell anemia, malarial parasites inside erythrocytes).

Elements of a case history include (1) *presentation*, the primary complaints and relevant history that caused the patient to seek medical attention; (2) *physical examination*, the clinical condition of the patient on admission or at the start of hematological studies; (3) *initial laboratory data*; (4) *clinical course and additional laboratory studies*, including outpatient and inpatient progress; and (5) *final diagnosis and disposition*.

ALGORITHMS FOR DISEASES AND LABORATORY PROTOCOLS

There exists a formidable selection of laboratory procedures that can be utilized for the diagnosis and periodic monitoring of medical conditions. New techniques are continually introduced, and their merits are evaluated with respect to the information they provide. A number of factors must be considered in a decision to add a new method or replace an old one, not the least of which is cost. Clinical pathologists and laboratory scientists utilize protocols for test sequences that help standardize the di-

agnostic process yet maintain flexibility to meet the particular requirements of an individual medical problem.

In general, most laboratory evaluations commence with screening tests to ascertain the general physiological state of the patient. Blood cell counts, packed cell volume (hematocrit), hemoglobin, and observation of cell morphology on a smear are common initial tests. Coagulation screening, prior to major surgery and for initial investigation of bleeding symptoms, usually consists of a bleeding time and partial thromboplastin time. These tests are done first because they are inexpensive, require little time or patient preparation, and they can be done in large batches on automated instruments (bleeding times are still an exception to this).

Depending on the initial findings and the clinical manifestations in the patient, the physician may request more detailed studies designed to eliminate (rule out) some possibilities or specifically investigate others. It is not an efficient use of laboratory resources to perform expensive electrophoretic separations for hemoglobinopathies before screening tests indicate the presence of anemia. A standardized sequence of decisions for evaluating disorders or for performing laboratory assays can be organized as an **algorithm.** This type of approach is especially efficacious when incorporated with computerized data retrival systems. A generalized algorithm is shown in Fig. 15-2. Those presented in the following chapters are suggestions for organizing data and sequencing test protocols, but each testing facility must organize its own protocol, based on the unique needs of the local patient population and the limitations of laboratory staffing and equipment.

SUMMARY

- A professional approach to clinical laboratory hematology entails a good knowledge of the normal physiology of the hematopoietic system, familiarity with the pathological processes that affect blood

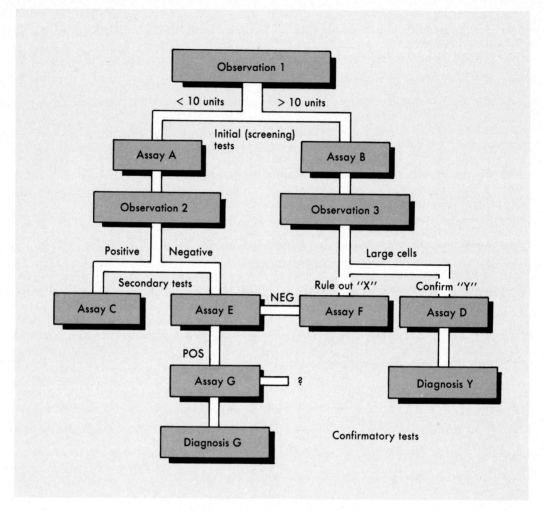

Fig. 15-2.   Sample algorithm.

cells and hemostatic mechanisms, and a thorough knowledge of the technical procedures available to the laboratory and their application to medical practice.

- Hematological disorders can be classified as genetic (hereditary) or acquired (environmental), primary or secondary, according to time of onset (congenital or prenatal, childhood, adult, etc.), and by degree of severity or extent of tissue and organ involvement.

- Expression of genetic information (genotype) as phenotypic characteristics depends on the relationship between the maternal and paternal alleles: dominant alleles are expressed preferentially over recessive alleles, others are codominant. The alleles can be the same (homozygous) or different (heterozygous) at a particular gene locus.

- Genes are paired as alleles on homologous chromosomes, 22 pairs of autosomes and an additional pair that specifies sex-related characteristics (XY = male and XX = female). Some recessive abnormal genes, present on the single X chromosome of males, are sex-linked, affecting males but carried by females.

• Case histories are utilized to integrate clinical and laboratory information, permitting a sequential view of pathological processes. Algorithms are used as a means of organizing protocols determining additional laboratory studies for diagnostic workups.

16

Abnormalities of Red Blood Cells

INTRODUCTION TO RED CELL DISORDERS

The inability to deliver sufficient oxygen to the tissues results in **hypoxia.** When the deficit is severe, tissue damage and death can result. Causes can be external to the body (e.g., low oxygen pressure at high altitudes), internal but nonhematological (cardiopulmonary disorders that diminish ventilation and circulation efficiency), or a result of a quantitative or qualitative deficiency of the red blood cells. Red cell deficiencies that result in hypoxia are collectively termed **anemias,** usually manifested by a decreased red cell mass, decreased or dysfunctional hemoglobin content, or both. Too much of a good thing is also abnormal: uncontrolled growth of the red cell mass increases blood viscosity and results in increased cardiovascular stress.

Anemia is associated with clinical symptoms that are indicative of a decreased red cell mass and impaired oxygenation of tissues:

1. Weakness and loss of breath, especially after physical exertion
2. Dizziness or fainting (syncope)
3. Gastrointestinal disturbances, loss of appetite, indigestion
4. Confusion, insomnia, hallucinations
5. Increased pallor (paleness), especially at mucous membranes and at the nail beds

The severity of clinical signs varies from none to life-threatening, depending on the severity of the red cell deficiency, the rate of onset of the disorder, and the age and general health of the patient. Mild anemias, especially those that develop slowly, may go undetected until revealed during investigation of an unrelated medical condition or crisis. The body possesses a remarkable ability to adapt to hypoxia, as can be seen in ambulatory patients with hemoglobins of 3 and 4 g/dL that finally seek medical advise because "they have been feeling less energetic lately." When the patient happens to be a 90-year-old woman, her family is not as likely to be alert to an underlying anemia as they would in a younger, more active individual. On the other hand, a traumatic, sudden drop in red cell mass and hemoglobin content (e.g., from a normal level of 15 g/dL to 5 g/dL) produces hypotensive shock and may result in cardiac failure. Patient age is an important determinant: newborn babies, particularly premature infants, are already struggling with a new environment, and the presence of anemia places additional stress on delicate lung and heart function. Geriatric patients may also be at increased risk from anemia, since some functional impairment may already be present in association with chronic disease and age-related tissue degeneration.

It is important to emphasize that anemia is not a primary disease per se but a secondary manifestation of another disorder, deficiency, or process. In other words, there is a reason for the red cell deficiency, one that can be investigated clinically and in the laboratory. Obviously, the ideal way to resolve the anemia is to identify and correct the underlying cause. Although this is not always realized, the erythrocytes provide a number of indications to help establish the cause, or **etiology,** of the anemia. Two traditional sources of evidence are the appearance of the red cells on peripheral blood smears (**red cell morphology**) and the numerical values (**red cell indices**) calculated from measurements of hemoglobin, hematocrit, and red cell count, previously described in Chapter 2.

RED CELL MORPHOLOGY: SIZE

Normal red blood cells are biconcave discs that measure 7.4 to 8.2 μm in diameter and contain about 85 to 95 fL of volume. These cells are known as **normocytes,** and their predominance in a blood sample is referred to as **normocytosis** (Fig. 16-1). Smaller or larger erythrocytes are produced by the bone marrow in states of nutritional deficiency or in association with other disorders. Moderate to severe iron deficiency, for example, results in cells that are predominantly smaller than 7.0 μm or 80 fL;

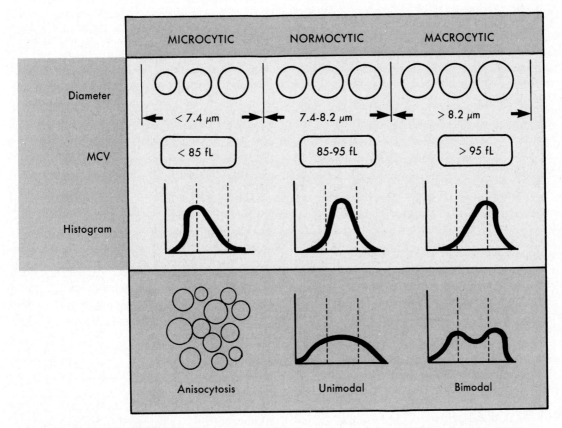

Fig. 16-1. Red cell size.
Correlation of relative size on the peripheral smear, volume (MCV) determined electronically, and an idealized histogram showing the red cell distribution for microcytes, normocytes and macrocytes. Dashed lines indicate the limits for normal MCV. Bottom row: anisocytosis and two different histograms that would result in a large calculated red cell distribution width (RDW).

these are **microcytes,** and the blood picture is termed **microcytosis.** Conversely, a moderate to severe deficiency of folic acid or vitamin B_{12} produces cells that are larger than 100 fL in volume (**macrocytes**), or **macrocytosis.** Note the emphasis on the word "predominantly," indicating that the cell size distribution is clustered and unimodal (one peak). Typical histograms are shown in Fig. 16-1 for each condition. "Macrocytes," a general term for large cells, should be distinguished from the word **megalocytes,** referring to abnormally large normoblasts in the bone marrow that are associated with megaloblastic anemia (Chapter 17) and certain myelodysplastic syndromes (Chapter 20).

It was noted in Chapter 2 that a cell's diameter is rarely measured by direct means in clinical practice. Preparation of a blood smear produces spreading artifacts (cells appear larger at the thin, leading edge of the smear), and optical calibration can be laborious because it must be done for each lens combination of each microscope. Even with an accurate optical system, measuring the diameters of a representative population of RBCs would be a time-consuming chore. Mean cell volume (MCV), on the other hand, is easily and accurately calculated from red cell counts and hematocrits or by direct electronic cell sizing by automated instruments (Chapter 26). Using the normal range of the MCV, blood cells can thus be classified as microcytic, normocytic, or macrocytic, providing one morphological basis for classifying anemias (see below).

Cell size predominance should not be confused with cell size variance. When cells of different sizes are present, producing either a broad distribution or two or more peaks (bimodal or polymodal), the condition is termed **anisocytosis.** This cell size variation is quantified by a calculation called the **red cell distribution width (RDW),** essentially the coefficient of variation of the MCV:

$$RDW = \frac{\text{Standard Deviation of MCV}}{\text{Mean MCV}} \times 100$$

The normal range for RDW is typically 11.5% to 14.5%, but blood cells are rarely so uniform in size that the RDW is less then 9% and no significance to a low RDW is indicated. RDWs greater than 15% should correlate with abnormal size variation on the blood smear, but examination of the formula above indicates that the magnitude of the RDW depends on the absolute value of MCV. Macrocytic cells (large MCV) result in a small RDW, whereas as microcytic cells magnify the RDW. The actual histogram, available as part of the data printout of many instruments, is a more reliable indicator of anisocytosis, in conjunction with the blood smear, than the RDW value alone. The histogram also distinguishes between a broad unimodal and bimodal distribution. The latter can occur following a large volume blood transfusion or after therapeutic response in a severe microcytic or macrocytic anemia.

RED CELL MORPHOLOGY: COLOR

The relative hemoglobin content of red cells on smears can be estimated by the extent of the central pallor, the clear zone representing the thin part of the biconcave disc (Fig. 16-2). Normal cells have a mean corpuscular hemoglobin concentration (MCHC) of about 32% to 36%, the ratio of the cell volume occupied by this essential protein. Such cells are **normochromic** (plate 1F), showing a small area of pallor that gradually increases in color toward the thicker cell periphery. When hemoglobin production is deficient but cell production is normal or increased, the MCHC decreases and the zone of pallor visibly increases, leaving only a thin rim of peripheral color in severe anemias. These cells are **hypochromic,** and this descriptor can further define anemias based on morphology. Cells do not contain more hemoglobin than their cell volumes will permit; only so many molecules can be packaged. However,

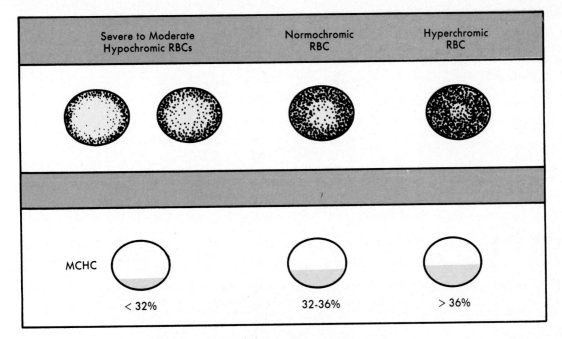

Fig. 16-2.   Red cell hemoglobin content.
Comparison of central pallor of cells on smears to MCHC.

macrocytic cells may occasionally appear "hyperchromic" on blood smears due to distortion of the biconcave disc, but the MCHC will be normal or decreased. Cells that have assumed a spherical shape (see below) also lose their central pallor and appear to be hyperchromic; because these cells may pack tightly when centrifuged and produce a low hematocrit, the calculated MCHC may exceed 36%.

Immature red cells (reticulocytes) contain enough RNA to react with Wright's stain, resulting in cells that are diffusely bluish-gray **(polychromasia)**. The presence of increased numbers of these larger, darker cells is an indication of accelerated marrow erythropoiesis; the reticulocyte count should be similarly increased. Polychromasia is seen in cases of hemolytic anemias, recovery from acute blood loss (non transfused), and the blood of newborn infants.

RED CELL MORPHOLOGY: SHAPE

The most dramatic morphological findings associated with anemias and other red cell conditions involve changes in cell shape or the presence of intracellular inclusions. The presence of aberrant cell shapes, exclusive of sampling or methodological artifacts, is termed **poikilocytosis**. There are many different terms that have been assigned for shape variants associated with particular diseases or conditions (Fig. 16-3 and Table 16-1). Some of these may be normal stages in the deformability of red cells under different conditions of fluid osmolality, whereas other shapes represent specific defects in cell membrane structure or abnormalities of cell contents. The mechanism underlying the shape variation is discussed in conjunction with each specific red cell disorder.

Discocytes is the term applied to normal

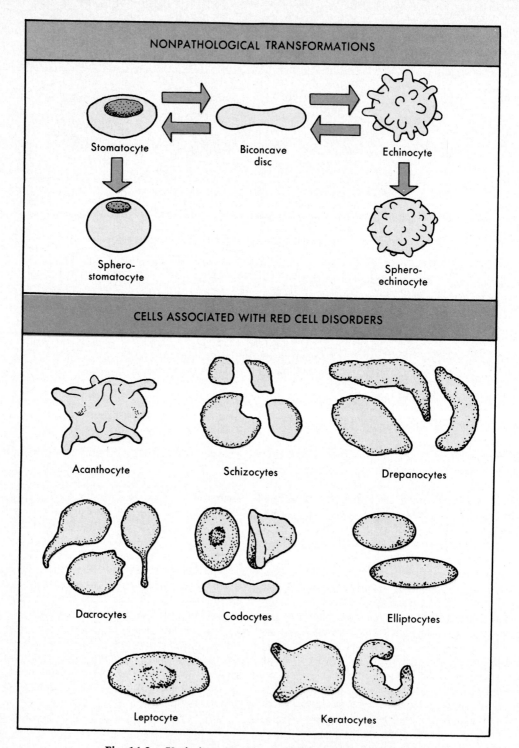

Fig. 16-3.   Variations in red cell shape (poikilocytosis).
See Table 16-1 for descriptions of each of these red cell forms.

Table 16-1. Variations in red cell shape (poikilocytosis)

Term	Appearance	Associated conditions
Discocyte	Biconcave disc	Normal
Stomatocyte (cup)	Uniconcave disc or sphere	Normal reversible response: low pH, cationic drugs Pathology: hemolytic anemia
Echinocytes (burr)	Many short regular spines	Normal reversible response: high pH (glass) Pathology: uremia, neonatal liver disease, pyruvate kinase deficiency
Spherocytes	Partial or full sphere	Irreversible, prior to lysis; hemolytic anemia, hereditary spherocytosis, severe burns
Schizocytes	Large to small fragments, different shapes	DIC, thrombotic disorders, myeloid metaplasia, severe burns, damaged heart valves, runner's anemia
Keratocytes (horns)	1-2 irregular projections from one side of cell	Same as for schizocytes
Codocytes (hat or bell)	Targets with central color and ring of pallor	Thalassemia, sickle cell anemia, hemoglobin C, iron deficiency, obstructive jaundice
Drepanocytes (sickle)	Sickle, boat, or squash-shaped	Sickle cell anemia (homozygous), can be demonstrated in trait
Dacrocytes (teardrop)	Pear-shaped, pointed at one end	Thalassemia, myeloid metaplasia, Heinz body anemia
Elliptocytes (oval)	Slightly oval to rod-shaped	Hereditary elliptocytosis, other anemias
Leptocytes (thin)	Flattened discs, large central pallor	Thalassemia, sickle cell anemia, iron deficiency, sideroblastic anemia, some liver conditions

biconcave erythrocytes. During their circulation through vessels of different diameters, fluid velocities and pressures, red cells deform and change shape to conform to the changing environment. In larger vessels, the discs may form stacks, called **rouleaux,** also seen on thick parts of smears and in wet preparations on slides. The amount of rouleau formation is increased when plasma protein concentration increases (e.g., during inflammation and in monoclonal gammopathies), resulting in large aggregates that fall rapidly in a sedimentation tube. The **erythrocyte sedimentation rate** is a widely used, nonspecific screening test for protein changes associated with infection, autoimmune disorders, and malignancies such as multiple myeloma.

Discocytes may reversibly transform into **stomatocytes,** or cup cells, (*stomato,* mouth) that are uniconcave and semispherical. The presence of cationic drugs or an environment of low pH favors this change in shape, which has been classified by Bessis (1977) into three progressive stages, plus two additional stages of spherostomatocytosis. Stomatocytes are also associated with some forms of hemolytic anemia. Conversely, high pH (at the surface of glass) and anionic compounds, fatty acids, and lysolecithin can produce a reversible transformation into **echinocytes** (burr cells), advancing to spheroechinocytes. Contrary to what has been taught to generations of laboratory students, echinocytes or crenated cells do not result from hypertonicity of the surrounding fluid; the cell shape (disc, cup or burr) is merely enhanced as water leaves the cell. However, hypotonic fluids will cause cells to swell and become unicon-cave, then spherical, before bursting. Although most burr cells on smears are probably due to contact with the alkaline surface of the glass slide, echinocytosis can also occur in vivo in association with uremia and pyruvate kinase deficiency and in neonates with liver disease. Patients on heparin therapy that have increased levels of fatty acids in their blood and blood that has been stored may exhibit echinocytosis in vitro, but this is readily reversible. Both of the transformations, from discocyte to either stomatocyte or to echinocyte, are believed to be due to differential changes in the composition of the membrane lipid bilayer, involving activity of the enzyme, lecithin-cholesterol acyl transferase (LCAT).

Spherocytes are cells that have attained a spherical or near-spherical form prior to lysis. This can occur because of hypotonicity of the surrounding fluid, membrane changes associated with antibody attachment, or as the terminal stage in marked stomatocytic or echinocytic transformation. Bessis (1977) distinguishes three types of spherocytes: (1) macrospherocytes are associated with hemolytic anemia, especially those with an immune basis; (2) microspherocytes that are sometimes seen in severe burn cases or as a result of incomplete phagocytosis; and (3) a variety of spherical forms seen in hereditary spherocytosis. All of these forms are removed by the spleen, presumably because the cells have lost their ability to deform and pass through the narrow capillaries. When the condition is inherited, such as the membrane defect associated with hereditary spherocytosis (Chapter 19), extravascular hemolysis can only be limited by removing the spleen, but the spherocytes persist and their fragility nevertheless results in some hemolysis.

Schizocytes are cell fragments (*schizo*, cut) that result from membrane damage encountered during passage through vessels that contain microthrombi or by contact with artificial surfaces, such as damaged heart valves or implanted needles and catheters. The fragments are usually removed by splenic phagocytes or they transform into spheroschizocytes and hemolyze. Incomplete phagocytosis of red cells can also produce schizocytes, sometimes referred to as "bite cells" because they lack a semicircular portion of the periphery. Schizocytes are associated with thrombotic diseases, disseminated intravascular coagulation (DIC), myeloid metaplasia, and other conditions that exhibit increased fibrin deposition on blood vessel walls. Osmotic, mechanical (runner's anemia, march hemoglobinuria), and thermal (severe burns) injuries also produce fragmented red cells.

Keratocytes have one or more irregular horn-like projections (*kerato*, horn) at one end of the cell. They form as a result of the same processes that produce schizocytes, namely, by interaction with fibrin strands deposited in blood vessels. This may produce an injured area or pseudovacuole in the cell. When this ruptures, the opposing ends of the membrane are left as projections. Their survival, like that of schizocytes, is short; they form spherokeratocytes and hemolyze.

Codocytes or, as they are more popularly known, **target cells,** are bell or hat-shaped cells that result from an abnormal ratio of membrane to internal contents (increased membrane or decreased hemoglobin). Because of this, they can withstand osmotic stress (hypertonic and hypotonic) to a greater extent than normal cells. Several different forms are classified by Bessis (1977). Codocytes with excess membrane are seen in obstructive jaundice, whereas hemoglobin-deficient forms are typically seen in thalassemia, iron deficiency anemia, and some hemoglobinopathies (sickle cell and hemoglobin C). They can be distinguished from stomatocytes by the thinness of the cup wall.

Drepanocytes or **sickle cells** (*drepano*, sickle) are deformed discocytes associated with the polymerization of abnormal hemoglobin, most commonly hemoglobin S (see Chapter 18). Sickle cells usually appear only in those patients that are homozygous for the abnormal S genes, but the blood of heterozygous individuals will also sickle under appropriate conditions of low oxygen. Most of the drepanocytes seen in peripheral smears are boat or squash-shaped, with only one end pointed, the other blunt. During acute crises, very aberrant forms may appear (Plate 5). Other hemoglobins can also crystallize inside erythrocytes: **hemoglobin C** forms tetragonal rods: others may result in precipitation of hemoglobin as Heinz bodies. Once formed, the crystals are irreversible, and the cells lose their ability to deform during passage through the microcirculation. Considerable damage is done to the kidneys and spleen when a large number of cells contain crystals. Although the cells are mechanically more fragile than normal cells, they are osmotically more resistant to lysis. True drepanocytes are diagnostic of sickle cell anemia, but fusiform cells (pseudosickle cells) can result from the artifactual polymerization of other hemoglobins.

Dacrocytes, or teardrop cells (*dacro,* tear), are pointed at one end or pear-shaped. They are believed to form as a result of stretching when splenic phagocytes attempt to remove inclusions, such as Heinz bodies. They are irreversible and are seen in conditions such as thalassemia, myeloid metaplasia, after stress produced by oxidant drugs, tuberculosis, and metastatic carcinomas of the bone marrow.

Elliptocytes or **ovalocytes** are elongated cells that vary from slightly oval to rod-like (up to 1:5 width to length ratio). They may be found in various anemias, but they are characteristic of mature erythrocytes (but not reticulocytes) of hereditary elliptocytosis (Chapter 19). The cells may be essentially normal with respect to hemoglobin content and osmotic fragility or, in other types of elliptocytosis, the cells may be fragile and hemolyze easily.

Leptocytes (*lepto,* thin) are flattened discs that contain less intracellular fluid, either hemoglobin or water, than normal. Thus they can result from dessication or from impaired hemoglobin production, as in iron deficiency anemia and thalassemia. They may also appear as thin codocytes (target cells) on smears. Typically, they are seen as ghost-like cells with large areas of central pallor and thin rims of peripheral hemoglobin (hypochromic). Leptocytes are also seen in sickle cell anemia, sideroblastic anemia, biliary obstruction and in some types of cirrhosis and steatorrhea.

RED CELL INCLUSIONS

Red cell inclusions (Fig. 16-4) are indications of deposits or precipitations of cell constituents, remnants of nuclear material, or the presence of parasites, such as malaria (Plate 5 F). Some inclusions are only visible with certain stains, such as the RNA precipitations of reticulocytes seen with brilliant cresyl blue or new methylene blue. Cell inclusions are compared in Table 16-2.

Howell-Jolly bodies are spherical granules of 1 to 2 μm in diameter consisting of DNA (Plate 5 D). In the mature RBC, they represent chromosomal fragment(s) of mitotic divisions that remain after nuclear expulsion, but they can also be found in the various normoblastic stages. Some of these inclusions may result from abnormal fragmentation of the nucleus itself. H-J bodies usually occur as single granules, occasionally two are present, rarely more. They are often located eccentrically and they stain distinctly dark purple with Wright's stain. The spleen normally removes H-J bodies as the RBCs pass through the macrophage-lined sinuses by a process called "pitting". They are not seen (or very rarely) in normal individuals, but they are found in those with nuclear maturation abnormalities (megaloblastic anemias), severe hemolytic anemias and thalassemias where red cell turnover rate is greatly increased, and after splenectomy or in the presence of a dysfunctional spleen.

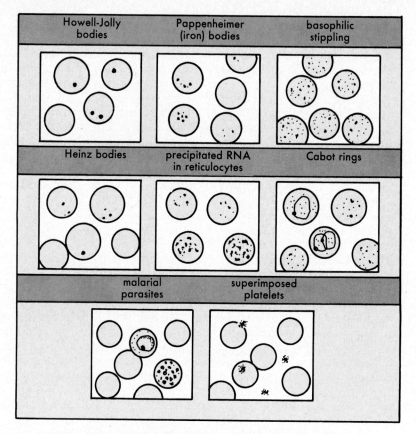

Fig. 16-4. Distribution and size of red cell inclusions.
See Table 16-2 for descriptions of these inclusions.

Siderosomes are granules or aggregates of ferritin, the cytoplasmic storage pool of iron intended for incorporation into heme during hemoglobin synthesis. They usually appear as small clusters near the periphery of normoblasts and, less often, reticulocytes. As the cell matures, the excess iron is utilized and there should be an absence of siderosomes in the circulating erythrocyte. Siderosomes stain with Prussian blue (Perls' reaction) and their presence is used to confirm adequate iron stores during marrow evaluation. Most of the cellular ferritin is finely dispersed and can only be demonstrated by electron microscopy. Abnormally large aggregates, seen in association with mitochondria and bordering the nucleus, form a **ringed sideroblast**, indicating sideroblastic anemia (Plate 8 B). **Pappenheimer bodies** are irregular deposits of iron in mature erythrocytes. They are associated with lysosomes, seen mainly near the peripheral border of the cell. On Wright-stained smears, they may appear as faint violet or magenta specks (azurophilic), often in small clusters, due to staining of the associated protein. Staining with Prussian blue confirms the presence of iron. They are always abnormal, usually associated with severe anemias and thalassemias.

Table 16-2. Red cell inclusions

Inclusion	Appearance	Composition	Staining reactions	Associated conditions
Howell-Jolly bodies	Spherical granules, 1-2 μm diameter	Nuclear remnant (DNA)	Wright's: dark blue-purple	Megaloblastic anemia, thalassemia, hemolytic anemia, after splenectomy
Sidero-somes	Few to many fine granules, near cell periphery	Ferritin (iron) deposits	Wright's: not stained* Prussian blue: light blue	Normal in normoblasts; ringed forms in sideroblastic anemia; increased in thalassemia and severe anemias; hemochromatosis
Heinz bodies	Spherical, 0.3-3.0 μm diameter, attached to cell membrane	Denatured hemoglobin	Wright's: not stained Supravital stains: positive	G-6-PD and pyruvate kinase deficiency, thalassemia, unstable hemoglobins, exposure to oxidizing drugs, after splenectomy
Cabot rings	Thin loops or double loops	Spindle microtubules	Wright's: reddish-violet	Severe anemias, dyserythropoiesis, after splenectomy
Basophilic stippling	Fine to coarse irregular granules	Aggregated ribosomes and polyribosomes (RNA)	Wright's: dark blue to black	Normal in fetal and neonatal RBCs; lead poisoning, some anemias, thalassemia, pyrimidine 5'-nucleotidase deficiency
Reticulofilamentous substance	Irregular granules, in clusters and strings	Ribosomal RNA	Wright's: not stained directly Supravital stains: positive	Normal RNA precipitate in reticulocytes and normoblasts

*Pappenheimer bodies in mature RBCs stain with Wright's because of the associated lysosomal protein.

Heinz bodies are spheres of denatured or precipitated hemoglobin that are attached to and distort the cell membrane. They vary greatly in size, 0.3 to 3 μm in diameter and they do not react with Wright's stain. Heinz bodies can be viewed in living cells (wet preparations of blood) by phase contrast microscopy or stained with brilliant cresyl blue, Nile blue, or crystal violet. Hemoglobin denaturation occurs in some enzyme deficiencies (G-6-PD and pyruvate kinase), in the presence of some types of unstable hemoglobin, after exposure to certain oxidizing drugs (e.g., phenylhydrazine), in thalassemia, and after splenectomy.

Cabot rings are mentioned and illustrated in every textbook, but they are very rarely seen in actual practice. They appear as one or more thin loops or double loops (invariably described as "figure-eights") in a cell, often in association with basophilic stippling. Bessis (1977) interprets these structures as remnants of fused microtubules, remaining from the spindle apparatus of mitosis. They are reddish-purple on Wright-stained smears and are most often associated with severe anemias, disturbed erythropoiesis, and following splenectomy. They should not be confused with the thicker ring forms of malarial parasites.

Basophilic stippling consists of fine, diffuse to coarse, irregular granules dispersed throughout the cell. They stain dark blue to black with Wright's stain and their presence can be induced as an artifact of smear preparation. Examination by electron microscopy reveals that the granules consist of aggregated ribosomes and polyribosomes, sometimes including siderosomes and mitochondria. They are especially prominent in fetal and neonatal blood and that of individuals exposed to lead and other toxic metals. They may or may not be seen in patients with thalassemia, other anemias resulting from impaired hemoglobin synthesis, and pyrimidine 5′-nucleotidase deficiency.

Reticulofilamentous substance is an artifact of supravital staining that characterizes normal reticulocytes, but is also present in normoblasts. The stain, usually brilliant cresyl blue or new methylene blue, precipitates ribosomal RNA, resulting in irregular granules or stringy clusters of granules throughout the cell (Plate 8 A). The relative amount of reticulum has been used by some investigators as an indication of cell maturity. The cells can also be counterstained with Wright's stain (Plate 1 E), during which the reticulum is decolorized by the alcohol and restained with the methylene blue component. In hemolytic anemias, when red cell turnover increases dramatically, both the number and relative immaturity of reticulocytes increases.

CLASSIFICATIONS OF ANEMIA

Anemia is most often classified on the basis of etiology (underlying cause), morphological characteristics of the red cells, and pathological manifestations (course of disease). The first two systems will be discussed in this textbook as a means of organizing information; a brief description of

pathophysiology is presented with each disorder in Chapters 17-19. As was stated previously, anemia is not a disease, but a manifestation of any of numerous other disorders that either increase red cell destruction or adversely affect one or more phases of red cell production. These changes are observed in the peripheral blood and bone marrow elements and associated with the underlying "cause" along with other physical and clinical observations. Once again, it must be emphasized that tables of classification and algorithms for laboratory procedures are devices for organizing information, they are not short cuts for instant diagnoses of complex pathological conditions.

Morphological classification

The availability of descriptive and quantitative criteria for classifying red blood cells by stage of maturation, shape, size, and hemoglobin content permits the establishment of a scheme for associating red cell morphology with different forms of anemia (see box below). Size, based on the MCV de-

---

MORPHOLOGICAL CLASSIFICATION OF ANEMIAS

I. Macrocytic Normochromic Erythrocytes
   A. Vitamin B_{12} and folic acid deficiencies
   B. Liver disease
II. Microcytic Hypochromic Erythrocytes
   A. Iron deficiency anemia (IDA)
   B. Thalassemia
   C. Sideroblastic anemias
III. Normocytic Normochromic Anemias
   A. Hemoglobinopathies
   B. Immune hemolytic anemias
   C. Aplastic and hypoplastic anemias
   D. Erythropoietin deficiency in renal disease
   E. Association with inflammatory disease
   F. Marrow replacement by neoplastic cells or fibrotic processes

---

termination and correlated with the appearance of the cells on the smear and examination of the volume histogram, is the primary criterion. The *mean* cell volume cannot be trusted by itself, since it may not represent the blood picture, for instance, when more than one population of abnormal cells is present. An equal number of microcytes and macrocytes, each significant as a cell population, will produce an averaged MCV that is normal. However, the bimodal peaks of the histogram should correlate with the blood smear morphology.

The second criterion is hemoglobin content (normochromic or hypochromic), based on MCH and MCHC indices. Again, the indice value may be misleading if a heterogeneous RBC population is present. With either measure, it is important to realize that the degree of morphological abnormality is a function of the severity of the disorder and that mild deficiencies may not exhibit morphological manifestations. Therefore, iron deficiency anemia is characteristically microcytic hypochromic in moderate to severe states, but this only occurs when marrow iron stores are depleted and hemoglobin synthesis is dramatically impaired. Likewise, patients with histories of alcohol abuse may be nutritionally deficient in iron and folic acid, producing microcytic and macrocytic manifestations.

A cost effective protocol for identifying the probable cause of anemia is beneficial to the patient and the medical care professionals (physician, clinical staff, and laboratory personnel). An example of a sequential workup, based initially on morphological criteria, is shown in Figure 16-5, in which examination of the smear reveals microcytic RBCs, confirmed by an MCV value of less than 84 fL. It is important to emphasize that other laboratories may have different limits for "normal" MCV values, based on experience with their instruments and patient populations. Microcytic, by their criteria, may be defined at MCV values of less than 80 or 78 fL, for example.

Similar algorithms can be constructed for other morphological results; examples can be found in the textbooks of McKenzie (1988) and Thorup (1987). The principles for developing such sequential protocols include: 1) utilizing screening tests that are rapid and inexpensive to obtain initial results; 2) avoid invasive procedures, such as bone marrow aspiration or biopsy, until initial results warrant the risk, expense, and patient discomfort that occurs; and 3) use secondary tests to both confirm the initial results and to rule out other diagnostic solutions to the clinical problem. An increased reticulocyte count, for example, signifies an active bone marrow response and effectively eliminates marrow failure as a factor in anemia. Simple tests for the presence of inflammation may establish this as a probable cause for moderate anemia without the need for specialized marrow studies or red cell chemistry procedures.

Etiological classification

This method of classification focuses on the mechanisms that result in decreased hemoglobin or red cell mass (see page 205). Three possibilities are considered: 1) marrow production is impaired, resulting in fewer cells or defective cells reaching the peripheral circulation; 2) production is normal or accelerated, but circulating cells are destroyed or lost; and 3) red cell production and survival is normal, but expansion of the plasma volume dilutes the apparent red cell mass and corresponding hemoglobin, mimicking anemia.

This approach is modified in organizing and presenting the anemias in the following chapters. Chapter 17 discusses those disorders that result from production failures, either due to pathological process primarily affecting the marrow as a tissue or those that are dyserythropoietic, involving maturational disturbances. Also included are production disorders that result in an increased red cell mass. Abnormalities that primarily concern hemoglobin are grouped

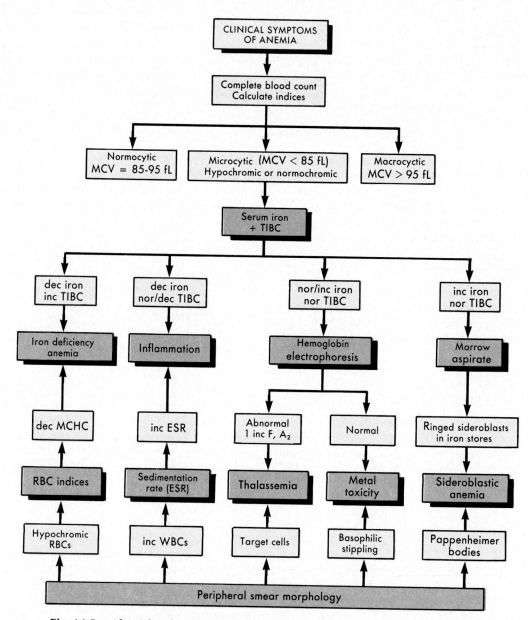

Fig. 16-5.   Algorithm for laboratory procedures to resolve a microcytic anemia.

ETIOLOGICAL CLASSIFICATION OF ANEMIAS

I. Decreased Red Cell Production
  A. Decreased erythropoietin levels
    1. chronic renal disease
    2. inflammation
    3. hypothyroidism
    4. reduced oxygen needs of tissues or increased oxygen pressure available
  B. Marrow damage or displacement of erythropoietic elements
    1. aplasia after exposure to toxic chemicals or radiation
    2. stem cell disorders leading to hypoplasia, aplasia, or dyserythropoiesis
    3. myelofibrosis
    4. displacement by neoplasms of other cell lines
II. Ineffective Red Cell or Hemoglobin Production
  A. Nuclear maturation disorders
    1. Vitamin B_{12} deficiency
    2. Folic acid (folate) deficiency
    3. Ascorbic acid (vitamin C) deficiency
  B. Iron deficiency
    1. nutritional deficiency
    2. chronic hemorrhage
    3. pregnancy
    4. inflammation
  C. Deficiency in globin production: thalassemia
  D. Deficiency in heme synthesis
    1. congenital porphyrias
    2. acquired porphyrias and heavy metal poisoning
    3. sideroblastic anemias
III. Increased Red Cell Destruction or Loss
  A. Hemorrhage
    1. acute, due to trauma
    2. chronic mucosal, gastrointestinal or menstrual
  B. Intravascular hemolysis
    1. thermal, chemical, osmotic or mechanical damage
    2. hereditary enzyme deficiencies (especially G-6-PD and pyruvate kinase)
    3. autoimmune and isoimmune antibodies
    4. exposure to bacterial toxins or specific venoms
    5. malarial parasites
    6. damage due to intravascular thrombus formation
  C. Extravascular hemolysis
    1. membrane deficiencies
    2. unstable hemoglobins, Heinz body anemias
    3. hemoglobinopathies (especially sickle cell and hemoglobin C disease)
    4. removal of antibody-coated cells by splenic phagocytes
    5. liver disease
IV. Pseudo-anemia as a Result of Increased Plasma Volume
  A. Edema (fluid retention)
    1. during the last trimester of pregnancy
    2. treatment with steroid drugs
    3. salt:water imbalance
  B. Hyperproteinemia
    1. monoclonal gammopathies (especially multiple myeloma)
  C. Sequestration as a result of severe splenomegaly

in Chapter 18. This treatment is somewhat unconventional in that iron deficiency anemia, enzyme deficiencies, hemoglobinopathies, and porphyrias are presented together. All of these involve hemoglobin production or function and therefore they can be considered as related defects in a continuous synthetic process, as discussed in Chapter 4. Finally, anemia resulting from red cell loss (hemorrhage) and destruction are reviewed in Chapter 19.

SUMMARY

- Hypoxia is defined as a decreased oxygen content of tissues and anemia is defined as a decreased hemoglobin content or red cell mass that impairs oxygen transport.
- Anemia is a clinical condition, not a laboratory result. Considerable variation exists between individuals, according to age and state of health, with regard to red cell parameters. Anemia is a manifestation of other conditions and disorders.
- Laboratory observations that assist in identifying an anemia include red cell morphology on blood smears (size, color, shape, and presence of intracellular inclusions) and red cell indices that establish cell volume and hemoglobin content.
- Anisocytosis is defined as variation in cell size and it is quantified by the red cell distribution width (RDW). Poikilocytosis is variation in red cell shape from a biconcave disc or discocyte. Some changes in shape are normal, reversible responses to environmental conditions and others are permanent, reflecting pathological disturbances in red cell metabolism, blood vessel structure, and other disorders.
- Red cell inclusions indicate abnormalities of iron use, hemoglobin stability, nuclear maturation and expulsion, or exposure to toxic chemicals.
- Classifications of anemia are generally based on morphological criteria or on the etiological mechanisms that result in decreased production and release or increased removal from the circulation.

17

Disorders of Red Cell Production and Maturation

The first major category of red cell disorders to be discussed includes those involving the hematopoietic tissues directly, conditions that disturb the marrow's architecture, disrupt replication and differentiation of blood cell precursors, or prevent maturation of stem cells to normal erythrocytes. Many of these disorders are secondary effects of other processes, such as invasion of the marrow by tumorous cells from other tissues, damage to stem cells from radiation or toxic chemicals, and maturational abnormalities caused by deficiencies of nutrients. The causes are heterogeneous, but the result is a change in the erythrocyte production rate or production of defective erythrocytes. Excluded from this chapter are diseases that affect hemoglobin synthesis or function (see Chapter 18).

APLASIA AND HYPOPLASIA (APLASTIC ANEMIA)

Anemias occur with or without corresponding changes in other blood cell lines (granulocytes and thrombocytes), depending on the types of marrow cells affected. A decrease in all peripheral blood cell types is called **pancytopenia (pan,** widespread, all), a condition that implies failure of hematopoietic production. The marrow's state is **hypoplastic** (or hypoproliferative) if production or cellular content is decreased, and **aplastic** if it has ceased or if hematopoietic cells are absent. Whether complete or partial, conditions of decreased production are

collectively defined as **aplastic anemia.** It is a term that embraces genetic, congenital, acquired, primary and secondary disorders (see p. 208). However, in about 60% of aplastic anemia cases investigated, an etiological agent or familial basis is not identifiable.

Two general patterns of manifestations occur. The first is dose-dependent, and the severity of the anemia is a function of exposure to the offending agent. Most individuals will react similarly to the same conditions. This is often reversible following removal of the offending agent. A second manifestation is not dose dependent, and the anemia is often irreversible. Chloramphenicol, for example, can produce a dose-dependent marrow response in some individuals and a dose-independent response in others. In the latter, the marrow may not show adverse effects for weeks or months after exposure to the drug, but it continues toward aplasia after the antibiotic is discontinued. The marrow may be permanently damaged, and even small doses of the antibiotic can be fatal. These individuals may be genetically predisposed for sensitivity to the toxic agents. A third pattern, which may operate in combination with either of the first two, involves an immunological response to the toxic agent. The agent could act as a hapten, or incomplete antigen, producing a response in conjunction with a protein carrier (e.g., chloramphenicol) or it could stimulate formation of an immune

ETIOLOGY OF APLASTIC ANEMIA

Secondary to toxic agent exposure
1. Ionizing radiation
2. Antimetabolic compounds
   a. Antifolate compounds
   b. Analogues of purines and pyrimidines (6-mercaptopurine; cytosine arabinoside; thioguanine)
3. Benzene, benzene derivatives, and related compounds (kerosene; trinitrotoluene; and the insecticides chlorophenothane or DDT, parathion, lindane or benzene hexachloride, and pentachlorophenol)
4. Antimitotic drugs (colchicine)
5. Dichlorovinylcysteine (byproduct of soybean extract)
6. Arsenic (inorganic and organic compounds)
7. Estrogens, in larg doses
8. Antibiotics (especially chloramphenicol, but also daunorubicin hydrochloride and adriamycin)
9. Sulfur and nitrogen mustards (busulfan, melphalan, and cyclophosphamide)
10. Phenylbutazone (an analgesic)
11. Gold compounds (used as antiarthritics)
12. Trimethodione (an anticonvulsant)

Secondary to infections
1. Viral hepatitis, especially non-A, non-B
2. Measles
3. Infectious mononucleosis
4. Influenza

Secondary to other conditions
1. Paroxysmal nocturnal hemoglobinuria
2. Myeloproliferative disorders

Idiopathic or congenital origins
1. Fanconi's anemia
2. Familial aplastic anemia
3. Amegakaryocytic thrombocytopenia

complex. Agents that attach to hematopoietic stem cells or that modify the stem cell membrane may initiate an autoimmune response to the "foreign" material. Other immunological proccesses may involve direct modification of responses by regulatory lymphocytes so that stem cells are suppressed or attacked. These pathophysiological mechanisms are sometimes called the seed (stem cell), soil (marrow microenvironment), and worm (lymphocytes and immunological products) hypotheses.

Marrow response to radiation has been examined as a result of exposure to the atomic bombs at Hiroshima and Nagasaki in 1945, accidental exposures to industrial and medical sources, and during the course of radiation therapy for malignant tumors. A total body dose of 300 to 500 rad results in generalized stem cell death and rapid aplasia. A localized dose of 4000 to 5000 rad will also produce an area of marrow aplasia, but this may gradually resolve over a period of several years, presumably by recruitment from nonirradiated tissue. Interestingly, aplastic anemia has not been observed in long-term survivors of exposure to the atomic blast at Hiroshima, but it is observed in radiologists that are exposed occupationally and in patients irradiated for treatment of ankylosing spondylitis, a condition associated with certain human leukocyte antigens (HLA B27).

Clinically, aplastic anemia usually presents three symptoms: bleeding (due to thrombocytopenia), a normocytic normochromic anemia with associated fatigue and weakness, and infection (due to granulocytopenia). The onset can be rapid or gradual and the manifestations mild or severe, depending on the degree of pancytopenia. Enlargement of the spleen is occasionally seen, but in most cases in which lymph node or splenic hypertrophy is present, the pancytopenia is not a result of aplastic anemia. As red cell production slows, iron stores and serum iron increase, eventually accumulating in histiocytes. The reticulocyte counts, corrected for anemia and expressed in absolute terms, are usually decreased. This reflects the inability of marrow to respond to the peripheral anemia, although the uncorrected reticulocyte count (percentage) may actually be normal or slightly elevated.

The marrow is usually fatty, showing little blood cell activity, although "hot" spots of hypercellular activity may be present. Sample sites must be chosen carefully and a biopsy is preferred over an aspiration technique so that relationships between cellular and acellular regions are structurally preserved. Hyperproliferation of lymphocytes and plasma cells is considered to be a poor prognosis. The median survival time after diagnosis of aplastic anemia is about 3 months; children have a mortality rate of about 50% and adults have rates of 65% to 75%.

Removal of the offending agent, if known, is obviously the first consideration for treating aplastic anemia. If the anemia is severe and appears to be irreversible, bone marrow transplantation offers the only resolution. Candidates for a transplant are usually less than 40 years old and they have not received blood transfusions or had children; thus they have a minimal risk of immunological sensitization. They must be compatible or minimally incompatible with the marrow donor for HLA antigens. Schumacher, Garvin and Triplett (1984) indicate that two of the following conditions should be present in the transplant recipient: a platelet count of less than $20,000/\mu L$, a neutrophil count of less than $500/\mu L$, and a corrected reticulocyte count of less than 1%.

Fanconi's anemia

Fanconi's anemia is a congenital form of aplastic anemia associated with several other abnormalities. These include the absence or rudimentary development of thumb and radius, abnormalities involving the heart and kidneys, retarded growth and skeletal abnormalities, albinism or hypopigmentation, and atrophy of the spleen. Males with this condition outnumber females by about 2 to 1, and a recessive gene is believed to be involved. Moderate to severe pancytopenia is present, and the anemia is either normocytic or slightly macrocytic.

Cytogenetic studies indicate that chromosomal breaks are numerous. These may be further associated with development of acute leukemias, hepatoma, or esophageal carcinoma. Because of the extensive systemic abnormalities, bone marrow transplants and other therapeutic measures are usually not successful. Although androgen (testosterone) maintenance appears to help some patients, most die by their mid to late teens.

Pure red cell aplasia (PRCA)

Hypoproliferation of the erythroid elements, without corresponding decreases in other blood cells, is characteristic of **pure red cell aplasia (PRCA)**. Three forms are generally recognized, although a number of variants and intermediate forms have been described.

Congenital hypoplastic anemia (Diamond-Blackfan syndrome) is a moderate to severe anemia associated with retarded sexual maturity and growth, osteoporosis, and portal hypertension. Although females predominate, the disorder is believed to be caused by an autosomal dominant gene. The condition is usually first seen in infants, some with hemoglobins of less than 2 g/dL. Marrow examination reveals a dearth of erythroid precursors, but plasma erythropoietin levels are usually elevated. A number of mechanisms have been proposed to account for the anemia, including an innate deficiency in the erythroid stem cells (CFU-E), a selective defect of DNA synthesis, presence of an inhibitor for heme synthesis, and a T lymphocyte mechanism that inhibits erythropoiesis. The disease is usually progressive, although some cases have been reported to remit spontaneously. Therapy usually consists of steroid administration and bone marrow transplantation (limited by considerations of HLA compatability) and occasional transfusions to alleviate the anemia. Unfortunately, transfusions accelerate the rate of iron accumulation, culminating in hemosiderosis unless iron chelating agents are also administered.

Acute acquired erythroblastopenia is a transient form of PRCA found mostly in children in association with infections or as a result of treatment with certain drugs (sulfonamides, chloramphenicol). It is also occasionally associated with malnutrition. In either case, it is usually reversible.

Chronic acquired erythroblastopenia is a refractory anemia seen most often in middle aged to elderly patients, especially in females with benign thymomas (3 to 4 times that of males). In contrast, there is a 2 to 1 male to female preference in patients that do not have a thymoma. Some females with this form of PRCA also have myasthenia gravis, an autoimmune disorder involving degeneration of muscle cell acetylcholine receptors. Therapy includes administration of androgens, other steroids, antithymocyte serum (removal of the thyoma is reported to help a few patients), and plasmapheresis.

STROMAL DISEASE: DISORDERS OF THE MARROW MICROENVIRONMENT

Disruption of the marrow architecture and displacement of hematopoietic elements results in a **myelophthisic** blood picture. This consists of a mild to moderate pancytopenia in association with immature leukocytes (especially myelocytes), large platelets, and increased numbers of reticulocytes and normoblasts. The immature elements are normally retained by the marrow tissue and endothelial lining of the marrow sinuses. When the stromal reticulum is disturbed, large platelet strands and nucleated red cells can be released. Stromal disease is usually associated with one of the myeloproliferative disorders, infiltration by metastatic tumor cells, or increased fibrous tissue formation (myelofibrosis). As the marrow structure deteriorates, compensatory extramedullary hematopoiesis by the spleen, liver and distal long bones is seen. Marrow aspiration may not be representative or even possible (fibrotic marrows often result in a "dry tap"), so that marrow bi-

opsy is the sampling technique of choice. Skeletal scans, using radioisotopes to label active areas of hematopoiesis in the marrow, can help identify favorable areas for biopsies.

DYSERYTHROPOIESIS

Dyserythropoiesis is a condition in which erythroid stem cells divide and differentiate, often at accelerated rates, to form abnormal cells with decreased survival times due to intramedullary destruction. Thus erythroid hyperplasia is seen in combination with a peripheral anemia that may be moderate to severe, a condition generally referred to as "ineffective erythropoiesis." Changes in red cell size are associated with an asynchrony of maturation between cytoplasm and nucleus: defects in cytoplasmic maturation often result in microcytic anemias, and defects in nuclear maturation are seen as macrocytic anemias.

Congenital dyserythropoietic anemia (CDA) is a group of related familial refractory anemias resulting from ineffective erythropoiesis, characterized by morphological abnormalities of the normoblasts. Incomplete mitotic division of the erythrocytic precursors results in multinucleated cells; other changes include asynchronous maturation between nucleus and cytoplasm, membrane alterations, and antigenic interactions with the immune system. Plasma iron turnover is accelerated, as measured by isotopic tracer methods, but iron uptake into red cells is decreased. A compensatory erythroid hyperplasia is present in response to intramedullary destruction and the shortened survival time of the immature red cells. The latter can be verified by measuring increases in carbon monoxide production and fecal stercobilin, products of heme catabolism.

The anemia may be moderate to severe and the absolute reticulocyte counts are usually normal or only slightly elevated, a further indication of poor red cell production or release. Three types of CDA are usually described, although a number of intermediate and variant forms are also known.

Type I is seen in infants and children and is characterized by megaloblastoid changes in the marrow and a mild to moderate macrocytic anemia peripherally (MCVs range from 93 to 155 fL). About 1% to 2% of the normoblasts are multinucleated or have segmented nuclei. Some of the binucleated forms have unequal lobes; others are connected by thin strands of chromatin. Erythrophagocytosis may be prominent. Unlike the megaloblastoid changes seen in folate deficiencies and in some myelodysplastic syndromes, only the erythroid series is affected. The anemia is usually moderate (hemoglobin = 8 to 12 g/dL), serum iron is usually normal to moderately elevated, bilirubin is slightly increased, and haptoglobin is decreased. This form of CDA is distinguished from type II by normal serological findings. Various abnormalities of red cell enzymes have been reported, but not consistently, in patients with type I CDA. Basophilic stippling and Cabot's rings, along with marked poikilocytosis and anisocytosis, characterize the peripheral red cells.

The disease is probably caused by an autosomal recessive gene. Jaundice may be present in some newborns, where others may not have clinically evident manifestations until late childhood or adolescence. The prognosis for survival is generally good, especially if transfusions can be avoided. Tissue iron overloading is a problem in any condition in which marrow hyperplasia is combined with peripheral anemia not due to hemorrhage.

Type II CDA is also referred to as hereditary erythroblastic multinuclearity with positive acidified serum test **(HEMPAS)**. This is the most common form of CDA, probably a result of an autosomal recessive gene which is encountered most often in northwestern Europe, Italy, and North Africa. The anemia is normocytic and quite variable in severity. Onset can be detected in infancy to late adulthood. Peripheral red cells show anisocytosis, poikilocytosis, basophilic stippling, a normal to slightly elevated reticulocyte count, and occasional contracted spherocytes. The marrow is characterized by the presence of multinucleated normoblasts (2 to 7 nuclei are present in 10% to 40% of the last two stages of normoblasts) and prominent signs of erythrophagocytosis. The cells are not megaloblastoid, however. Electron microscopy reveals abnormalities of the red cell membrane and increased amounts of endoplasmic reticulum near the cell periphery. As with other forms of CDA, serum and tissue iron concentrations are increased. Secondary complications can include hemochromatosis (deposition of excessive iron in tissues) and gallbladder dysfunction.

The distinguishing feature of HEMPAS is abnormal serological findings. An antigen (HEMPAS) is present on the red cells that reacts with antibodies in acidified serum, similar to the mechanisms responsible for paroxysmal nocturnal hemoglobinuria (PNH). Unlike PNH, HEMPAS red cells yield a negative test for lysis in sugar water (Chapter 27). Red cells containing the HEMPAS antigen also have an unusually high concentration of i antigen, which reacts with anti-i. In addition, HEMPAS red cells lyse in the presence of anti-I antibodies. Normal fetal red cells also contain i antigen, but this is converted to I antigen during postfetal maturation. Naturally occurring antibodies to both i and I antigens can be found in most people's serum, but these rarely cause problems in vivo. In addition, various abnormalities in red cell enzymes have been described in association with HEMPAS. This disorder is usually not progressive and transfusions should be avoided to prevent iron accumulation. Splenectomy has been used to limit immunological destruction of red cells in some patients, but this is controversial since infections often result.

Type III CDA or hereditary benign erythroreticulosis is an autosomal dominant form that combines features of types I and II. Giant, multinucleated normoblasts (up to 12 nuclei in cells of up to 50 μm diameter!) are seen but the anemia is normocytic or only slightly macrocytic and the presence of clinical symptoms and signs of anemia vary greatly. Increased agglutination reactions of type III red cells to anti-i and lysis and anti-I are seen, but the acidified serum acid test is negative.

ANEMIAS OF CHRONIC DISORDERS (ACD)

Anemias due to hypoproliferation in association with chronic disorders are relatively common. Most are the result of mechanisms that either interfere with iron metabolism (e.g., inflammation) or with erythropoietin production (e.g., renal disease).

Acute or chronic inflammation often results in development of a mild anemia (hemoglobin greater than 9 g/dL) that could be attributed to several factors. First, inflammation is associated with changes in the membranes of reticuloendothelial macrophages and the release of iron. As senescent red cells are removed from the circulation (lysed by macrophages of the liver and spleen), hemoglobin is catabolized and the heme iron is stored and eventually transported to the marrow for incorporation into developing normoblasts. Inflammation interferes with iron release, resulting in accumulation of ferritin within the macrophages. Thus the presence of increased ferritin stores in combination with low levels of serum iron helps distinguish ACD from true iron deficiency anemia (Chapter 18).

Some evidence shows that iron uptake by marrow normoblasts is also reduced during inflammatory states. The survival time of red cells may be slightly reduced in ACD, possibly due to changes in erythrocytic membranes that result from fever and from interaction with inflammatory response mediators. Macrophages of the spleen and liver appear to be hyperactive during inflammation and remove cells showing minimal abnormalities. Increased intermedullary destruction may also be a factor, involving immunological responses to therapeutic drugs or to altered red cell membranes.

Finally, the role of erythropoietin has been investigated. A normal marrow should be able to compensate for a slowly developing anemia, but patients with chronic inflammation or inflammatory connective tissue diseases produce less erythropoietin than normally occurs in the presence of anemia. Patients with some forms of malignancies produce adequate amounts of erythropoietin but the marrow fails to respond. The reasons for these altered responses are not clear, but dietary and metabolic changes associated with illness, especially those involving protein metabolism, may be partly responsible.

Some endocrine disorders are also associated with mild anemias. Hypothyroidism results in lower metabolism and oxygen demand by tissues, erythropoietin levels decrease accordingly, resulting in hypoproliferation by the bone marrow. Patients with hypopituitarism may display a more severe anemia (hemoglobin decreased by 3 to 6 g/dL) and associated leukopenia caused by secondary effects on thyroid and adrenal gland function. The adrenals produce hormones that stimulate erythropoietin production and affect erythroid stem cell activity. Testosterone, produced by the testes, also stimulates erythropoietin and a deficiency is associated with a mild decrease in hemoglobin levels.

Uremia associated with renal disease also produces a progressive decrease in erythropoietin production. Reticulocyte production remains normal and the hemoglobin concentration drops, stabilizing at 7 to 9 g/dL. Blood urea nitrogen will usually be above 40 mg/dL, and the serum creatinine level is above 3 mg/dL. Nitrogen retention probably affects the survival of circulating red cells, accounting for part of the anemia.

The typical course of ACD is mild and manifestations occur 1 to 2 months after onset of inflammation or connective tissue disorder or following hospitalization for malignancy. ACD presents as a normocytic to microcytic, normochromic to hypochromic red cell picture. Reticulocyte production remains low and iron studies indicate the presence of normal to increased levels in tissue stores. Poikilocytosis and anisocytosis may be noted with some forms of ACD, especially those associated with renal disease. Acanthocytes and schistocytes are often seen and triangle-shaped cells may be present when uremia is marked.

Treatment is directed at the underlying disorder and—in most cases—the anemia is not severe. Hormone therapy to relieve endocrine disturbances often corrects the hypoproliferative state. Dialysis to alleviate uremia, however, poses additional problems. Blood is lost during the procedure and iron deficiency can occur, producing a microcytic pattern. Folate deficiency can also occur during dialysis, unless folic acid supplements are given. If not corrected, a macrocytic anemia can add to the complications of the peripheral blood picture.

MEGALOBLASTIC ANEMIAS

Megaloblastic (megalo = large) hematopoiesis results from a defect in nuclear maturation that is manifested by nuclear-cytoplasm asynchrony and a number of morphological abnormalities, the most prominent being the large size of the blood cell precursors affected. It is important to define terms that are used interchangeably. **Megaloblastic** refers to an abnormal maturation process in any cell line, including blood cells. Thus, in some early stages of leukemia or myelodysplastic syndrome, granulocytes, megakaryocytes, and erythroblasts are often described as "megaloblastic". A **megaloblast,** however, refers specifically to a megaloblastic erythroid precursor and a maturation series can be described for megaloblasts with stages analagous to normoblasts (Fig. 17-1 and box on p. 215). In fact, when cells associated with megaloblastic anemia were described in the last century, they were believed to comprise a separate cell series. They are now known to be the maturational products of precursors that have undergone megaloblastic transformation. The maturational defect is most commonly acquired as a result of either vitamin B_{12} or folic acid deficiency, both of which are required for normal DNA synthesis during nuclear division.

A further distinction must be made between megaloblastic anemia and macrocytic anemia. The former term is reserved for disorders in which DNA synthesis and nuclear maturation abnormalities result in production of large blood cell precursors with mature cytoplasms and immature nuclei. As megaloblasts mature, they are released into the peripheral blood as large cells (macrocytes) with distinctive oval shapes (**ovalo-macrocytes**) (Fig. 17-2). However, macrocytes also occur as a result of other processes. The normal marrow response to severe anemia (sickle cell crisis, autoimmune hemolytic anemia, or acute hemorrhage) is to release immature ("shift") reticulocytes and to accelerate erythrocyte maturation. These larger cells, with volumes of 100 to 130 fL, are associated with polychromasia and an increased reticulocyte count (10% to 25%, depending on the severity of the anemia and vigor of the marrow response). Macrocytes are also observed in some liver diseases (MCV averages 105 to 115 fL), but the cells are often thin or occur as target cells. Primary causes for macrocytic anemias are summarized in Table 17-1.

The macrocytes and ovalo-macrocytes derived from megaloblastic processes have volumes of 100 to 140 fL and contain normal amounts of hemoglobin. Because of their size, some may appear to be hyperchromic and the MCHC may be slightly higher than normal. In addition, reticulocyte counts are normal or low normal, indi-

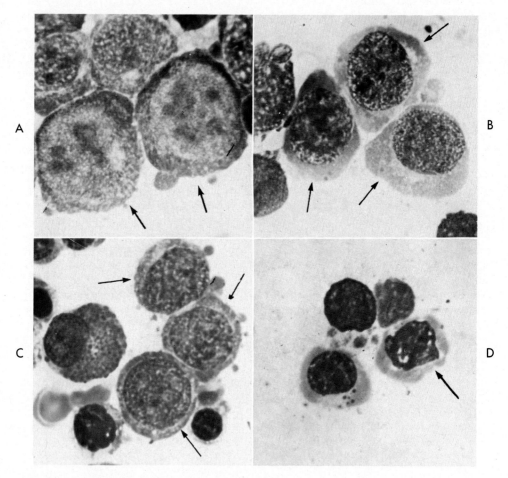

Fig. 17-1.   Maturation stages of megaloblasts.
Bone marrow from a patient with pernicious anemia. **A,** Promegaloblasts. **B,** Basophilic megalo-blasts. **C,** Polychromatophilic megaloblasts. **D,** Orthochromic megaloblasts. (From Miale, JB: Laboratory medicine: Hematology, ed 6, St Louis, 1982, The CV Mosby Co.)

MATURATION STAGES OF MEGALOBLASTS

Promegaloblast (megalocytic rubriblast) (Fig. 17-1, *A)*
Size and shape: 19 to 27 μm in diameter; round to oval, often irregular.
Nucleus: Very fine, delicate chromatin, approaching that of marrow reticulum cell. One or two nucleoli contrast sharply with chromatin. Parachromatin is abundant and stains relatively lighter than that of corresponding normoblasts. Nucleus is slightly oval to round, centrally or slightly eccentric in the cell.
Cytoplasm: Mottled, deeply basophilic. Nucleus to cytoplasm ratio is smaller than in corresponding normoblasts.

Basophilic megaloblast (megalocytic prorubricyte) (Fig. 17-1, *B)*
Size and shape: 15 to 22 μm diameter; often irregular in outline, round to cuboidal.
Nucleus: Abundant parachromatin, demarcated from chromatin material. A single nucleolus may be seen with difficulty, most often none are visible. Chromatin is coarser than in promegaloblast, but finer than that of basophilic normoblast. Nucleus is round to slightly oval, usually eccentric in cell.
Cytoplasm: Deep basophilia, royal blue in color. More abundant than that of corresponding normoblast. Often mottled with nonbasophilic areas, especially near nuclear membrane.

Polychromatophilic megaloblast (megalocytic rubricyte) (Fig. 17-1, *C)*
Size and shape: 10 to 18 μm in diameter; the cell outline may be very ragged and the shape irregular.
Nucleus: Shape is round or slightly oval and it is eccentric in location. The nuclear membrane appears thick compared to previous stages. Nucleoli are not present. Parachromatin is still abundant, but arranged in blocks and centrifugal pattern typical of late stage normoblasts. Chromatin is coarser than that of preceding stage, but nucleus is still immature compared to corresponding normoblast.
Cytoplasm: Color varies considerably, depending on severity of anemia and degree of nuclear-cytoplasm asynchrony, from uniform pink-orange to mottled pink-gray to basophilic.

Orthochromic megaloblast (megalocytic metarubricyte) (Fig. 17-1, *D)*
Size and shape: 8 to 15 μm in diameter; cell irregularity about the same as that of metarubricytes.
Nucleus: Condensation of chromatin is nearly complete, but nucleus may be segmented or the cell may show evidence of several irreguarly sized and shaped nuclei, indicators of dyserythropoiesis. Occasionally, the nucleus may be very large and retain features of an earlier stage, despite the maturity of the cytoplasm.
Cytoplasm: Orange-pink in color, fully hemoglobinized. More abundant than that of the corresponding metarubricyte.

---

cating the presence of ineffective erythropoiesis instead of a normal marrow response to the presence of an anemia that can be moderate to severe (hemoglobin less than 7 g/dL). Maturational changes are also seen in other blood cells and iron turnover studies confirm an increased rate of intramedullary and extravascular destruction. Indirect bilirubin may also be elevated. Examination of the marrow reveals an eryth-

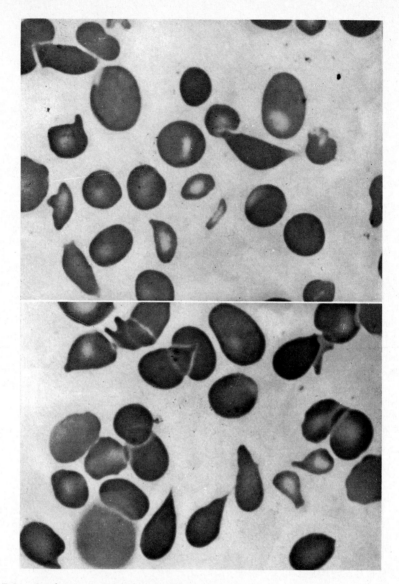

Fig. 17-2. Ovalo-macrocytes in pernicious anemia.
Peripheral blood: note the degree of poikilocytosis and anisocytosis. (From Miale, JB: Laboratory medicine: Hematology, ed 6, St Louis, 1982, The CV Mosby Co.)

roid hyperplasia (the myeloid/erythroid ratio may be 1 or less), but the cells are megaloblastic.

In addition to deficiencies in vitamin B_{12} and folic acid, other causes of impaired DNA synthesis have been identified with megaloblastic anemia. Some of the chemotherapeutic drugs used for malignancies interfere with DNA synthesis by blocking steps in nucleic acid metabolism. Rare, he-

Table 17-1. Laboratory results in macrocytic anemia

Determination of blood loss	Normal	Vitamin B_{12}	Folate deficiency	Response to deficiency
Mean cell volume (fL)	85-95	100-140	100-140	100-130
Reticulocyte count (%)	0.5-1.5	0.1-1.2	0.1-1.2	5.0-20+
Serum cobalamin (pg/mL)	160-800	5-100	50-500	—
Serum folate (ng/mL)	5-20	5-40	>3.0	—
Red cell folate (ng/mL)	160-650	25-400	>100	—
Marrow morphology	Normal	Megaloblastic	Megaloblastic	Erythroid hyperplasia
Blood morphology	Normal	Macrocytic	Macrocytic	Polychromatophilia

reditary deficiencies in these pathways are also known, producing megaloblastic anemia in neonates and infants.

VITAMIN B_{12} METABOLISM

How does a vitamin deficiency result in the megaloblastic changes of blood cell maturation? Vitamin B_{12} (cyanocobalamin) is synthesized only by certain microorganisms. Animals either harbor the microbes (e.g., the rumen of herbivorous mammals) or acquire the vitamin secondarily by eating other animal products (meat, fish, liver, eggs, and milk are sources). Adult humans require about 1 μg per day. A typical western diet contains 5 to 30 μg/day, of which about 3 to 5 μg are absorbed. Pregnant women, growing children, and persons with increased cell production have increased needs for B_{12}. Strict vegetarians often show a vitamin deficiency, as measured by serum B_{12} levels, but they rarely develop a clinically significant anemia. Because the daily intake and retention exceeds usage by a comfortable margin, a deficiency of vitamin B_{12} occurs only after a prolonged interruption in supply. Normal body stores, concentrated primarily in the liver and kidneys, ranges from 1 to 5 mg. The body loses about 0.1% of the total body stores each day, thus the required net total intake is from 2 to 5 μg per day. Thus, depletion of the body pool of B_{12}, even with increased loss or demand, may take several years after a drastic change in diet or onset of a malabsorption disorder.

Vitamin B_{12} is bound to protein in most foods; this is ingested and passed into the stomach where pepsin and hydrochloric acid frees the vitamin from the protein (Fig. 17-3). Two proteins, one a rapidly-moving component on electrophoresis (**R protein** or haptocorrin) and the other a slow-moving component (S protein or **intrinsic factor, IF**), are present in the gastric fluid. Either can combine with the vitamin, but only the IF-B_{12} complex can be absorbed in the small intestine. Intrinsic factor is a glycoprotein, weight 44 to 45 kd, produced by the parietal cells of the gastric mucosa. The R protein binds most of the B_{12} and this complex, along with free IF, passes into the duodenum where pancreatic enzymes release the vitamin for uptake by the intrinsic factor. The IF-B_{12} complex passes into the ileum to bind with specific receptors on the microvilli. B_{12} is released and transported across the mucosal cell to complex with a beta plasma protein, **transcobalamin II (TC II)**, for transport to either the hematopoietic

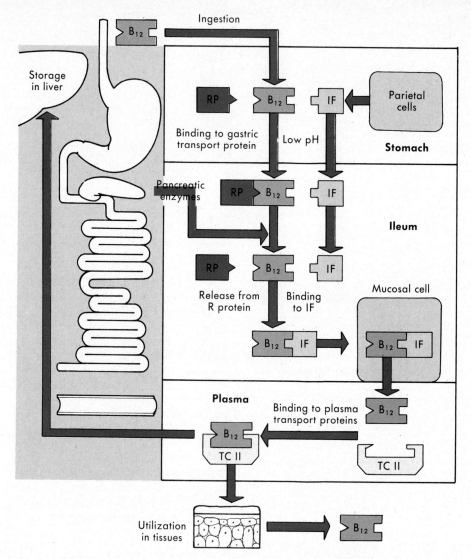

Fig. 17-3 Pathways of vitamin B$_{12}$ absorption, transport, and storage.
Transport through the digestive system involves binding of cobalamin to R protein (RP), release
in the ileum, and transport across the mucosa by intrinsic factor (IF). Transport to tissue usage
and storage sites is accomplished by transcobalamin (TC).

tissues or to tissue storage sites. The TC II-
B$_{12}$ complex is rapidly cleared from the
plasma. Storage occurs mainly in the parenchymal cells of the liver and most of the
B$_{12}$ remaining in the plasma (measured in

serum) is eventually bound to a similar protein, transcobalamin I (TC I).

Vitamin B$_{12}$ weighs 1335 daltons and has
a complex structure consisting of tetrapyrrole ring plane (called a corrin) that resem

bles the porphyrin ring of hemoglobin, and a nucleotide plane (Fig. 17-4). The center metal atom is cobalt, thus the molecule is also called **cyanocobalamin** (note the CN group = cyano). Several types of cobalamins exist, named after other groups in place of CN. Cobalamin and vitamin B_{12} will be used interchangeably in this text. The pyrrole structures shared by hemoglobin and cobalamin are not coincidental: both are synthesized from aminolevulinic acid (ALA).

Vitamin B_{12} participates indirectly in DNA synthesis by acting as a methyl receptor for **methyltetrahydrofolate** (MTHF). The methyl group is transferred to homocysteine, which converts this amino acid to methionine, an important step in protein synthesis (Fig. 17-5). When B_{12} is deficient, MHTF is "trapped," preventing its conversion into an active coenzyme of DNA synthesis. This will be discussed in a following section on folate metabolism.

Vitamin B_{12} deficiency

A number of diverse problems can affect cobalamin metabolism and availability, from dietary restriction and absortion to tranport and utilization. When the deficit is sufficiently severe, DNA metabolism in all cells of the body is disrupted. Blood cells, because of their rapid turnover rates, are among the first and most obvious to show abnormalities. Deficiencies can be grouped by mechanism or site of disturbance, most of which involve formation of the IF-B_{12} complex or absorption of the vitamin (see box on p. 221).

Since only 1 or 2 µg of cobalamin per day are required for metabolic activities, it is unusual for deficiencies to occur solely as a result of diet, unless the individual has been a strict vegetarian for an extended time. A deficiency in both hydrochloric acid and production of intrinsic factor is likely in disorders that affect the gastric mucosa, such as damage from ingestion of caustic materials, or diseases for which total or partial gastrectomy is required. Vitamin B_{12} is supplied by injection to patients following permanent damage or removal of large portions of the stomach.

Disorders that involve intrinsic factor can be caused by: (1) the secretion of an abnormal IF molecule that does not facilitate ileal absorption, (2) a congenital lack of IF, or (3) insufficient secretion of IF by the parietal cells of the gastric mucosa. The first two conditions are rare. A hereditary deficiency of IF due to an autosomal recessive gene with an accompanying megaloblastic anemia is observed in homozygous infants. The deficiency is specific for IF since the structure of the mucosal cells and the ability to secrete hydrochloric acid are normal. A dysfunctional IF molecule is known from a single case.

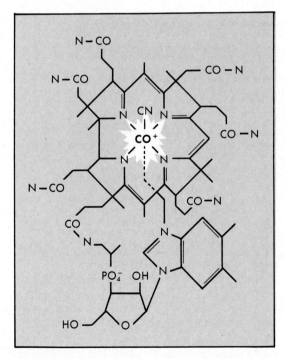

Fig. 17-4. Structure of cyanocobalamin (vitamin B_{12}).

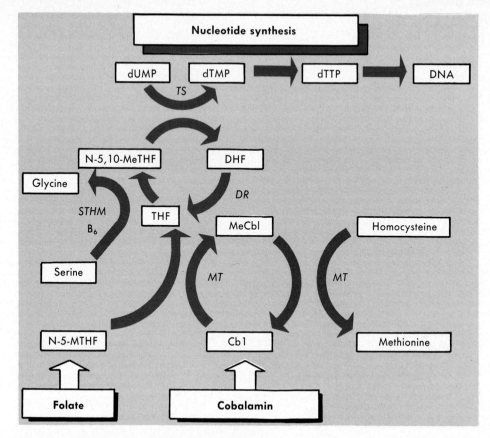

Fig. 17-5.   Metabolism of cobalamin and folate.
Vitamin B_{12} and methyltetrahydrofolate (MTHF) conversions require an exchange of a methyl group. A deficiency of cobalamin results in MTHF being "trapped" so that it is unavailable for conversion to a coenzyme in nucleotide metabolism.

PERNICIOUS ANEMIA

The remaining intrinsic factor disorder was described in the late 1800s with the name **pernicious anemia (PA),** because of the unknown and insidious nature of its clincal course (pernicious = dangerous). This term has been applied to a variety of megaloblastic anemias, but its proper use is confined to a relatively common anemia resulting from intrinsic factor deficiency. Other causes of cobalamin deficiency, as well as other megaloblastic and macro-cytic anemias, are excluded from this definition.

PA is the most common cause of cobalamin deficiency. It affects both sexes and all races, usually occurring after the age of 40 and rarely in individuals younger than 25. The relationship between a progressive, fatal anemia and the presence of megaloblasts in the marrow was established by Ehrlich in 1910. Subsequently, the association of PA with **achlorhydria,** the lack of gastric acid secretion, was also clarified.

CAUSES OF VITAMIN B$_{12}$ DEFICIENCY

Problem	Effect on B$_{12}$
A. Dietary	
1. Alcohol abuse and poor dietary habits	Not ingested
2. Restrictive diet (e.g., vegetarians)	Not ingested
B. Gastric	
1. Gastric injury, surgical removal	Not released from protein
2. Lack of intrinsic factor or antibody to IF	IF-B$_{12}$ complex not formed
C. Intestinal	
1. Ileal inflammation, sprue	Not absorbed
2. Certain bacterial and helminth infections of ileum	Utilized by organisms
3. Certain drugs; neomycin, KCl, colchicine, para-aminosalicylic acid	Not absorbed
4. Chronic pancreatitis	Not released from R-protein
D. Transport and utilization	
1. Deficiency of transcobalamin II	Not transported
2. Nitrous oxide inhalation	Oxidized and inactivated
3. Certain inborn errors of metabolism	Folate-DNA path blocked
E. Increased demand	
1. Pregnancy	Less available to mother
2. Hyperthyroidism, infancy, certain neoplasms	Insufficient supply

Early attempts to treat this disease focused on dietary factors, and liver was found to be a source of a corrective factor, especially when extracted and given by intramuscular or intravenous injection. In 1948, this factor was identified as vitamin B$_{12}$ (cyanocobalamin), leading to its synthesis in 1973. Unfortunately, this was only part of the deficiency. It became apparent that assimilation of this *extrinsic* dietary factor also required participation of an *intrinsic* gastric factor, something other than hydrochloric acid. Although administration of cobalamin via parenteral (nonoral) routes corrected the megaloblastic anemia, oral administration did not. The state of achlorhydria and associated degeneration of the gastric mucosa seen in advanced cases of PA had been noted and used as diagnostic criteria. Some evidence has suggested a familial occurrence for PA, but the genetic contribution is not clear. If it exists, it is probably complex and dependent on other factors that are not understood.

The identification of intrinsic factor as a specific glycoprotein necessary for absorption of cobalamin provided an understanding for the basic pathogenesis of PA, but it is still not clear what produces the deficiency of intrinsic factor. Several immunological mechanisms have been investigated. About 90% of PA patients have autoantibodies in their sera that react with their parietal cells, but 5% to 10% of the normal adult population (up to 15% of normal women) possess similar antibodies. Furthermore, over 50% of PA patients possess a different autoantibody, directed against intrinsic factor, which is rarely seen in individuals without PA. This is commonly known as a blocking antibody, since it prevents binding of IF to B$_{12}$. A third autoantibody, known as a binding antibody, is expressed against the IF-B$_{12}$ complex in some individuals. These immunological results are further complicated by finding a high incidence of antiparietal cell antibodies in patients with other autoimmune diseases, such as Hashimoto's thyroiditis and rheumatoid arthritis. The reverse is also true: patients with PA have a high incidence of antithyroid antibodies.

In addition to the nuclear maturation defects of megaloblastic anemia, a condition that is reversible with vitamin B_{12} therapy, neurological manifestations occur. Early signs include a numbing of feet and hands and disturbances of balance and vibration reception. If the condition is not treated, a progressive degeneration of the dorsal and lateral columns of the spinal cord ensues. The first lesions involve only a few myelinated fibers, but these spread and form larger areas of irreversible damage. The patient becomes increasingly disoriented and irritable. Before recognition of cobalamin deficiency and its neurological consequences, many older patients with pernicious anemia were undoubtably institutionalized for mental retardation or insanity. Death can eventually result from severe deterioration of neural tissues.

Laboratory findings in pernicious anemia are relatively specific. A peripheral macrocytic anemia is associated with a megaloblastic marrow (Plate V-A) and a low reticulocyte count. The marrow may show an increased number of mitotic figures and giant metamyelocytes with bizarre, lobed nuclei. Megakaryocytes may have few granules and a loosely connected ("exploded"), multilobed nucleus. Hypersegmented neutrophils are characteristic in the peripheral blood (Fig. 17-6). Red cells are ovalomacrocytic and they may contain Howell-Jolly bodies and Cabot's rings (Fig. 17-7). Serum iron levels may be elevated, due to ineffective hemoglobin production, unless iron deficiency anemia is also present. Serum cobalamin levels are low (often less than 100 pg/mL, as measured by radioimmunoassay techniques) and tests for gastric secretion show a decreased fluid volume and lack of hydrochloric acid. Assays for autoantibodies in serum or gastric juice often reveal anti-parietal cell and/or anti-intrinsic factor specificities. Biopsy examination of the gastric mucosa usually shows degenerative lesions characteristic of PA.

The classic procedure to distinguish PA from other causes of cobalamin deficiency is the **Schilling test.** The patient is given 0.5 to 1.0 µg of radioactive cyanocobalamin (^{57}Co) orally followed by an intramuscular injection of 1 mg of unlabelled cobalamin to saturate the tissues and plasma. If the patient can process B_{12} normally, about 25% of the oral dose will be absorbed in the ileum and a fraction of this will be excreted in the urine during the next 24 hours. Most laboratories report an excreted value of greater than 7% in 24 hours as normal. If

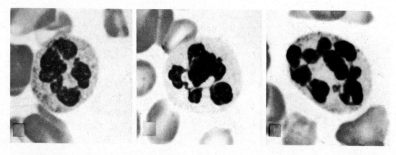

Fig. 17-6.   Hypersegmented neutrophils in pernicious anemia.
Hypersegmented neutrophils have more than 5 nuclear lobes. They are usually larger than normal (macropolycytes) and result from abnormal granulopoiesis. (From Miale, JB: Laboratory medicine: Hematology, ed 6, St Louis, 1982, The CV Mosby Co.)

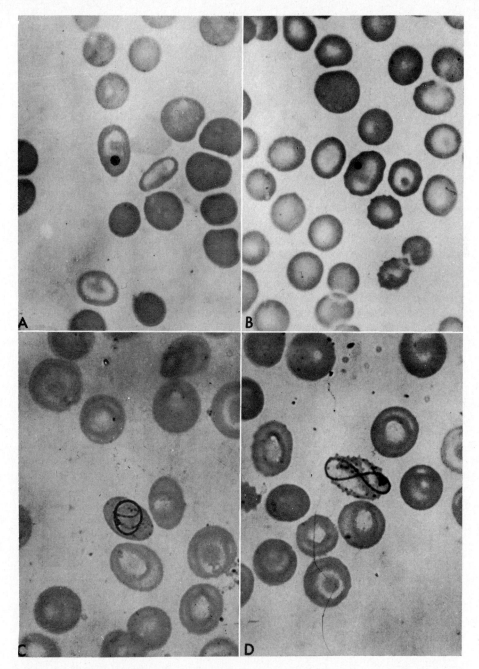

Fig. 17-7.   Peripheral red blood cells in pernicious anemia.
Howell-Jolly bodies and Cabot's rings may be seen in some of the macrocytes. Note the differences in hemoglobin content of various cells. (From Miale, JB: Laboratory medicine: Hematology, ed 6, St Louis, 1982, The CV Mosby Co.)

Table 17-2. Results of the Schilling test in megaloblastic anemia[*]

Condition		B_{12} only	B_{12} + IF
Normal	Urine[†]:	7-35% of dose	7-35% of dose
	Plasma[‡]:	0.3-2.4% of dose/L	0.3-2.4% of dose/L
Malabsorption	Urine:	0-10% of dose	0-10% of dose
Pernicious anemia	Urine:	0-3% of dose	6-30% of dose
	Plasma:	0.02-0.15% of dose/L	0.2-0.6% of dose/L

[*]Based on an oral cobalamin dose of 0.5 μg.
[†]Reported as percent of dose excreted in 24 hours.
[‡]Reported as percent of dose circulating per liter of plasma at 8 hours.

this initial result is less than 7%, a second test is run. This time, the oral radioactive dose is given with intrinsic factor. If the poor initial excretion is due to a deficiency of IF (true pernicious anemia), the second test should show an increase in the urinary excretion of labelled cobalamin (see Table 17-2). However, if the poor absorption and excretion of cobalamin is due to an absorption problem other than IF, addition of intrinsic factor should not significantly change the results. If the latter occurs, the patient must be evaluated with respect to small bowel disease, parasitic infection, pancreatitis, or bacterial infection.

The Schilling test can also be performed by measuring fecal excretion of labelled cobalamin, in which the results will be reciprocal to those for urine. Patients with severe renal disease can be evaluated by plasma determinations, but this requires a measurement of plasma volume to compare patient results with reference values. Obviously, urine is easier to process than fecal material to obtain representative sample and the urine assay is easier to perform and interpret than the plasma assay. A modification of the two-stage technique, for any specimen, is also commercially available. The two cobalamin doses, one with and one without a bound intrinsic factor component, are given simultaneously. One is labelled with [57]Co (bound to IF) and the other with [58]Co (unbound). The energy spectra of the two isotopes are separated electroni-

cally with a discriminator and a ratio of the concentrations is calculated. Patients with PA will have a ratio of [57]Co/[58]Co that is greater than 1.7, whereas normal patients will have a ratio of about 1 (no difference between the two presentations). Despite improvements in direct assays for serum cobalamin concentration, the Schilling test is still considered a definitive test for pernicious anemia.

Treatment of pernicious anemia is by parenteral administration of vitamin B_{12} in long-term doses that exceed the likely requirements. The response to successful therapy is dramatic (Fig. 17-8), transforming the megaloblastic marrow to normoblastic in a few days. A marked increase in the reticulocyte count occurs within 5 to 10 days, marking the end of ineffective erythropoiesis. Plasma iron levels fall as hemoglobin production increases. The hemoglobin level, red blood cell count, and MCV require weeks or months to return to normal, since the abnormal cells persist and contribute to these relative erythrocyte measures. Thorup (1987) summarizes information on treatment strategies and dosages.

COBALAMIN DEFICIENCY: OTHER MECHANISMS

Malabsorption of vitamin B_{12} can result from a number of diseases affecting the samll bowel. Tropical sprue can produce a severe cobalamin deficiency, as can diseases and abnormalities of the ileum that result

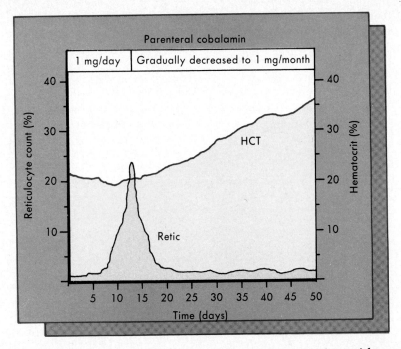

Fig. 17-8 **Erythropoietic response to vitamin B$_{12}$ therapy in patient with pernicious anemia.**
Patient was started on 1000 μg of cobalamin per day and continued on 1000 μg per month after reticulocyte response peaked (see case history). Hemoglobin, RBC count, and MCV returned to normal as macrocytic cells were replaced.

in an overgrowth of bacterial populations. These microorganisms assimilate cobalamin before it can be absorbed by the ileal microvilli. This type of competitive utilization is also seen in some individuals infected with a tapeworm *(Diphyllobothrium latum)* found in fish.

A deficiency of the transport protein, transcobalamin II, is relatively rare but a megaloblastic anemia develops despite normal absorption and serum levels. Since most of the serum pool of cobalamin is bound to transcobalamin I, the presence of anemia and a normal serum level of cobalamin help rule out IF and absorption deficiencies. Low levels of TC I do not appear to be associated with megaloblastic anemia; only a deficiency of TC II results in anemia.

Patients with this disorder are usually diagnosed early in life and they respond to parenteral vitamin B$_{12}$. Other patients have been found to have a dysfunctional transport protein, with little or no capability for binding with cobalamin.

A familial form of cobalamin malabsorption is known, believed to be caused by a recessive gene that results in a deficiency of ileal receptors for the vitamin. Assays for gastric acid and intrinsic factor are normal. The condition is associated with proteinuria.

Cobalamin use is abnormal in children with certain inborn errors of protein metabolism, such as homocystinuria and methylmalonic aciduria. These normally act as methyl receptors for cobalamin, permitting conversion of folate to its active coenzyme form. As a result of the abnormal amino acidurias, methyltetrahydrofolate is not able to participate in DNA synthesis. Urinary levels of methylmalonic acid can increase from 0-3.5 mg/day in normal individuals to as much as 300 mg/day in these patients.

FOLATE METABOLISM

Green leafy vegetables (aspargus, spinach, broccoli), liver, and mushrooms are good sources of dietary folate or folic acid. The minimum daily allowance of 50 µg/day is easily provided in a diet of 150 to 250 µg, of which 50% to 75% is absorbed. Folate (pteroylmonoglutamic acid, Fig. 17-9) is ingested as a reduced folate polyglutamate, which is converted by a carboxypeptidase into folate monoglutamate (Fig. 17-10). The monoglutamate is absorbed in the proximal portion of the jejunum, where it is converted to N-5-methyltetrahydrofolate monoglutamate (MTHF-G) by a reductase in the mucosal cells. MTHF-G is transported through the plasma for delivery to

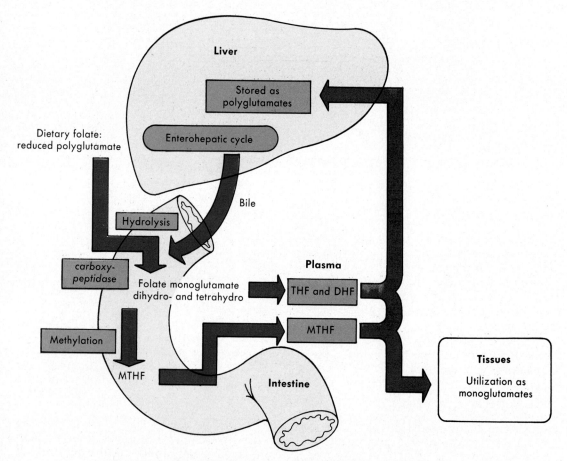

Fig. 17-9 Pathways of folate absorption, transport and storage.
EHC = entero-hepatic cycle.

the erythropoietic marrow and other tissues, to be incorporated into the DNA synthesis pathway as a coenzyme. The liver stores 5 to 10 mg, enough reserve for several months, in parynchemal cells. A constant circulating supply is maintained by release of stored amounts from the liver to the intestines via the entero-hepatic cycle (EHC).

Folate is bound to plasma proteins in the monoglutamate form and it is delivered to intracellular sites by passive and active uptake mechanisms. Folate in the liver and in red cells exists primarily as polyglutamates. A small portion of the total body folate content is excreted by the kidneys, mainly as degradation products. Because of the many forms of folate in the body and the relative reactivity of these molecules to assay systems, determinations of total folate have been largely unsuccessful.

Methyltetrahydrofolate (MTHF) transfers a methyl group to cobalamin (Fig. 17-5 and Fig. 17-11) to become tetrahydrofolate (THF), a conjugated form that is retained by the cell. A deficiency of cobalamin (vitamin B_{12}) blocks this step, the so-called "methylfolate trap". THF is converted to N−5, 10−methylene THF (MeTHF) during a coreaction of serine to glycine that is catalyzed by pyridoxine (vitamin B_6). MeTHF serves as a coenzyme in the conversion of deoxyuridylate (dUMP) to thymidylate (dTMP), one of the two pyrimidine nucleotides of DNA.

MeTHF becomes dihydrofolate (DHF) as a result and is subsequently reduced to THF to begin a new cycle. THF also participates in the transformation of formiminoglutamic acid (FIGLU) to glutamic acid in the pathway of histidine catabolism.

FOLIC ACID DEFICIENCY

A deficit of body folate can occur through decreased dietary intake, particularly during times of increased demand (pregnancy, lactation, and conditions requiring accelerated cell turnover), in malabsorption syndromes similar to those producing cobalamin deficiencies, and as a result of interference by drugs (see box on p. 229).

Dietary deficiencies have often been noted in tropical regions where poor economic conditions result in consumption of starches and grains to the exclusion of fresh vegetables and meat products. Obviously, poverty and poor eating habits, even in those that can afford a better diet, are not confined to the third world. Food fads, particularly those associated with extreme dietary restrictions, can result in a serum folate deficiency and a mild macrocytic anemia within a few months. Food preparation can also be a factor, since over cooking, especially boiling, removes the folate content of many vegetables. A dietary deficit becomes more pronounced in patients with conditions that are accompanied by marked increases in cell production (DNA synthe-

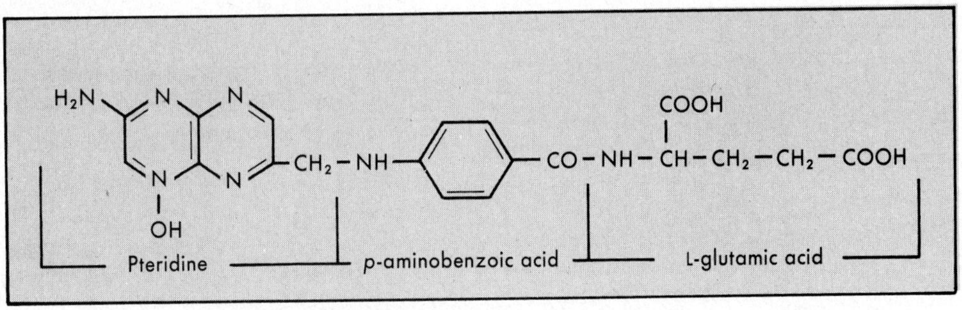

Fig. 17-10. Molecular structure of pteroylmonoglutamic acid (folic acid).

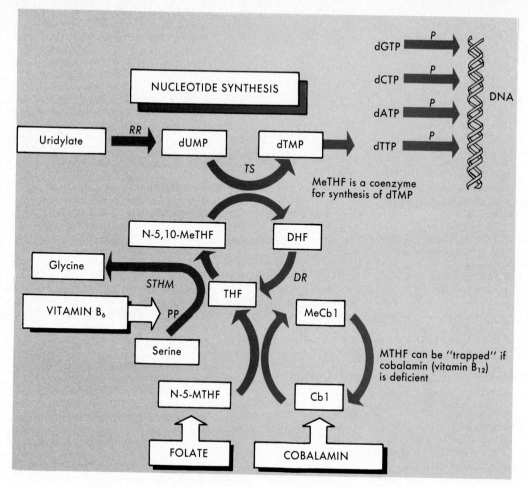

Fig. 17-11   Interaction of folates with nucleotidyl metabolism.

sis) and during the last few months of pregnancy. Whereas vitamin B_{12} stores may take years to deplete, folate stores only provide a 2 to 4 month reserve. Alcohol abuse can result in megaloblastic anemia within a few weeks because of the many mechanisms of disturbance associated with liver damage, poor diet, and malabsorption.

Malabsorption disorders may adversely affect the availability of cobalamin and iron, in addition to folate. As a result, microcytic and macrocytic processes may both exist and the MCV of peripheral red cells may be normal. Examination of the smear, however, often reveals a dimorphic population of small and large cells, including hypochromic macrocytes.

Megaloblastic anemia of hereditary disorders

Deficiencies of enzymes of the purine and pyrimidine pathways of DNA synthesis can produce megaloblastic anemias. These are rare, but often severe, disorders due to the

CAUSES OF FOLATE DEFICIENCY

Dietary deficiency

Lack of green leafy vegetables ("foliage") and animal foods with high folate content

Disorders affecting absorption

Tropical sprue
  Possibly an infectious disease, endemic in some tropical regions; disrupts intestinal absorption of dietary folate and that recycled via the EHC pathway.
Celiac disease
  Nontropical sprue: inability to absorb certain fats and carbohydrates, intolerance to glutens of grains; primarily seen in children, may persist into adulthood; iron deficiency is also often present.
Idiopathic steatorrhea
  Nontropical sprue: gluten intolerance in adults, may be hereditary.
Competitive use of folates due to overgrowth of intestinal bacteria

Interference by drugs and alcohol

Administration of anticonvulsant drugs:
  Diphenylhydantoin (Dilantin), phenobarbital, primidone (Mysoline)
Drugs that inhibit dihydrofolate reductase and DNA synthesis
  Methotrexate, trimethoprim, triamterene (a diuretic)
Alcohol abuse
  Especially in association with cirrhosis of liver; interferes with absorption, storage of folate in liver, EHC cycle, and use by cell.

Increased demand for folate

Pregnancy
  Especially during third trimester and immediately post partum; fetal needs increase maternal dietary demands up to ten fold.
Increased cell turnover
  Some malignancies and hematopoietic responses to chronic hemorrhage or hemolytic anemias (e.g., sickle cell crisis, thalassemia, immune destruction)

generalized deficit in cell replication: mental and physical retardation are usually present. **Orotic aciduria** is an autosomal recessive disorder resulting in a deficiency of one or two enzymes that convert orotic acid to uridine-5-phosphate (pyrimidine nucleotide pathway). The excess orotic acid is excreted in the urine, a diagnostic indicator in megaloblastic anemias that do not respond to folate of vitamin B_{12} therapy. The disease may also be accompanied by severe, fatal infections; an impairment of cell mediated immunity and decreased number of T helper cells has been noted in a few patients.

Other hereditary disorders may result in megaloblastosis that is unresponse to vitamin therapy. Lesch-Nyhan syndrome is a sex-linked disorder of purine synthesis manifested by severe mental and neurological disturbances, including self-mutilating behavior. These children have a deficiency of hypoxanthine-guanine phosphoribosyl transferase. Deficiencies of dihydrofolate reductase, N-5-methyl tetrahydrofolate transferase, and formiminotransferase have also been reported (Wintrobe, 1981).

ERYTHROCYTOSIS

Production of red blood cells increases as a response to hypoxia or blood loss, provided that the raw materials for synthesis of hemoglobin and other cell constituents are available. This response is appropriate as a compensatory (homeostatic) mechanism to maintain adequate red cell and hemoglobin concentrations. **Erythrocytosis** is identified in the marrow as a relative hyperplasia of erythroid elements (decrease in marrow M:E) and in the peripheral blood with the appearance of reticulocytes and polychromatophilic red cells. This normal erythrocytic response is *secondary* to the condition that caused the anemia and it is manifested as an *absolute* increase in the red cell mass, mediated by erythropoietin. The term **secondary polycythemia** is also used for this normal response, seen in acclimation to high altitudes (Chapter 3) and in response to conditions that decrease oxygen availability (chronic pulmonary diseases and circulatory abnormalities, carbon monoxide poisoning; see box below). Note that the response is normal, but the condition that stimulated it is most often pathological. Some forms of hemoglobin have an abnormally high affinity for oxygen, resulting in tissue hypoxia that is compensated by erythrocytosis (Chapter 18).

Erythropoietin can also be elaborated in inappropriate circumstances, that is, when tissue hypoxia is absent. Most instances involve tumors or cysts of the kidneys: Wilms' tumor (a sarcoma), hypernephroma,

renal adenoma, and polycystic kidney disease. Neoplasms of other tissues are also known to possess erythropoiesis-stimulating activity: liver (hepatoma), uterus (leiomyoma), adrenal glands (pheochromocytoma), ovaries (luteoma), and cerebellum (hemangioblastoma). Cushing's syndrome, involving hyperactive secretion of steroids by the adrenal glands, is often associated with a mild erythrocytosis. Administration of androgens or androgen-producing tumors also exerts and erythropoietin-like effect. Some of these tissues, such as the liver, secrete erythropoietin identical to the molecule derived from the kidneys and it is presumed to act directly on marrow red cell precursors. The biochemical mechanisms of products derived from other tissues are less clearly understood.

Familial erythrocytosis describes a heterogeneous collection of disorders that appear to be inherited. Autosomal recessive and dominant means of transmission are known or suspected from studies of affected siblings. Most of these disorders are benign, requiring intervention only to relieve symptoms of high blood pressure or cardiac stress. Many cases, described decades ago, can now be attributed to inheritance of hemoglobins with increased oxygen affinities. The abnormal amino acid substitutions associated with these hemoglobinopathies are listed in the next chapter. Other congenital forms of erythrocytosis involve deficiencies of the erythrocyte glycolytic pathways affecting 2,3-DPG production (increasing hemoglobin oxygen affinity), excess production of erythropoietin independent of hypoxia, and idiopathic cases for which no mechanisms have been identified.

Relative erythrocytosis

A decrease in the plasma volume *relative* to a normal red cell mass will result in an *apparent* increase in the hemoglobin and red cell concentration. This type of **relative erythrocytosis** or polycythemia is seen in patients suffering from dehydration, burns, and those undergoing aggressive diuretic

---

CONDITIONS ASSOCIATED WITH SECONDARY ERYTHROCYTOSIS

Decreased atmospheric oxygen (high altitudes)
Pulmonary diseases
   Chronic obstructive pulmonary disease (COPD)
   Diffuse pulmonary infiltration
   Chronic cor pulmonale
Cardiac and circulatory abnormalities
   Right to left shunt of cardiac circulation
   Abdominal circulatory shunting due to cirrhosis of the liver
   Hereditary hemorrhagic telangiectasia (Chapter 22)
   Idiopathic pulmonary arteriovenous aneurysms
Hypoventilation syndromes
   Intermittent alveolar hypoventilation in normal males
   Central alvolar hyperventilation: barbiturate toxicity, encephalitis, Parkinson's disease, Pickwickian syndrome
   Peripheral alveolar hypoventilation: poliomyelitis, severe spondylitis, muscular dystrophy
Disorders involving hemoglobin
   Carbon monoxide poisoning (mild erythrocytosis)
   Some forms of hemoglobin M (Chapter 18)
   Abnormal hemoglobins with high oxygen affinity (Chapter 18)

therapy. Middle-age, overweight males, particularly those with heavy cigarette smoking habits, histories of chronic alcohol consumption, and stress-producing occupations, may have a relative erythrocytosis that has been referred to as "stress polycythemia", pseudopolycythemia, or Gaisböck's syndrome. These men may hypoventilate while asleep or lying recumbent. Hypertension and cardiovascular disease are often associated conditions. Smoking continuously for 2 hours or more can elevate carboxyhemoglobin levels to 15%, but neither this nor the other findings provide a satisfactory explanation for the syndrome. The red cell mass is usually normal or slightly elevated and the absolute plasma volume is usually decreased. The hematocrit rarely exceeds 60%, but it may be necessary to differentiate this condition from erythrocytosis of an absolute nature.

MYELOPROLIFERATIVE DISORDERS

Increased red blood cell production due to mechanisms inherent in erythrocytic precursors constitute one or more forms of **myeloproliferative disorder,** analogous to leukemia in white cells and essential thrombocythemia in platelets (see Chapter 20). These diseases are thought to be clonal neoplasms, on the basis of chromosome markers and isoenzyme studies. They can be classified on the basis of the hematopoietic abnormalities and the course of the disease. Primary polycythemia or **polycythemia vera (PV)** is an autonomous increase in red cell mass that is not associated with tissue hypoxia. **Erythroleukemia** or Di Guglielmo's syndrome is a form of erythroid and myeloid neoplasm that is related to acute myelocytic leukemia. Other myeloproliferative disorders (myeloid metaplasia, refractory anemia, sideroblastic anemia) may be intermediate stages or specific manifestations in a complex of preleukemic and leukemic conditions. These conditions are discussed and compared in the sections on myeloproliferative disorders and myelodysplastic syndromes in Chapter 20.

Polycythemia vera (PV)

Primary polycythemia, or erythremia, occurs mainly in older adults, with peak occurrence at 50 to 80 years of age. The incidence is estimated to be between 0.6 and 1.8 per 100,000, with a slight bias for males and caucasians. Like other myeloproliferative disorders, the etiological basis remains controversial. Up to half the patients display chromosomal abnormalities, such as trisomy of 8, partial deletion of 20, and morphological abnormalities in number 1. Several lines of evidence point to a neoplasm of clonal origin, most likely involving the pluripotential stem cell that preceeds the erythrocytic, granulocytic, and thrombocytic blast cells. As the disease progresses, the marrow becomes increasingly hypercellular, involving the three cell lines (panmyelosis) and the peripheral cell concentrations may increase accordingly. Basophils are often increased, a feature shared with chronic myelocytic leukemia (CML). Leukocyte alkaline phosphatase activity (LAP) increases in PV but is decreased in CML. Eventually, the marrow may become fibrotic and the patient develop the classic features of myeloid metaplasia. Because this compromises cell production, the magnitude of erythrocytosis may decrease, but immature elements (nucleated red cells, metamyelocytes) may increase. Iron deficiency may occur, moderating red cell production. The disease may progress to acute myelogenous leukemia, especially in those treated with myelosuppressive drugs or radiotherapy.

Extramedullary hematopoiesis is a common feature and splenomegaly is seen in about 75% of the patients with PV. The increased amount of cell reproduction is partly offset by ineffective erythropoiesis; increased nucleotide catabolism results in elevated serum uric acid levels and the onset of gout in many patients. Over 90% of the patients with PV tested show an increase in serum histidine levels.

The increased red cell mass causes an increase in blood viscosity, especially appar-

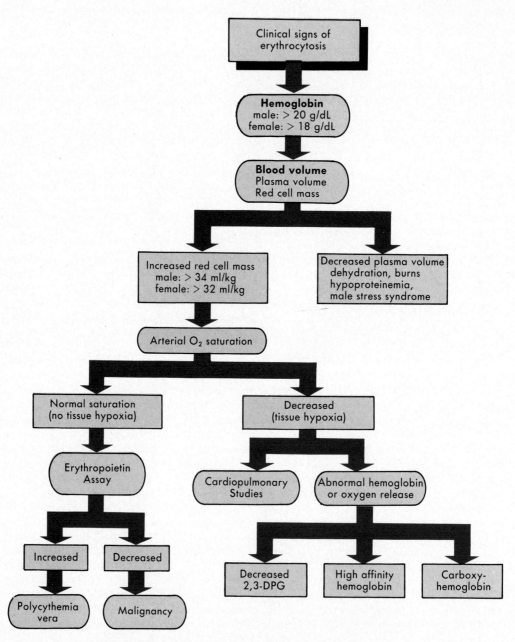

Fig. 17-12   Laboratory characterization of erythrocytosis.

ent in the microvasculature. Tissue hypoxia can result, leading to cerebral stroke and cardiac damage. In older or weakened individuals, the increased workload required to pump thicker blood can result in congestive heart failure. Systolic hypertension is a common feature in advanced disease that is untreated. Distension of vessels by the increased blood volume leads to formation of thrombotic deposits and stimulation of hypercoagulative activity.

One of the major problems for the physician is distinguishing the clinical symptoms of PV from those of secondary erythrocytosis. Laboratory studies are helpful and a typical sequence is illustrated in Fig. 17-12. Symptoms, such as ruddy complexion and high blood pressure, associated with hypervolemia and hyperviscosity are confirmed by a hemoglobin determination. A persistent hemoglobin value of greater than 20 g/dL in males or greater than 18 g/dL in females indicates erythrocytosis. Ruling out dehydration and determining total protein concentration eliminates decreased plasma volume in most cases, but an isotope-based determination of plasma volume or red cell mass can establish the presence of absolute polycythemia. Arterial oxygen saturation studies distinguish secondary erythrocytosis due to hypoxia from other causes. If hypoxia is present, exami-

nation of the patient for circulatory anomalies or pulmonary disease is made. Laboratory studies for abnormal hemoglobins, increased carboxyhemoglobin, or 2,3-DPG deficiency may also be indicated. If oxygen saturation studies are normal, an assay for erythropoietin can be used to distinguish PV (decreased erythropoietin) from tumors and other conditions associated with increased erythropoietin production. Marrow studies will confirm the presence of myeloproliferative processes. Future diagnostic workups will probably include more reliable assays for erythropoietin and biochemical studies of pluripotent stem cells. Table 17-3 compares laboratory findings for relative, secondary and primary mechanisms of erythrocytosis.

Therapy for polycythemia depends on the etiological mechanism involved. Secondary types of erythrocytosis are usually corrected by removing or correcting the source of disturbance: excising a tumor, compensating for hypoventilation, repairing circulatory anomalies, or successfully treating pulmonary disease. Polycythemia vera usually requires phlebotomy to relieve the hypervolemia and reduce the hemoglobin concentration. The frequency of phlebotomy and the volume of blood removed depends on the age and health of the patient. Since the removal of one or two units (about 500

Table 17-3. Comparison of laboratory results in erythrocytosis

Observation	Relative	Secondary	Primary (PV)
Character of disorder:	Decreased plasma volume	Hypoxia	Clonal neoplasm
Hemoglobin	Increased	Increased	Increased
Red cell mass	Normal	Increased	Increased
Marrow cellularity	Normal	Erythroid hyperplasia	Panmyelosis
Tissue iron stores	Normal	Normal	Decreased
Erythropoietin	Normal	Increased	Decreased
Arterial oxygen saturation	Normal	Decreased	Normal
Leukocyte alkaline phosphatase	Normal	Normal	Increased

to 600 mL/unit) of blood could have an adverse consequence in an older patient with relative erythrocytosis, a diagnosis of PV must be made with care. The goal of sequential phlebotomies, conducted over several months, is to induce a state of iron deficiency that helps limit red cell production. Hoewver, as PV progresses and panmyelosis becomes manifest, myelosuppres-

Gastric analysis (pH):	5.1	(normal = 1.4 to 4.4)
after histamine stim.:	4.9	(normal = 0.8 to 3.8)
Serum vitamin B_{12}:	67 pg/mL	(normal = 160-740 pg/mL)
Serum folate:	14.6 ng/mL	(normal = 2.5-15.0 ng/mL)
Ova and parasites (stool):	negative	

sive chemotherapy or radiotherapy is usually necessary.

Case History

PRESENTATION:

R.C., a 52-year-old white female, was seen by her physician because of numbness in her hands and feet for the past 3 weeks. She had also felt weak and dizzy for about 6 months, but she attributed it to ageing and occasional periods of heavy drinking. The dizziness had grown progressively worse and she often felt disoriented.

PHYSICAL EXAMINATION:

The patient is somewhat underweight, she is pale in complexion, and she appears ill at ease, but is otherwise not in acute distress. Her blood pressure and other vital signs are normal. Examination of neurological, pulmonary, cardiac, and other organ systems were unremarkable.

INITIAL LABORATORY DATA:

WBC: 3.1 X 10^3/μL	HCT: 23%
Seg. Neut.: 40%	HGB: 10.4 g/dL
Band Neut.: 11%	RBC: 1.81 X 10^6/μL
Lymph.: 46%	MCV: 127fL
Mono.: 3%	MCH: 40.9 pg
PLT: 124 X 10^3/μL	MCHC: 32.2%
Retic.: 0.4%	

Smear: macrocytosis (4+), ovalo-macrocytes, Howell-Jolly bodies, hypersegmented neutrophils (6 of 40).

BUN, glucose, electrolytes, and total protein were normal. Urinalysis was normal.

FURTHER STUDIES:

The patient was admitted to a local hospital for additional study of macrocytic anemia. Radiographs of the chest and gastrointestinal tract were normal. Further questioning revealed a 10-year history of sporadic alcohol abuse, but she denied poor or unusual eating habits.

ADDITIONAL LABORATORY STUDIES:

The findings of achlorohydria and decreased serum cobalamin level was followed by performance of a two-stage Schilling test. After an oral dose of 0.5 μg of radioactive cobalamin and 1000 μg of stable cobalamin I.M., a 24 hour urine assay yielded 2.2% of the dose. Three days later, the test was repeated with radioactive cobalamin and 60 mg of hog intrinsic factor, resulting in 8.5% of the dose excreted in 24 hours. A lack of intrinsic factor and a diagnosis of pernicious anemia was established.

TREATMENT:

The patient was started on parenteral vitamin B_{12}, 1000 μg per day and discharged with instructions to return every 5 days for a hematocrit and reticulocyte determination.

Day	Retic count	Hematocrit	
5	0.3%	22%	
10	12.3%	24%	
15	20.1%	25%	Vitam. B_{12} reduced to 1 mg/mo.
20	0.9%	30%	
30	0.8%	36%	

The patient continues to do well 2 years later as she continues to receive parenteral cobalamin. The macrocytic anemia has disappeared and no neurological symptoms are present.

SUMMARY

• Disorders of red cell production include disturbances in the stem cell population (destruction, displacement, suppression), disruption of the marrow tissue architecture, deficiencies in enzymes or nutrients that disrupt DNA synthesis and nuclear maturation, and hyperproliferative disorders.

- Aplastic anemia is a failure of blood cell production that can be congenital, acquired or idiopathic. Exposure to toxic drugs and radiation damage are common acquired causes.

- Failure of red cell production only is termed pure red cell aplasia (PRCA). A congenital form (Diamond-Blackfan syndrome) and two acquired forms of PRCA are generally recognized.

- Stromal disease is a disruption of the marrow tissue structure, producing a myelophthisic blood picture (pancytopenia, immature WBCs, large platelets, nucleated RBCs) and fibrotic marrow.

- Dyserythropoiesis results in the hyperplastic production of abnormal marrow RBC precursors, anemia due to intramedullary destruction (ineffective erythropoiesis) and peripheral hemolysis. Nuclear-cytoplasmic asynchrony and bizarre morphological red cells are characteristic. Several forms of congenital dyserythropoietic anemia (CDA) have been described, some involving immunological mechanisms of pathology.

- Anemias may be associated with certain chronic diseases (mainly infections), renal and hepatic diseases, malignancies, and endocrine disorders. Changes in erythropoietin production, oxygen consumption in body tissues, and dietary factors have been proposed as pathogenetic mechanisms.

- Macrocytic anemias are defined on the basis of decreased RBC or hemoglobin levels in combination with increased MCVs (>100 fL). Megaloblastic anemias are characterized by giant blood cell precursors in the marrow, a nuclear maturation deficit, and peripheral macrocytosis. A megaloblast is a stage in the maturation sequence of giant red cell precursors, analogous to the stages of the normoblastic (rubricytic) series.

- The two most common causes of megaloblastic anemia are vitamin B_{12} (cobalamin) and folate deficiency. Either may be caused by decreased dietary intake, by malabsorption, or by metabolic deficiencies in transport or use.

- Pernicious anemia is defined as a cobalamin deficiency due to a lack of intrinsic factor, associated with achlorhydria (deficiency of gastric acid). Autoantibodies to IF, parietal cells, and other tissues are often present. The Schilling test, comparing cobalamin absorption and excretion with and without IF, is a definitive test for PA.

- Cobalamin and folate interact in pathways of protein metabolism and nucleotide synthesis. Both are required for nuclear maturation. The body has a cobalamin reserve of several years and a folate reserve of several months. Pregnancy increases folate demand; alcohol abuse interferes with folate metabolism at several points.

- Erythrocytosis or polycythemia are general terms for increased red cell production. Most increases are adaptive secondary responses to tissue hypoxia, stimulating erythropoietin and RBC production. Tumors of some tissues can stimulate erythropoietin inappropriately.

- Familial forms of erythocytosis are often associated with inheritance of hemoglobins with high affinities for oxygen, others are idiopathic.

- Relative erythocytosis, measured as an increased hemoglobin or RBC count, is caused by a decreased plasma volume. This can be due to dehydration, burns, low plasma protein, or a stress syndrome peculiar to middle-aged males.

- Primary erythrocytosis or polycythemia vera is a myeloproliferative disorder resulting from a clonal neoplasm. The disease often progresses to myeloid metaplasia and acute myelocytic leukemia.

18

Disorders Involving Hemoglobin

PROBLEMS WITH HEMOGLOBIN SYNTHESIS AND FUNCTION

Hemoglobin is the molecule responsible for transporting respiratory gases to and from the tissues. If hemoglobin is not present in sufficient quantities or if the molecule's structure does not facilitate normal oxygen uptake and release, anoxia (anemia) results. As with disorders involving other blood cells, hemoglobin problems can be inherited or acquired.

Manifestations of these disorders provide clues to their cause. Red cells on a peripheral smear that appear to be deficient in hemoglobin content (decreased MCH and MCHC) indicate an impairment in the production process. Microcytic hypochromic cells are typically associated with deficiencies of iron and with impaired globin production. The former is confirmed by serum and tissue iron studies, the latter by protein electrophoresis. Hemoglobins with congenital abnormal molecular sequences may form crystals under certain conditions of low oxygen saturation. In addition to impaired oxygen carrying capacity, the cells have a shortened survival time. These cells can be tentatively identified by their morphological appearance, and definitively identified by their electrophoretic pattern. The presence of basophilic stippling in mature RBCs and increased amounts of heme precursor molecules in plasma or urine is typically found in enzyme defects caused by lead poisoning, specific hepatic diseases, or as a result of a genetic abnormality in the enzyme structure. Fig. 18-1 summarizes the major steps in hemoglobin synthesis at which abnormalities occur.

Other problems in hemoglobin function are acquired as a result of exposure to materials that compete with oxygen for transport. Carbon monoxide, for example, irreversibly binds to hemoglobin at 210 times the rate of oxygen. Exposure to significant amounts of carbon monoxide or to certain sulfurous compounds can produce immediate and serious consequences, including cyanosis (blue color from lack of oxygen), tissue anoxia, and death. All of these problems involve the hemoglobin molecule, but the mechanisms and underlying etiologies are quite diverse (Table 18-1). Following the same sequence, we will look first at disorders of iron metabolism, examine defects of heme and globin synthesis, and, finally, review problems occurring after hemoglobin production is complete.

DISORDERS OF IRON METABOLISM

The pathways and mechanisms of iron metabolism were briefly introduced in Chapter 4. Disorders can be attributed to problems with ingestion (dietary intake and gastric reduction), absorption, transport, storage, and utilization. Measurements of plasma iron and transferrin, the transport protein, are widely used to assess iron status. Plasma iron concentrations are dependent on the amount of iron released from ferritin stores of the reticuloendothelial system (RES) and the amount incorporated into the erythropoietic and other heme-synthesizing tissues of the body (Fig. 18-2).

Synthesis and release of transferrin is reciprocal to plasma iron levels: hepatocytes produce less transferrin when iron levels are high and more transferrin when levels are low. The sum of transport protein that is saturated by iron (plasma iron) and that which is unsaturated equals the **total iron binding capacity (TIBC)** of the plasma. The amount of transferrin associated with iron is often expressed as percent saturated. These parameters can be informative in the

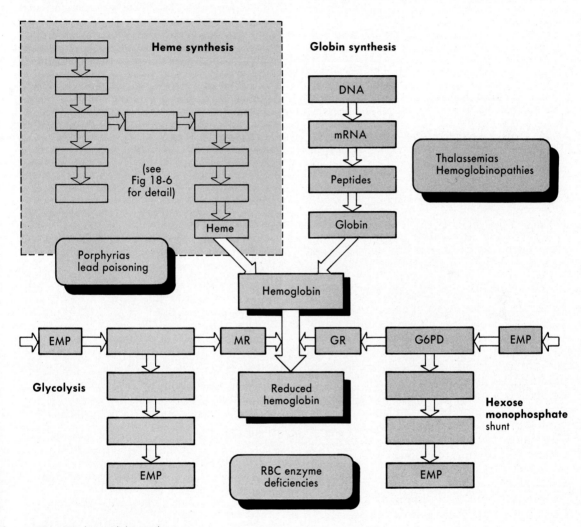

Fig. 18-1.   Disorders of hemoglobin production and function.

MR = Methemoglobin reductase
GR = Glutathione reductase
G6PD = Glucose-6-phosphate dehydrogenase
EMP = Embden-Meyerhof pathway

Table 18-1. Summary of hemoglobin disorders

Disorder	Etiology	Critical laboratory tests
Iron deficiency anemia	Gastrointestinal blood loss	Serum iron, TIBC, ferritin; fecal occult blood
	Insufficient dietary iron	Serum iron, TIBC, ferritin
Sideroblastic anemia	Neoplastic transformation	Marrow cell examination, iron stain
Porphyria	Hereditary or acquired	Free erythrocyte protoporphyrin; urinary porphyrins
Thalassemia	Hereditary; deficiency in globin production	Hemoglobin electrophoresis
Sickle cell anemia and other hemoglobinopathies	Hereditary: abnormal amino acid sequence in globin	Hemoglobin electrophoresis
Unstable hemoglobins	Hereditary: amino acid substitution	Heinz bodies; electrophoresis; spectral analysis
G-6-PD and other enzyme deficiencies	Hereditary: decrease in EMP HMS, or HRP enzymes	Enzyme spot tests; Heinz bodies on smears

differential diagnosis of anemias and disturbances of iron metabolism (Fig. 18-3). Assessment of stored iron is made either by staining deposits of iron in marrow and RES tissues or by measuring serum ferritin levels.

Iron deficiency is defined as a decrease in plasma iron concentration below that of reference values (each laboratory should establish its own limits). **Iron deficiency anemia (IDA)** occurs when the plasma and storage pools of iron are insufficient for hemoglobin production. Unless other red cell disorders or deficiency processes (such as cobalamin or folate) are present to confuse the morphological picture, untreated IDA is eventually manifested by the appearance of microcytic, hypochromic red blood cells.

Dietary iron can be ingested in a form associated with heme, from meat sources as hemoglobin and myoglobin, or in a nonheme form, from vegetables and eggs, as ferritin and hemosiderin. Iron ingested in a nonheme form requires vitamin C (ascorbic acid) for optimal absorption, whereas iron incorporated into heme does not. Gastric pepsin releases the iron and it is bound to chelators and carried into the lower intestine. Most iron absorption occurs in the upper duodenum, although some is transported across mucosal cells in the rest of the gastrointestinal tract.

Poor dietary intake is rarely a cause of iron deficiency anemia in developed countries, except in infants, rapidly growing adolescents, and pregnant women. In these instances, demand is increased above normal maintenance levels. However, in the latter, iron deficiency is common, with about one-fourth of pregnant women in developed countries experiencing IDA. Whelby (1984) determined the following amounts of iron are used during a full term pregnancy:

200-600 mg	expanded maternal red cell mass
200-370 mg	fetal red cell mass (80 mg/kg of fetal weight)
90-310 mg	lost during parturition
30-170 mg	contained in placenta and umbilical cord

These amounts can be compared with the usual amount of iron lost during menstruation (10 to 45 mg per month). Supplements

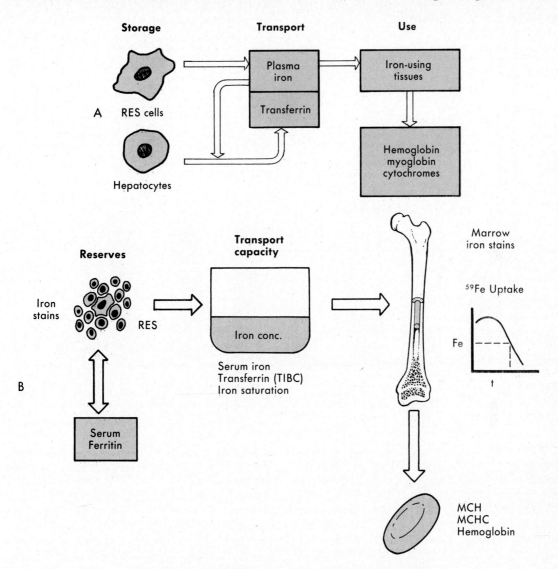

Fig. 18-2 Ferrokinetic compartments in iron disorders.

of oral iron, especially during the last trimester, are usually sufficient to meet the increased demand during pregnancy and the loss of blood at delivery. In nondeveloped countries, iron deficiency, with or without anemia, may be common. It is estimated that up to one-third of the world's population may not ingest sufficient dietary iron. The actual magnitude of the problem is difficult to evaluate, since most studies are based on nutritional data and hemoglobin measurements rather than iron studies. Insufficient dietary iron is further compounded by bacterial and parasitic infections (especially hookworm) that disrupt intestinal absorption.

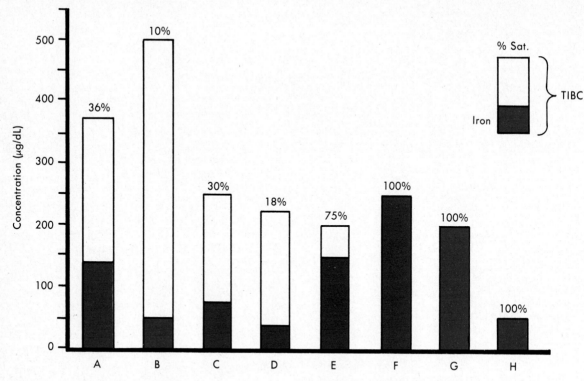

Fig. 18-3   Serum iron, TIBC, and ferritin in iron disorders.

By far the most prevalent cause of iron deficiency, particulary in adult men, is related to chronic bleeding, especially from the gastrointestinal tract. Each 2 mL of blood contains about 1 mg of iron. Thus, even a moderate hemorrhage of 10 to 20 mL of blood per day can offset the amount of iron ingested (10 to 15 mg) and absorbed (1 to 2 mg). Additional blood loss results in iron deficiency and signs of anemia appear as the iron stores are exhausted. A loss of 100 mL/day (50 mg of iron) would lead to complete exhaustion of a 1500 mg store in only 1 month. Losses of this magnitude may be associated with ulcerous lesions, malignancies, and esophageal varices and they may be exacerbated by alcoholism and aspirin ingestion. In women of childbearing age, excess menstrual losses or depletion during pregnancy results in IDA, unless replenished by good dietary sources or oral iron supplements.

Iron loss can also occur as a result of malabsorption caused by sprue, infestation by hookworms and other parasites, some gastrointestinal bacterial infections, or following partial to total gastrectomy. Iron deficiency may be associated with pernicious anemia (achlorohydria and parietal cell dysfunction or loss) and other conditions that disturb gastrointestinal integrity.

Intravascular hemolysis can result in the loss of iron through the kidneys. When the red cell destruction is massive or prolonged, haptoglobin and other protein carriers of hemoglobin are exhausted and the excess is excreted in the urine (hemoglobinuria). Some hemoglobin is reabsorbed in the tu-

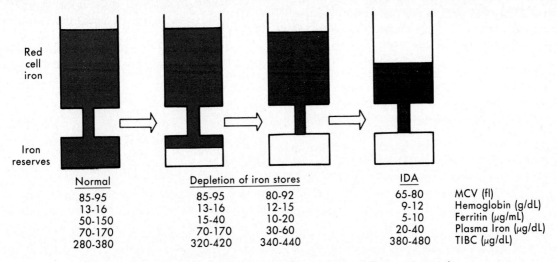

	Normal	Depletion of iron stores		IDA	
	85-95	85-95	80-92	65-80	MCV (fl)
	13-16	13-16	12-15	9-12	Hemoglobin (g/dL)
	50-150	15-40	10-20	5-10	Ferritin (μg/mL)
	70-170	70-170	30-60	20-40	Plasma Iron (μg/dL)
	280-380	320-420	340-440	380-480	TIBC (μg/dL)

Fig. 18-4   Changes in laboratory values in iron deficiency anemia.

bules and stored as hemosiderin. This is lost as the tubular cells are routinely shed into the lumen of the nephron and passed into the urine. Similar mechanisms of iron loss occur during hemolysis associated with paroxysmal nocturnal hemoglobinuria (PNH, see Chapter 19) and mechanical hemolysis caused by prosthetic heart valves.

An interesting form of iron deficiency has been noted in long distance runners. Many do not have anemia whereas others have a typical picture of IDA with microcytic, hypochromic red cells (**runner's anemia**). Although several mechanisms were initially proposed to account for the low hemoglobin and iron concentrations, most evidence points to loss of blood from the gastrointestinal tract. During intense exertion, such as that required for fast marathon times, blood is shunted from the gut for prolonged periods (hours), producing ischemia and damage to the mucosal layer. Iron is lost with the sloughed mucosal cells and in the red cells that pass into the bowel. The bleeding can be detected up to 2 days later by a positive test for fecal occult blood. Fortunately, the GI bleeding is transient and the iron deficiency responds to oral ferrous sulfate, but

this condition must be distinguished from other causes of GI hemorrhage, such as gastrointestinal lesions and malignancies.

The appearance of hypochromic microcytic red blood cells, along with the classic signs of anemia (pallor, fatigue, bradycardia and weak, fluttering pulse), is the last stage in development of iron deficiency. It is important to note the sequence of changes in laboratory values commonly employed to ascertain iron status (Fig. 18-4). As the deficiency develops, iron stores are depleted first and serum ferritin levels drop below normal. With further depletion of stored iron, serum iron levels may decrease slightly and transferrin (TIBC) levels may be slightly increased, but saturation levels may be only slightly decreased or low normal. Free erythrocyte protoporphyrin (FEP) can also be measured and this will remain normal until iron is no longer available in sufficient amounts to accommodate hemoglobin synthesis. Prior to development of laboratory-defined anemia (low hemoglobin and changes in red cell morphology), accumulations of porphyrin compounds can be detected by exposing red cells to ultraviolet light. Although increased FEP is not diagnostic of iron deficiency (many other types of disturbance in porphyrin synthesis can produce similar findings, which will be described later), it can be used to monitor iron status before anemia is apparent. FEP can be used to distinguish IDA from thalassemia, since the latter is also manifested as a hypochromic microcytic anemia. However, thalassemia results from defective globin synthesis, the heme molecule is completed, and FEP is normal (values are usually less than 50 µg/dL of whole blood). In the presence of increased FEP, serum iron should be decreased and TIBC should be increased. Serum ferritin values should be extremely low. Iron saturation should be very low (<15%) and an examination of marrow or RES tissue stained with Prussian blue should reveal no iron granules. Hemoglobin values should be only minimally depressed, unless bleeding is the underlying cause of the pending IDA. Microcytic changes probably precede hypochromia, but as the deficiency becomes more acute, hemoglobin values fall below 11 g/dL (MCH <25pg) or less and the MCV decreases to less than 75 fL. FEP may exceed 100 µg/dL of whole blood and serum iron may be less than 30 µg/dL. Examination of the marrow reveals a mild to moderate erythroid hyperplasia, often accompanied by signs of dyserythropoiesis (abnormal nuclei, scanty cytoplasm, intramedullary phagocytosis, etc.) The low to normal reticulocyte count and decreased red cell count are further indications of the marrow's inability to produce mature red cells despite the hyperplastic response of the stem cells.

As clinical manifestations of anemia become pronounced, some individuals acquire abnormal appetites for substances such as ice, chalk, and dirt. **Pica** is a term for this behavioral change, but this must be distinguished from the practice of some cultures in which clay eating or similar habits occur as a learned ritual. Interestingly, most of these substances are not compensatory sources of iron, but the behavior seen in IDA may be part of an evolutionary response for dealing with dietary deficiencies in general.

Treatment for IDA is often empirical, provided that underlying causes have also been ruled out. Oral iron is usually given as ferrous sulfate for routine supplementation and replacement, but parenteral iron is given when a rapid response is required, persistent bleeding requires additional amounts, the patient is unable to tolerate oral iron, or gastrointestinal disorder prevents digestion and absorption. The response to therapy is monitored, using clinical manifestations as an immediate indicator. Patients usually begin feeling better within a week from the onset of treatment, although the hemoglobin or hematocrit may not return to normal for 1 to 3 months. Reticulocyte counts may increase to levels of 3% to 10%, depending on the severity of the anemia, within a week of beginning therapy. Marrow cellularity and reticulocyte count return to normal as the peripheral manifestations of hypoxia are relieved.

Iron overload and hemochromatosis

It has been noted that the body can dispose of iron only by loss of blood cells or by losing mucosal cells containing iron. Excess iron can accumulate as a result of increased intake or absorption. Persons with adequate iron stores that ingest large amounts of oral iron supplements may accumulate increased amounts of tissue iron stores. This can also occur in areas of the world where people use iron cookware to prepare all of their food. The administration of multiple blood transfusions in patients that are not hemorrhaging (hemolytic anemias, marrow production failures) will produce an iron overload unless iron chelating agents (e.g., desferrioxamine) are also given. Some types of anemia (thalassemias, sideroblastic anemias) also result in iron accumulation because iron absorption increases in response to the anemia, but iron use is poor because of abnormal hemoglobin formation.

Idiopathic **hemochromatosis** is a hereditary disorder that leads to an increase in absorption of iron by the intestine. The patient experiences some symptoms of anemia (weight loss, fatigue). However, the skin color is usually darker than normal and more serious signs appear, such as abdominal and joint pain, hepatomegaly, and cardiac failure. Increased iron stores are preferentially distributed in the parenchymal cells of the liver, whereas the spleen and marrow macrophages store the excess iron in thalassemia and sideroblastic anemia. Serum iron, TIBC, and ferritin levels are increased, as expected. If family studies indicate a probable genetic basis and other causes have been ruled out (alcoholic cirrhosis may also be associated with increased stores of iron in the liver), many patients benefit from diets to restrict iron intake and periodic phlebotomy to reduce the accumulated iron.

Sideroblastic anemias

Sideroblastic anemia is characterized by **ringed sideroblasts** in the bone marrow, a finding associated with several hereditary, acquired, and idiopathic disorders. Ringed sideroblasts are erythroblasts containing several large aggregates of nonferritin iron located around the periphery of the nucleus (Fig. 18-5). These deposits, associated with the perinuclear mitochondria, indicate either a state of iron overload or ineffective erythropoiesis. In either case, iron transported to the developing erythroblast is not

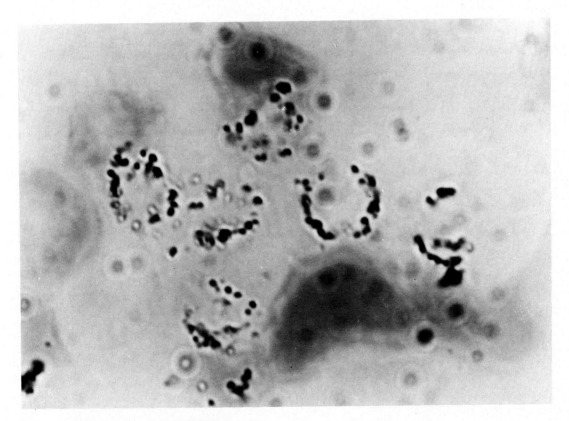

Fig. 18-5. Ringed sideroblasts.
(From Miale, JB: Laboratory medicine: Hematology, ed 6, St Louis, 1982, The CV Mosby Co.)

incorporated into protoporphyrin to form heme and the accumulating iron store can be stained, especially in metarubricytes, with Prussian blue. Ringed sideroblasts (RS) must be distinguished from normal sideroblasts, that is, erythroblasts that contain up to 5 small granules of ferritin. Normally, from 20% to 80% of the marrow erythroblasts will display evidence of cytoplasmic iron, the percent varying directly with the saturation level of transferrin. The presence of more than 6 granules in a cell is indicative of a pathological condition, whether arranged in a perinuclear pattern or diffuse.

Regardless of cause, most forms of sideroblastic anemia (SA) are characterized by hypochromic cells (low MCH and MCHC) and a state of iron overload (high plasma and tissue iron content with normal or low TIBC). Depending on the underlying mechanisms (see box below), the peripheral red

cell morphology may also be dimorphic, consisting of normochromic normocytic (occasionally macrocytic) cells and hypochromic microcytic cells. FEP may be increased, reflecting a defect in the latter stages of heme synthesis. The marrow picture is often hyperplastic and indicative of ineffective erythropoiesis, reflected in a normal or subnormal reticulocyte count. Because of the heterogeneity in underlying mechanisms and causes, sideroblastic anemia should be regarded as a descriptive term rather than the designation for a particular disorder. Until more information is available on acquired and hereditary forms, however, they can be grouped as such for discussion.

The congenital forms of SA are usually recognized in young adults or older children, and occasionally in infants. The severe forms most often involve males, although partial expression of the anemia may be seen in some female relatives. A form of familial SA is less commonly found that is manifested equally in males and females. Iron overload and a dimorphic blood picture characterize these congenital forms.

The acquired forms of SA are more common and, in some cases, better understood. Some authors group these anemias into those that are responsive to pyridoxine or pyridoxal phosphate (PP or vitamin B_6) therapy and those that are not. PP is a cofactor in the formation of delta-aminolevulinic acid in the heme synthesis pathway. SA may result after treatment with isoniazid and other antituberculosis compounds, and chloramphenicol. The latter has been shown to inhibit heme synthase activity, but it doesn't produce anemia in every patient. SA occurs in about 30% of chronic alcoholics due to interference by ethanol metabolites with pyridoxine metabolism. The anemia is reversible within 1 week of discontinuing alcohol or therapy with PP. Megaloblastoid changes, caused by folic acid deficiency, sometimes accompanies alcoholic SA, further exaggerating the

---

TYPES OF SIDEROBLASTIC ANEMIA

Hereditary

Congenital sideroachrestic (sideroblastic) anemia: sex-linked recessive
Sideroblastic anemia: autosomal recessive pattern

Acquired

Secondary to toxic drugs and substances
  Isoniazid and other antituberculosis drugs
  Chloramphenicol: inhibits activity of heme synthase
  Chronic alcohol ingestion: interferes with pyridoxal phosphate activity
  Cytotoxic drugs used for treating leukemia and other malignancies
  Lead poisoning: interferes with ALA dehydrase and heme synthase activities
Secondary to other disorders: malignancies, infections, inflammatory states

Idiopathic

Sideroblastic anemia with ringed sideroblasts (RARS), a form of myelodysplastic syndrome

dimorphic pattern of red cell size. Treatment of neoplasms with alkylating agents and other cytotoxic drugs can also produce SA, but this is usually irreversible and represents a poor prognosis for the disease.

Lead poisoning can occur from inhalation of industrial compounds (adults) or ingesting lead-based paints (young children). The peripheral erythrocytes characteristically display **basophilic stippling,** coarse, dark-staining inclusions that represent aggregated ribosomes and the remnants of mitochondria (Fig. 16-4). Lead poisoning can also be regarded as a form of acquired porphyria, as described later.

SA may also be associated with some malignancies and as a transient condition secondary to infection or acute inflammation. Treatment of the underlying condition usually resolves the anemia. Another form, often called "primary acquired sideroblastic anemia", appears in adults without other known associations (idiopathic). This form appears to represent a clonal change that affects one or more hematopoietic cell lines, often culminating in acute leukemia. For this reason, this form of SA is now classified as a preleukemic or myelodysplastic disorder, **refractory anemia with ringed sideroblasts (RARS)** (see Chapter 20).

DEFICIENCIES OF HEME PRODUCTION: THE PORPHYRIAS

Porphyrias are disorders affecting enzymes of the heme biosynthesis pathway with increased excretion of porphyrin molecules. Several types of porphyria are known. Most are congenital deficiencies of a specific enzyme that result in accumulation of a heme precursor in the tissues (Table 18-2). A few types of porphyria are acquired as a result of drug intoxication, liver damage related to alcoholism, or lead poisoning. Deposition of porphyrins in the skin result in a photosensitive reaction characterized by formation of lesions and scarring. In certain porphyrias, deposition occurs in the nervous system, resulting in an acute attack

Table 18-2. Enzyme deficiencies associated with porphyrias

Enzyme	Clinical disorder
δ-ALA synthase	Increased excretion in several types of porphyria
δ-ALA dehydrase	Lead poisoning; unnamed ALA dehydrase deficiency
UPG I synthase	Acute intermittent porphyria
UPG III cosynthase	Congenital erythropoietic porphyria
UPG decarboxylase	Porphyria cutanea tarda
CPG oxidase	Hereditary coproporphyria
PPG oxidase	Variegate porphyria
Heme synthase	Erythropoietic protoporphyria; lead poisoning

syndrome that includes psychological disturbances and, in some cases, death. The key to understanding these disorders is found in the pathway for heme synthesis (Fig. 18-6).

Acute intermittent porphyria (AIP) is an autosomal dominant deficiency of uroporphyrinogen (UPG) I synthase. Porphobilinogen (PBG) accumulates, since conversion to either UPG I or UPG III products requires UPG I synthase. An increased excretion of PBG accompanies acute attacks of AIP. Neurological manifestations are present in many instances, but cutaneous photosensitivity does not result since PBG is a colorless, nonfluoresecent compound. Other products that may be detected in the urine in increased amounts during acute attacks include delta-aminolevulinic acid (δ-ALA) and uroporphyrin. Assays for the specific enzyme, UPG I synthase, reveal decreased amounts. Much of the time, patients with AIP and the other acute attack types of porphyria (variegate porphyria and hereditary

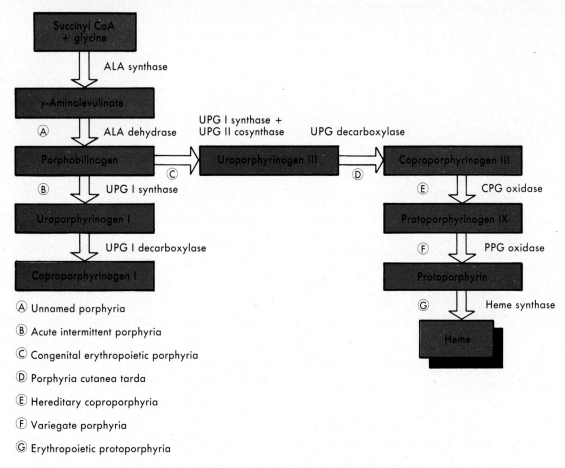

A Unnamed porphyria

B Acute intermittent porphyria

C Congenital erythropoietic porphyria

D Porphyria cutanea tarda

E Hereditary coproporphyria

F Variegate porphyria

G Erythropoietic protoporphyria

Fig. 18-6.   Porphyrias resulting from disturbances in heme synthesis.

coproporphyria) do not display clinical signs of the disorder. During these periods of remission, the urinary PBG and uroporphyrin levels may be normal (UPG I synthase will be decreased in AIP, however). The problem is related to the production of δ-ALA synthase in the liver. This enzyme is responsible for the conversion of succinyl CoA and activated glycine into δ-ALA, a step that is normally controlled by the concentration of heme, the end product of the pathway. During acute attacks, heme repression of the enzyme is blocked (usually by drugs, sex hormones, or specific steroid compounds)

and large amounts of δ-ALA are produced. The lack of UPG I synthase creates an obstacle downstream in the pathway, thus δ-ALA and PBG accumulate in the urine and tissues. Similar manifestations result from a rare, congenital deficiency in δ-ALA dehydrase, except that PBG is not formed and only δ-ALA is excreted in increased amounts.

Congenital erythropoietic porphyria (CEP) is an extremely rare but dramatic disorder caused by a deficiency of UPG III cosynthase. This enzyme is believed to be responsible for a molecular rearrangement in an intermediate product during the conversion of PBG to UPG III, the normal route for heme production. If UPG I synthase acts by itself, PBG is converted to UPG I and subsequent metabolites that are excreted. The disorder is an autosomal recessive trait that is manifested during infancy or early childhood. Lack of the enzyme results in accumulation of large amounts of the I-type isomers, molecules that fluoresce and impart a red color to urine, skin, and tissues. Even bones and teeth will fluoresce a bright red wine color (erythrodentia) when exposed to an ultraviolet lamp. Deposition of these pigments in the skin, followed by exposure to the ultraviolet radiation of sunlight, result in severe cutaneous lesions. Disfigurement and hirsutism (abnormal growth of hair) are characteristic of these young patients. Match these clinical manifestations (abundant facial and arm hair, extensive scarring, red teeth) with behavioral adaptations (avoidance of sunlight) and one can understand why some investigators have speculated on a relationship between CEP and various folk legends of werewolves and vampires.

The next enzyme in the heme pathway is UPG decarboxylase, active in converting UPG III to coproporhyrinogen (CPG) III. A deficiency of this enzyme results in **porphyria cutanea tarda (PCT)**, a form occurring in adults that also is manifested by skin lesions. The symptoms are not as severe as those of CEP and the lesions occur primarily on the outer (dorsal) surface of the hands, face, and ears. The disease is confined to cutaneous signs, often in association with sun exposure. Acute attacks do not occur (no neurological involvement), but PCT has been associated with chronic alcoholic intoxication. Metabolic byproducts of the uroporphyrins and porphyrins that accumulate can be detected in the feces as isocoproporphyrin. An acquired form of PCT can result from ingesting hexachlorobenzene.

Hereditary coproporphyria (HCP) results from a deficiency of coproporphyrinogen oxidase and an accumulation of CPG, detected in increased quantities in feces and urine. It is one of the acute attack porphyrias, with cutaneous and neurological involvement. **Variegate porphyria (VP)** is caused by a deficiency of protoporphyrinogen (PPG) oxidase, resulting in increased fecal and urinary excretion of CPG and increased urinary excretion of PPG. Finally, a deficiency of the last enzyme in the heme pathway, heme synthase or ferrochelatase, results in **erythropoietic protoporphyria (EPP)**. The accumulation of protoporphyrin, a molecule that is less water soluble than the previous porphyrin compounds, is excreted via the bile into the gut. Therefore, fecal protoporphyrin is increased, but urinary protoporphyrin is not. Increased protoporphyrin concentrations in red blood cells are characteristic of this disorder.

Lead poisoning is an acquired form of protoporphyria that is associated with basophilic stippling of red blood cells and accumulation of unused iron. Photosensitivity does not occur, however. Lead inhibits the activity of both δ-ALA dehydrase and heme synthase, but the disturbance is reversible. Urinary δ-ALA and coproporphyrin are increased and erythrocytic protoporphyrin is increased, as measured by a zinc chelation technique. Likewise, in hereditary tyrosinemia, accumulation of a metabolite (succinyl acetone) inhibits PBG synthase. In both of these secondary conditions, δ-ALA excretion is increased, whereas PBG is normal or only slightly increased (compare this to AIP, which also involves the initial part of the heme pathway).

THALASSEMIAS

Thalassemias are hypochromic microcytic anemias that result from hereditary defects in the synthesis of globin chains. The term is derived from the Greek word *thalassa* (sea) because the first cases were described in patients from the Mediterranean region. In fact, evidence of skeletal changes, believed to represent prehistoric

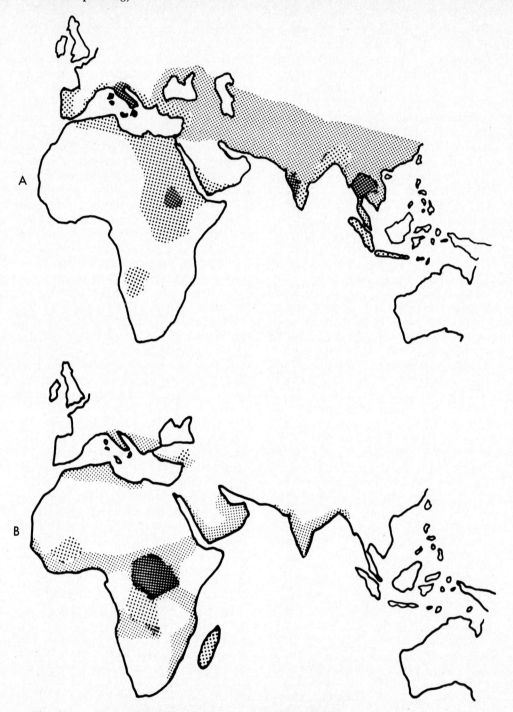

Fig. 18-7. Geographical distribution of hemoglobinopathies.
A, Distribution of thalassemia in the Old World. **B,** Distribution of the sickle cell gene in the Old World. **C,** Distribution of hemoglobin C gene in the Old World. (From Miale, JB: Laboratory medicine: Hematology, ed 6, St Louis, 1982, The CV Mosby Co.)   *Continued.*

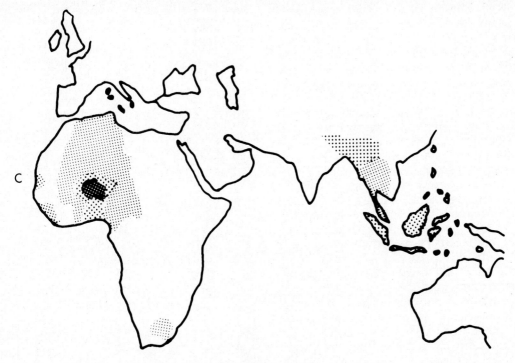

Fig. 18-7. cont'd

examples of thalassemia, are found in human remains that are 50,000 years old. These have been excavated from submerged sites south of Italy and Greece (Zaino, 1964). Although thalassemia is still associated primarily with this region, forms of it are found throughout Africa and Asia (Fig. 18-7).

Severe and mild forms of the disease have been designated **thalassemia major** and **thalassemia minor,** based on the degree of anemia and systemic complications. The degree of severity is related to the number of genes controlling production of the defective globin chain. Defects in production of the alpha chain or beta chain of hemoglobin are classified as **alpha thalassemia** or **beta thalassemia.** Defects in other types of globin chains are also known, as well as conditions in which more than one chain type is involved. Combined hemoglobinopathies result from a globin defect and an-

other type of hemoglobinopathy (e.g., sickle cell/thalassemia).

Genetic mechanisms underlying the manifestations of thalassemia have been investigated extensively in recent years. A number of defects have been proposed to account for the decreased production of globin chains: (1) a partial or total deletion of a structural gene, (2) a mutation in the mRNA strand that encodes the globin, or (3) a mutation that results in either a premature or delayed completion of the peptide sequence. Any of these mechanisms can result in an imbalance between the production rates of alpha and nonalpha chains. Excess chains, produced at the normal rate, accumulate in the cell. These may eventually precipitate as cytoplasmic inclusions, resulting in destruction of the erythrocyte by RES macrophages. Globin structural genes are found on chromosomes 11 and 16

(Fig. 18-8). The alpha chain and its embryonic counterpart, the zeta chain, are located on chromosome 16. Two genes on each homologous chromosome (4 per diploid cell) specify the alpha globin sequence, whereas only one gene per chromosome (two per diploid cell) specifies most of the nonalpha chains on chromosome 11 (the gamma chain is also represented by two sites per chromosome). This is an important difference for understanding the genetic basis of alpha versus beta thalassemia.

Alpha thalassemia results from production deficiencies in the alpha globin chain. The severity of the disease depends on how many of the four structural genes are abnormal. Several genetic mutations have been well characterized:

1. Deletion of a single gene is defined as the α-thal-2 genotype ($\alpha\alpha/-\alpha$);
2. deletion of two genes from the same chromosome defines the α-thal-1 genotype ($\alpha\alpha/$);
3. mutation in a DNA sequence that codes for termination of the alpha chain, resulting in an elongated peptide (172 amino acids instead of the normal 141), defines hemoglobin Constant Spring (Hb CS). Functionally, this mutation behaves like the α-thal-2 genotype. This genotype is most often encountered in southeast Asia and less often in Africa and the Mediterranean area.

The alpha thalassemias can be classified on the basis of these genotypes and the total number of abnormal genes that result (Table 18-3). When alpha chain production is severely restricted (3 genes deleted), **hemoglobin H**, a tetramer of beta chains (β_4), forms. In the absence of alpha chain production (4 genes deleted), **hemoglobin Bart's** forms as a tetramer of gamma chains (γ_4). A single gene deletion (alpha thalassemia minor) represents the **silent carrier** state in that no clinical problems are evident. Family studies and DNA hybridization techniques are usually necessary to identify this

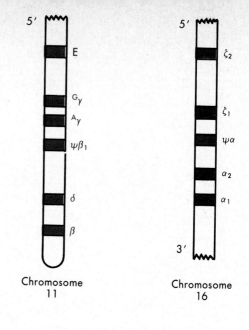

Chromosome 11   Chromosome 16

ψ-Pseudogene

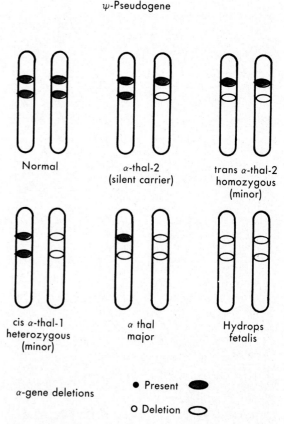

Normal

α-thal-2 (silent carrier)

trans α-thal-2 homozygous (minor)

cis α-thal-1 heterozygous (minor)

α thal major

Hydrops fetalis

α-gene deletions

● Present ⬤

○ Deletion ⬭

Fig. 18-8. Arrangement of structural genes for globin chains.

Table 18-3. Classification of alpha thalassemias

Name	Gene	Deletions	Hemoglobin
Thalassemia minor (silent carrier)	heterozygous α-thal-2	1	1%-2% Hb Bart's (cord)
Thalassemia trait	heterozygous α-thal-1 or homozygous α-thal-2	2	5%-10% Hb Bart's (cord)
Thalassemia major (Hb H disease)	double heterozygous α-thal-1 and α-thal-2	3	20%-30% Hb Bart's (cord) 5%-40% Hb H (adult)
Hydrops fetalis	homozygous α-thal-1	4	99% Hb Bart's; trace of Hb Portland
Hb Constant Spring	mRNA termination defect	1	1%-2% Hb Bart's (cord)

genotype (α-thal-2). Note that the ratio of beta to alpha chains is almost normal, but that a small amount of Hb Bart's may be detected in cord blood at birth.

Alpha thalassemia trait can result from either a heterozygous α-thal-1 genotype (two deletions on the same chromosome) or from a homozygous α-thal-2 genotype (both chromosome have one deletion). The red cells are usually hypochromic and microcytic and some target cells may be present, but hemoglobin levels are essentially normal to slightly decreased. Red cell inclusions can sometimes be detected after supravital staining. The beta/alpha globin ratio is slightly increased and 5% to 10% of the cord blood hemoglobin is Hb Bart's, enough to establish trait in newborns. Despite the mild red cell abnormalities, clinical manifestations are absent and the main concern is to identify individuals with trait and carrier status for genetic counseling.

Alpha thalassemia major or **hemoglobin H disease** occurs as a double heterozygous genotype of α-thal-1 and α-thal-2. Hemoglobin Bart's occurs at birth and is replaced by Hb H (5% to 40%) as beta chain production increases during infancy. Erythrocytes are moderately hypochromic and microcytic; poikilocytosis is apparent and target cells

are common. Both Hb Bart's and Hb H have increased affinities for oxygen, resulting in poor tissue oxygenation and both are unstable, precipitating as large Heinz bodies. These red cell inclusions result in a decreased red cell survival time and mild to moderate hemolytic anemia. Hepatosplenomegaly usually develops in an older child or young adult, especially if transfusions result in immune sensitization. Splenectomy is often necessary to control the hemolytic anemia, but this increases the risk of infections in young children. Superficial ulcers of the lower extremities are not uncommon. Frequent maintenance transfusions result in iron overload, usually by early adulthood. Iron toxicity leading to cardiac failure and infection with gram positive cocci are the usual causes of death. Compensatory expansion of the marrow space of the long bones can be detected in radiographs and about one third of the patients show marked changes in the facial bones ("mongloid facies").

Hydrops fetalis, a lack of alpha chain production (α^0 thalassemia), is incompatible with life. About 50% of those affected die in utero, the others expire within an hour after birth. The fetus is extremely anemic and edemic, the liver is greatly enlarged and splenomegaly is moderate. This condition results from a homozygous α-thal-1 genotype. Cord blood contains mostly Hb Bart's and small amounts of Hb H and Hb Portland. The latter may be responsible for fetal survival, since it has a normal oxygen dissociation curve. Interestingly, the α-thal-1 genotype is rare among black populations and hydrops fetalis has not been reported.

Beta thalassemia would appear to be simpler in genetic terms, since the beta chain is structurally represented by a single gene on each chromosome 11. However, the molecular defects are heterogenous and two major types of abnormal gene has been described. The β^+ gene is the most common, characterized by a reduced rate of mRNA synthesis. This is not a deletion, only an allele of the normal gene that results in a slow rate of beta globin production. Conversely, the β^0 gene results in no beta chain production. Because either of these genes can be inherited in a homozygous or heterozygous fashion, a spectrum of clinical manifestations and anemias can result.

Beta thalassemia minor results from inheriting a single abnormal gene. This rarely results in a clinical disorder. Target cells and some poikilocytosis may be present but hemoglobin levels are normal or slightly decreased. The MCH and MCV are slightly to moderately reduced. If hemolysis does occur, the bilirubin may be elevated and the reticulocyte count may be slightly increased. Erythrocytes are more resistant to osmotic stress than normal cells (decreased osmotic fragility). Hb A_2 levels are increased (3% to 7%) and Hb F is normal to slightly increased. A few patients have a reversed pattern, with normal Hb A_2 and elevated Hb F. Serum iron levels may be slightly increased, but tissue iron is usually normal.

Beta thalassemia major results from a homozygous or double heterozygous abnormal gene. Less severe variations have been described as thalassemia intermedia. Beta chain production can vary from zero (β^0/β^0) to moderately decreased (β^+/β^+). Gamma chain production compensates for beta chain loss, resulting in increased Hb F (20% to 90%); Hb A_2 may be normal or increased. The resulting anemia is usually severe (hemoglobin <8 g/dL) and the erythrocytes display marked anisopoikilocytosis, hypochromia, microcytosis, tear drop and target cell shapes, and basophilic stippling due to increased iron accumulation. Hemolysis is moderate to marked, the indirect bilirubin is elevated and the reticulocyte count usually exceeds 5%. Intracellular Hb F can be detected with the Kleihauer-Betke technique and the electrophoretic pattern reveals little or no Hb A. The full symptoms of anemia, skeletal abnormalities and iron overload appear in early childhood. The skull radiographs may display a vertical pattern of striations known as "hair-on-end". Hepatosplenomegaly is usually severe and liver disease may be complicated by cirrhosis. Death often occurs during childhood from recurrent infections and iron overloading resulting in cardiac failure. Generally, the clinical manifestations of homozygous beta thalassemia are more severe than those of Hb H disease.

Ineffective erythropoiesis is evident in all of the severe thalassemias, but especially in beta thalassemia. Intramedullary destruction of erythroblasts probably occurs because of the overproduction of normal chains that result in cytoplasmic precipitates. Erythoird hyperplasia occurs in compensation for the peripheral anemia and the marrow space expands, producing the thin hollow bones that are characteristic of the disease. Iron overloading occurs as a result of increased absorption and from transfusions used to manage the anemia.

F thalassemia is a combined defect of delta and beta chain synthesis, seen in patients of Greek or Sicilian origin. Fortunately, gamma chain production compensates almost fully for the deficient globins so that a good ratio of alpha to nonalpha chains is maintained. The homozygous condition is known as F thalassemia, since 100% of the hemoglobin tetramers are composed of alpha and gamma chains. **Hb Lepore** is another structural abnormality affecting nonalpha chain production. The proximity of the delta and beta gene loci on chromosome 11 (Fig. 8-8) can result in an abnormal crossover during meiosis. The amino acid end of the delta chain gene is fused to the carboxy end of the beta chain. Two of these hybrid chains plus two alpha chains form Hb Lepore. Hb anti-Lepore results from the other product of the abnormal meiosis. The amount of Hb Lepore formed varies from 0% to 30%; the rest is comprised of Hb F. Hb Lepore has a slightly increased affinity for oxygen. Excess alpha chains form precipitates, similar to those seen in beta thalassemia. The clinical manifestations can vary from mild to severe, including skeletal and systemic changes like those of beta thalassemia major.

Hereditary persistence of fetal hemoglobin (HPFH) is a term given to a heterogenous group of anomalies characterized by retention of Hb F into adult life (15% to 30% of total hemoglobin) and dysfunctional or absent delta and beta chain production. Some of the cases traditionally described as HPFH probably represent β or F thalassemia. About 0.1% of American blacks have HPFH, but two other types are also known, based on the presence of alanine (A) or glycine (G) at position 136 of the γ chain:

Black type	Equal amounts of $^G\gamma$ and $^A\gamma$, homogeneous red cell distribution
Greek type	$^A\gamma$ is the predominant form, homogeneous distribution
Swiss type	$^G\gamma$ and $^A\gamma$ are equal but cell distribution is heterogeneous

The Kleihauer-Betke technique reveals one of two patterns, either all of the cells contain equal amounts of Hb F, or it is confined to a subpopulation of the cells. The latter pattern is also seen in conjunction with double heterozygous Hb S and thalassemia syndromes. Excess alpha chains are not produced in this condition and clinical manifestations do not occur, even in the homozygous state. The peripheral blood picture may show some slight hypochromia and microcytosis. Because Hb F has a higher oxygen affinity than Hb A, the red cell count may be elevated and the marrow may display a mild hyperplasia.

HEMOGLOBINOPATHIES

Inherited abnormalities in the amino acid sequence of the globin chains that result in hematological disorders are collectively known as **hemoglobinopathies.** The genetic defect is most often a substitution of a single amino acid for another at a critical site in one of the peptide chains (usually the beta chain). Adverse effects include: (1) an unstable form of hemoglobin that precipitates during oxidative stress, (2) altered binding sites for oxygen resulting in increased affinity and tissue hypoxia, or (3) altered binding sites resulting in decreased oxygen affinity and decreased transport to tissues. Over 350 substitutions, deletions, and other alterations in the amino acid sequence have been documented, but over half of these do not result in clinically significant disorders. About twice as many detectable variants involve the beta chain compared to alpha chain, even though there is only one beta gene locus and there are two alpha gene loci.

Sickle cell anemia

Sickle cell disease or anemia is a hereditary defect in the beta chain of hemoglobin that results in formation of intracellular crystals, distorting the cells and culminating in their destruction by RES macrophages. The genetic defect is expressed as a substitution of valine for glutamic acid at position 6 in the peptide sequence, written $\beta^{6Glu \rightarrow Val}$ (Table 18-4). Incorporation of a single abnormal peptide into a tetramer with two normal alpha chains and one normal beta chain results from the heterozygous condition, sickle cell trait (Hb AS).

Table 18-4. Genetic defects in major hemoglobinopathies

Hemoglobin	Chain	Position	Amino acids	Disorder
Hemoglobin S	Beta	6	glu→val	Sickle cell anemia, trait
Hemoglobin C	Beta	6	glu→lys	Hb C disease, trait
Hemoglobin D	Beta	Various	Various	Mild hemolytic anemia
Hemoglobin E	Beta	26	glu→lys	Mild hemolytic anemia
Hemoglobin O$_{Arab}$	Beta	121	glu→lys	Mild to moderate hemolytic anemia

The homozygous condition, Hb S, results from the production of two abnormal beta chains. The genetics of single gene beta chain variants is diagrammed in Fig. 18-9.

Homozygous **sickle cell anemia** (SS) is a severe hemolytic anemia that affects about one in every 1900 American blacks that survive the first year of life. The red cells at birth are essentially normal, containing large amounts of Hb F. During the first year of life, when beta chain synthesis normally results in production of Hb A, only Hb S is produced. Polymerization of hemoglobin occurs when oxygen tensions drop below 85% saturation, when blood pH falls or 2,3-DPG concentrations increase. These conditions occur normally in the red pulp of the spleen (pH = 6.4 to 6.8) at the same time that blood viscosity increases and oxygen levels are low. Hemoglobin polymerization results in the formation of stiff rods in the red cells, producing the "sickle" or elongated shape of the drepanocyte (Fig. 18-10 and Plate V-B). Chronic sickling of SS red cells results in occlusion in the microvasculature of the spleen, producing tissue damage and mechanical destruction of the red cells. As circulation to the affected tissue is disrupted, oxygen levels and the pH drop further, enhancing the conditions for additional sickle cell formation. These episodes or crises affect other tissues as well: the lungs, kidneys, liver, ocular and cerebral circulation, bones, and joints are especially prone to circulatory interruption. An early sign of the anemia in young children is "hand and foot syndrome" a form of dactylitis in which the feet and hands undergo painful swelling. The head of the femur and head of the humerus are often affected in older children and adults. Necrosis of bone tissue is usually followed by repair, including revascularization and reossification. If repair does not occur or necrosis persists as a result of continuous sickling crises, the joint may collapse, causing a permanent disability.

The spleen is progressively damaged by the sickled cells, leading to functional asplenia as the child matures. This is indicated in the peripheral blood by an increase in the number of red cells containing Howell-Jolly bodies. Immune function is also compromised, including the production of antibodies, chemotactic responses of phagocytes, and activation of the alternate complement cascade. Most deaths in young children occur because of severe bacterial infections. Pneumonia and meningitis are particularly troublesome: *Streptococcus pneumoniae*, *Staphylococcus* and *Haemophilus influenzae* are prevalent. Other infections prominent in sickle cell patients include urinary tract infections, osteomyelitis (from *Salmonella* and *Staphylococcus*), and skin lesions.

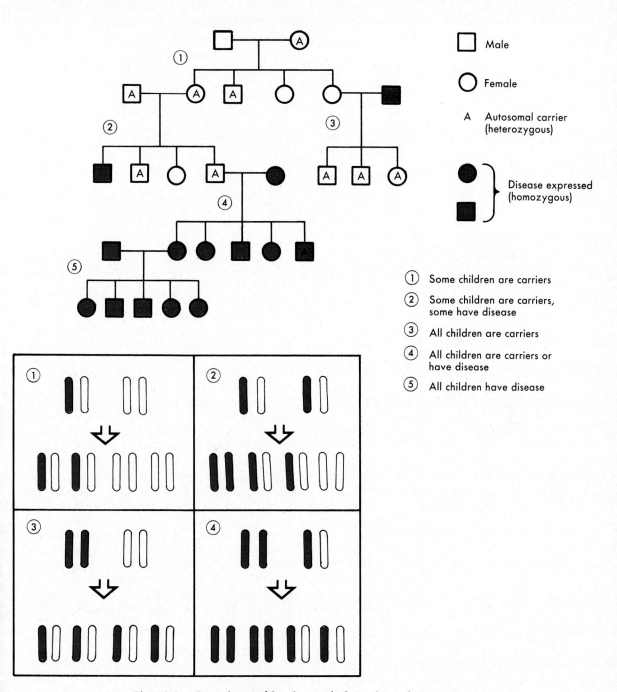

Male

Female

A Autosomal carrier
   (heterozygous)

Disease expressed
(homozygous)

① Some children are carriers

② Some children are carriers,
   some have disease

③ All children are carriers

④ All children are carriers or
   have disease

⑤ All children have disease

Fig. 18-9. Genetic combination underlying beta chain variants.

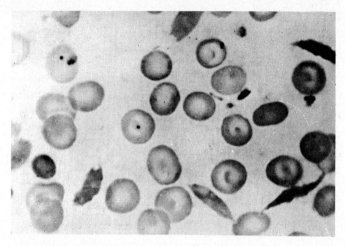

Fig. 18-10.   Sickle cell anemia.
Drepanocytes, codocytes (target cells), and Howell-Jolly bodies are evident. (From Miale, JB: Laboratory medicine: Hematology, ed 6, 1982, The CV Mosby Co.)

Destruction of circulating red cells causes a compensatory erythroid hyperplasia in the marrow and reticulocyosis in the peripheral blood. Reticulocyte counts can exceed 25% following a hemolytic crisis and increased red cell turnover can lead to a folate deficiency if the diet is deficient or vitamin supplements are not provided. In some patients, an aplastic crisis can develop: marrow red cell production ceases and the peripheral hemoglobin concentration falls to 2 to 3 g/dL. The crisis is usually self-limiting, but the ensuing anemia requires supportive treatment. A large number of transfusions at an early age inevitably produces immune-related problems later.

Diagnosis is based on family history and the occurrence of joint pain with anemia at an early age. Although the disease is largely restricted to persons of black ancestry, Hb S is found in some populations of southern India, the Arabian peninsula and among peoples of the eastern Mediterranean and Turkey. Screening tests for sickle cell anemia and trait are based on the polymerization of Hb S under conditions of low oxygen tension (Chapter 27).

Solubility tests are based on the fact that lysed red cells release hemoglobin into a solution: Hb S is opaque and Hb A is clear. The test is economical for screening family members and large populations at risk, but some other hemoglobinopathies and artifacts can produce false positive results. Sickling tests are done by sealing a drop of blood under a cover slip with a reducing agent, such as sodium metabisulfite, and observing sickle cell formation directly under the microscope. Positive results by either of these methods must be confirmed by hemoglobin electrophoresis, the definitive test for identification of any hemoglobinopathy. Homozygous patients will have 85% to 100% Hb S (Hb F comprises most of the remainder) when blood is separated on cellulose acetate at pH 8.4. Representations of typical patterns are shown in Fig. 18-11.

Other laboratory findings in patients with SS include: decreased osmotic fragility (sickled cells tolerate more water influx before forming spherocytes and lysing), decreased sedimentation rate (rouleaux formation is minimal for drepanocytes), increased

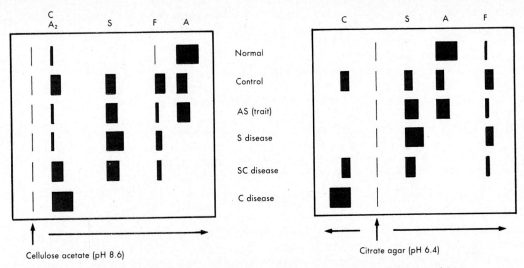

Fig. 18-11. Hemoglobin electrophoresis patterns of hemoglobinopathies.

MCV (folate deficiency in some patients, sporadic reticulocytosis in most others), and increased platelet counts. Microvascular thrombus formation may affect a number of hemostatic parameters, including an increase in factor VIII activity.

Amniocentesis provides prenatal detection of carriers of an Hb S gene. A restriction endonuclease, MST II, cleaves the DNA sequence for a normal beta chain between the codons for amino acids 6 and 7. However, this cleavage does not occur between the codons that specify the Hb S chain, so that different DNA segments are obtained after enzyme treatment. Since the test uses the genetic material of any fetal cell, it is possible to identify fetuses with the homozygous S condition before hemoglobin is formed!

Treatment has progressed greatly during the past few decades, although it is largely supportive in nature. Prevention of infections in children is a major concern. Some authorities advocate prophylactic antibiotics, others rely on close monitoring and rapid intervention to minimize problems. Several studies are in progress to determine the effect of periodic transfusion in fore-stalling hemolytic crises. Partial exchange transfusions are given to children and young adults to reduce the amount of hemoglobin S below 60%. If joint damage and spleen infarction can be minimized, disability and the danger from infections can be greatly reduced. Hemolytic crises and infections do not occur as often after childhood, so that the rationale for this aggressive therapy is one of "buying time". Future possibilities include the insertion of normal DNA sequences into the marrow red cell precursors of sickle cell patients to convert production to normal beta chains.

The heterozygous state (AS) is **sickle cell trait,** a carrier condition that results in clinical manifestations only when the patient is exposed to conditions of low oxygen tension. Administration of oxidant drugs, general anesthesia, or exposure to high altitudes (10,000 feet above sea level or higher) are typical circumstances that can produce a hemolytic crisis in an otherwise normal patient. In contrast to SS, red cell sickling occurs in AS patients only when oxygen saturation falls below 40%. These conditions exist in the loop of Henle and AS individuals may experience hematuria and hyposthenuria (inability to concentrate urine) on occasions. About 8% to 10% of American blacks are believed to carry at least one gene for Hb S, but the incidence increases to about 40% in East African Bantus and it ranges from 20% to over 30% for tropical Africa as a whole. Although homozygous sickle cell anemia (SS) is just as devastating in Africa as it is in America, the heterozygous state (AS) confers protection from another deadly disease, falciparum malaria. The parasite, *Plasmodium falciparum*, invades circulating red cells but it is apparently less successful in red cells containing Hb S. Whether this is due to abnormal metabolic activities of the AS cell or whether the RES system is able to remove parasites more effectively because the AS cells have a shorter survival time than normal cells is still not known. Some other hemoglobinopathies, forms of thalassemia, and enzyme deficiencies (e.g., G-6-PD) are also known to confer an advantage for resistance to malaria. Considering the number of deaths and abortions attributable to malaria infection, the genetic selection for sickle cell trait in tropical areas is not surprising.

Individuals with sickle cell trait usually have red cells with less than 40% Hb S when tested by hemoglobin electrophoresis. Hb F levels are normal and the remainder is Hb A and A_2. Screening tests for Hb S are usually positive, depending on the quantity of Hb S present. As with thalassemia, the value of detecting the trait condition is to offer genetic counseling and help avoid conditions of low oxygen tension.

Other hemoglobinopathies

Other single amino acid substitutions can result in the formation of peptide chains with adverse effects on hemoglobin function. **Hemoglobin C** occurs when the glutamic acid of beta chain position 6 is replaced by lysine (replacement by valine produces Hb S, as previously stated). In the homozygous state (CC), **hemoglobin C disease** is manifested as a mild to moderate hemolytic anemia, often accompanied by splenomegaly. Mild to moderate joint pain may be present in some patients, but most are asymptomatic. The peripheral smear is often characterized by the presence of target cells and folded cells (Plate 5, *C*). If the smear is dried slowly or the blood is mixed with a hypertonic solution, rhomboid crystals may form inside some of the RBCs. These inclusions have been described as obelisks or "Washington monuments" and they result in shortened survival times (30 to 60 days) for the red cells that contain them (Fig. 18-12). Thus, a mild erythroid hyperplasia and peripheral reticulocytosis is seen in this disease, as seen in other mild forms of hemolytic anemia. Osmotic fragility is also decreased, in common with sickle cell anemia and thalassemia. Electrophoresis reveals about 85% to 90% Hb C and a slight increase in Hb F (up to 8%). Despite the fact that neither of the two beta chains are normal in persons with Hb C disease, the cells do not form rigid inclusions in vivo as readily as do the cells containing Hb S. Therefore, tissue damage is minimal and splenomegaly is mainly a function of red cell destruction.

Hemoglobin C trait (AC) is present in about 3% of American blacks but it produces no clinical symptoms. A slight increase in target cells may be noted on peripheral smears, but crystal formation is often difficult to demonstrate. Hemoglobin electrophoresis reveals about 30% to 40% Hb C and no increase in Hb F.

Hemoglobin E is especially prevalent in Orientals and some black populations. It results from a substitution of lysine for glutamic acid at beta chain position 26. This hemoglobin has a slightly reduced affinity for oxygen and it tends to be mildly unstable, leading to a shortened red cell life span. The anemia in homozygous persons (EE) is mild and slightly microcytic, characterized

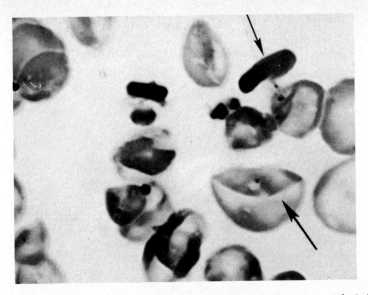

Fig. 18-12. Crystal formation and red cell folding in homozygous Hb C disease.
(From Bauer, JD: Clinical laboratory methods, ed 9, St Louis, 1982, The CV Mosby Co.)

by target cells. Heterozygotes (AE) experience no clinical manifestations.

Hemoglobin D results from a substitution of glutamine for glutamic acid at beta chain position 121. Both the homozygous and heterozygous states are essentially normal with respect to anemia and clinical manifestations, but Hb D in combination with Hb S does produce a mild to moderate sickling type of anemia with decreased red cell survival. In American populations, the gene is most often seen in blacks, thus the possibility of SD must be entertained in black patients with moderate anemia.

Double heterozygotes for hemoglobinopathies

The world's distribution of the Hb C gene overlaps with that for Hb S, thus the double heterozygous condition **hemoglobin SC** is not uncommon. Hb C is less damaging than Hb S, but SC persons lack a normal beta chain, so that the resultant clinical manifestations are moderately severe. The combination of the S chain with any other abnormal chain produces anemia and clinical

manifestations that are more severe than most other double heterozygous states:

Severe	Moderate	Mild	None
SS	SC	AS	AC
E-thal	S-thal	CC	AD
SO	SD	EE	AE
		SE	

Interestingly, the SC cells contain about 10% more Hb S than do AS cells. Alpha chains combine preferentially with normal beta chains to form tetramers. When beta chains are produced (as in AS persons), alpha chain-S chain tetramer formation is correspondingly reduced. This is why abnormal hemoglobin of heterozygotes does not exceed 50% of the total when quantitated by electrophoresis. In the absence of a normal beta chain (SC, SE, etc.), alpha chains form tetramers with both abnormal peptides, resulting in a higher Hb S content. Target cells are especially prevalent and Hb C crystals may be readily demonstrated. Almost equal amounts of Hb S and Hb C are seen with electrophoresis, along with 5% to 8% Hb F.

Sickle cell/β thalassemia combines ab

normal beta chain production with decreased rate of beta chain synthesis. The hypochromic microcytic anemia is moderate in severity (it is usually milder in blacks), but it produces less sickling and tissue damage than sickle cell disease (SS). The spleen is enlarged in about 75% of the patients and red cell survival is shortened. Because the thalassemia gene results in a slow rate of beta chain production, the majority of tetramers form as Hb S (60% to 90%). Hb A may be present (10% to 25%) or this may be replaced by Hb F, depending on the nature of the thalassemia defect. Hb A_2 is usually increased as well.

A number of other double heterozygotes have been described, with variable clinical manifestations. The degree of anemia depends on the rate of erythrocyte destruction, marrow response, and oxygen affinity of the hemoglobin. Most hemoglobin variants are asymptomatic or mild with respect to symptoms. Many are discovered during research on population genetics and they are of interest to anthropologists or to biochemists for information on the assembly and function of hemoglobin as a molecular entity.

HEMOGLOBINEMIAS

Hemoglobinemias are disorders of abnormal hemoglobins that are unstable, have abnormal oxygen affinities, or have structures that result in the formation of methemoglobin. Most of these disorders are hereditary and almost all cases are heterozygous (homozygous expression of these abnormalities are apparently lethal). Unstable hemoglobins, better known as **Heinz body anemias,** result from amino acid substitutions that affect the stability of the molecule. Most occur in the beta chain in the inner surface facing the heme molecule. The destabilized molecule oxidizes to methemoglobin, the globin separates from the heme to attach to the inner surface of the erythrocyte membrane as a Heinz body. These structures cannot be visualized with Wright's stain but they are seen with supravital stains, such as brilliant cresyl blue. The inclusion is removed by RES macrophages, resulting in pitting of the red cell, appearing in the peripheral smear as a "bite cell". The inclusions also impair the cell's capability to deform during their passage through the microcirculation. Thus, these cells have a shortened survival time and a hemolytic anemia results. The heme molecule is catabolized into dipyrrole compounds and excreted through the kidneys to form a dark-colored urine.

The anemia is normochromic normocytic, although all of the indices may be slightly decreased as RES pitting increases, removing the concentrated globin inclusions. Reticulocytosis is a function of red cell destruction, but it is usually mild. Laboratory confirmation of an unstable hemoglobin is made by performing the heat instability test: a lysate of red cells in Tris buffer solution is heated to 50°C for an hour. Development of a fine precipitate is positive evidence for an unstable hemoglobin.

Hemoglobins with abnormal oxygen affinities result from specific amino acid substitutions that affect heme-heme interacting sites, especially at points of contact between the alpha-1 and beta-2 globin chains and at 2,3-DPG binding sites. At the carboxyl terminal of the beta chain, amino acid substitutions affect the conformational changes of the molecule during oxy- and deoxyhemoglobin transformation (Table 18-5).

About 20 hemoglobin variants are known that result in increased oxygen affinity, producing a shift to the left in the dissociation curve. The inability to release oxygen at the tissues results in hypoxia, increased erythropoietin production and erythroid hyperplasia. A congenital erythrocytosis (hematocrit ranges from 55% to 65%, hemoglobin from 18 to 21 g/dL) occurs, producing a ruddy complexion in the person. The condition is inherited as an autosomal dominant,

Table 18-5. Data on selected hemoglobinemias

Hemoglobin	Chain	Position	Amino acids	Disorder
Hb Torino	Alpha	43	phe→val	Decreased O_2 affinity; unstable
Hb M Boston	Alpha	58	his→tyr	Decreased O_2 affinity; met-Hb
Hb M Iwate	Alpha	87	his→tyr	Decreased O_2 affinity; met-Hb
Hb Chesapeake	Alpha	92	arg→leu	Increased O_2 affinity
Hb E Saskatoon	Beta	22	glu→lys	Unstable
Hb Austin	Beta	40	arg→ser	Increased O_2 affinity; dissociation
Hb Hammersmith	Beta	42	phe→ser	Decreased O_2 affinity; unstable
Hb Zurich	Beta	63	his→arg	Increased O_2 affinity; unstable
Hb M Saskatoon	Beta	63	his→tyr	Increased O_2 affinity; met-Hb
Hb M Milwaukee-1	Beta	67	val→glu	Decreased O_2 affinity; met-Hb
Hb Mobile	Beta	73	asp→val	Decreased O_2 affinity
Hb M Hyde Park	Beta	92	his→tyr	Increased O_2 affinity; met-Hb
Hb Kempsey	Beta	99	asp→asn	Increased O_2 affinity
Hb Kansas	Beta	102	asn→thr	Decreased O_2 affinity

so that entire families may be affected. Otherwise, clinical manifestations are minimal and the red cells have normal survival times. About half of the variants can be detected on the basis of abnormal electrophoresis patterns, but the definitive procedure is to establish increased oxygen affinity.

Hemoglobin variants that result in decreased oxygen affinity (oxygen dissociation curve shifts to the right) are classified into four types:

1. Autosomal recessive deficiency of NADH diaphorase
2. Autosomal dominant amino acid substitution resulting in tetramer dissociation
3. Autosomal dominant amino acid substitution that results in Hb M
4. Acquired oxidation of hemoglobin iron to the ferric state

NADH diaphorase is the enzyme that reduces methemoglobin as it forms normally in red cells (methemoglobin reductase pathway, Chapter 4). A deficiency of this enzyme permits methemoglobin to accumulate. Methemoglobin contains heme iron in the ferric state; therefore, it is unable to combine with oxygen. Cyanosis is clinically evident when the methemoglobin concentration exceeds 1%. The increased availability of oxygen to the tissues results in decreased red cell production and a mild erythropenia, which could be misinterpreted as an anemia. The condition is diagnosed by quantitative assays for the enzyme. Some substances can also produce oxidation of heme iron: aniline dyes, nitrates and nitrites. Formation of methemoglobin can be reversed in both the congenital and acquired forms by administration of methylene blue or ascorbic acid (vitamin C).

Dissociation of the hemoglobin tetramer into subunits occurs in a few hemoglobin variants (e.g., Hb Kansas and Hb Beth Israel) in which the amino acid substitution affects an alpha 1-beta 2 interface site. Lists of known hemoglobin variants can be found in the comprehensive hematology textbooks (Miale; Thorup; Williams et al.; Wintrobe).

Hemoglobin M results from substitutions of tyrosine for histidine at critical sites in the alpha or beta chain (see Table 18-5). Tyrosine binds to the heme iron, stabilizing it in the ferric state, producing methemoglobin. Some forms of Hb M are somewhat unstable so that a mild hemolytic anemia may also be present. Babies with variants of the alpha chain are cyanotic at birth, whereas children with beta chain variants slowly develop cyanosis around the sixth month after birth. The blood is a characteristic chocolate-brown and the absorption spectrum is unique (Fig. 18-13). Hemoglobin electrophoresis is done at pH 7.1 to separate Hb M from Hb A. Unfortunately, Hb M variants cannot be treated with reducing agents.

ENZYME DEFICIENCIES AFFECTING HEMOGLOBIN FUNCTION

Several red cell enzymes indirectly affect hemoglobin function. Recalling the role of the hexose monophosphate shunt (HMP) presented in Chapter 5, the production of reduced glutathione provides a mechanism to clear cells of oxidizing metabolites, helping to maintain hemoglobin in its functional reduced state. Deficiencies of enzymes in the HMP pathway lead to an accumulation of oxidants, resulting in the formation of methemoglobin and the formation of Heinz bodies. The inclusions are removed, as in the anemias previously discussed, by RES macrophages, producing abnormal red cells with short life spans.

Glucose-6-phosphate dehydrogenase deficiency is the most common type of red cell enzyme deficiency. The enzyme is expressed as a sex-linked trait in more than 150 molecular forms. G6PD-B is the most

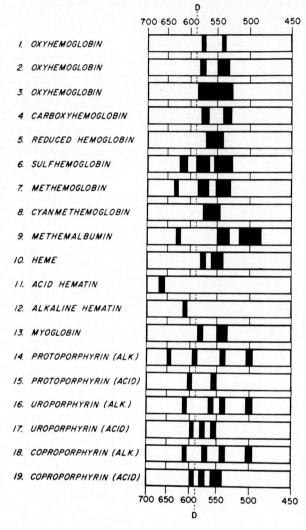

Fig. 18-13. Absorption spectra of hemoglobin precursors and variants.
1-3, Three different concentrations of oxyhemoglobin, in increasing order; 4-8, functional derivatives of hemoglobin; 9-12, byproducts of hemoglobin breakdown; 13, myoglobin; 14-19, heme precursors. (From Miale, JB: Laboratory medicine: Hematology, ed 6, St Louis, 1982, The CV Mosby Co.)

common normal isoenzyme, present throughout the world in about 70% of black populations and over 99% of white populations. It catalyzes the conversion of NADP to NADPH, generating the formation of reduced glutathione (Fig. 18-14). About 20% of American blacks possess a different normal variant, G6PD-A$^+$. It has the same enzymatic activity as the B isoenzyme, but it displays faster mobility with electrophoretic separation.

About 10% of American black males have a different isoenzyme, G6PD-A$^-$, which possesses only about 10% of normal activity. This amount is sufficient for cellular metabolism under normal conditions, but exposure to infection or to certain oxidizing drugs can overwhelm the decreased quantity of enzyme and produce a hemolytic episode. The disorder was discovered in the 1950s in Korea when a large number of black soldiers were given the antimalarial drug, primaquine. Many experienced the classical signs of hemolytic anemia. Fortunately, the enzymatic activity is greater in young red cells, especially reticu-

locytes, and declines as the cells mature. When hemolysis occurs, abnormal cells are destroyed and the release of many young red cells with increased enzyme activity maintains hemoglobin in its reduced state. The hemolysis reoccurs, however, if reexposure to the adverse conditions occurs after the RBCs mature in the circulation. For this reason, testing for enzyme activity in blacks should be delayed for 2 to 3 months after hemolysis or false normal results may be obtained.

Severe forms of hemolytic anemia are found in people with other variants: G6PD-Mediterranean (affecting whites) and G6PD-Canton (present in Orientals). These migrate with the same electrophoretic mobility as the normal B isoenzyme but less than 1% of the enzyme activity is present. These variants also differ from the A$^-$ isoenzyme in that young RBCs are as deficient

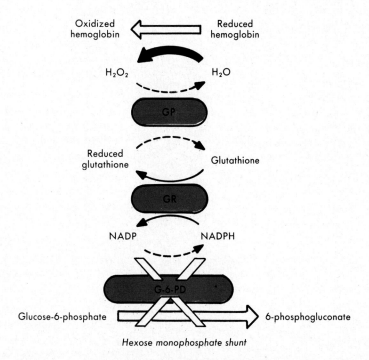

Fig. 18-14. Glucose-6-phosphate dehydrogenase deficiency.
Deficiency of G6PD produces a sequential metabolic disturbance and accumulation of oxidants, resulting in oxidation and precipitation of hemoglobin and eventual red cell hemolysis.

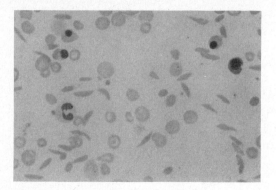

Fig. 18-15. Hemoglobin electrophoresis pattern.

as older cells. Red cells must be capable of dealing with routine oxidant stress, because chronic hemolytic anemia is usually not present in the populations with these abnormal enzymes. However, when a source of oxidation is encountered, the hemolytic anemia is not self-limiting, and life-threatening episodes are well documented. One source of oxidation, for some individuals, results from eating fava beans or inhaling the pollen (favism).

Females can express a heterozygous form of the deficiencies which, as expected, is milder than that seen in males. Red cells from heterozygous females have a dual population of the enzyme because only one of the two X chromosomes is expressed in a given red cell (the Lyon hypothesis). Affected cells can be damaged to the same extent as the affected cells of males, but the overall degree of hemolysis reflects the smaller population of cells involved.

Some widely used drugs and other substances have been implicated in hemolytic episodes associated with G6PD deficiency: antimalarials, sulfonamides, chloramphenicol, nalidixic acid, nitrofurazone, some common pain killers (aspirin and acetophenetidin), and vitamins K and C. Some of these are probably risks only when taken in high concentrations or in persons with the severe forms of enzyme deficiency.

Screening tests for G6PD deficiency use activity of the enzyme to generate NADPH, detectable directly by fluorescent light (filter spot test) or by ability to reduce brilliant cresyl blue to a colorless solution. Quantitative procedures measure the conversion of NADP to NADPH spectrophotometrically.

Deficiencies of glutathione synthetase and glutamylcysteine synthetase are known, each of which leads to a reduction in reduced glutathione and a Heinz body type of hemolytic anemia. Other red cell enzyme deficiencies, not directly involving hemoglobin function, are included in Chapter 19.

Case history (sickle cell anemia)

The patient is a 34-year-old black male referred from a local county hospital after being diagnosed with anemia. He has three brothers with documented sickle cell anemia. The patient's primary complaints are those of intermittent episodes of severe and sharp pain of the anterior tibias bilaterally, intermittent cramping abdominal pain, and intermittent chest pain.

Physical examination revealed slight dehydration, a blood pressure of 122 over 80, a pulse of 110 and a temperature of 39°C. A high embossed forehead was noted, as was severe gingival hyperplasia. In addition, there was pallor of the oral mucosa and conjunctivae. Other physical findings were long and slightly deformed fingers with fusiform swelling and pallor of the nailbeds. A systolic ejection murmur was also present. No hepatosplenomegaly was detected. The patient demonstrated marked tenderness of the anterior tibial surfaces, abdomen, and sternum.

Laboratory evaluation revealed a white cell count of 15,200/μL, a hemoglobin of 9.2 g/dL, and a hematocrit of 25.9%. The platelet count was 350,000/μL. The reticulocyte count was 4.8%. A biochemical screening survey was normal except for a total bilirubin of 3.2 mg/dL. Hemoglobin electrophoresis was ordered and the pattern is shown in Fig. 18-15. A peripheral blood smear revealed sickle cells, target cells, and marked aniso/poikilocytosis

The diagnosis is homozygous sickle cell anemia and sickle cell vaso-occlusive (infarctive) crisis. The patient, on this particular occasion, also demonstrated mild hemolysis, but not a hemolytic crisis.

The treatment was hydration, oxygenation by nasal canullae, analgesics, folic acid supplement, and instructions regarding adequate home hydration and refraining from activities likely to induce undue acidosis.

SUMMARY

- Hemoglobin disorders have been described for virtually every step in the synthesis of the molecule. Major steps that are affected involve iron metabolism, synthesis of the heme structure, and production of the globin chains. Other disorders affect hemoglobin functions, especially those concerned with oxygen binding and hemoglobin reduction.
- Iron deficiency anemia is the most common form of anemia, characterized by low serum iron, increased iron binding capacity, and decreased or absent tissue iron stores. IDA is common in pregnant women, growing children with insufficient diets, and in adults with chronic gastrointestinal bleeding.
- Deficiencies of hemoglobin production are commonly manifested as hypochromic microcytic anemias (iron deficiency, sideroblastic anemia, and thalassemia).
- Iron overloading is a problem in some anemias because the body absorbs additional iron during increased red cell production but it cannot excrete excess amounts. Accumulating tissue damage from iron deposition is called hemachromatosis.
- Sideroblastic anemias are characterized by perinuclear iron deposits in erythroblasts, indicating ineffective erythropoiesis and iron overloading. Some forms are associated with myelodysplastic syndromes and may develop into acute leukemia.
- Deficiencies of enzymes that catalyze production of the heme molecule lead to the accumulation and excretion of porphyrin compounds (porphyrias). Some are congenital forms that include symptoms of severe photosensitivity and skin lesions. Lead poisoning is a reversible disturbance of heme synthase and ALA dehydrase that

also results in basophilic stippling of red cells.
- Thalassemias are congenital defects of globin chain production. Beta chain defects are the most common. Heterozygous conditions (minor = trait) are mild and homozygous conditions (major = disease) are usually severe. Red cells are hemolyzed due to the accumulation of normal chains. From 1 to 4 genes can be deleted in alpha thalassemias, 1 or 2 genes are missing in beta thalassemias.
- Hemoglobin F is present as a compensatory oxygen carrier in many hemoglobinopathies. A failure to switch off gamma chain production can result in hereditary persistence (HPFH) through adulthood, without medical consequences.
- Sickle cell anemia is a common amino acid substitution (valine for glutamic acid at position 6) involving the beta chain. Hb S polymerizes under conditions of low oxygen saturation or low pH, forming a rigid cell that occludes the microvasculature and causes tissue necrosis. The spleen is destroyed and immune function is compromised. Recurrent, severe infections are the leading cause of death.
- About 10% of American blacks carry at least one gene for a hemoglobinopathy, and double heterozygotes for SC, S-thal, and other combinations are well known. Frequencies of S trait are especially high in tropical Africa, where it confers resistance against one form of malaria.
- Hemoglobin electrophoresis is the definitive procedure for characterizing hemoglobinopathies and thalassemias. Various techniques are used to separate hemoglobin variants, using different substrates and buffers of varying pH.
- Hemoglobin variants are known with unstable molecular forms, resulting in precipitation as Heinz bodies. These inclusions are removed by macrophages, producing a hemolytic anemia. Other variants have increased or decreased affinities for oxygen. The former usually result in familial erythrocytosis and the latter may

display a mild anemia. Hb M is an irreversible methemoglobin, producing chocolate-brown blood with a unique absorption spectrum. All of these exist as heterozygotes; homozygote expression is believed to be fatal.

- G6PD deficiency is a common, mild to severe sex-linked disorder that affects hemoglobin stability, producing Heinz bodies and hemolytic episodes. Most occurrences are acute, associated with infections or the administration of oxidant drugs.

19

Anemias of Hemorrhage and Hemolysis

BLOOD LOSS BY HEMORRHAGE

A normochromic normocytic anemia results from chronic or acute hemorrhage. The anemia's severity depends on the rate of blood loss and the marrow's capability for erythropoietic response. A patient who is otherwise healthy can tolerate a blood volume loss of 10% to 20% (up to 1 liter in an average-sized adult) with only minimal difficulties (dizziness when standing suddenly, etc.). Losses of 20% to 40% result in hypovolemic shock, characterized by rapid heartbeat (tachycardia), shallow and irregular pulse, shallow and rapid breathing, pallor, restlessness, profuse sweating while feeling cold, and a sense of impending doom. Cyanosis may develop around the nail beds and lips. The patient may eventually become unconscious.

Sudden loss of whole blood represents two problems: shock induced by hypovolemia (low total fluid) and hypoxia due to decreased oxygen transport by hemoglobin. Extravascular fluid begins to move into the vascular compartment within a few hours after blood loss and this compensatory adjustment is usually complete by 72 hours after bleeding stops. The hematocrit/hemoglobin/red blood cell count will, of course, continue to be normal until this fluid shift occurs. In the stabilized patient, the hematocrit falls as fluid dilutes the remaining blood. Depending on the health, metabolism, and activities of the patient, an erythropoietic response to decreased oxygen de-

livery usually occurs at hemoglobin concentrations of 10 to 12 g/dL. Increased erythropoietin levels are usually evident within a few hours after blood loss, but evidence of hyperproliferation in the marrow does not appear until 7 to 10 days later. Reticulocytes begin to increase to 3 or 4 times the nonstimulated (basal) level at 4 to 7 days, achieving maximum concentration by 10 days after stimulation (Fig. 19-1).

Reticulocyte response depends on adequate iron stores. Liver and other RES stores of iron vary considerably with health, age, and sex of the patient (Chapter 18), but depleted iron stores will inhibit the erythropoietic response and reticulocytes will increase only slightly or not at all. A slight increase in MCV reflects the presence of young, large cells; reticulocytosis is accompanied by polychromatophilia on stained smears. In iron-poor patients, cell production may be manifested by the appearance of microcytic hypochromic red cells. Iron conservation and reuse is possible when hemorrhaging is internal, that is, into the tissues. In this case, tissue macrophages are able to catabolize the hemoglobin and recycle the iron and depletion is less likely. External bleeding results in irreversible loss of iron.

Therapeutic intervention depends on the rate and amount of blood loss. Plasma expanders are used to restore blood volume and counteract the potentially fatal effects of shock. Red cell replacement is necessary when the hemoglobin content falls to a

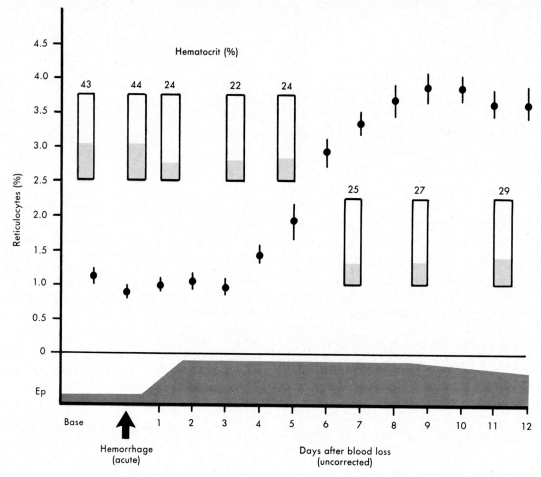

Fig. 19-1   Responses to acute and chronic hemorrhage.

level that places the patient under hypoxic stress. If bleeding has been chronic and the patient is in otherwise good health, transfusion may not be necessary at hemoglobin levels greater than 8 g/dL. Most patients can tolerate a mild to moderate anemia without undue risk and the mild hypoxia stimulates production by their own marrow, a much safer supply of new red cells than any nonautologous donor source. Whole blood is rarely given since volume replacement is easier with albumin, saline, and other fluid components. One unit of concentrated (packed) red cells elevates the hemoglobin concentration by about one gram/dL (about 3% increase in hematocrit). Obviously, the situation is more complicated in a patient who continues to bleed and experience shifts in fluid compartments.

HEMOLYTIC ANEMIAS

An anemia due to red cell destruction, either by intravascular or extravascular mechanisms, is defined as a **hemolytic anemia.** There are a number of ways to classify hemolytic disorders. They include immune versus nonimmune, congenital versus acquired, intravascular versus extravascular, and so forth. The box below is not comprehensive, but it does include most of common hemolytic disorders, including the hemoglobin disorders (Chapter 18) that result in red cell destruction.

Almost any event that alters the internal (cytoplasmic) or external (outer membrane) structure of the erythrocyte may result in a phagocytic response by macrophages lining the microvasculature as the red cells pass through the spleen and other RES tissues. The formation of cytoplasmic inclusions (hemoglobin precipitation, iron overloading and aggregation, retention of DNA remnants, for example) subjects red cells to phagocytic scrutiny. In this context, the normal changes that accompany senescence should also be noted: various components that increase and decrease as the erythrocyte ages have been investigated as contributing factors to red cell destruction (see box below). Any of these factors may also be apparent in red cells prematurely destroyed by a hemolytic process.

One group of hemolytic disorders is associated with membrane defects, usually expressed as a deficiency in the amount of a structural protein, a qualitative abnormality in the interactions of structural molecules, or as an imbalanced ratio of lipid constituents. Many of these defects are also characterized by morphological aberrations of the red cells that can be demonstrated on peripheral smears.

HEREDITARY SPHEROCYTOSIS

Loss of cell membrane occurs during the life span of normal circulating erythrocytes. As macrophages remove cytoplasmic accumulations and membrane bound IgG, the surface to volume ratio decreases and the cell becomes gradually more spherical (Fig. 19-2). These **microspherocytes** are less deformable and are more likely to be removed

---

HEMOLYTIC ANEMIAS

Nonimmunological hemolytic anemias

Membrane defects
  Hereditary spherocytosis
  Abetalipoproteinemia
  Rh null and other membrane deficiency
    phenotypes
Red cell enzyme deficiencies
  Glucose-6-phosphate deficiency (Chapter 18)
  Pyruvate kinase deficiency
  Methemoglobin reductase deficiency
Hemoglobin production deficiencies and defects
    (Chapter 18)
  Thalassemia
  Sickle cell anemia and other
    hemoglobinopathies
Anemias caused by infectious agents
  Malaria and other blood parasites
  Hemolysis due to bacterial agents and toxins
Red cell destruction caused by toxins, venoms,
    and chemicals

Immune-mediated hemolytic anemias

Autoimmune hemolytic anemias (AIHA)
  Drug-induced hemolytic anemias
  Paroxysmal cold hemoglobinuria (PCH)
  Cold hemagglutinin disease (CHD)
Alloimmune hemolytic anemias
  Hemolytic disease of the newborn (HDN)
  Hemolytic transfusion reactions

AGE-RELATED CHANGES IN RED BLOOD CELLS

Increases	Decreases
Intracellular sodium	Intracellular
Methemoglobin	potassium
content	Membrane sialic acid
Membrane-bound	Cholesterol
IgG	Adenosine triphos-
Mean cell hemoglo-	phate (ATP)
bin concentration	Mean cell volume
(MCHC)	(MCV)
Cell viscosity (less	Glycolytic pathway
water)	enzymes

by RES macrophages. One form of hemolytic anemia is characterized by large numbers of spherical red cells that circulate in the peripheral blood of considerably shorter intervals. **Hereditary spherocytosis (HS)** is inherited most often as an autosomal dominant trait, affecting about 1 in 5000 persons in the United States. The disease is rarely found in blacks. The disorder may be present from birth, producing neonatal jaundice and anemia, or it may appear late in adult life.

The pathophysiological mechanism underlying the decreased red cell survivability has been somewhat elusive. Recent investigations have focused on a structural gene abnormality that results in a deficiency of spectrin, the major cytoskeletal protein of the RBC membrane (Chapter 5). Spectrin levels of 75% to 90% of normal are correlated with a mild spherocytosis and anemia, levels of 50% to 75% with moderate manifestations, and less than 50% with a severe anemia. Patients in the latter catagory are presumably homozygous. In addition, some patients with HS also have a qualitative de-

fect: spectrin binds abnormally to protein 4.1 As a result of these cytoskeletal abnormalities, the membrane is more resistant to deformation during passage through the microvasculature. The cells may spend an increased amount of time in the splenic cords, an acid environment in which glucose is rapidly depleted. The membrane changes also permit sodium influx to occur at an increased rate. The ATP-driven sodium pump must compensate and this requires additional glucose use. As the ability to pump sodium out of the cell decreases, water enters the cell and spherocyte formation results, enhancing splenic retention still further. Membrane loss occurs in the spleen as a result of retention, a process called "splenic conditioning". Although some of the microspherocytes pass into the peripheral blood, many are destroyed by RES macrophages. This manifests as a hemolytic anemia.

The severity of the anemia depends on the degree of red cell membrane abnormality and the extent of erythropoietic compensation. The marrow should display a

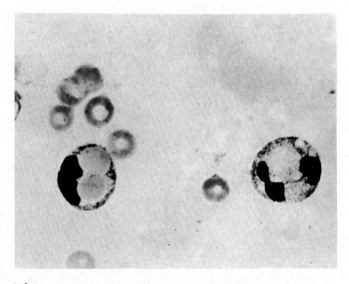

Fig. 19-2.   Spherocytes.
(From Miale, JB: Laboratory medicine: Hematology, ed 6, St Louis, 1982, The CV Mosby Co.)

mild to moderate erythroid hyperplasia and the reticulocyte count often ranges from 7% to 15%. Splenomegaly may be slight to marked and symptoms characteristic of anemia (pallor, weakness, etc.) may be present, especially during the sporadic hemolytic bouts or "crises." Such crises are especially common in children after infections; viruses may also supress marrow cell production, manifesting as an aplastic crisis. Increased red cell production can produce a folic acid deficiency in some patients, eventually distorting the blood cell pattern with a megaloblastic component, unless folic acid supplements are provided. The problem with susceptability to infection creates a problem for managing the hemolytic anemia. Young children (less than 5 years old) are more susceptible to serious infections if the spleen is removed, but splenectomy does alleviate much of the red cell destruction. The red cells still form spherocytes and they remain osmotically fragile, but they are not subjected to the splenic microenvironment of low glucose, extremely narrow sinus passageways, and concentrations of RES macrophages.

The **osmotic fragility test (OF)** is the classic means of establishing HS as the cause of anemia (see box below). However, the routine procedure is relatively insensitive and only those persons with moderate deficiencies and hemolysis are likely to be detected (about 1 in 4 patients with HS will have normal OF results.) When the red cells are incubated in a low glucose medium, simulating in vivo conditions of the spleen, pa-

tients with milder expressions of HS are also detected (Chapter 27). The test simply measures the ability of red cells to withstand water influx in a series of dilute saline solutions. Hemolysis is measured when it is first apparent and when all red cells are destroyed (complete). Osmotic fragility curves are compared in Fig. 19-3. Note that most hemoglobinopathies result in *decreased* osmotic fragility (increased resistence to lysing) because cells in these disorders do not form spherocytes readily.

The **autohemolysis test** can help distinguish hereditary spherocytosis from other membrane defects, particularly acquired disorders or those secondary to other conditions (uremia, pneumonia, some forms of leukemia, myelofibrosis, and drug-induced autoimmune hemolytic anemia). Patient and normal control red cells are individually incubated under sterile conditions for 48 hours. About 2% of the red cells of normal patients hemolyze during this time, whereas 20% to 30% of the RBCs of HS patients are destroyed. When the test cells are incubated with glucose, survivability increases in HS patients (only 5% to 10% are lysed), but glucose addition does not lessen the destruction of red cells from patients with acquired and secondary hemolytic anemias.

Confirmation of changes in membrane protein components is made by lysing the red cells, denaturing the membrane with sodium dodecyl sulfate (SDS) and separating the proteins by polyacrylamide gel electrophoresis (PAGE). The separated products are stained with materials like Coomassie brilliant blue and periodic acid-Schiff reagent (see Chapter 5 for PAGE patterns). Although this technique is not routinely used by clinical laboratories, it is widely employed in research and reference laboratories.

Unfortunately, HS and other membrane defects appear to be heterogeneous, displaying a variety of manifestations and possible pathophysiological mechanisms. Newer techniques may be able to discriminate

OSMOTIC FRAGILITY TEST (UNINCUBATED)		
	Start of hemolysis	Complete hemolysis
Normal	0.45 − 0.55% NaCl	0.30% NaCl
HS	0.50 − 0.75% NaCl	0.40% NaCl

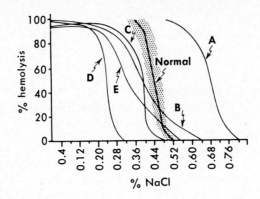

Fig. 19-3.   Osmotic fragility.
Osmotic fragility of erythrocytes (method of Dacie). **A,** Hereditary spherocytosis. **B,** Thalassemia major. **C,** Thalassemia minor. **D,** Hb E disease. **E,** Thalassemia.

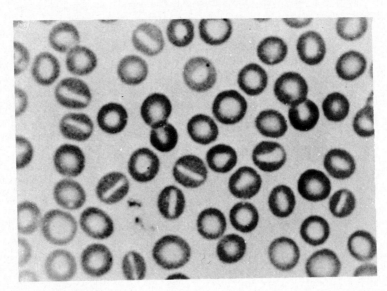

Fig. 19-4.   Stomatocytes.
(From Miale, JB: Laboratory medicine: Hematology, ed 6, St Louis, 1982, The CV Mosby Co.)

between forms of HS. For example, a radioimmunoassay (RIA) procedure can quantitate the number of spectrin dimers present on the red cell surface. Normal RBCs contain about 240,000, but the RBCs of HS patients have only 75,000 to 200,000.

OTHER HEREDITARY MEMBRANE DEFECTS

Hereditary elliptocytosis (HE) is an autosomal dominant disorder characterized by oval or rod-like erythrocytes (Plate 5, *E*). From 2 to 5 persons per 10,000 have some form of HE and about 10% of these experience hemolysis. Typically, 25% to 90% of the red cells on blood smears from persons with HE will be elliptical. True elliptocytosis can be partly distinguished from artifacts of smear preparation by homogeneous dispersion (all areas of the slide should contain relatively constant proportions of oval RBCs) and random orientation (the cells are not all aligned in the same direction). The pathophysiological mechanism is poorly understood and a number of defects have been proposed:

1. A defect in the ability of spectrin to interact with other spectrin molecules
2. Abnormal interaction of spectrin with actin
3. Aggregations of hemoglobin at the poles of the elliptocyte
4. A defect in protein band 4.1

Newborn infants may have jaundice and an anemia severe enough to necessitate transfusion. This form of HE, most often seen in black patients, may be accompanied by red cell budding (resembling yeast cells), red cell fragmentation, and various aberrant cell shapes. The anemia's severity usually declines as the child matures, unless hypersplenism becomes a problem. As with hereditary spherocytosis, infection can be a complicating factor, especially in young children.

Hereditary stomatocytosis is characterized by cells on smears with slits (Fig. 19-4). On wet preparations, these cells have the typical bowl shape of stomatocytes (Fig. 16-3). Although stomatocytes are also a normal transitional stage of erythrocyte shape in response to hydration-dehydration conditions, they are also characteristic of a congenital membrane defect that is occasionally accompanied by a moderate hemolytic anemia. Increased ion passage across the RBC membrane has been seen in some cases, but not others. **Hereditary xerocytosis** is characterized by target cells and dehydrated, spiculated forms with an increased MCHC. The structural and functional defects have not been identified, although a decreased concentration of intracellular potassium has been noted (loss of cell water would accompany ion efflux).

Hereditary pyropoikilocytosis (HPP), as the prefix pyro indicates, involves red cells that are unusually sensitive to heat in association with bizarre shapes and fragmented forms. Some destruction occurs at normal body temperature, but the laboratory procedure tests for hemolysis at 45° C (normal cells lyse at about 50°C). HPP is probably a variant of elliptocytosis, either a double heterozygote of two abnormal genes or a homozygous expression of a mild form of HE. Red cells of these patients, like those of some but not all HE patients, have a defect in spectrin to spectrin interactions. Most patients with HPP are black and a mild form of HE is usually present in one or more close relatives.

Abnormalities in the lipid content of the red cell membrane can also result in shortened survival times. A deficiency in **lecithin-cholesterol acyltransferase (LCAT),** the enzyme that regulates the concentration ratio of these two major membrane lipids, is associated with a mild anemia. The cholesterol content is increased; sphingomyelin and lecithin components are decreased and the cell contains an excess membrane surface area compared to volume. Actually, the anemia may be more a function of decreased marrow production than of increased destruction. Other patients have been identified with red cells having an increased lecithin content, also resulting in hemolytic anemia.

Patients with rare phenotypes in which no antigens of a particular blood group system are expressed also have a moderate to severe hemolytic anemia. This is especially true of those cell antigens that are integral structural components of the membrane, such as the Rh, Kell, and Kidd determinants. Lack of antigenic expression is referred to as a "null" phenotype (e.g., **Rh null syndrome**); lack of Kell antigens constitutes the McLeod phenotype. Patients with Rh_{null} red cells have an increased osmotic fragility and autohemolysis tests. Peripheral smears are characterized by stomatocytes.

HEMOLYTIC ANEMIAS ASSOCIATED WITH ENZYME DEFICIENCIES

Deficiencies of enzymes involved in the glycolytic pathway and those that maintain hemoglobin reduction can result in shortened red cell life spans, especially under conditions of oxidative stress. Glucose-6-phosphate dehydrogenase and methemoglobin reductase deficiencies were described in Chapter 18.

The most common disorder of the glycolytic pathway, **pyruvate kinase (PK) deficiency,** is very rare in comparison with the incidence of G-6-PD deficiency. PK deficiency is inherited as an autosomal recessive pattern and a number of variants have been described. Heterozygotes rarely exhibit clinical manifestations, but homozygotes (or double heterozygotes) express a mild to severe anemia. The latter requires frequent transfusion therapy. Since the glycolytic pathway generates the cellular ATP needed to maintain membrane repair and ion regulation, enzyme deficiencies result in membrane lesions or inability to retain potassium ions or both. As with other hemolytic anemias, splenectomy helps control the extent of extravascular destruction, but the relative concentration of reticulocytes (5% to 15% before splenectomy) actually increases following spleen removal. Levels of 50% or more are not uncommon.

Pyruvate kinase regulates glycolysis at a late step in the pathway. Therefore, a PK deficiency results in an accumulation of 2,3-DPG in the Rapaport-Luebering pathway, increasing the red cell concentrations of 2,3-DPG from normal levels of about 5 mmol/L to 10 to 15 mmol per L. The increased 2,3-DPG facilitates oxygen release

to the tissues from hemoglobin and thus partly compensates for the low hemoglobin levels (5 to 12 g/dL).

Laboratory findings for PK deficiency and G-6-PD deficiency are quite different. Whereas the latter results in the formation of Heinz bodies, PK deficiency does not. Spherocytes are frequent findings in G-6-PD deficiency, but dehydration and echinocyte formation are characteristic of PK deficiency. The osmotic fragility test is usually normal for the latter, unless incubated. A positive autohemolysis test is partly corrected (return to a lower percent of cells lysed) by addition of the deficient substance, ATP. Specific diagnosis of the disorders is difficult because the most abnormal cells (lowest ATP levels) are the ones that are most rapidly removed by the spleen. A screening test for PK deficiency uses phosphoenolpyruvate (PEP), the substrate that PK converts to pyruvate. Red cells incubated in PEP generate pyruvate which is then exposed to NADH for conversion to lactate. NADH is converted to NAD during this process. Since NADH is a fluorescent compound with ultraviolet light, persistence of NADH in the red cell mixture is an indicator of PK deficiency.

Other enzymopathies associated with hemolytic anemias are rarer still. **Glucose phosphate isomerase (GPI) deficiency** results in hemoglobin precipitation during oxidant stress because products of the hexose monophosphate shunt are recycled through the step involving GPI. Hemolytic anemia is also associated with deficiencies of hexokinase (HK), phosphoglycerate kinase (PGK), phosphofructokinase (PFK), aldolase, diphosphoglycerate mutase (DGM), and triosephosphate isomerase (TPI). All of these but PGK deficiency exhibit autosomal recessive patterns of inheritance. PGK is sex linked and females have a very mild form, whereas hemizygote males have a severe anemia and experience mental retardation.

Other enzyme deficiencies that directly

affect ATP metabolism can also result in a hemolytic anemia. The most common of these is **pyrimidine 5-nucleotidase (P5N) deficiency.** The appearance of basophilic stippling in red cells is similar to that seen in lead toxicity (lead inhibits 5PN in the acquired form of this anemia). The enzyme splits pyrimidine nucleotides into smaller molecules that diffuse from the red cell. P5N deficiency results in accumulation of the pyrimidines as aggregates, the stippling visualized with Wright's stain. Increased **adenosine deaminase** activity of 50 to 70 times that of normal results in ATP depletion and a clinical picture similar to pyruvate kinase deficiency.

ACQUIRED HEMOLYTIC ANEMIA

Intravascular hemolysis can follow exposure to a number of environmental conditions and agents. Red cell destruction usually ceases when the responsible agent is withdrawn, a distinction from the continuing problems associated with congenital membrane defects. Enzyme deficiencies have composite characteristics in that the underlying pathology is a congenital molecular defect, but hemolysis occurs in most heterozygotes only during oxidant stress or after exposure to specific substances (e.g., fava beans in some forms of G-6-PD deficiency).

A major distinction is made between hemolytic anemias involving immunological responses and those caused by agents that damage red blood cell directly. Some nonimmune causes of acute hemolysis are listed in the following box.

Consumption coagulopathies (DIC) involve depositions of microthrombi in the blood vessels, providing surfaces that damage circulating erythrocytes. Fragmented RBCs are often seen in association with hypercoagulation syndromes. March hemoglobinuria is named after a mild anemia that was diagnosed in soldiers following strenuous marches. Repeated impact to capillary beds produces the red cell damage. The

---

NONIMMUNE ACQUIRED HEMOLYTIC ANEMIAS

Mechanical (physical) damage caused by:
  Prosthetic heart valves and blood vessel catheters
  Vasculitis secondary to autoimmune disorders
  Microthrombus formation in association with DIC syndrome
  March hemoglobinuria, seen in runners, soldiers, and martial arts practitioners
Thermal (heat) damage caused by severe burns
Osmotic damage from:
  Intravenous administration of distilled water
  Vascular contamination by amniotic fluid
Chemical damage after exposure to:
  Metals, such as lead, arsenic, and copper
  Animal venoms (rattlesnakes, certain spiders)
Destruction by infectious agents:
  Intraerythrocytic protozoans (malaria, *Babesia*)
  Hemolytic toxin from bacteria *(Clostridium perfringens)*
  Extravascular hemolysis due to *Bartonella* (Carrion's disease)

---

same phenomenon is seen in some long distance runners and individuals involved in high impact sports, such as karate. Proper foot padding prevents most of the hemolysis in marchers and runners. Incidentally, this form of intravascular hemolysis is not to be confused with runner's anemia, attributable to iron loss via the gastrointestinal tract (Chapter 18).

Hemolysis occurs within 24 hours of suffering severe burns. The red cells are mechanically and osmotically fragile, forming microspherocytes and fragments. These are removed quickly by the spleen and the hematocrit drops accordingly. Direct intravascular destruction is associated with decreased haptoglobin, and increased plasma hemoglobin (the serum or plasma is visibly reddish-orange).

Exposure to lead from paint, gasoline, or industrial products directly interferes with ATP production as well as inhibits heme synthesis. Arsine gas (AsH$_3$) may be inhaled by workers in the forestry and metal smelting industries. As with lead exposure, the red cells may show basophilic stippling, intravascular hemolysis is severe, and red cell fragments may be numerous. Inorganic copper release into the blood stream is seen in Wilson's disease and as a contaminant from hemodialysis equipment. Low levels of phosphates (hypophosphatemia) in some diabetic patients, alcoholics, and in dietary disturbances producing serum phosphate levels of less than 0.5 mg/dL, are associated with a hemolytic anemia, presumably due to interference with ATP and 2,3-DPG production.

Some snake venoms, especially those of certain cobras and pit vipers, contain hemolysins that, in sufficient amounts, can produce intravascular hemolysis. Snake venom can also initiate DIC, resulting in additional red cell destruction. Spider bites, particularly those of the recluse spiders *(Loxosceles)*, are associated with a mild to moderate hemolytic anemia in some individuals.

Bacterial infections rarely result in hemolysis in vivo, despite the presence of hemolysing agents that are demonstrable in vitro. An exception is *Clostridium perfringens*, the causative agent of gas gangrene. This anaerobic organism produces powerful toxins and enzymes that break down tissue. One of these, the so-called alpha toxin, is a lecithinase that attacks the red cell membrane lipid structure, producing intravascular hemolysis. The peripheral blood shows microspherocytes, red cell fragments, thrombocytopenia, and leukocytosis with a granulocytic shift to the left.

Bartonella bacilliformis is a flagellated bacterium transmitted by sand fly bites. It causes Oroya fever (bartonellosis), the hemolytic phase of Carrion's disease, in Peru, Ecuador, and Columbia. Giemsa or Wright's stains of peripheral blood smears reveal the small bacterial rods on and in the red cells (Fig. 19-5). The disease is also characterized by a skin lesion phase and systemic manifestations (lymphadenopathy, hepatosplenomegaly). Bartonellosis has a high fatality

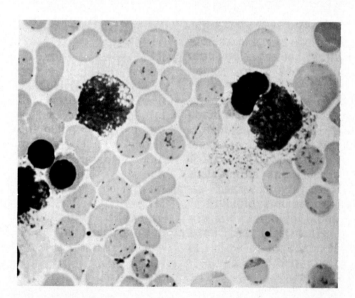

Fig. 19-5. Bartonella infection.
(From Miale, JB: Laboratory medicine: Hematology, ed 6, St Louis, 1982, The CV Mosby Co.)

rate if untreated, but antibiotics (penicillin, streptomycin and tetracycline) are usually effective.

Malaria is the most common infectious disease in the world. It is caused by a protozoan parasite, *Plasmodium*, that is transmitted from mosquitos to man (Fig. 19-6). The sporozoite stage of the malarial parasite enters the blood stream in the mosquito's saliva. The sporozoite circulates to the liver to invade parenchymal cells, where asexual reproduction produces the merozoite stage. After several days, the liver cells rupture and the merozoites enter the blood stream to invade red blood cells. Again, asexual reproduction occurs, filling the infected RBC with 16 to 32 merozoites (the red cell is now referred to as a schizont). The infected red cells lyse, releasing the merozoites to infect additional cells. The intracellular lysis is approximately synchronous and results in the clinical manifesta-

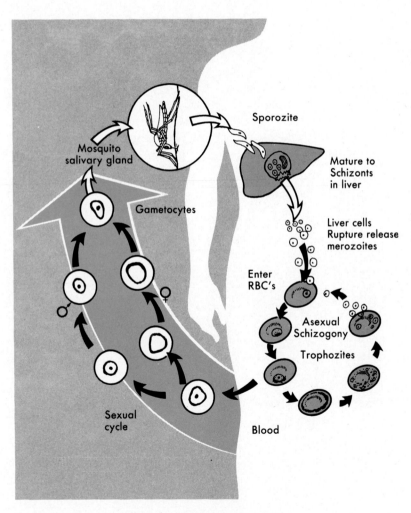

Fig. 19-6   Malaria cycle in man.

tions of chills, a spiking fever, and pain. "Blackwater fever" is a rare but particularly severe hemolytic episode associated with infection by *P. falciparum*, resulting in significant hemoglobinuria.

Red cell destruction is usually multifactoral. Invaded red cells produce less ATP for cell membrane function and thus may be subject to osmotic lysis. An immunological component is also involved; the red cell membrane is altered during infection and antimalarial antibodies fix complement. Many of these cells are removed in the extravascular cords of the spleen, destroying additional red cells in the process. Patients taking quinine as an antimalarial agent may also be subject to hemolytic reactions from the drug, particularly if they have a G-6-PD or other enzyme variant that is sensitive to oxidizing drugs. In addition, the marrow erythropoietic response is depressed, slowing compensatory red cell replacement. Increased RES macrophage activity slowly culminates in splenomegaly, which in turn is associated with a progressive thrombocytopenia. The total white cell count is usually normal or reduced, but eosinophils may be increased.

Four species of *Plasmodium* have been identified as human parasites and each has unique morphological and functional characteristics (Table 19-1). *P. vivax* is the most common and it characteristically invades younger red blood cells, including reticulocytes. On the other hand, *P. malariae* prefers older cells and *P. falciparum*, the most devastating, invades cells of all ages. The hematocrit is usually only mildly decreased, but about 1 in 5 persons with *falciparum* malaria have a severe anemia.

Persons of tropical origin have red cell phenotypes that have been related to increased resistance to malarial infestation. Heterozygotes for S hemoglobin (sickle cell trait) have a lower incidence of vivax infection than normal Hb A/A individuals. The Duffy blood group phenotype Fy(a−b−) confers almost complete resistance to the same species. Blacks with the G6PD mutant A+ are less susceptible to *falciparum* infection. Each of these otherwise disadvantageous genes is maintained at high frequencies in a population by the principle of heterozygote superiority. Thus red cells with a minor deficiency are protected from a more serious threat because their metabolism or membrane structure is not optimal for malarial entry or reproduction.

Additional information on malaria identification can be found in the suggested readings for this chapter or in any book on parasitology. The intracelluar protozoans are easily stained with Giemsa or Wright's stain, but they are not always easy to locate on routine peripheral smears. The search can be enhanced, especially with light infections, with preparation of thick smears, lysing the red cells and staining the residual parasites. Timing is also important since lysis and release of the merozoites occurs in distinct episodes, preceeding the febrile spikes (Chapter 27).

Babesiasis is another protozoan infection transmitted to humans by ticks. *Babesia* in-

Table 19-1. Characteristics of malaria

Species	Incubation period	Fever cycle	Red cells infected	Special features
P. vivax and ovale	8-27 days	48 hours	Young cells	Most common
P. malariae	19-30 days	72 hours	Older cells	Nephrotic syndrome
P. falciparum	10-12 days	Continuous	All cells	Most severe

vades the red cells and produces hemolytic episodes similar to those of malaria. The disease appears to be more severe in patients without spleens, but it can be treated with antibiotics (clindamycin) and quinine. The parasites can be identified on Wright's or Giemsa stained smears.

IMMUNE HEMOLYTIC ANEMIAS

Destruction of red cells by antibodies or antibodies and complement components can also be intravascular or extravascular. The antibodies can be directed against foreign proteins (**alloimmune hemolytic anemia**) or against the host's own antigens (**autoimmune hemolytic anemia, AIHA**). The antibodies are demonstrated by in vitro testing under a variety of conditions (parameters include type of medium, ion content, temperature, and use of enhancing agents). Antibodies that are primarily reactive at body temperature are referred to as "warm" and those that are best demonstrated at less than body temperature (usually at 4° to 30° C) are called "cold" antibodies. Exposure of a functioning immume system to non-self antigens results in formation of specific immunoglobulins by plasma cells (Chapter 9 and 10). The antigens may be in the form of microbial coat proteins, complex chemicals or therapeutic drugs, or red cell antigens resulting from transfusion or transplacental bleeding during delivery. The hemolytic anemia resulting from these alloimmune processes is limited by the presence of the antigens. Removal of the offending drug or clearance of the incompatible red cells stops the hemolysis.

Autoimmune hemolytic anemia (AIHA)

Autoantibodies against host tissue antigens are associated with a number of connective tissue diseases, such as rheumatoid arthritis and systemic lupus erythematosis. Autoantibodies also occur naturally, usually as cold-reacting IgM agglutinins to red

blood cell antigens such as I, H, and IH. Autoimmune hemolytic anemia occurs when autoantibodies are produced against red blood cell antigens, most often as a result of drug interaction, following an infection or secondary to a myeloproliferative disorder.

Antibodies that cross react against the I antigen of the Ii blood group, almost universally present on the red cells of adults, are sometimes seen after infections with *Mycoplasma pneumoniae.* Similar antibodies occasionally react with the i antigen following infectious mononucleosis (Chapter 21). These antibodies are cold reacting but active over a broad thermal range. They are usually IgM and they bind complement, occasionally producing in vivo hemolysis. The cold agglutinins associated with infections are transient, and the anemia is usually mild, but splenomegaly and jaundice may be evident in some patients. Similar antibody specificities are seen in lymphoproliferative disorders.

Cold hemagglutinin disease (CHD) is idiopathic in nature, occurring primarily in older adults during the winter, the antibodies are most commonly IgM with anti-I, less often anti-i, and rarely anti-Pr specificities. The antibody titer in CHD tends to be much higher than that seen in normal persons or in those with secondary cold agglutinins (**agglutinins** are antibodies that produce cell aggregations). Coating of red cells by the antibodies, a process called **sensitization**, can be detected with the **direct antiglobulin test (DAT)**. This is one of the most important procedures for distinguishing immune from nonimmune mechanisms underlying hemolytic anemia. The DAT test is almost always positive in CHD when the antisera contains complement (C3b) components, but it is usually negative if only IgG is present in the antisera. Because the antibodies bind to the red cells at cool temperatures, a blood sample may show signs of autoagglutination, interfering with attempts to obtain reliable cell counts or make smears with well dispersed red cells.

Paroxysmal cold hemoglobinuria (PCH) is a specific type of cold AIHA that occurs when an autoantibody binds to red cells at cool temperatures, fixes complement to the red cell surface, and then hemolyzes the cell at normal body temperature. Unlike the cold antibodies previously described, those associated with PCH are IgG. The dual temperature response and hemolytic manifestation gives these antibodies the term "biphasic hemolysin." They are also known as Donath-Landsteiner antibodies, the investigators that described them, and they demonstrate anti-P specificity, occasionally anti-IH.

PCH occurs most often in young children following viral infections (viral flu, chicken pox, measles, mumps, and infectious mononucleosis are common examples), but the disorder was originally described in association with syphillis. Fortunately, the disease is usually self-limiting, occurring as a sequalae to the viral infection. The hemolytic anemia can be severe, however, producing all the classic signs of intravascular hemolysis. These include chills, fever, low back pain, and hemoglobin in the urine. A chronic form of the disease may persist in older adults in which exposure to a cold environment is followed by an episode of hemolysis. Exposure of hands and face is sufficient to produce cooler capillary blood temperatures, antibody binding, and complement fixation. As the blood returns to the center of the body and warm temperatures, hemolysis results. Persons suffering from the chronic form must avoid cold temperatures and some must forsake the comforts of air conditioning.

Warm autoimmune hemolytic anemia, as the name implies, occurs at body temperature and usually involves an IgG antibody. Most cases are idiopathic, secondary to another disease, or associated with administration of drugs. The red cells are sensitized (coated) by the antibodies and the cells are destroyed during passage through the spleen. Removal is especially rapid if complement has also been fixed to the erythrocyte. The DAT should be positive for IgG or complement, or both. Warm autoantibodies often have specificities that cross react with Rh antigens, especially hr'' (e).

Drug-induced AIHA involves an immunological response to a particular drug (contrast this with adverse reactions seen in some enzyme deficiencies). Hemolysis occurs as a result of one of three mechanisms (Table 19-2). Recognition of a drug induced AIHA often depends on obtaining a good medication history and ruling out other potential causes. A partial list of common drugs that have been implicated in immune-mediated hemolytic anemia are listed in the accompanying box.

From 10% to 20% of acquired immune hemolytic anemias may be drug induced, with methyldopa by far the drug most often implicated. The autoimmune mechanism of AIHA is associated with a positive direct antiglobulin test (DAT), not only during administration of the inducing drug, but for months to years after drug discontinuation. The anitbody that coats the red cells is most often IgG, usually with Rh specificity. IgM and complement are also present on RBCs in patients experiencing severe hemolysis. Because a number of other autoantibodies have also been found after methyldopa therapy, it has been suggested that the drug interferes with tolerance discriminating mechanisms of the immune system, probably by inhibiting suppressor T lymphocyte function.

Many patients receiving penicillin form antibodies to the drug or its metabolic derivatives. Most of these are IgM antibodies and they cause no clinical problems. However, in some patients the derivatives are adsorbed to erythrocyte membranes and act as antigenic stimuli (the red cell acting as a carrier for the hapten metabolite) to produce high titers of IgG antibodies. The DAT

Table 19-2. Drug-induced AIHA

Mechanism	Ig type	DAT result	Example
Adsorption (Hapten)	IgG	IgG positive	Penicillin
Autoimmune	IgG	IgG positive	Methyldopa
Immune complex	IgM	C' positive	Quinidine
Immune complex	IgG	IgG positive	Insulin

DRUGS IMPLICATED IN AIHA

Drug	Therapeutic use
Induction of autoantibodies	
Methyldopa (Aldomet)	Anithypertensive
Levodopa	Parkinson's disease
Mefenamic acid	Rheumatoid arthritis
Absorption onto red cell membrane (Hapten type)	
Penicillin	Antibiotic
Tetracycline	Antibiotic
Cephalothin	Antibiotic
Streptomycin	Antibiotic
Formation of immune complexes	
Acetaminophen	Analgesic and antipyretic
Chloropromazine (Thorazine)	Sedative and antiemetic
Phenacetin	Analgesic and antipyretic
Isoniazid (NIH)	Antibiotic
Quinidine	Cardiac arrhythmias

result is positive and intravascular hemolysis can be severe if complement is fixed.

Some drugs bind readily to plasma proteins and this circulating drug-protein complex serves as an antigen, invoking an antibody response. The antibody forms a complex with the antigen and the complex attaches to the red cell membrane. Either IgM or IgG may be produced. The former is more likely to attach to red cells, fix complement, and produce a hemolytic anemia, whereas the latter is usually directed against platelets, producing an immune thrombocytopenia. Some patients may produce both antibodies and suffer both types of destruction. IgG rarely remains on the cell so that the DAT is positive only when using anticomplement antisera.

Paroxysmal nocturnal hemoglobinuria (PNH)

Paroxysmal nocturnal hemoglobinuria is an acquired hemolytic anemia in which the red cells are extremely sensitive to complement components. Several factors enhance the complement sensitivity, including lower pH and increased concentrations of glucose. These conditions are realized during sleep, resulting in a hemolytic episode (usually at night or in the morning after rising) and the release of hemoglobin in the urine. The condition is chronic but sporadic in severity. The intravascular hemolysis is often associated with activation of the coagulation pathway and thrombotic complications, some of which can be fatal.

The etiological basis for PNH is still unknown, but evidence points to a disturbance of the hematopoietic stem cell, because all blood cells show evidence of a similar membrane defect. PNH has often been correlated with aplastic anemia and pancytopenia preceeds the appearance of PNH in about one fourth of the cases. The disorder may terminate in acute leukemia and myelofibrosis may also be present.

Three distinct cell populations are known to be present in PNH patients, based on their sensitivity to complement:

Type I cells: normal complement binding

Type II cells: show increased complement binding (C3 fixation to cell surface)

Type III cells: increased binding plus enhanced penetration of the membrane by the C5-9 complex

Complement activation is thought to occur via the alternate pathway, since antibody production has not been demonstrated. Overall, type II cells are about 2 to 5 times more sensitive to complement than normal cells and type III cells are 20 times as sensitive. Reticulocytes are especially vulnerable to lysis, thus the reticulocyte count may be normal or decreased despite the hemolytic process. Other abnormalities include a depressed neutrophil alkaline phosphatase content and a secondary decrease of acetylcholinesterase in erythrocytes.

Although the disease occurs in patients as young as 5 years old, most cases appear in adults 30 to 50 years old, affecting both sexes. The relationship of hemolysis to sleep is also not fully understood. Carbon dioxide is retained to a slightly greater extent when a person is at rest, producing a small drop in pH. Magnesium levels also change during sleep, enhancing the potential to activate the alternate complement pathway. In addition, one of the regulatory proteins that inhibits complement activation (decay accelerating factor) is known to be deficient.

Three tests are especially helpful in diagnosing PNH. The acidified serum (Ham) test is a simple procedure: pH of the patient's serum/red cell mixture is lowered with 0.2N HCI and checked for hemolysis in comparison to a normal control serum. The sugar water (sucrose hemolysis) test is similar, looking for increased complement activation as the ionic strength of the serum is decreased. A third finding is the presence of hemosiderin in the urine. Other hemolytic anemias may also show positive results with some of these procedures. HEMPAS (Chapter 17) gives a positive Ham test, but only with normal sera (containing antibodies). Autologous serum will be positive by Ham test in patients with PNH and negative in patients with HEMPAS. Although most of the hemolytic anemias may exhibit hemosiderinuria, it is so characteristic of PNH that a negative result essentially rules out PHN.

Hemolytic crises are brought on by a variety of events, including administration of certain drugs, use of antisera, and infections and inflammatory processes. Even menstruation can precipitate a severe hemolytic episode. The median survival time after diagnosis is less than 5 years, with death attributable to the anemia, infection, or thrombotic complications. The disease is refractory to most forms of therapy. Supportive therapy for the anemia consists of transfusions, using washed red cells or deglycerated (frozen then thawed) cells to avoid sensitization and additional complement activation.

Hemolytic disease of the newborn

Red cell antigens carried by the human fetus reflect the genetic contributions (genotypes) of the father and mother. Therefore, a fetus always has a genetic constitution that differs from its mother. Although the placenta effectively separates the cellular components of the maternal and fetal circulatory systems, some transplacental bleeding is inevitable during delivery. Bleeding may also occur during the pregnancy because of trauma or due to a defect in the membranes. The mother is thus exposed to the foreign antigens of her baby and her immune system has the potential to respond to those antigens that she lacks. The more babies and deliveries, the greater the risk of immunological response.

Actually, most mothers do not respond to most of the antigens to which they are exposed. Some antigens are weak and do not stimulate the immune system. Some women simply do not respond to certain red cell antigens, even to those red cell determinants that are very antigenic in other people. The response potential is also dependent on the amount of blood that passes from fetus to mother.

Before the late 1960s **hemolytic disease of the newborn (HDN)** was a frequent and serious problem. Babies were born with severe hemolytic anemia and rapidly developing jaundice. Their peripheral blood displayed a marked increase in nucleated red blood cells, thus the condition was also known as **erythroblastosis fetalis.** Severity varied from mild, self-limiting anemia to severe conditions manifested by cardiac failure, pulmonary congestion, edema (hydrops fetalis, see Thalassemia, Chapter 18), and systemic pathology. Some women gave birth to several of these "yellow" babies (named for the jaundice that developed soon after birth), often after having one or two normal or mildly affected infants.

The nature of the disease was realized when antibodies in the mother's serum were discovered that reacted to the red cells of the infant. The discovery coincided with development of the antiglobulin test by Coombs and his associates in the late 1930s and early 1940s, making it possible to detect and identify the antibodies responsible for destruction of the fetal erythrocytes. Red cells and accompanying antigens pass into the mother's bloodstream during delivery (Fig. 19-7). In most cases, this amounts to 20 mL of blood or less, but it is enough for some antigens to stimulate the maternal immune system. The mother produces antibodies against the red cell antigen and forms memory cells that will recognize the determinants if reexposure occurs. If she carries a second baby with the same antigenic determinant, the circulating IgG antibodies can cross the placenta and attack the fetal red cells. This occurs during the last trimester, since the fetal red cells do not express most antigens until then. Depending on the titer of maternal antibody and the nature of the antigen, intravascular hemolysis can produce a mild to severe anemia.

Released hemoglobin is metabolized mainly by the mother's liver (the fetal liver is unable to conjugate bilirubin until well after birth), so that the main problem for the fetus is the anemia and cardiovascular complications associated with it.

After delivery, red cell destruction is limited to the residual concentration of maternal antibody. With time, this is cleared from the circulation and the infant's hematopoietic tissue struggles to replace the red cell mass. This isn't easy, since the demands of growth place a severe strain on red cell production even in normal infants. The other major problem, however, is the accumulation of bilirubin in the neonate's tissues as red cell destruction continues. Without the support of the maternal liver, the unconjugated bilirubin is deposited in central nervous tissue, particularly in the basal ganglia. This results in a condition called **kernicterus.** The damage is irreversible, producing mental retardation or death. Thus the prenatal problem is one of anemia, the postnatal problem is one of bilirubin accumulation. Exchange transfusion, using blood compatible with the mother (but lacking antibodies), is often required to elevate the neonate's hemoglobin, remove maternal antibodies, and reduce the bilirubin concentration. A bilirubin level that rises by more than 0.5 mg per dL each hour or by 10 mg/dL in 24 hours warrants consideration of a transfusion. The bilirubin should not exceed 18 mg/dL and several transfusions may be necessary before the baby is stabilized.

The most common and severe forms of HDN were due to the D (Rh$_o$) antigen, the factor that designates a person as "Rh positive" (D antigen present) or "Rh negative" (D antigen absent). Rh positive babies carried by Rh negative mothers produced the greatest risk of HDN. However, during the 1960s a technique was developed to prophylactically treat Rh negative women during and/or after pregnancies with Rh positive babies. Rh immune globulin (RhIg) is given

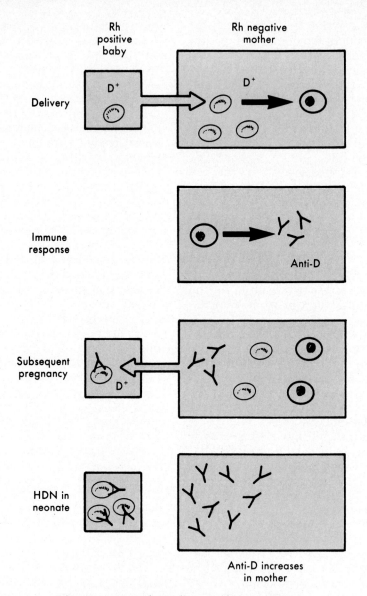

Fig. 19-7 Hemolytic disease of the newborn.

antenatally (28 weeks gestation) and/or within 72 hours after delivery. The RhIg binds to the circulating fetal cells and enhances their removal by the spleen, but without stimulating the immune response.

How this is accomplished is uncertain, since the spleen is quite capable of acting as a mediator for immune responses during extravascular destruction. RhIg may bind to sufficient D antigen sites to inhibit the splenic macrophages, or the Rhlg may act directly on the central immune response processes.

Whatever the mechanism, it works. HDN due to Rh incompatability (D antigen specifically) is now relatively rare in developed countries where prenatal care is readily available. Rhlg must be given with each incompatible pregnancy and it is of no use if an anti-D titer has already developed. Prior sensitization can occur by transfusion as well as pregnancy, so that an indirect antiglobulin test on the mother's serum is required before administering Rhlg. Because of these preventative measures, HDN due to Rh incompatability is now less than one third of total HDN cases.

The most common form of HDN is now due to ABO incompatability, when an O group mother carries a group A or, less commonly, a group B fetus. Group O individuals produce antibodies to A and B antigens, including a complex antibody, anti-A,B. The latter is often an IgG antibody that is capable of crossing the placenta and attacking the red cells of a group A or B fetus. Since these maternal antibodies are naturally occurring (they do not require stimulation by pregnancy or transfusion), the first pregnancy can be affected. Contrast this with the first pregnancy for women with Rh incompatability where the fetus is rarely affected, although a low titer anti-D occurs in a small fraction of such women at the time of their first delivery. Fortunately, ABO incompatability results in a much milder form of HDN than does Rh incompatability. The postnatal bilirubin level usually remains within safe limits and treatment is often confined to exposing the infant to an ultraviolet light which degrades the bilirubin passing through superficial blood vessels. Because the ABO system antibodies occur naturally, prophylactic therapy like that used for the Rh factor is not possible. Other antigens may also produce HDN, such as other Rh spe-

cificities, Kell system antigens, etc. However, these account for less than 3% of cases.

Additional progress has been made in treating HDN. Cell products and metabolites from the fetus are detectable in the amniotic fluid and this can be sampled by a technique called **amniocentesis.** Bilirubin passes from the fetus into the amniotic fluid en route to the maternal blood stream. Increased amounts of bilirubin can be detected spectrophotometrically and compared to normal values for the gestational age of the fetus. Abnormally high concentrations, along with a rising maternal antibody titer, may indicate the need for labor induction (if the pregnancy is near term) or for an intrauterine exchange transfusion (if fetal development is not sufficient for a safe delivery and postnatal survival). This technique can also obtain evidence of thalassemia and other hereditary disorders.

Laboratory findings in HDN include indications of hemolytic anemia (increased reticulocyte count, increased erythroblasts, low hematocrit), increased unconjugated bilirubin, positive DAT (the responsible antibodies can be eluted from the red cells and identified), and leukocytosis due to a stress-related increase in neutrophils. The amount of transplacental bleeding can be determined with the **Kleihauer-Betke test** for fetal hemoglobin. When maternal blood on a smear is exposed to an ~~alkaline~~ acidic solution, the normal maternal cells (Hb A) wash out and appear as "ghosts", whereas the fetal cells (Hb F) resist elution and stain with a counterstain (Fig. 19-8). The relative proportion of fetal to maternal RBCs can be determined and the amount of fetal blood volume calculated. The mother's red blood cell volume is also calculated, based on her body size and hematocrit. The dosage of prophylatic Rhlg is proportional to the volume of fetal cells present (300 μg of Rhlg per 15 mL of fetal red cells).

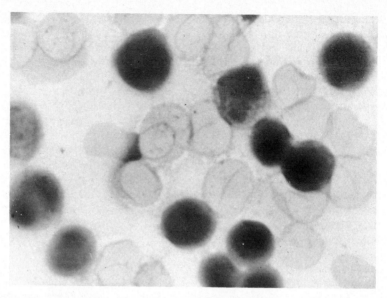

Fig. 19-8.   Kleihauer-Betke stain for fetal hemoglobin.
(From Miale, JB: Laboratory medicine: Hematology, ed 6, St Louis, 1982, The CV Mosby Co.)

Hemolytic transfusion reaction

Donor blood cells that are imcompatible with a recipient's blood cells can also result in a host immune response. As is the case with HDN, some antigens are more likely to elicit a response than others and recipients show varying degrees of responsiveness. ABO incompatabilities are by far the most dangerous because the antibodies are already present in high titer and the red cells contain a large number of antigenic sites. ABO antibodies fix complement and produce a devastating intravascular hemolysis. For instance, if a donor's group A cells are mistakingly transfused to a group B patient, they will be destroyed by the patient's anti-A antibodies. The hemolysis is often accompanied by chills, fever, pain at the site of destruction, low back pain as the kidneys filter the hemoglobin from the plasma, and a sense of impending doom. Renal failure, cardiovascular shock, and death can occur within a few minutes if active intervention does not occur.

Investigation reveals an increased plasma hemoglobin (often visible by merely looking at the plasma of a pre- and posttransfusion blood sample), decreased serum haptoglobin, and hemoglobinuria. Transfusion reaction due to other blood group incompatabilities usually occurs as a result of prior sensitization by pregnancy or earlier transfusion. Alloantibodies should be present in the recipient's serum, and are detected by the indirect antiglobulin test.

SUMMARY

- Acute or chronic hemorrhage is manifested as a normocytic normochromic anemia. Severity is a function of rate of bleeding and the capability of the bone marrow to respond. Hypovolemic shock and hypoxia are the major problems associated with massive blood loss.
- A normal response to blood loss includes an erythropoietin increase within a few hours, reticulocytes increase at 7 to 10 days, and hemactocrit levels return to

normal within a few weeks. The ability to respond depends to a large extent on iron reserves and whether the blood loss is internal (into the tissues) or external.

- Hemolytic anemias can be catagorized by origin (acquired and hereditary), mechanism (immune and nonimmune), and site (intravascular and extravascular). Nonimmunological hemolytic anemias can be caused by membrane defects, deficiencies of red cell enzymes, defects in hemoglobin production, and acquired anemias from exposure to malaria, infections, venoms, and toxic chemicals.

- Immune hemolytic anemias include autoimmune and alloimmune mechanisms. Autoimmune hemolytic anemias can be idiopathic or triggered by infections, malignancies, and other autoimmune disorders. The most common forms are induced by drugs, such as methyldopa and penicillin. Alloimmune hemolytic anemias include hemolytic disease of the newborn and transfusion reactions, both occurring as a result of imcompatible blood group antigens between two individuals.

- In general, hemolytic anemias are characterized by signs of red cell destruction (falling hematocrit, short RBC survival time), the appearance of hemoglobin derivatives (bilirubin increases, jaundice may be clinically evident), and a compensatory production response (erythroid hyperplasia, increased reticulocyte count).

- Extravascular hemolysis is often accompanied by splenomegaly. Intravascular hemolysis may show depleted haptoglobin and hemoglobinuria. Immune mechanisms may show a positive direct antiglobulin test for lgG or complement and evidence of circulating antibodies (indirect antiglobulin test).

- Membrane defects may be accompanied by increased osmotic or mechanical fragility (increased fragility test, red cell fragments on smears). Enzyme deficiencies may result in formation of Heinz bodies or be detectable by assays for enzyme activity.

20

Primary Disorders of White Blood Cells

LEUKOCYTE DISORDERS: AN OVERVIEW

Diseases and abnormalities involving white blood cells, as with disorders of other blood elements, can be classified in a variety of ways. These different approaches are neither mutually exclusive nor do they satisfy all of the needs to organize and understand relationships between diseases. The box on p. 289 indicates some of these approaches to classification:

This textbook arbitrarily separates leukocyte disorders into two groups: this chapter describes the hematopoietic neoplasms; Chapter 21 presents other, non-neoplastic conditions, including reactive states and various anomalies. Disorders of platelets and thrombocytic precursors are discussed in Chapter 23.

MORPHOLOGICAL AND FUNCTIONAL FEATURES OF WHITE CELL DISORDERS

It is not always easy to correlate the degree of morphological abnormality with functional deficiency. Neutrophils that appear normal in terms of shape, size, granule content, and routine staining pattern may be unable to respond to chemotactic stimuli or to mount an oxidative response to phagocytic events. On the other hand, white cells that appear atypical, even immature, by morphological criteria may function normally. Distinguishing between cells that appear immature because they are **reactive**, that is, responding to inflamma-

tory stimuli as part of normal host defense, and cells that are immature products of abnormal uncontrolled growth, is both a diagnostic and technical problem of some importance.

Before the advent of biochemical and immunological methods, the morphological appearance of white cells on smears and marrow sections provided the primary laboratory evidence for the presence of a pathological state. Some reactive conditions were easy to confuse with neoplastic processes. This was particularly true for conditions involving lymphocyte responses: a knowledge of lymphocyte development and recirculation was necessary to evaluate the nature of blast transformations in response to viral antigens. Although various white cell surface antigens can now be specified and some of these are diagnostically characteristic of certain blood cell tumors and leukemias, morphological studies are still widely used to identify abnormal cells and provide a definitive diagnosis.

CHROMOSOMAL CHANGES

Chromosomal abnormalities have been found in several types of leukemia and at times they may be prognostic indicators of response to therapy. For this reason, cytogenetic studies are routinely included in many protocols. Most chromosomal changes involve **translocations** of genetic material from one autosome to another, as in Burkitt's lymphoma where material from

VARIOUS CLASSIFICATION APPROACHES FOR DISORDERS OF WHITE BLOOD CELLS

Classification based on nature of abnormality

1. Quantitative: based on numbers of cells in marrow, peripheral blood, or both
   a. Leukocytopenias: decreased numbers of cells (e.g., neutropenia)
   b. Leukocytoses: increased numbers of cells (e.g., reactive lymphocytosis)
2. Qualitative: based on a defect or deficiency in a cell component
   a. Morphological: defect is observed primarily as a structural abnormality (e.g., Pelger-Huët anomaly)
   b. Functional: defect is primarily functional (e.g., myeloperoxidase deficiency)
   c. Combined: most disorders involve structural and metabolic changes (e.g., lipid storage diseases)

Classification based on etiological origin

1. Hereditary basis: genetically passed as an allele from generation to generation
   a. Recessive: disease expressed in homozygous and hemizygous conditions (e.g., Chediak-Higashi syndrome)
   b. Dominant: disease expressed in heterozygous as well as homozygous condition (e.g., May-Hegglin anomaly)
2. Acquired basis: disorder occurs to individual, not included in genome
   a. Congenital: present at birth, often involves developmental abnormalities Some of these may have a genetic basis which has not yet been demonstrated (e.g., DiGeorge's syndrome)
   b. Postnatal: acquired during childhood or as an adult. May be primary, attributable to an environmental agent (e.g., drug-induced cytopenia) or secondary to another disease process (e.g., myeloid displacement due to a metastatic carcinoma)
3. Idiopathic: cause unknown Although a number of different factors have been investigated as potential causative agents for different leukemias, most cases cannot be attributed to specific environmental or hereditary origins

Classification based on progression of symptoms and outcome

1. Acute: onset of symptoms and rate of disease progress is rapid. Morphological changes in the blood cell picture are often dramatic (e.g., immature cells seen in acute leukemias)
2. Chronic: onset of symptoms may be gradual, sometimes insidious (unrecognized), progression may occur over many years, and morphological changes may be slight to moderate (e.g., chronic leukemias)

These manifestations are not mutually exclusive; they may undergo transitions from chronic to acute or back as a result of therapy or relapse following failure of therapy (e.g., many of the myeloproliferative disorders begin as chronic disorders but may terminate as acute leukemias)

Classification by cell lineage (Table 20-1)

Disorders are classified on the basis of the cell line most obviously affected. Several diseases involve precursors of more than one cell line (e.g., pluripotential stem cells), so that abnormalities appear in two or more of the myeloid and erythroid elements

chromosomes 8 and 14 are rearranged, written as t[8;14][q24;q32]. The symbol, t, indicates a translocation between the two indicated chromosomes at the respective regions or bands (q24 of chromosome 8 and q32 of chromosome 14), symbolized by the letters p and q. Indeed, some investigators believe that these translocations may be the reason for the neoplastic changes that occur. In the example given above, an oncogene is known to be located at each of the two regions involved. Translocation brings the two genes in proximity, causing an as yet unspecified change in regulation of cell proliferation. What is responsible for the translocation? Some bands of chromosomes are naturally "weaker" than others, and these sites apparently are subject to breakage. This process may be accelerated by a number of environmental agents, such as

Table 20-1. Leukocyte disorders

Disorders of granulocytes
Quantitative: neutropenias
  Congenital neutropenias
  Acquired neutropenias
  Granulocytic leukemias
Qualitative: dysfunction
  Mobility and chemotactic disorders
  Metabolic disorders
  Immunophagocytic disorders
Morphological: benign conditions
	Disorders of lymphocytes
	Lymphopenias
	Lymphoid leukemias and lymphomas
	Monoclonal gammopathies
	
	Disorders of histiocytes
	Lipid storage diseases
	Histiocytoses

Disorders of monocytes Monocytic leukemias Mobility and chemotactic disorders	**Multiple cell lines** Acquired leukopenias Stem cell leukemias Myeloproliferative syndromes Myelodysplastic syndromes

toxic chemicals, radiation, and intracellular activities of some viruses. Some individuals may also be genetically more susceptible to certain translocations than others.

CORRELATION OF MARROW AND PERIPHERAL BLOOD PATTERNS

Regardless of the etiological basis, the establishment of a genetically abnormal clone of hematopoietic precursors changes the marrow and, ultimately, peripheral blood composition. How much and how soon depends on a number of factors. If the new cells are recognized as abnormal by the immune surveillance system (especially the killer T cells), they may be attacked and removed either by lymphocytic lysis or as a result of phagocytosis by marrow macrophages. To what extent this occurs and why it fails is the focus of much oncological research.

Growth rate and replication time determine whether the abnormal clone replaces normal marrow elements. Interestingly, evidence from tissue cultures of neoplastic cells indicates that the abnormal cells reproduce *slower* than their normal counterparts. In addition, most abnormal clones fail to reach maturation, some aborting during replication. Yet, these cells can compete and eventually overcome the normal marrow elements. Most of these cells do not leave the marrow, especially during the earliest stages of the disorder; their continued presence and reproduction assures a gradual increase in the number of abnormal stem cells, whereas the normal stem cell population remains relatively constant (Fig. 20-1). The neoplastic cells undoubtedly compete with normal cells for nutrients and they may release substances that actively inhibit neighboring stem cells, both which serve to widen the competitive advantage. The extent to which neoplastic cells respond to feedback mechanisms (i.e., colony-stimulating factors and leukopoietins) that regulate stem cell reproduction is also under investigation.

Neoplastic processes vary greatly in course and manifestations. Essentially, two types of disorder can be defined. **Myeloproliferative disorders (MPD)** are autonomous (uncontrolled) expansions of cell clones involving one or more hematopoietic cell lines: granulocytic, monocytic, lymphoid, erythroid, thrombocytic, histiocytic, and fibroblastic. Used generally and loosely, myeloproliferative diseases include the acute leukemias, which are clearly malignant states. Most references restrict the use of

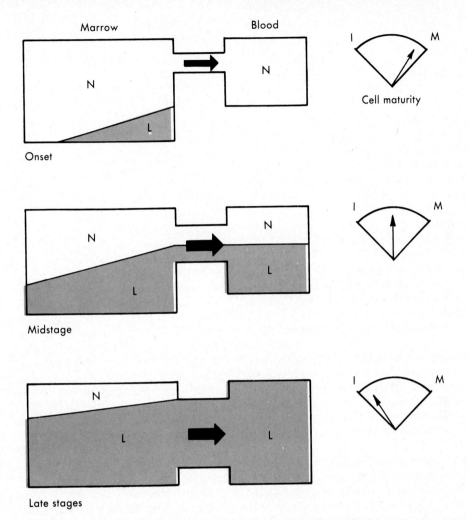

Fig. 20-1.   Relationship of neoplastic and normal cells in the bone marrow.

MPD to chronic leukemias and to three other conditions characterized by neoplastic, but not necessarily malignant, growth. MPDs are contrasted with **myelodysplastic syndromes (MDS)** or dysmyelopoietic syndromes, in which blood cell precursors exhibit abnormal, usually ineffective, maturation. Although the marrow may be hypercellular in both MPD and MDS, the peripheral blood usually has an increased cell concentration in the former but it is decreased in the latter. Cytopenia and cellular abnormalities associated with MDS reflect the inability of the marrow cells to mature and assume normal function (analagous to dyserythropoietic anemias; see Chapter 17).

Terms associated with changes in cell proliferation

The proliferation and differentiation of blood cells as a tissue are described by a variety of terms and a few of these are compared at this time.

Hyperplasia describes an increase in cell numbers, such as the reactive proliferation of normoblasts in response to hypoxia or that of white cells in response to infection.

Hypertrophy is an increase in the size of cells and the tissue or organ that the cells comprise. Usually, expanded volume of the cytoplasm is the reason for cellular enlargement, but in some cases it is the nucleus that expands. Most mechanisms for hypertrophy are reactive.

Dysplasia is an abnormal or atypical increase in cell number due to a pathological process.

Metaplasia is a change of one cell type to another type, a process that may be benign or malignant. Genetic mechanisms underlie the change in identity, expressed morphologically, biochemically, or immunologically.

Neoplasia is defined as an abnormal growth or expansion of tissue, one that is progressive and persistent, uncontrolled by the normal cellular mechanisms that regulate reactive processes. Neoplasms (meaning *new growths*) are commonly referred to as tumors.

Benign tumors are characterized by slow growth (decreased mitotic rate) of well differentiated mature cells that do not invade surrounding tissues nor do they migrate to other sites (they are not metastatic). They are surrounded, usually by a capsule of fibrous tissue. Most benign tumors are non-reoccurring and in most cases, they are not directly life threatening.

Malignant tumors are characterized by the expansion of cells into adjacent tissues, displacing normal cells and becoming progressively life threatening. They may grow rapidly or slowly and the state of cell differentiation varies. Malignancies are further-subdivided by tissue of origin:

Sarcomas are derived from mesenchymal tissues

Carcinomas are derived from epithelial tissues

LEUKEMIA

Leukemia is defined as an unregulated malignant proliferation of hematopoietic tissue that progressively displaces normal blood cell elements. Leukemias are traditionally classified by the predominant cell type involved and the degree of maturity or immaturity that characterizes the peripheral blood cell pattern. A general scheme of leukemia types is presented on p. 293, emphasizing the differences between acute and chronic forms.

Although morphological criteria (cell size, nuclear and cytoplasmic features) provide the traditional bases for classifying leukemias, the use of cytochemical staining techniques during the past few decades has made it possible to identify abnormal hematopoietic precursors with more confidence. A battery of special staining studies of the bone marrow and peripheral blood is part of a complete workup for a patient with leukemia (see Chapter 27 and below). The combination of morphological and cytochemical characteristics of leukemic cells is utilized by special study groups to compare data and treatment results of patients from various parts of the country and world.

The various oncology groups (e.g., SWOG, the Southwest Oncology Group, and CCSG, the Children's Cancer Study Group) follow a strict protocol for laboratory studies and specimens of marrow and blood are submitted for review by criteria established by each group. Thus, several clinics and hospitals, representing hundreds of physicians, can analyze the diagnostic and therapeutic data of a large number of patients. This cooperative effort makes it possible to establish differences between therapeutic regimens and arrive at statistical conclusions that would be impossible on the basis of isolated cases at each medical facility.

MANIFESTATIONS OF LEUKEMIA

Acute leukemia

Acute myelogenous leukemia, AML (acute non-lymphoid, ANLL)
    Undifferentiated leukemia (stem cell; acute myeloblastic)
    Acute myelocytic leukemia (differentiated AML)
    Promyelocytic leukemia (hypergranular promyelocytic; progranulocytic)
    Myelomonocytic
    Monocytic
    Erythroleukemia (erythroblastic; DiGuglielmo's disease)
    Megakaryocytic
Acute lymphocytic leukemia, ALL
    T cell ALL
    B cell ALL
        Pre-B cell ALL
    Null cell ALL (non-T, non-B cell ALL)
        Acute lymphoblastic leukemia of childhood
        Null cell ALL of adults

Chronic leukemia

Chronic myelogenous leukemia, CML
    Granulocytic leukemia, CGL
    Eosinophilic leukemia
    Basophilic leukemia
    Myelomonocytic leukemia (see myelodysplastic syndromes)
    Chronic lymphocytic leukemia, CLL
    T cell CLL
    B cell CLL
    Hairy cell leukemia, HCL (leukemic reticuloendotheliosis)
    Plasma cell leukemia, PCL (see multiple myeloma)

Other leukemia

Mast cell leukemia (systemic mastocytosis)

FAB Classifications

An international cooperative effort to generate data resulted in the formation of the **French-American-British (FAB) Cooperative Group** and the publication of a scheme for classifying acute leukemias

Table 20-2. FAB classification of acute leukemia

FAB Number	Name
M1	Acute myeloblastic leukemia without maturation
M2	Acute myelocytic leukemia with differentiation
M3	Hypergranular promyelocytic leukemia
M4	Myelomonocytic leukemia
M5	Monocytic leukemia
	M5a Monoblastic (poorly differentiated)
	M5b Promonocytic-monocytic (differentiated)
M6	Erythroleukemia (erythroblastic)
M7	Megakaryocytic leukemia
L1	Acute lymphoblastic leukemia, small blast
L2	Acute lymphocytic leukemia, heterogenous
L3	Acute lymphocytic leukemia, Burkitt type

based on morphological characteristics (Table 20-2). Currently, the FAB system recognizes seven types of nonlymphoblastic leukemia (M1 to M7) and 3 types of lymphoblastic leukemia (L1 to L3). The criteria are reviewed periodically in order to incorporate additional data. Much new information about cell lineage has been provided by studies using immunological markers to identify specific stages of precursors that may share common morphological or cytochemical features. This information has not been incorporated into the FAB classification, nor has it been applied with universal success to predicting treatment outcomes. In fact, cell identities classified according to FAB criteria do not agree with those based on cell surface antigens. Interestingly, many oncologists believe that clinical courses and responses to treatment protocols show a better correlation to FAB criteria than to the more specific identities

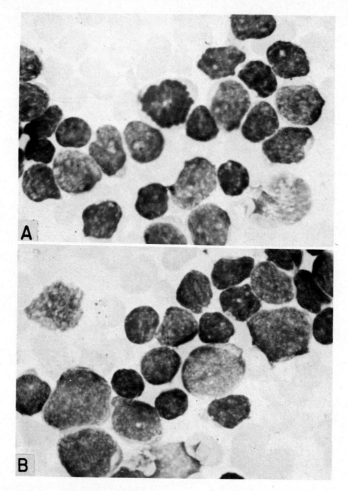

Fig. 20-2.   Acute lymphocytic leukemia.
A, Bone marrow smear; **B,** peripheral blood smear. (From Miale JB: Laboratory medicine: Hematology, ed 6, St Louis, 1982, The CV Mosby Co.)

provided by immunological methods, although noted exceptions occur. Until the discrepancies between the two systems are explained, most clinicians continue to use the data bases provided by the FAB system.

Lymphoid leukemia

Acute lymphoblastic leukemia (ALL).
Acute lymphocytic or lymphoblastic leukemia is characterized by increased numbers of immature lymphocytes in the peripheral blood and infiltration of these cells into the bone marrow. ALL remains the most prevalent form of malignancy in children. Despite considerable progress in chemotherapeutic remission of this disease over the past two decades, the mortality rate has remained at 30% to 70%, depending on the stage of the disease at first diagnosis and several parameters of clinical presentation.

Acute lymphoblastic leukemia occurs most commonly in young children, peaking at ages of three to seven years old. The clinical presentation typically includes a rapid onset of fatigueability, infection with associated fever, and various signs such as gum bleeding, easy bruising, petechial hemorrhage, and bone or joint pain. Physical examination often reveals an enlarged liver and/or spleen, lymphadenopathy, and various manifestations of bleeding and anemia.

The white cell count usually exceeds 10,000/μL, but 25% of the cases are **aleukemic,** with counts of less than 5000/μL. Lymphocytes predominate in the peripheral blood, varying from occasional blasts to almost 100% occurrence of immature cells (Fig. 20-2). As a result of marrow infiltration by the lymphocytes, displacement of other elements leads to neutropenia (increased susceptability to infections), thrombocytopenia (bleeding manifestations) and varying degrees of anemia. Direct inhibition of normal marrow cells by leukemic cells is also a topic of recent research. Cytochemical procedures for cases of ALL includes the periodic acid Schiff (PAS) reaction, which stains granules in lymphoblasts red (Plate 8, C and D). Unfortunately, other precursors also show some affinity for the stain (Table 20-3), and only about 70% to 80% of ALL cases show a positive reaction. If the red granules occur in a characteristic "block" pattern, the identification of the cell as a lymphoblast is more certain, although abnormal erythroblastic precursors may also display this pattern. Peroxidase and Sudan black B stains are usually negative for lymphocytes.

The FAB classification of ALL includes the following subtypes.

L1 (Fig. 20-3)—Small cells predominate, characterized by a scant amount of cytoplasm of slight to moderate basophilia and a nucleus of regular shape. The nuclei of a few cells may have clefts or indentations and the nucleoli are usually indistinct or not visible. Vacuoles are uncommon. This is the most common type of ALL (about 85% of cases in children) and the one with

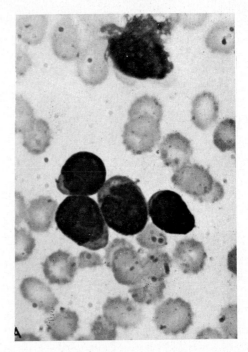

Fig. 20-3.   L1 subtype of ALL, peripheral blood.
(From Miale JB: Laboratory medicine: Hematology, ed 6, St Louis, 1982, The CV Mosby Co.)

the most favorable prognosis. Immunological studies indicate that L1 cases include undifferentiated, T cell and null cell forms, but not those of B cell identity (Table 20-4). Unfortunately, T cell leukemias do not respond well to therapy, thus the prognosis for L1 depends on the immunological subtype.

L2 (Fig. 20-4)—This form is characterized by the presence of large and small lymphocytes (heterogeneous size distribution) containing a moderately abundant amount of cytoplasm of variable, occasionally intense, basophilia. Vacuolization is uncommon. The nuclei are commonly irregular in shape and nuclear clefts and indentations are common. The chromatin is often variable and nuclei are prominent and often large. Like the L1 type, L2 consists of cells carrying CALLA, T cell, and null cell markers,

Table 20-3. Histochemical reactions for acute leukemias

	FAB leukemia designation					
Histochemical method	M1	M2-3	M4	M5	M6	L1-3
Myeloperoxidase or Sudan	+	+++	+++	±	+/++	−
Nonspecific esterase (NAE)	+	+/++	++	+++	+++	−
Specific esterase (NCE)	+	+++	+++	+++	+/++	−
Periodic acid Schiff	+	+	++	++	+	++/+++
Muramidase	−	+	++	+++	+	−
Acid phosphatase	+	+	++	+++	+/++	−/+
Alkaline phosphatase (LAP)	−	−	−	+	+/++	+/++

Table 20-4. Features of acute lymphocytic leukemias (FAB)

Feature	L1	L2	L3
Cell morphology			
Cell size	Small	Variable	Large
Nucleus: shape	Round	Irregular, clefted	Round, oval
Chromatin	Homogenous	Heterogenous	Homogenous
Nucleoli	Indistinct	One or more	One or more
Cytoplasm: amount	Scant	Moderate	Moderate
Color	Mod. basophilic	Variable basophilic	Deep basophilic
Vacuoles	Variable	Variable	Prominent
Cytochemistry			
TdT activity	Marked	Marked	Absent

but not those for B cells. About 14% of the children with ALL in one large study were assigned L2 as an FAB catagory.

L3 (Fig. 20-5)—The rarest form (less than 1% of childhood cases) of ALL is also the most distinct morphologically and immunologically. The cells are homogeneous and large, containing regular round to oval nuclei that have finely stippled chromatin. Nuclei are prominent. The cytoplasm is abundant and deeply basophilic, containing prominent vacuoles. Antigenic markers indicate that these cells are 100% B lymphocytes, none of which show a positive PAS reaction. This type is also commonly referred to as the lymphoma type of ALL and it has the worse prognosis for response to treatment.

Further definition of ALL with monoclonal antibody testing (Table 20-5) has characterized **pre-B cell leukemia** as a separate entity, based on more than 10% of the lymphoblasts containing cytoplasmic immunoglobulin (μ heavy chains). Pre-B leukemia is one of the forms included in the null cell catagory, comprised of FAB types L1 and L2, but Pre-B ALL is associated with a higher incidence of central nervous sys-

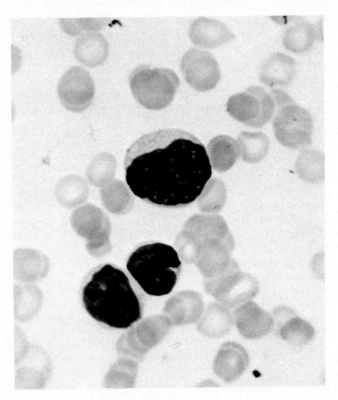

Fig. 20-4. L2 subtype of ALL, peripheral blood.
(From Bauer JD: Clinical laboratory methods, ed 9, St Louis, 1982, The CV Mosby Co.)

tem involvement and bone marrow relapse than other null types.

Regardless of the FAB or immunological subtype, outcome of the disease has been found to correlate, in most studies, with one or more clinical findings. Clinical and hematological remissions, maintained for three years or longer, were most prevalent in children that were at least 2 but less than 10 years old. White children fared far better than black children, but differences were not seen with regard to sex. The racial difference was largely attributed to a greater dissemination of the disease at first presentation, however, rather than to genetic differences per se. Patients presenting with WBC counts of less than 10,000/μL responded best and those with WBCs greater than 50,000/μL did very poorly. Other indicators for a poor prognosis included early CNS involvement (leukemic cells in spinal fluid), the presence of a mediastinal mass (seen in T cell ALL), or a greatly enlarged liver or spleen. The poorer prognosis of both T cell and B cell leukemia may be due to the origin of these neoplasms outside of the bone marrow. As a result there is less compromise of other marrow elements and a delay in the clinical manifestations. When the child is brought to medical attention, the leukemia is usually disseminated to a greater extent and therapy is less effective.

About 10% of the acute leukemias in adults are of lymphoid origin, whereas 80% of the childhood leukemias are ALL. The most common FAB type in adults is L2

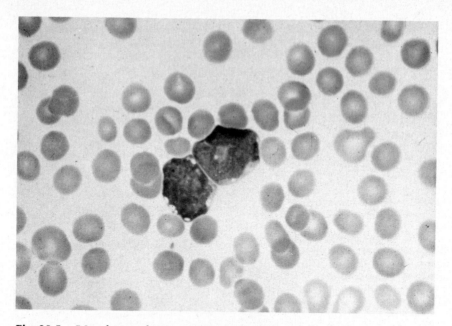

Fig. 20-5.   L3 subtype of ALL, peripheral blood.
(From Bauer JD: Clinical laboratory methods, ed 9, St Louis, 1982, The CV Mosby Co.)

Table 20-5. Features of acute lymphocytic leukemias (immunological)

	Predominant lymphocyte present				
Immunological marker	T cell	Pre-B cell	B cell	Undiff.	Null cell
Common ALL antigen (CALLA)	−	+/−	+/−	+	+/−
Sheep RBC rosette	+	−	−	−	−
Cytoplasmic Ig	−	+	−	−	−
Surface Ig	−	−	+	−	−

(67%), but the prognosis for all adults with ALL is less favorable than that for children with similar FAB types and clinical manifestations.

Chronic lymphocytic leukemia. Chronic lymphocytic leukemia (CLL) is characterized by proliferation of small lymphocytes in the bone marrow, lymph nodes, and spleen, appearing eventually in the peripheral blood (Plate 6, *A*). It is primarily a ma-lignancy of older adults (more than 40 years of age) and it is very rare in children or adolescents. In over 90% of the cases, B cells represent the abnormal clone. Since these cells do not display normal maturation, immunoglobulin production is limited and hypogammaglobulinemia often occurs in the late stages of the disease. However, autoimmune hemolytic anemia (AIHA) with an associated positive direct antiglobulin test is

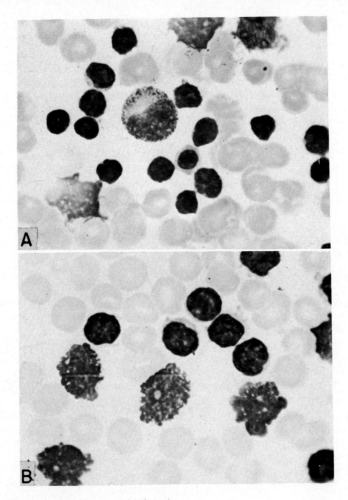

Fig. 20-6.   Chronic lymphocytic leukemia.
A, Bone marrow smear; **B,** peripheral blood smear. (From Miale JB: Laboratory medicine: Hematology, ed 6, St Louis, 1982, The CV Mosby Co.)

not uncommon. The T cell form, although rarer, is more malignant, progresses rapidly and responds poorly to chemotherapy.

In contrast to acute leukemia, most patients with CLL have increased leukocyte counts: about 20% of patients exceed 100,000/µL, and more than 90% of patients exceed 10,000/µL. The percentage of lymphocytes on the differential count typically ranges from 60% to 85%, most of which are small, mature appearing cells (Fig. 20-6). A few lymphocytes may be larger, have indentations or nuclear clefts, and show signs of immaturity. **Smudge cells,** fragile lymphocytes that are ruptured during the preparation of the wedge smear, are typical in CLL. Anemia and thrombocytopenia are often present, but they are rarely severe unless other contributing factors are present. Marrow displacement of normal elements by leukemic cells is not as pronounced as it is in the acute leukemias or in chronic myelogenous leukemia.

CLL does not progress as rapidly as other forms of leukemia. The median survival time after first diagnosis is about 10 years, but this is difficult to establish accurately because many cases are diagnosed incidentally, during a physical examination or as a result of laboratory studies done for other reasons. Initial complaints, if any, are usually related to fatigueability or lymph node enlargement. Splenomegaly is often present, but usually not severe. Most patients die of complications related to infection or other chronic conditions associated with the elderly. Therapy is often conservative and aimed at relieving symptomatic problems (hepatosplenomegaly, infection, anemia, or bleeding) rather than attempting to achieve remission.

Prolymphocytic leukemia (PPL) is characterized by large numbers of small lymphocytes in the peripheral blood with scant cytoplasm and the immature features of prolymphocytes (Fig. 20-7). Splenomegaly is usually very severe and the disease progresses rapidly, not responding well to chemotherapy.

Plasma cell leukemia. The extent to which **plasma cell leukemia (PCL)** exists as a distinct disease or represents the fulminant conclusion of multiple myeloma is debatable. Both conditions are characterized by the appearance of large numbers of plasma cells in the marrow and peripheral blood (Fig. 20-8). In general, a few plasma cells are present in the peripheral blood in all cases of multiple myeloma (examination of the buffy coat will usually reveal that they comprise up to 2% of the peripheral cell differential). When the peripheral differential count exceeds 10% plasma cells, a diagnosis of PCL is justified. In the marrow, the plasma cells often occur in clumps or sheets and a few small aggregates may also be seen in the peripheral blood. Binucleated forms are not uncommon (Plate 6, *B*).

Patients with PCL often display a hypergammaglobulinemia that is composed of IgD and IgE, whereas multiple myeloma plasmas are more typically composed of increased IgG or IgA. The clinical course is also typical for that of a leukemia, displaying signs of anemia and bleeding manifestations as plasma cells displace normal marrow hematopoietic elements. PCL responds poorly to chemotherapy and the disease often terminates in a blast crisis.

Hairy cell leukemia. **Hairy cell leukemia (HCL)** or leukemic reticuloendotheliosis is a chronic lymphoid malignancy characterized by cells with fine, irregular pseudopods and immature nuclear features (Fig. 20-9). In 90% of the cases, a proliferation of B cells is involved. At various times, investigators believed that the monocytoid cells with the "hairy" appearance were monocytes, histiocytes, or T lymphocytes. The delicate cytoplasmic projections can be seen by staining with Janus green. The cells are not plentiful, but they can be found in the peripheral blood, bone marrow, spleen, liver, and lymph nodes. Splenomegaly is a common feature of the disease, although lymphadenopathy is an infrequent finding.

HCL is now believed to comprise about 2% of all leukemia cases, confined exclusively to adults (median age is 50 to 60 years of age). Curiously, several studies indicate a male to female preponderance that is slight or absent in other studies but 4:1 or more in some series. The clinical course of the disease is slow and relatively benign, with about 50% of the patients surviving 10 years and one third living 10 years after diagnosis. Considering the advanced age of many of these patients, most die from secondary conditions or unrelated causes.

Despite the chronic nature of HCL, the disturbances to normal hematopoietic function are considerable. A marked pancytopenia is almost always a feature and the peripheral blood differential count may be almost entirely monocytoid, even though typical "hairy cells" may be uncommon.

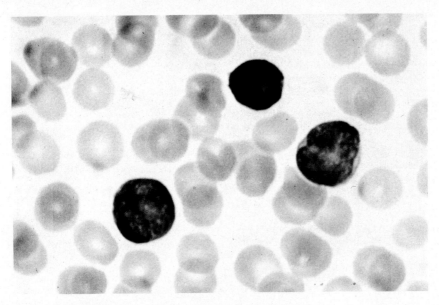

Fig. 20-7. Prolymphocytic leukemia, peripheral blood.
(From Bauer JD: Clinical laboratory methods, ed 9, St Louis, 1982, The CV Mosby Co.)

Bone marrow aspiration is often unsuccessful because of complete infiltration by hairy cells, resulting in a dispersed spongy web of cells in an increased meshwork of reticulin fiber. Splenomegaly is usually marked, with weights of 20 times normal. The traditional method of histochemical confirmation involves a two-step acid phosphatase procedure. Hairy cells contain an isoenzyme of acid phosphatase that is not inhibited by tartaric acid, whereas other cells, except eosinophils, have an isoenzyme that is inhibited. Unfortunately, some hairy cells show poor reactions with this technique, and some other types of malignant lymphoid cells may display positive reactions.

Death typically occurs from infection, involving organisms such as *Pseudomonas, Staphylococcus aureus, Streptococcus pneumoniae, Escherichia coli, Proteus, Klebsiella*, and atypical mycobacteria. Secondary malignancies have been noted in about 10% to 15% of the cases, and autoimmune disorders are also prevalent. Treatment is usually conservative and symptomatic.

Myelogenous leukemia

The term "myelogenous" refers to the bone marrow and in the context of leukemia it is used to describe the malignancies that are not lymphoid in origin. In the past, "granulocytic" was often used interchangeably with "myelogenous," describing acute or chronic leukemias of the neutrophilic series. Increases in peripheral eosinophils and basophils often accompany the chronic type, so the term granulocytic seemed appropriate. With the adoption of the FAB system of classification for acute leukemia, the term **acute nonlymphocytic leukemia (ANLL)** has attained widespread use. Chronic forms of myelogenous leukemia are not included in the FAB classification of leukemia, although chronic myelomonocytic leukemia is included in the FAB system describing myelodysplastic syndromes.

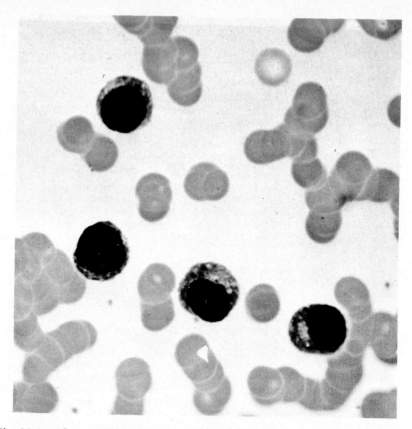

Fig. 20-8. Plasma cell leukemia, peripheral blood.
(From Bauer JD: Clinical laboratory methods, ed 9, St Louis, 1982, The CV Mosby Co.)

Acute nonlymphocytic leukemia. ANLL is characterized by the appearance of blasts and other early precursors in the peripheral blood and excess amounts of these cells in the bone marrow. The disease may appear suddenly and progress rapidly or it may have a slower onset, progressing through a chronic phase before terminating in a blast crisis. Hepatosplenomegaly and lymphadenopathy are usually less remarkable than that seen in ALL. A moderate to severe normocytic normochromic anemia and thrombocytopenia develop as the leukemic cells progressively displace normal blood cell precursors. Using the revised (1985) FAB classification, the seven major types of ANLL are described below, but it should be

remembered that these working classifications, based on morphological and histochemical criteria, do not necessarily reflect the molecular and cellular mechanisms underlying the various manifestations. Thus individual cases may not fit neatly into this scheme, and the cellular patterns may not always correlate well with histochemical reactions and immunological studies.

Acute myeloblastic leukemia without maturation (M1). Little or no differentiation of the blastic cells is evident and the cells may not exhibit myeloperoxidase activity. Some of these cases have probably been included within another form of leukemia, by exclusion of other identifiable types, as **acute un-**

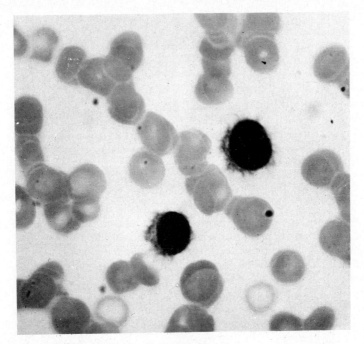

Fig. 20-9.   Hairy cell leukemia, peripheral blood.
(From Bauer JD: Clinical laboratory methods, ed 9, St Louis, 1982, The CV Mosby Co.)

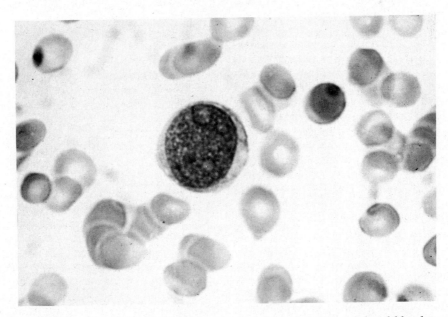

Fig. 20-10.   Undifferentiated (M1) myeloblastic leukemia, peripheral blood.
(From Bauer JD: Clinical laboratory methods, ed 9, St Louis, 1982, The CV Mosby Co.)

differentiated leukemia (AUL), but techniques are now available to assign many of these cases to one of the FAB types. Both the marrow and peripheral blood display few cells of the intermediate stages of granulocyte development (Fig. 20-10). Monoclonal antibodies for myeloid antigens are useful for confirmation. The formal FAB criteria state that blast cells in the marrow (the sum of types I and II as defined in the 1982 FAB criteria for myelodysplastic syndromes) must comprise 90% or more of the nonerythroid cells, and at least 3% of these blasts must be positive with either Sudan black or myeloperoxidase staining.

Acute myeloblastic leukemia with differentiation (M2). Myeloperoxidase activity (or a positive reaction to Sudan black) is clearly present and the blasts have the characteristic, irregular outlines of myeloblasts. Promyelocytes and myelocytes may also be present in the peripheral blood, further evidence of the myeloid character of the disease (Fig. 20-11). In about 50% of the patients with M2 acute myeloblastic leukemia, azurophilic rods or needles (**Auer rods**) can be observed in the cytoplasm of the myeloblasts or promyelocytes (Plate 6, *C,* and Fig. 20-12), although they may be evident in only 2% or fewer of the cells in any patient. The Auer rods are composed of lysosomal material, essentially fused primary granules, and there is a strong correlation between the presence of these inclusions and positive staining with myeloperoxidase and specific esterase. The myeloblasts comprise from 30% to 89% of the nonerythroid cells, and 10% or more of the cells are maturing granulocytes (promyelocytes and later stages). Monocytic cells are less than 20% of the nonerythroid cells, and erythroid cells should be less than 50% of all marrow blood cells. One variant of this disease is characterized by the presence of **micromyeloblasts** (Fig. 20-13) rather than the usual, large cells. Fig. 20-14 presents a karyotype from a patient with a third representative of chromosome 8 present.

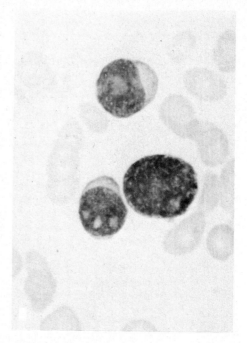

Fig. 20-11. Differentiated (M2) myeloblastic leukemia, peripheral blood.
(From Miale JB: Laboratory medicine: Hematology, ed 6, 1982, The CV Mosby Co.)

Treatment for both types of acute myeloblastic leukemia require symptom-related administration of transfusions and broad spectrum antibiotics, plus a regimen of cytotoxic chemicals to supress the proliferation of leukemic cells. Remissions are more difficult to achieve than in cases of ALL and the interval of remission is usually shorter. Cytosine arabinoside and daunorubicin are given in large doses to achieve marrow aplasia (the inductive phase of therapy), from which about 75% of the patients recover by regenerating normal marrow elements. Maintenance therapy, utilizing smaller but still potent doses, is designed to inhibit the return of neoplastic cells, but only about 25% of the patients are still in remission, as confirmed by marrow examination, after 5 years. Marrow transplanta-

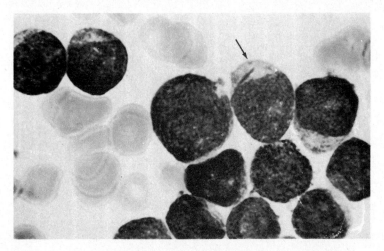

Fig. 20-12.   Auer rod in a myeloblast, AML, bone marrow smear.

(From Bauer JD: Clinical laboratory methods, ed 9, St Louis, 1982, The CV Mosby Co.)

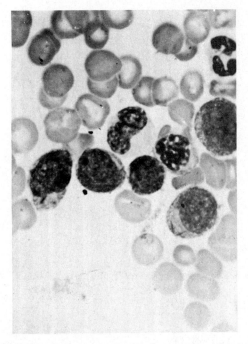

Fig. 20-13.   Micromyeloblasts in bone marrow, AML.

(From Miale JB: Laboratory medicine: Hematology, ed 6, St Louis, 1982, The CV Mosby Co.)

tion, requiring virtually identical HLA haplotypes between donor and recipient, offers better chances for survival, but only a few patients have siblings or other donors with a compatible haplotype.

Hypergranular promyelocytic leukemia (M3). Domination of the cell pattern by promyelocytes is characteristic of this rare but very malignant form (Fig. 20-15). The promyelocytes contain an increased concentration of large lysosomal granules, often fused to form Auer rods. In some cases, the Auer rods may be so greatly concentrated and fused that the cells appear to be hypogranular. The nuclei are often more immature in appearance and irregular in shape than those of normal promyelocytes. In about half of the cases, a chromosomal translocation, t(15; 17), is evident.

The lysosomal contents are able to induce procoagulant activity, especially after chemotoxic therapy produces massive cell lysis and release of the granular material. As a result, disseminated intravascular coagulation is a common manifestation of this form of leukemia, resulting in additional bleeding problems due to coagulation

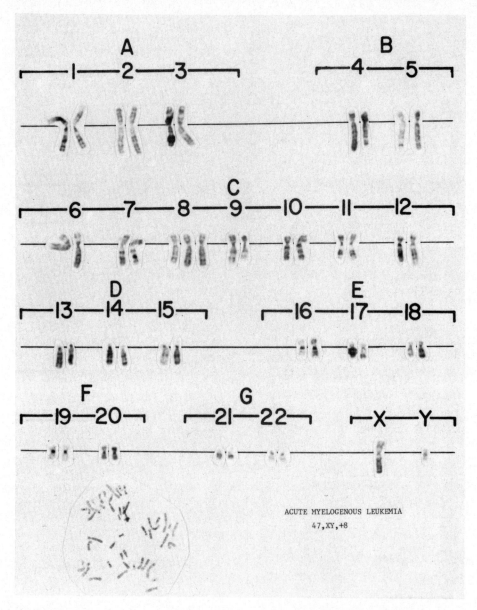

Fig. 20-14. Karyotype of a patient with acute myelogenous leukemia.

factor and platelet consumption and the presence of increased concentrations of fibrin degradation products. Therapeutic administration of intravenous heparin may be required to control the extent of DIC while risking further hemorrhage. Frequent replacement therapy (platelets, frozen plasma, and packed red cells) may be required to control the disease. Although the chemotherapeutic regimen is similar to that of the

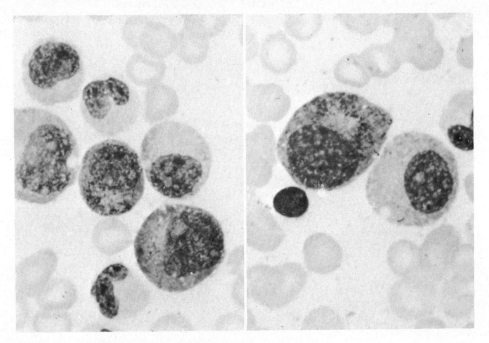

Fig. 20-15.   Promyelocytic leukemia (M3), bone marrow.
Coarse granules are characteristic in these atypical, hypergranular promyelocytes. (From Miale
JB: Laboratory medicine: Hematology, ed 6, St Louis, 1982, The CV Mosby Co.)

myeloblastic leukemias, remissions are more difficult to achieve and they persist for shorter intervals.

Myelomonocytic   leukemia   (M4). This type, formerly named the Naegeli type of monocytic leukemia, features the presence of monocytoid blasts that have folded, lacy or reticular nuclei with 2 to 5 nucleoli (Plate 6, *D*, and Fig. 20-16). Histochemical studies reveal a weakly positive nonspecific esterase activity, increasing as the monocytoid cells mature. The Sudan black reaction may be more diffuse and finer than that seen in typical myeloblasts. Other esterase reactions, including the test for fluoride inhibition, is variable. The abundant cytoplasm is often vacuolated and it may contain azurophilic granules and Auer rods. Over 20% of the nonerythroid cells of the marrow and peripheral blood must be monocytic and in the marrow over 30% of the nonerythroid cells must be blasts. If the

monocytic cells exceed 80% of the nonerythoid cells, a diagnosis of monocytic leukemia (M5) is made. About 25% of all adult ANLL can be assigned to the M4 class.

Increased concentrations of eosinophils (5% to 30% of the nonerythroid cells) are present in a fraction of the cases of myelomonocytic leukemia. These eosinophils are abnormal, being positive for chloroacetate esterase and PAS; some have an unsegmented nucleus and large basophilic (immature) granules. Tissue infiltration by monocytes is a common finding, especially in the gingivae, other mucosal surfaces, the meningal linings of the central nervous system and in lymph nodes. Serum and urinary lysozyme levels are usually elevated.

Monocytic leukemia (M5). When 80% or more of the nonerythroid cells of the bone marrow are identified with the monocytic series, a diagnosis of monocytic leukemia (formerly called the Schilling type of mono-

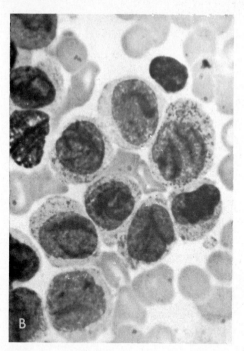

Fig. 20-16. Acute myelomonocytic leukemia (M4), peripheral blood.
(From Miale JB: Laboratory medicine: Hematology, ed 6, St Louis, 1982, The CV Mosby Co.)

cytic leukemia) can be made (Fig. 20-17). If most of the monocytic cells (80% or more) are monoblasts, a further distinction (M5a) is made, whereas a better differentiated cell pattern is defined as M5b. Less than 20% of the nonerythroid cells belong to the granulocytic series. The monoblasts in the poorly differentiated form are large, containing nuclei with 3 to 5 nucleoli and a distinct, folded nucleus. Serum and urinary lysozyme concentrations are typically elevated, up to three times normal, in the differentiated form. Bleeding and hypercoagulation manifestations are not uncommon, especially during chemotherapy. Fig. 20-18 is a karyotype from a patient with AML exhibiting a variety of chromosome abnormalities, including an extra autosome (chromosome 8), an inversion (chromosome 1) and

two translocations (from 3 to 9 and from 11 to 17).

Erythroleukemia (Di Guglielmo's disease) (M6). All blood cell lines exhibit some abnormalities or disturbances in proliferation, but normoblasts (all stages) account for more than 50% of the marrow cells (Fig. 20-19). Many of these cells have bizarre morphological features, such as multinuclearity and clover-leaf shaped nuclei; megaloblastoid changes are common. Ringed sideroblasts, gigantic megakaryocytes, and Auer rods are seen in many cases.

Erythroleukemia is distinguished from some of the myelodysplastic syndromes (MDS) in that 30% or more of the nonerythroid cells are also blasts (type I and II, by FAB criteria). However, when erythroblasts predominate (>50% of all marrow cells) but there is less than 30% of blasts among the non-erythroid elements, a diagnosis of MDS is appropriate. This type of leukemia can also occur in a more chronic form, but it eventually terminates in an acute phase. Anemia is usually present due to the dyserythropoiesis associated with abnormal marrow precursors. Increased red cell hemolysis is associated with a greatly increased serum lactic dehydrogenase content and increased fecal urobilinogen. Leukocyte counts vary, from slightly decreased to moderately elevated, and thrombocytopenia may be severe. The PAS stain is positive, often with a block pattern, in erythroleukemia, whereas normal erythroblasts are PAS negative. The PAS reaction will also be positive in some cases of thalassemia and sideroblastic anemia. As the disease progresses, increasing numbers of myeloid precursors appear in the marrow and peripheral blood, along with undifferentiated blast cells. The prognosis for this type of leukemia is always poor, and response to chemotherapy is often minimal.

Megakaryoblastic leukemia (M7). MKC leukemia is a relatively rare form characterized by a proliferation of atypical megakary-

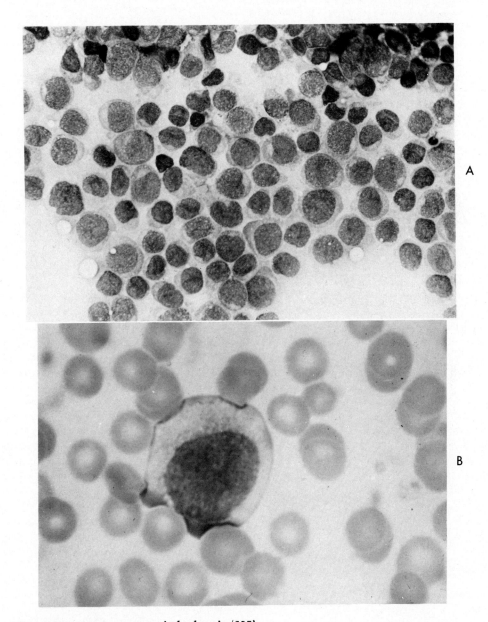

Fig. 20-17.   Acute monocytic leukemia (M5).
A, Bone marrow; **B,** peripheral blood. (From Bauer JD: Clinical laboratory methods, ed 9, St Louis, 1982, The CV Mosby Co.)

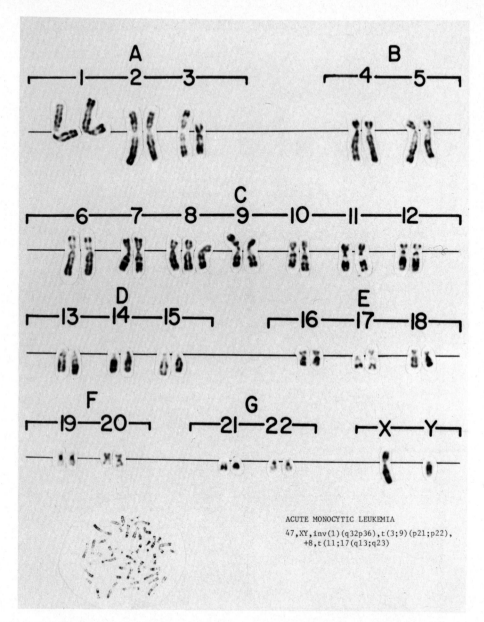

Fig. 20-18.   Karyotype of a patient with acute monocytic leukemia.

ocytes and the appearance of large poorly differentiated blasts in the peripheral blood. The leukemic MKCs are typically smaller than normal MKCs, with a high nucleus-to-cytoplasm ratio. Vacuoles are often present in the cytoplasm and blunt pseudopods may be seen on the periphery of the cell. The blasts typically stain negative for Sudan black and myeloperoxidase, but they often show a localized positive reaction to non-

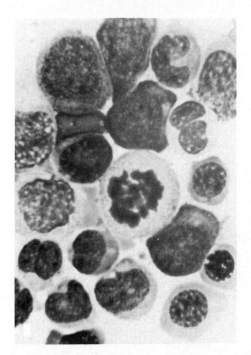

Fig. 20-19. Erythroleukemia (M6), bone marrow.
(From Miale JB: Laboratory medicine: Hematology, ed 6, St Louis, 1982, The CV Mosby Co.)

specific esterases (monocytes are also positive but with a diffuse pattern). However, when butyrate is used as a substrate, the reaction is almost always negative, ruling out monocytic blasts. The marrow often shows an increase in the presence of fibrous tissue and aspiration may be unsuccessful in advanced cases, necessitating a biopsy. Identification of the atypical blasts can be made by using an assay for platelet peroxidase, an isoenzyme distinct from myeloperoxidase, or with the aid of monoclonal antibodies directed against MKC glycoproteins or factor VIII–related antigen.

The peripheral blood is characteristically pancytopenic and a severe thrombocytopenia is usually associated with bleeding manifestations. The disease may be easily confused with the changes seen in myelodysplastic syndromes and many early cases have probably been classified as preleukemic, using the same criteria. The disease progresses rapidly, terminating within days to a few months in acute leukemia characterized by widespread infiltration of the tissues.

Chronic myelogenous leukemia. The most dramatic white cell disorder, in terms of leukocyte counts, is chronic myelogenous leukemia (CML). Although the marrow and peripheral blood contains fewer of the early myeloid precursors than will be found in the acute leukemias, the capability of the marrow to effectively produce and release a large number of cells results in WBC counts of 50,000 to more than 500,000/μL. CML is also distinguished from AML with a longer clinical course, typically lasting 1 to 4 years, rather than a few months. Splenomegaly is a common finding and may be the cause of initial presentation for medical examination. The increased rate of cell production and turnover produces a hypermetabolic state characterized by night sweats, fever, weight loss, and fatigueability. Increased cell turnover manifests by an increased uric acid concentration in the plasma. Displacement of MKC and erythroblastic precursors in the marrow eventually produces anemia. Platelet counts are most often increased, accompanied by large forms. Bleeding manifestations may result from abnormal platelet function.

The increased leukocyte count can often be seen in the hematocrit tube as a greatly expanded buffy coat, with each 1% of leukocrit approximating 15,000 WBCs/μL (Beck, 1985). On peripheral smears, blasts should account for less than 10% of the differential count, except during the terminal phase or blast crisis. Myelocytes and later forms of neutrophils predominate and the relative percentage of eosinophils and basophils is increased. Nucleated red cells may also be present, displaying anisocytosis and basophilic stippling. The marrow shows a generalized hyperplasia of the granulocytic series, focusing on increased numbers of intermediate stages (Fig. 20-20). The M:E ra-

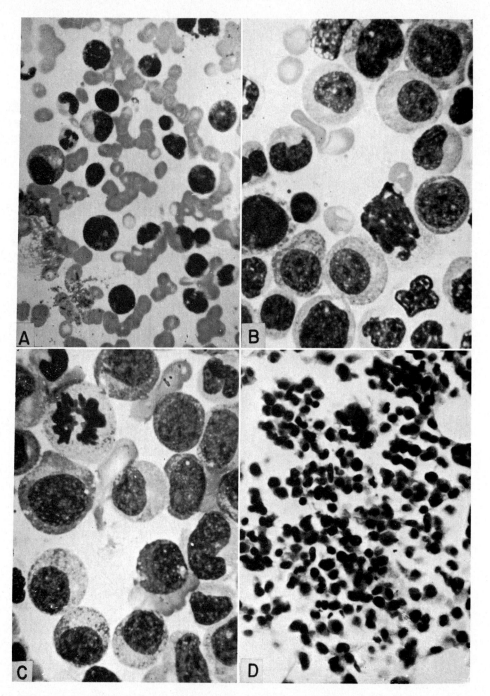

Fig. 20-20.   Chronic myelogenous leukemia, bone marrow.
(From Miale JB: Laboratory medicine: Hematology, ed 6, St Louis, 1982, The CV Mosby Co.)

tio may be as high as 25:1! Megakaryocytes may also be increased, but much of the remaining cell pattern is similar to that seen in the peripheral blood.

About 90% to 95% of CML patients possess a somatic cell mutation commonly referred to as the Philadelphia chromosome (Ph[1]), a translocation t(9; 22) shown in Fig. 20-21. Ph[1] is present at first in the myeloid precursors, but as the leukemia progresses and the abnormal clone displaces normal elements, other cell lines begin to express the abnormality, eventually occurring in distantly related cells such as B lymphocytes. Interestingly, patients that do not exhibit Ph[1] fare considerably worse in response to treatment than those that are positive.

CML can be distinguished, in the absence of blasts and promyelocytes, from severe leukmoid reactions by leukocyte alkaline phosphatase activity (LAP). LAP activity is diminished or absent in over 90% of the cases of CML and typically increased in benign responses to infections. The disease is not as common as the acute forms and it usually occurs in older adults. Therapy is most often accomplished with cytotoxic drugs, such as busulfan (Myleran), hydroxyurea, or 6-mercaptopurine. Unfortunately, eradication of the abnormal clone and complete remission are rarely possible without complete destruction of the marrow and replacement by transplantation. An acute phase marked by a rapid increase in the percentage of blasts signals the terminal phase, often exhibited by features suggestive of acute lymphoblastic leukemia (negative peroxidase, the presence of TdT enzyme activity).

Other rare forms of leukemia have also been described that are characterized by the proliferation of particular cells. Eosinophilic leukemia, basophilic leukemia, and mast cell leukemia may be chronic or acute, depending on the associated percentages of blasts and the time course of the disease.

Other myeloproliferative disorders

In addition to chronic myelogenous (granulocytic) leukemia, a number of other proliferative disorders involving marrow elements have been described (see p. 315). These disorders are nonmalignant neoplasms that usually affect a pluripotent hematopoietic stem cell and the descendant blood cell lines derived from it. Most disorders are characterized by the absence of the normal physiological mechanisms that regulate cellular kinetics, so that the disorders are often regarded as autonomous.

Polycythemia vera (primary polycythemia). Uncontrolled proliferation of blood cells can also occur as a non-malignant process. An absolute increase in the red cell mass in the absence of hypoxic stimulation is characteristic of **polycythemia vera (PV)** or primary polycythemia. In addition to erythroid hyperplasia, this disorder also exhibits an increased production of leukocytes and platelets. PV occurs almost exclusively in older adults, and its etiology is unknown. The abnormality underlying the neoplasm probably arises in a pluripotent stem cell, as evidenced by using isoenzyme markers in heterozygous females to show that all of the cell lines exhibiting the hyperproliferation are derived from one allelic set.

Clinically, polycythemia vera is characterized by an absolute increase in red blood cell mass and volume, increased viscosity and a high blood pressure. The patients typically appears erythemic, presenting a ruddy complexion. Hepatosplenomegaly is common in these patients, and peptic ulcers are frequent occurrences. As with other myeloproliferative disorders, increased cell metabolism results in an elevated plasma uric acid level. The increased platelet count may lead to the formation of microthrombi and activation of the intrinsic coagulation pathway. Distension of capillaries due to the increased viscosity and pressure often produces localized bleeding problems. As the disorder progresses and all cell lines exhibit increased hyperplasia (panmyelosis), the

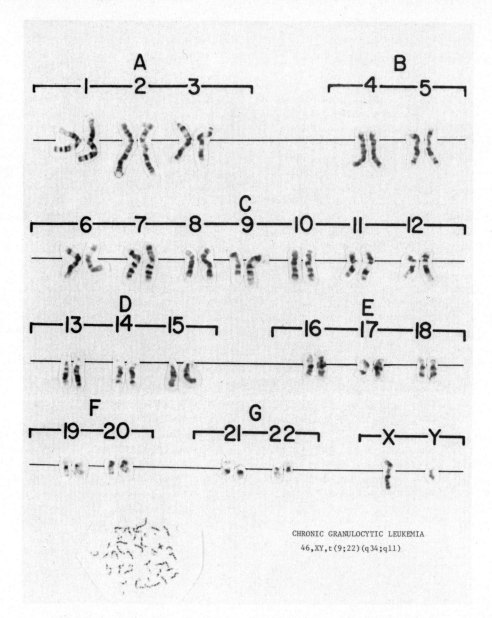

Fig. 20-21.   Karyotype of a patient with chronic granulocytic leukemia.

normal morphological features of the peripheral red cells are replaced by the appearance of "teardrop" cells and other poikilocytes. Fibrotic replacement of the normal marrow architecture leads to myeloid metaplasia and myelofibrosis, eventually culminating in aplastic anemia. Patients treated with cytotoxic chemicals or radiation often terminate with chronic or acute myelogenous leukemia.

CLASSIFICATION OF MYELOPROLIFERATIVE DISORDERS

Acute myeloproliferative disorders
Acute myelogenous (nonlymphoid) leukemias
   (see p. 301)

Chronic myeloproliferative disorders
Chronic granulocytic (myelocytic) leukemia
   (CGL or CML)
Polycythemia vera (primary polycythemia)
Agnogenic myeloid metaplasia
Essential thrombocythemia (primary
   thrombocythemia)

The erythropoietin levels are decreased, distinguishing PV from reactionary forms of erythrocytosis (see Table 17-3 for comparisons). Reticulocyte counts are mildly to moderately increased and nucleated red blood cells may appear in the peripheral blood, along with immature granulocytes. Leukocyte alkaline phosphatase activity is usually increased, further distinguishing PV from reactive erythrocytoses and CML. Because one form of symptomatic therapy involves periodic phlebotomies to remove excess red cell mass, iron deficiency is a potential complication. Intestinal absorption is decreased, in contrast to that of anemic states, so that sufficient iron may not be available to provide for the increased production of hemoglobin. Therapeutic bleeding does relieve some of the symptoms associated with hyperviscocity, but if blood volume is decreased too rapidly, an erythropoietin-mediated response occurs, just as if the patient were truly anemic.

Myeloid metaplasia. Myeloid metaplasia is defined by the occurrence of hematopoiesis outside of the marrow in adults, primarily in the spleen and liver, and an increased proliferation of leukocytic and erythrocytic elements. This is distinguished from reactive processes, such as extramedullary hematopoiesis in response to severe anemia or hemorrhaging. The underlying cause of my-

eloid metaplasia, like other myeloproliferative disorders, is unknown (another term is idiopathic or agnogenic myeloid metaplasia). Myelofibrosis, replacement of the marrow space by fibrotic tissue, often accompanies this disorder, but it does not appear to be the stimulating cause of the displaced hematopoiesis. It occurs primarily in older adults and it manifests clinically by the presence of a greatly enlarged spleen, a progressive anemia accompanied by dacrocytes (teardrop cells) and the presence of immature leukocytes on the peripheral blood smear.

Extramedullary sites of blood cell production are confirmed by needle biopsy. The presence of increased fibrosis is not diagnostic of myeloid metaplasia, but its extent is often a prognostic indication of the severity of the disease. The marrow may be too fibrotic for aspiration, so that needle biopsy is also required to obtain a medullary sample. Since fibrotic replacement frequently occurs in a heterogeneous fashion, multiple sampling sites may be necessary in order to obtain a representative picture.

The LAP score is usually elevated, assisting in separating the peripheral blood picture of immature white cells from that of CML. Platelet counts and WBC counts are usually elevated initially (Plate 6, *E*) and other signs of increased cell turnover are present: hyperuricemia and hypermetabolism. Unlike polycythemia vera, the red cell mass is progressively decreased and an erythropoietin-induced reticulocytosis occurs. Later phases of the disease exhibit thrombocytopenia and associated bleeding and bruising manifestations. Therapy is generally ineffective and may result in conversion of the metaplasia to leukemia. Splenectomy may relieve excessive red cell sequestration and symptomatic treatment for bleeding, anemia, and infection are used as needed.

Essential thrombocytosis (thrombocythemia). Thrombocythemia is another myeloproliferative disorder of older adults, characterized by a marked increase in platelet production (see Chapter 23). Unlike the other myeloproliferative disorders, other cell lines are not involved. The mechanism is autonomous, that is, not subject to the mechanisms that regulate platelet production in the bone marrow. The number and volume of megakaryocytes is increased and peripheral platelet concentrations can be as high as 20 million per microliter! The peripheral smear reveals platelets with a wide variation of size, including forms the size of lymphocytes.

Many of these platelets are functionally defective and both bleeding problems and thrombotic manifestations can occur. Gastrointestinal bleeding is a major problem, along with coronary and cerebral strokes induced by small clots. Anemia may occur as a result of blood loss and iron deficiency is a potential complication. Infection is also a frequent finding and WBC counts are often elevated with a high percentage of immature neutrophils present. Therapy, in the form of alkylating agents or radiation, is aimed at reducing the platelet count.

Myelodysplastic syndromes

Myelodysplastic, or dysmyelopoietic, syndromes are characterized by an abnormal or ineffective blood cell production in two or more cell lines, usually as a pattern of marrow hypercellularity coupled with peripheral blood cytopenia. Several forms of refractory anemia and a type of chronic leukemia are presently included with the disorders recognized by the FAB as myelodysplastic (see p. 317):

A number of factors are common to these varied manifestations of MDS. Most patients are older adults, usually over 50 years of age, but younger patients are also being diagnosed with MDS, especially those who have received prolonged therapy with cytotoxic drugs or radiation. The morphological and functional abnormalities are expressed in two or more of the granulocytic, erythroid, and megakaryocytic cell lines, but the abnormal clone coexists with normal cells.

In the erythroid line, this results in a peripheral blood dimorphic pattern of macrocytic and normocytic erythrocytes.

The bone marrow usually displays a hypercellular pattern, but it can also be hypocellular, especially if the dysplastic clone is suppressing proliferation by normal elements. Normal marrow cellularity varies with age, so that these patterns must be evaluated with respect to each patient. The erythroid population can vary from 5% to more than 60% of the cell population. In some disorders, the erythroid precursors exhibit a distinct shift toward immaturity; others are characterized by the presence of ringed sideroblasts, indicating defective erythropoiesis. The most consistent feature of the bone marrow is the presence of megaloblastoid normoblasts, resembling the changes seen in folate and vitamin B_{12} deficiencies. Multinuclear cells, normoblasts with coarsely clumped chromatin, nuclear fragments, giant forms, and cells with indented nuclei are frequently seen. Evidence of defective hemoglobinization may also be present. The peripheral blood may show obvious indications of anemia, but a low reticulocyte count confirms the dyserythropoietic process associated with MDS. Basophilic stippling and hypochromic, microcytic red cells are present in some forms.

Dysgranulopoiesis is evidenced by neutropenia and functional abnormalities of the PMNs. Many of the neutrophils are agranular or hypogranular (Plate 6, F) and in some an asynchrony of nuclear and cytoplasmic maturation results in a condition that has been termed *pseudo Pelger-Huët anomaly*. In other cases, the neutrophils may be large and bizarre in shape, occasionally hypersegmented. Myeloperoxidase or alkaline phosphatase activity may be decreased or absent and some cells show decreased chemotactic responsiveness. Granulocytic precursors may be increased in the bone marrow, but by FAB definition the number of blasts must be less than 30% or a diagnosis of leukemia is appropriate.

Ineffective production of platelets results in peripheral thrombocytopenia in most cases, although normal and increased counts are also seen. The megakaryocytes may be small or gigantic, some with only a single nuclear lobe and others that are hypersegmented. Granulation may be very coarse or entirely absent. Platelets reflect these abnormalities, varying in size and ultrastructural features. Many are dysfunctional as well, resulting in bleeding problems.

Although this description of myelodysplastic syndrome includes a wide variety of cellular changes and possible patterns of abnormalities, they share a common destination. Most, but not all, patients with MDS will eventually progress toward a form of leukemia, usually AML or ALL. The various features of MDS are often described as **preleukemia** or **preleukemic syndrome,** recognizing these marrow changes as the prodrome of a malignant state. In fact, the major difference between MDS and acute leukemia may be simply the rate at which the malignant clone displaces normal marrow elements and proliferates as a blastic marrow and blood picture. Furthermore, some cytotoxic agents, used to suppress the myelodysplastic changes, appear to stimulate the conversion to leukemia. In some cases, polycythemia vera or myeloid metaplasia precede the conversion to ALL or AML. The frequency of leukemia varies with the type of MDS: 10% to 15% in cases of refractory anemia and RA with ringed sideroblasts, greater than 25% for cases with excess blasts and cases of chronic myelomonocytic leukemia.

Refractory anemia (RA) is characterized by peripheral anemia that resists treatment with conventional approaches. The reticulocyte count remains low and the red cells may be dimorphic. Leukocytes and platelets are usually normal. Blast cells, when present, comprise less than 1% of the peripheral blood differential; in the marrow they account for less than 5% of the blood cells. Megaloblastoid changes are apparent, and ringed sideroblasts are usually minimal.

Refractory anemia with ringed sideroblasts (RARS). Peripheral blast counts remain below 1% and marrow blast counts are less than 5%, but ringed sideroblasts comprise more than 15% of the nucleated red cells. Granulocytic and platelet abnormalities are more evident than in cases of simple refractory anemia.

Refractory anemia with excess blasts (RAEB). Abnormalities are evident in all three cell lines and cytopenia is evident in at least two, usually as anemia and neutropenia. The marrow shows obvious signs of ineffective granulopoiesis and megakaryocytopoiesis. Peripheral blood blasts are less than 5% of the differential count, but the marrow blasts comprise 5 to 20% of the marrow cells, resembling acute leukemia. Abnormal promyelocytes with large coarse cytoplasmic granules may be present and peripheral neutrophils may be agranular or show pseudo Pelger-Huët anomaly.

Refractory anemia with excess blasts in transition (RAEBT). Excess numbers of blasts, from 20% to 30% of the marrow total, is considered to be MDS in transition to

---

CLASSIFICATION AND SYNONYMS OF MYELODYSPLASTIC SYNDROMES

Refractory Anemia (RA)
   Erythemic myelosis
   Refractory megaloblastic anemia
Refractory anemia with ringed sideroblasts (RARS)
   Acquired idiopathic sideroblastic anemia (AISA)
Refractory anemia with excess blasts (RAEB)
Refractory anemia with excess blasts in transition (RAEBT)
   Acute myeloproliferative syndrome
   Primary acquired panmyelopathy with myeloblastosis (PAMP)
Chronic myelomonocytic leukemia (CMMoL)

acute leukemia, the latter defined by FAB criteria as having 30% or more blasts. In many cases, myeloblasts and promyelocytes contain distinct Auer rods. Blasts in the peripheral blood often exceed 5% and abnormalities of the three cell lines are usually evident. This form of MDS usually evolves into AML within a few months of diagnosis.

Chronic myelomonocytic leukemia (CMML) is characterized by the presence of many monocytic precursors in the marrow and peripheral blood. Other cell lines are abnormal and cytopenia is usually present, although often mild. Peripheral blast counts are less than 5% and marrow blast counts are 5% to 20%. Many patients exhibit splenic and/or hepatic enlargement, but the mucosal infiltration typically seen in acute myelomonocytic leukemia is absent. Despite the absolute monocytosis of the peripheral blood, the bone marrow is dominated by immature myelocytic elements and Auer rods are found in some of the blasts.

Lymphoproliferative disorders

Proliferation of lymphoid elements can occur in the bone marrow and appear in the peripheral blood as a form of acute or chronic lymphocytic leukemia. Proliferation of lymphoid cells in the lymph nodes, spleen, or thymus results in the formation of a **lymphoma.** These disorders are not mutually exclusive, since lymphoma cells can invade the marrow and leukemias can infiltrate secondary lymphoid tissues. Furthermore, the terminal stages of lymphomas may be expressed as leukemias. The broad category of lymphoproliferative disorders also includes the **plasma cell dyscrasias (PCD)** or immunosecretory disorders, malignant proliferations of plasma cells resulting in hypergammaglobulinemias.

Lymphomas are classified into **Hodgkin's disease (HD),** one of several forms of neoplasm of the lymphatic system, and the malignant or **non-Hodgkin's lymphomas (NHL),** neoplasms of the immune system that are primarily located in the lymph nodes. A distinction between HD and NHL is the presence of **Reed-Sternberg cells** in the former, whereas the latter is characterized by a number of different cell types that form the basis of numerous classification schemes.

Hodgkin's disease occurs at any age but a bimodal distribution of age-related occurrence is evident with maxima involving young adults (20 to 30 years old) and older adults (50 to 65 years old). A bias for males (2:1) has also been demonstrated. Most patients present with enlarged lymph nodes, but other symptoms associated with hypermetabolism (night sweats, fever, weight loss, fatigueability) may also be present. The diagnosis requires demonstration of the large (50 to 100 μm) Reed-Sternberg (RS) cells in the affected tissues (Fig. 20-22). A lymph node biopsy is used to characterize HD into one of four subtypes, according to the Rye classification:

Lymphocytic predominance: small mature lymphocyte and mature histiocytes

Lymphocyte depleted: few lymphocytes; histiocytes common; atypical RS cells

Mixed cellularity: lymphocytes, plasma cells, histiocytes, eosinophils, RS cells

Nodular sclerosis: nodules defined by collagen bands, atypical histiocytes

The nodular sclerosing form is the most common type of HD, accounting for about one third of all cases, characterized by discrete nodules composed of atypical histiocytes (lacunar cells), plasma cells, lymphocytes, and a few RS cells, separated by bands of collagen. This form typically occurs in young women, often occurring as a mass in the mediastinum. The second most frequent subtype is the mixed cellularity type, also occurring primarily in young adults. RS cells are moderately abundant and the disease is usually well advanced when first diagnosed. The lymphocyte predominant form is relatively rare (7% to 8%

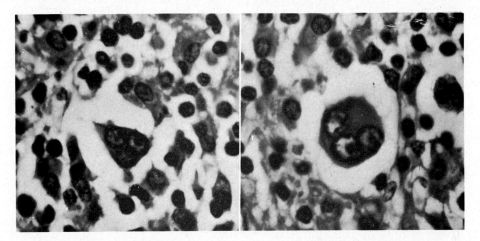

Fig. 20-22.   Reed-Sternberg cells in a lymph node section, Hodgkin's disease.
(From Miale JB: Laboratory medicine: Hematology, ed. 6, 1982, The CV Mosby Co.)

of HD) and occurs most frequently in young adult males. It is often localized to one or a few adjacent lymph nodes, particularly in the cervical area, so that treatment is often successful for this subtype. The lymphocyte depleted form is the rarest (less than 2% of HD cases) and the most malignant form, accompanied by fever and pancytopenia. Lymphadenopathy is frequently absent and the patient, usually an older adult male, may not seek medical attention until the malignancy has spread to several sites. The disease may also involve the spleen, liver, bone marrow, skin, and lungs, making effective treatment all but impossible.

Therapeutic results are related to the maturity of the cells involved and the relative spread of the disease at diagnosis. Confinement of the disease to one side of the diaphragm is an important criterion for successful treatment. Staging is a classification of disease progression that helps determine the mode of therapy, based on tissue biopsies, chest x-rays, and radiographic studies using dye injections of the lymph nodes:

Stage I: One node or localized area, located on same side of the diaphragm

Stage II: Two or more nodes or areas, lo-cated on the same side of the diaphragm

Stage III: Involvement of lymph nodes on both sides of diaphragm, may include spleen

Stage IV: Involvement of any tissue (disseminated)

Rates of survival decrease from 85% for stage I HD to 50% for stage IV. Survival is also more likely in young patients and in those with mature cell types predominating. Irradiation or multiple agent chemotherapy is given, depending on the stage of the disease.

Non-Hodgkin's lymphomas are classified morphologically (The Rappaport system is the traditional classification), using a combination of morphological and immunological features (Lukes-Collins system), and by comparing morphology and disease progression (international Working Formulation, IWF). A variety of other systems have been proposed (see Sun, Li, and Yam, 1985 for a review), but the IWF system is probably the most widely used. Although these disorders are largely confined to the lymph nodes and other lymphoid tissues, lymphoma cells may be observed on occasion in the periph-

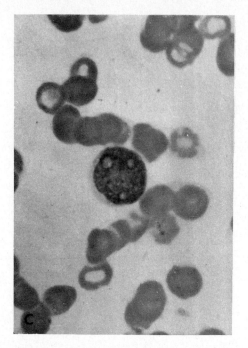

Fig. 20-23. Lymphoma cell in the peripheral blood.
(From Miale JB: Laboratory medicine: Hematology, ed 6, St Louis, 1982, The CV Mosby Co.)

eral blood (Fig. 20-23). Lymphomas of B cells, T cells, undifferentiated lymphocytes and histiocytes are among the many specific types that are described (McKenzie, 1988 provides an excellent summary for medical technologists).

Plasma cell dyscrasias. Multiple myeloma is a malignant neoplasm of plasma cells that occurs mainly in older adults. It is characterized by plasma cell proliferation within the bone marrow, resulting in osteolytic destruction of the bone material. Extreme pain and the occurrence of pathological fractures is often the complaint during initial presentation and the lesions are confirmed by radiography (see case history). The plasma cells may occurs as diffuse aggregates of mature and immature cells or as solid sheets (Fig. 20-24). Many of these so-

called myeloma cells are larger than normal plasma cells and some are multinucleated. As described previously (see plasma cell leukemia), the appearance of substantial numbers of plasma cells in the peripheral blood provides the basis for a diagnosis of PCL, probably the terminal phase of multiple myeloma.

The outstanding characteristic of the plasma cell malignancies is the production of massive amounts of immunoglobulin of a single class. Since the plasma cell neoplasm originates as a clone, only one Ig type is secreted, resulting in a distinct peak (M-spike) on a serum or urine electrophoresis pattern (Fig. 20-25). The gamma globulin fraction is the one usually increased, although the alpha or beta components can also be increased. When immunoelectrophoretic techniques are employed, using monoclonal antibodies for specific Ig classes, the specificity of the plasma protein as a **monoclonal gammopathy** is revealed. IgG is the most common class involved, followed by IgA and IgD. Myeloma cells associated with IgA secretion may have cytoplasms with a pink to red color (flame cells).

Immunoglobulins are composed of light and heavy peptide chains, but it is the light chains that are produced in such amounts that they appear in the urine as **Bence Jones protein.** In about 20% of the cases, only light chains are secreted and since these are rapidly cleared from the plasma by the kidneys, the abnormal protein pattern is seen only in the urine but not in the plasma. Therefore, a urine electrophoresis should always be run in conjunction with a serum pattern when myeloma is suspected. The increased globulin concentration produces a marked increase in rouleaux formation, accelerating the erythrocyte sedimentation rate dramatically. The abnormal proteins also interfere with the coagulation cascade and some of the clotting test results may be abnormal.

Therapy is often withheld in patients that

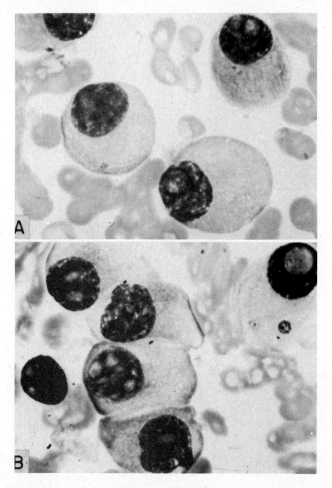

Fig. 20-24. Multiple myeloma, plasma cells in bone marrow.
(From Miale JB: Laboratory medicine: Hematology, ed. 6, St Louis, 1982, The CV Mosby Co.)

are clinically asymptomatic. The most frequent complication, because of the impaired immune system, is infection. Patients with aggressive forms of the disease are treated with alkylating agents and irradiation, along with symptomatic relief provided by fresh frozen plasma to aid coagulation and packed cells to correct anemia.

Waldenström's macroglobulinemia is characterized by the secretion of monoclonal IgM by proliferating B cells with a plasmacytoid appearance. The cells infil-

trate the bone marrow, but do not produce the osteolytic lesions that characterize multiple myeloma. The high concentrations of IgM create a hyperviscous plasma that results in cardiovascular complications, visual disturbance, and interference with coagulation proteins. Rouleaux formation is increased and the ESR is elevated. Most patients are elderly and they are usually male. Because of their age, it is difficult to assess survival intervals. Treatment by plasmapheresis to alleviate plasma hyperviscocity is combined with the use of alkylating agents to reduce the hypersecretory clone of lymphocytes.

Other gammopathies include the **heavy chain diseases,** manifestations of plasmacy- toid lymphocyte proliferations that produce only the heavy chain portion of immuno- globulins. Four types have been described, corresponding to the production of alpha (the most common), gamma, delta and mu

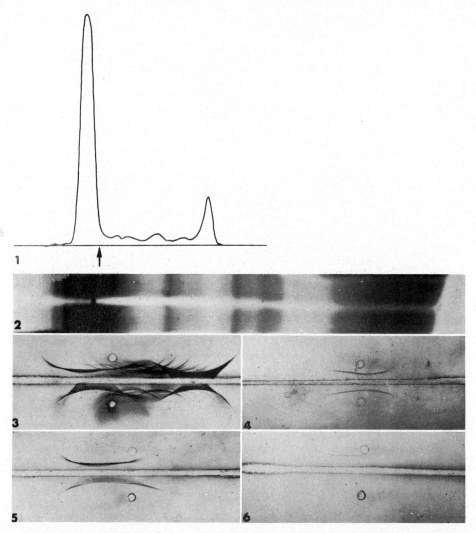

Fig. 20-25.   Multiple myeloma. 1, Electrophoresis showing abnormal peak in the γ area. **2,** Starch gel electrophoresis showing abnormal γ bands. **3-6,** Immunoelectro- phoresis, normal control at top, patient at bottom: **3,** polyvalent antiserum; **4,** anti- IgA serum; **5,** anti-IgG serum showing abnormal γ component; **6,** anti-IgM serum showing decrease of IgM. (From Miale JB: Laboratory medicine: Hematology, ed 6, St Louis, 1982, The CV Mosby Co.)

chains. The clinical features are similar to those of the malignant lymphomas and most cases are progressive, resulting in death from infection or bleeding complications.

Case Histories

CASE 1: CHRONIC MYELOGENOUS LEUKEMIA

The patient is a 57-year-old caucasian male previously in excellent health now presenting

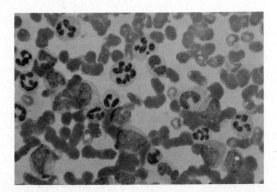

Fig. 20-26.   Chronic myelogenous leukemia, peripheral blood.

with a 5-month history of progressive weight loss and decrease in appetite. In addition, over the past 3 weeks he had noted night sweats and a persistent sharp pain and fullness in the left upper quadrant of the abdomen. He had also experienced left shoulder pain during the past 2 weeks. Physical examination was unremarkable except for the noting of a large tender mass in the left upper quadrant, a splenic rub on deep inspiration, and the presence of mild muscle wasting of the lower extremities bilaterally.

Laboratory evaluation revealed a white cell count of 185,700/μL, the differential count revealed 51% segmented neutrophils, 26% bands, 3% metamyelocytes, 10% myelocytes, 2% promyelocytes, 2% myeloblasts, 5% lymphocytes, and 1% monocytes. The peripheral smear is shown in Fig. 20-26. The hemoglobin was 11.7 g/dL, and the hematocrit was 41.7%; the platelet count was 175,000/μL. The biochemical survey was normal except for an elevated uric acid and elevated LDH. The leukocyte alkaline phosphatase score was 2 Kaplow units. A CT scan of the abdomen was performed (Fig. 20-27) and revealed massive splenomegaly. A bone marrow biopsy and aspirate was obtained and revealed marked marrow hypercellularity and marked myeloid hyperplasia. The marrow biopsy is shown in Fig. 20-28, and a marrow smear is shown in Fig. 20-29. The diagnosis is chronic myelogenous leukemia.

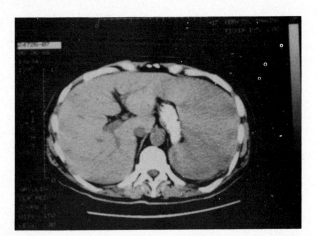

Fig. 20-27.   CML.
Computed tomography (CT) of the abdomen, showing an increased splenic mass on the left side of the body.

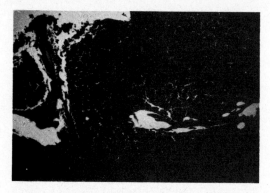

Fig. 20-28.   CML.
Bone marrow biopsy.

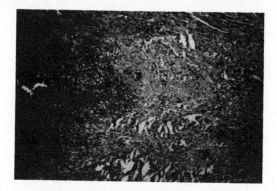

Fig. 20-30.   Hodgkins's disease.
Fibrous tissue in cervical lymph node.

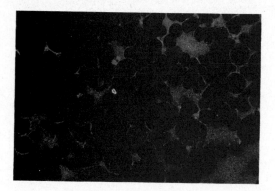

Fig. 20-29.   CML.
Bone marrow smear.

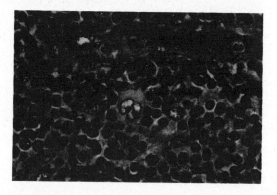

Fig. 20-31.   Lymph node biopsy.
Reed-Sternberg cell in nodular sclerosing type of Hodgkin's disease.

The patient was started on allopurinal and hydroxyurea, and his counts normalized over a 3-week period.

CASE 2: HODGKIN'S DISEASE

The patient is a 28-year-old caucasian female who was self-referred, seeking a second opinion regarding cervical lymphadenopathy. The patient had presented to her family physician 7 months previously complaining of bilateral cervical lymph nodes and fatigue; he recommended a course of antibiotics. After 6 weeks of antibiotics, the nodes continued to enlarge, and a heterophile test and Epstein-Barr and cytomegalovirus titers were ordered. The heterophile test and cytomegalovirus titer were negative; however, the Epstein-Barr titer was positive at 1:1280 to IgG and negative to IgM antibody. She was thus told by her physician that she had chronic Epstein-Barr virus syndrome and was advised to remain on antibiotics. After 7 months of continuous antibiotic therapy and progressive lymphadenopathy, she decided to seek further consultation. At the time of hematological evaluation, she denied any systemic symptomatology other than fatigue; in particular, she had experienced no anorexia, no weight loss, no fever, and no pruritis. Physical examination demonstrated bilateral cervical, infra-auricular and supraclavicular adenopathy, bilateral axillary adenopathy, and right inguinal adenopathy. There was no hepatosplenomegaly.

Laboratory and radiographic studies were ordered, and the patient was referred to a surgeon

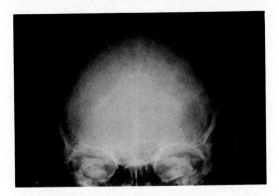

Fig. 20-32.   Multiple myeloma.
Radiograph of skull showing osteolytic lesions.

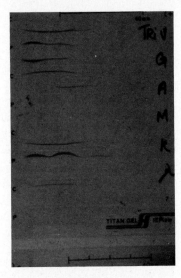

Fig. 20-34.   Multiple myeloma.
Immunoelectrophoresis of the serum identifies the IgG spike as a monoclonal kappa chain. *P*, patient, *C*, control.

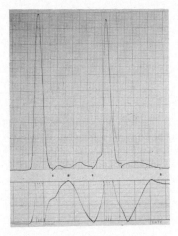

Fig. 20-33.   Multiple myeloma.
Serum protein electrophoresis, showing a prominent IgG spike.

for lymph node biopsy from the cervical and inguinal regions.

Laboratory studies revealed a total WBC count of 10,500/μL, with the differential count revealing 75% segmented neutrophils, 13% bands, 10% lymphocytes, and 2% eosinophils. The hemoglobin was 10.7 g/dL, and the hematocrit was 33.9%. The platelet count was 450,000/μL, and the sedimentation rate was elevated to 58 mm/hr. The only abnormality on a biochemical screening survey was a markedly elevated LDH (371 IU/L). CT scan of the thorax revealed medi-astinal adenopathy, and CT scanning of the abdomen revealed hepatosplenomegaly.

Lymph node biopsy revealed significant disease. Fig. 20-30 is a low-power view of a cervical lymph node and demonstrates destruction of the normal architecture by invasion of dense bands of fibrous tissue into the lymphoid areas. Fig. 20-31 is a high-power view showing a typical Reed-Sternberg cell. A diagnosis of nodular sclerosing Hodgkin's disease was made, and the patient immediately underwent staging laparotomy and splenectomy. Following the laparotomy, her pathological stage was 3A$_2$. The patient was treated with six cycles of MOPP chemotherapy and achieved complete remission.

CASE 3: MULTIPLE MYELOMA

At presentation the patient was a 43-year-old caucasian female with complaints of fatigue, fever to 39° C, weight loss, and rib pain of 2 months duration. She was admitted for evaluation and found to have pathological fractures of three ribs. Additional evaluation revealed massive hepatosplenomegaly. A rib biopsy and liver biopsy both revealed an infiltrate of abnormal-appearing plasma cells and extensive amyloid

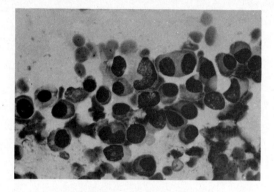

Fig. 20-35.   Multiple myeloma.
Bone marrow aspirate, showing plasma cell hyperplasia, including binucleated cells.

deposits. Following this, a bone marrow biopsy and aspirate were obtained which revealed a plasmacytosis of 40%, characterized by morphologically abnormal plasma cells; in addition, congo red staining of the marrow biopsy also revealed extensive amyloid deposits. A metastatic bone survey demonstrated extensive lytic lesions of the skull (Fig. 20-32), ribs, vertebrae, and proximal femurs.

Additional laboratory evaluation revealed elevated liver enzymes. The total protein was elevated to 14 gm/dL, and globulins were elevated to 6.5 g/L. Serum protein electrophoresis (Fig. 20-33) revealed a paraprotein spike, and quantitative immunoglobulins revealed an IgG of 6000 mg/dL, an IgA of < 20 mg/dL, and an IgM of < 20 mg/dL. Immunoelectrophoresis of serum revealed the paraprotein to be a monoclonal IgG kappa. IEP is shown in Fig. 20-34, and a bone marrow smear is shown in Fig. 20-35.

A diagnosis of IgG kappa myeloma, complicated by amyloidosis, was made and the patient was started on the Sloan-Kettering M-II protocol and achieved complete remission; 4 years later she remains in complete remission.

SUMMARY

- Leukocyte disorders can be divided into reactive patterns, such as responses to infections, proliferative disorders that are characterized by an autonomous, non-regulated nature, and dysplastic disorders that exhibit abnormalities of production or release from the marrow.

- Neoplasms are proliferations of cells that can be benign (slow developing and non-invasive growths) or malignant (rapid expansion and invasion of adjacent tissues). Malignancies are usually progressive and life threatening if not treated effectively.

- Leukemia is a malignancy of blood cell tissue, primarily of the bone marrow, that displaces normal elements and produces anemia, bleeding disorders, and loss of host defense capability. Acute leukemias develop rapidly and are characterized by the proliferation of very immature cells; chronic leukemias develop slowly and exhibit increases of intermediate and mature cells.

- Acute leukemias and myelodysplastic syndromes are classified by the French-American-British (FAB) system: 3 types of ALL, seven types of AML and 5 types of MDS are recognized, based on a combination of morphological and histochemical criteria.

- Acute lymphoblastic leukemia is the most common type in young children and the most easily treated. Chronic leukemias are most commonly seen in older adults. Chromosome abnormalities are associated with most white cell malignancies; the Philadelphia chromosome is a translocation seen in most cases of CML. CLL and hairy cell leukemia are chronic forms seen in older adults. Most leukemia patients die of complications due to displacement or suppression of normal blood cell production (infections, bleeding, and anemia).

- Other myeloproliferative disorders include polycythemia vera (a proliferation of marrow erythroblasts and the peripheral red cell mass), myeloid metaplasia (displacement of marrow blood cell production to other sites, often accompanied by myelofibrosis, a fibrotic infiltration of the marrow), and essential thrombocytosis (an autonomous expansion of platelet production).

- Myelodysplastic   syndromes   are   often

preleukemic changes that include dyshematopoiesis of two or more cell lines, megaloblastoid changes of the erythroid series, the presence of increased blasts in the peripheral blood and marrow, and a number of other abnormalities.

• Hodgkin's disease and non-Hodgkin's lymphomas are malignancies of the lymphatic system. They are classified on the basis of predominant cellular types and they are clinically staged by the extent of tissue dissemination and cellular maturity.

• Multiple myeloma, plasma cell leukemia, macroglobulinemia, and heavy chain diseases are plasma cell malignancies that result in the increased production of immunoglobulins or Ig chains. They can be detected by serum and urine protein electrophoresis and identified by immunoelectrophoresis, using monoclonal antibodies.

21

Metabolic Diseases, Deficiencies, and Responses of Leukocytes

LIPID STORAGE DISEASES OF MACROPHAGES

Collectively, lipid storage diseases are hereditary deficiencies of lysosomal enzymes that are involved in cellular glycolipid degradation. Lipids accumulate in macrophages of the spleen, liver, and bone marrow, resulting in cells with a characteristic foamy cytoplasm. A number of specific enzyme deficiencies have been described (Table 21-1), but only three of are considered here.

Gaucher's disease is a deficiency of beta-glucocerebrosidase, resulting in accumulation of **glucocerebrosides** in macrophages. The disorder is inherited as an autosomal recessive pattern and it is most prevalent among Ashkenazic (eastern European) Jews. Three forms of the disease are recognized. They are a chronic type which first appears in older children and adults and does not involve the nervous system (type 1); an acute, very progressive type that appears in neonates and young infants and involves severe neurologic pathology (type 2); and a progressive type in children between 1 and 8 years of age that involves bone destruction but minimal neurologic damage (type 3). The neonatal form is rare and does not display the ethnic prevalence of the other types. Death usually occurs within 2 years of onset. The adult form (type 1) is more common, with an estimated heterozygote (carrier) frequency of 1 out of 50 among Jewish populations. The prognosis is generally better with later age of onset and some

patients may live relatively normal lives. Splenomegaly is the most consistent finding and this may be accompanied by thrombocytopenia, associated bleeding and purpura, bone lesions and pain, pulmonary disease, skin hyperpigmentation, and signs of liver involvement.

The diagnostic and characteristic laboratory finding is the presence of **Gaucher cells** in the bone marrow and other organs. These cells are relatively large (20 to 80 μm in diameter) and contain a small, often eccentrically placed nucleus. The cytoplasm is pale blue and filled with lipid inclusions arranged in a fibrillar or "crinkled tissue paper" pattern (Fig. 21-1). Occasionally, the cytoplasm may appear to be sponge-like, with many fine to large vacuoles produced by incomplete lipid degradation. The cytoplasm stains strongly positive with PAS; weakly positive with Sudan black-B; and strongly positive for iron, nonspecific esterase, and acid phosphatase. In diseases involving massive cell proliferation, such as chronic myelogenous leukemia, the lipid degradation products cannot be catabolyzed adequately and the accumulation of lipids results in cells that are similar in appearance (pseudo-Gaucher cells).

Other laboratory findings may include a moderate normochromic, normocytic anemia with slight to moderate reticulocytosis. A moderate to severe panleukopenia may be present, especially if splenomegaly is marked. If splenectomy is used to relieve

Table 21-1. Lipid storage diseases

Enzyme (deficiency)	Substrate (accumulation)	Disorder
Beta-glucocerebrosidase	Glucocerebroside	Gaucher's disease
Alpha-galactosidase	Ceramide trihexoside	Fabry's disease
Beta-galactosidase	Monosialoganglioside G_{M1}	Generalized gangliosidosis
Beta-hexosaminidase A	Ganglioside G_{M2}	Tay-Sachs disease
Sphingomyelinase	Sphingomyelin	Niemann-Pick disease
Acid esterase	Triglycerides, cholesterol esters	Wolman's disease
Lipoprotein lipase	Triglycerides, phospholipids, etc.	Hyperlipidemia

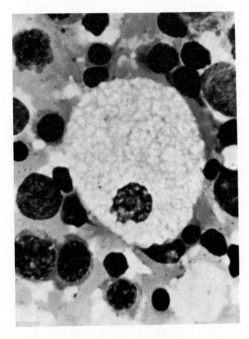

Fig. 21-1. Gaucher cells in bone marrow.
(From Miale, JB: Laboratory medicine: Hematology, ed 6, St Louis, 1982, The CV Mosby Co.)

bleeding manifestations, the white cell and platelet counts may be elevated and a variety of red cell abnormalities may be noted. These include Howell-Jolly bodies, target cells, peripheral normoblasts, marked an-isocytosis, and poikilocytosis. Serum acid phosphatase is usually elevated but lipid levels are within normal limits. The most sensitive test for establishing Gaucher's disease, including the presence of the heterozygote or carrier state, is measurement of leukocyte or cultured fibroblast beta-glucoside activity. This can also be extended to prenatal diagnosis by measuring the same activity in cultured cells obtained by amniocentesis.

Treatment is largely symptomatic, including splenectomy and management of bone pain and fractures. Enzyme replacement therapy has been attempted, but the techniques are experimental and the results are controversial.

Niemann-Pick disease is the second most common lipid storage disease and, like Gaucher's disease, it is inherited as an autosomal recessive pattern and it is most prevalent among Ashkenazic Jews. The occurrence of rare, physiologically-related disorders in a definable ethnic or geographic population raises questions about the adaptive selection of recessive genes (heterozygote superiority), such as has been documented for sickle cell trait and thalassemia minor in African and Mediterranean peoples, respectively. So far, a selective advantage has not been identified.

The typical form of disease occurs in

young infants (infantile or type A, about 85% of cases) with manifestations of hepatosplenomegaly and nervous system disturbances. These include severe mental retardation, delayed structural development, and, in many cases, retinal degeneration. The disease is progressive and death usually occurs by the age of 2 or 3. Other forms include an infantile form that is more chronic and without central nervous system signs (type B); a childhood onset form (type C) with later liver, spleen, and neurological involvement; and an adult form that is mild and without neurological disturbance (type E). All variants result from a deficiency of **sphingomyelinase** and the resulting accumulation of sphingomyelin in macrophages. These are the "foamy histiocytes" found in liver, spleen, bone marrow, and lymphatic tissues. Other lipoid materials may also be present, including cholesterol and ceroid. The latter may result in the appearance of a blue-green cytoplasm with Wright's or Giemsa staining, known as **sea-blue histiocyte syndrome,** which some workers have correlated with the adult type of Niemann-Pick disease.

Niemann-Pick cells are similar in size (20 to 80 μm diameter) and nucleus to cytoplasm ratio as Gaucher cells, but the lipoid deposits usually occur as globules or as foamy vacuoles. The nucleus is small, pyknotic, and often eccentrically located. Staining with PAS may give variable results, Sudan black-B gives a stronger reaction than in Gaucher cells, and acid phosphatase is negative. The lipoid droplets will fluoresce greenish-yellow in ultraviolet light and appear birefringent in polarized light. Identification of Niemann-Pick cells is accomplished by demonstrating the deficiency of sphingomyelinase in white blood cells or in cultured fibroblasts, and the commercially available methods can be applied to cells obtained by amniocentesis. Lipid-filled vacuoles may also appear in peripheral lymphocytes and a mild anemia may be present.

The prognosis in this disease is similar to that for Gaucher's disease in that later onsets are generally associated with milder, more chronic manifestations. Treatment is symptomatic, aimed at relieving pain from visceral disturbances and bone lesions.

It is not clear to what extent the appearance of numerous histiocytes with ultramarine cytoplasm constitutes a definable disorder. Many of the clinical symptoms of **ceroid storage disease** (sea-blue histiocyte syndrome) are similar to those seen in Gaucher and Niemann-Pick diseases and a deficiency of sphingomyelinase has been identified in some familial forms. A primary syndrome, consisting of splenomegaly and thrombocytopenia, usually with adult onset, is often mild and chronic. However, visceral involvement and an earlier age of onset carry a less favorable prognosis. The secondary syndrome is associated with myeloproliferative diseases, such as chronic myelogenous leukemia and myeloma, and idiopathic thrombocytopenic purpura. This may be due to excessive lipid catabolism which a normal enzyme system cannot complete, or to a mild enzyme deficiency, or both. These cells may also appear after treatment with certain tranquilizers, antileukemic drugs, or medications for anorexia and rheumatism.

HISTIOCYTOSIS (RETICULOENDOTHELIOSIS)

A group of diseases, characterized by the proliferation and infiltration of histiocytes or macrophages into various organs, have been collectively termed **histiocytosis.** Infiltration may be localized or systemic and may also include eosinophils. Etiological bases for these disorders are unknown, but they are suspected to be congenital and probably involve immunological responses. Three clinical types have been identified.

Letterer-Siwe disease. This occurs primarily in infants and young children. It is acute and systemic in nature, involving histiocyte infiltration of the spleen, liver, lymph nodes, and bone marrow. Hepatosplenomegaly, thrombocytopenia, diabetes insipidus, exophthalmos (eye protrusion), skin rashes, and bone lesions are among the manifestations. Many of the histiocytes appear foamy, but specific lipid abnormalities have not been identified. Leukopenia and a refractory anemia may be present. The course of the disorder is rapid and aggressive chemotherapy is required. Most patients under 2 years of age will die within weeks to a few months of onset of the disease.

Hand-Schüller-Christian disease. This variety is more benign and chronic. It is found in older children than those with Letterer-Siwe disease, but it is also systemic and the prognosis depends on the extent of organ involvement. Many of the clinical symptoms are similar, but the peripheral blood and bone marrow pictures are essentially normal. Osteolytic lesions of the skull are characteristic. Diagnosis and differentiation from other histiocytic disorders depends on histiological examination of the involved tissue. Eosinophils often accompany the macrophage infiltrate and fibrosis may occur during late stages of the disorder.

Eosinophilic granuloma. This is the most common variant, with onset in a wide range of ages but most common in adolescents and young adults. Osteolytic lesions appear in various parts of the skeleton, especially the skull and femur, resulting in bone pain. Pathological fractures are not uncommon. Bone biopsy reveals eosinophils and histiocytes, but the marrow and peripheral blood pictures are essentially normal. Treatment may be by surgical extrication of the lesion, low-level irradiation, or by chemotherapy if multiple sites are involved. Some cases remit spontaneously.

Other forms of histiocytosis are known, but their relationship to those previously described is uncertain. Diagnosis must be based on a biopsy of the involved area and the demonstration of histiocytic or histiocytic-eosinophilic infiltration. Some of the cells may fuse to form giant cells. Necrotic tissue, plasma cells, and fibrotic tissue may also be present at the lesion site.

DEFICIENCIES OF WHITE BLOOD CELL FUNCTION

The inability of phagocytic leukocytes to respond to or kill invading microorganisms will result in recurrent infections. The deficiency may be mild with the infections merely annoying or the defect may be severe with the infections life threatening. Some abnormalities are primarily morphological with little or no functional impairment, whereas others present a normal appearance but exhibit primary enzyme or bactericidal deficiency (Table 21-2).

Chédiak-Steinbrinck-Higashi syndrome is characterized by large azurophilic granules in most of the granule-forming cells of the body. They are especially prominent in neutrophils. The disorder is inherited in an autosomal recessive manner, affecting infants and young children. Most die in infancy or early childhood. The patients are subject to recurrent pyogenic infections because of several defects in leukocyte function. Investigators have reported deficiencies in chemotaxis, the ability of neutrophils to adhere to natural and artificial surfaces, microtubles associated with the plasma membrane, and formation of the phagolysosome. The patients also exhibit a pigment dilutional deficit (partial albinism) because of defective melanosomes, resulting in silvery hair and decreases in ocular and cutaneous pigment. Photophobia is a characteristic behavioral response in affected children. Platelets have a storage pool defect (Chapter 23) which is often associated with a bleeding tendency. The occasional patient that survives childhood or that does not initially present with severe manifestations usually shows an accelerated phase of symptoms during adolescence or as a young adult. Clinical signs may include lymphadenopathy, hepatosplenomegaly, peripheral neuropathy, pancytopenia, and infiltration of tissues by lymphocytes and macrophages.

The abnormal granules present in neutro-

Table 21-2. Leukocyte defects

Disorder or anomaly	Defect	Laboratory result
Chédiak-Steinbrinck-Higashi syndrome	Lysosomes	Decreased microbicidal capacity
Chronic granulomatous disease	Oxide production	Negative NBT
Lazy leukocyte syndrome	Motility, chemotaxis	Abnormal Rebuck skin window response
Myeloperoxidase deficiency	HOC1 and peroxide production	Decreased MPO staining
Diabetes	Chemotaxis, motility	Abnormal Rebuck skin window response
Alder-Reilly anomaly	Large azurophilic granules	Morphology only
May-Hegglin anomaly	Döhle-like inclusions	Morphology; bleeding and infection
Jordan's anomaly	Vacuolated WBCs	Morphology only
Pelger-Huët anomaly	Decreased nuclear segmentation	Morphology only

phils stain positively with Sudan black, peroxidase, and acid phosphatase, indicating derivation from lipid-containing and lysosomal granules. Ultrastructural and histochemical studies have determined that the granules consist of abnormally fused primary (azurophilic) and secondary (specific) granules. Some normal secondary granules may be seen in mature PMNs, but no normal primary granules are found.

Chronic granulomatous disease (CGD) is a heterogeneous group of disorders in which recurrent bacterial infections lead to an early death. Unlike Chédiak-Steinbrinck-Higashi syndrome, CGD does not exhibit obvious morphological abnormalities. The disease is seen primarily in males that suffer from chronic cutaneous and pulmonary infections, often from organisms that are only mildly to moderately pathogenic (*Serratia, Klebsiella*). Other clinical indications may include eczematous and granulomatous skin lesions, hepatosplenomegaly, and osteomyelitis.

The pathophysiological mechanism is uncertain, and a number of abnormalities of neutrophil function have been described:

1. Inability of bactericidal granules to release contents
2. Deficiencies of enzymes in or related to the respiratory burst
   a. Hexose monophosphate shunt enzymes (G6PD, glutathione reductase, glutathione synthetase)
   b. Oxidase associated with cell membrane (NADPH oxidase, NADH oxidase)
3. Defective cell membrane, not activated by bacterial factors, immunoglobulins, complement components, or other inflammatory stimuli

Most deficiencies have been related to the oxidative bactericidal mechanisms that are responsible for up to 90% of intracellular killing of ingested microbes. Other phagocytic cells (macrophages and eosinophils) are also defective. Although most cases are attributed to a sex-linked inheritance pattern (an autosomal recessive form has also been described), the actual defects are not known. Heterozygous females with the sex-linked form exhibit diminished bactericidal

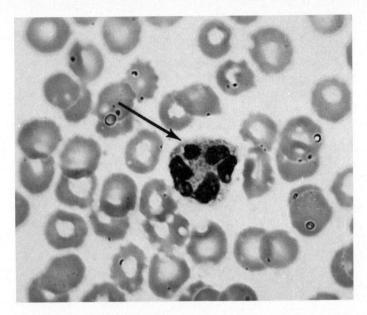

Fig. 21-2. Nitroblue tetrazolium (NBT) test.
Arrow points to a dark inclusion in a neutrophil incubated in NBT, constituting a positive result.
Defective cells are unable to reduce the NBT dye to formazon, and bluish inclusions are decreased or absent. (From Bauer, JD: Clinical laboratory methods, ed 9, St Louis, 1982, The CV Mosby Co.)

capacity with appropriate assays, but they do not manifest clinical problems.

The most widely used procedure to diagnose CGD is the **nitroblue tetrazolium (NBT) test** in which oxygen metabolites reduce the clear to yellowish NBT to formazon, a dark blue color. Normally, about 75% to 90% of the neutrophils incubated in NBT and exposed to microorganisms should show evidence of oxidative activity (respiratory burst) with the formation of blue intracellular inclusions (Fig. 21-2); defective neutrophils from patients with CGD show less than 25% positive cells. Heterozygous females have mixed populations of NBT-positive and NBT-negative cells.

Myeloperoxidase (MPO) deficiency is a benign, relatively common autosomal recessive defect that has no apparent clinical consequences, even in homozygous persons. Both the neutrophils and monocytes are deficient, whereas the eosinophils (different type of peroxidase) are normal. The fact that infections are not a problem in these individuals would seem to indicate that the generation of hypochlorites is not a critical step in bactericidal activity.

Lazy leukocyte syndrome is, as the name implies, a defect in the ability of white cells to respond to infections and inflammatory stimuli. Cells are less readily released from the bone marrow, resulting in a peripheral blood neutropenia, and a diminished chemotactic response. Patients suffer from recurrent infections, particularly of the respiratory system. This disorder is rare, but it can be diagnosed by various assays for neutrophil response, including the Rebuck skin window, described in Chapter 8.

HEREDITARY ANOMALIES OF LEUKOCYTES

Alder-Reilly anomaly is characterized by dark, coarse azurophilic granules in all white blood cells, (Plate 7 A). The granules contain acid polysaccharides and glycogen, they stain metachromatically with toluidine blue O and negatively with PAS stain. The granules are particularly evident in leukocyte precursors on bone marrow preparations. Although these inclusions may be occasionally seen as an inherited anomaly in otherwise healthy individuals, they are most often associated with genetic mucopolysaccharidoses, such as Hunter's syndrome and Hurler's syndrome. The leukocytes appear to be fully functional, despite the obvious morphological abnormality.

May-Hegglin anomaly is an autosomal dominant disorder characterized by large irregular inclusions in various white cells. The inclusions resemble Döhle bodies, they range in size from about 2 to 5 μm, and they contain glycogen and RNA, producing a positive reaction to methyl green pyronine stain. The major problems for patients with this disorder is an increased susceptibility to infections and a bleeding tendency. Platelets are larger than normal and thrombocytopenia is common (Chapter 23). Platelets have a survival time that is less than half of normal, the clot retraction test is prolonged, and the capillary fragility test (tourniquet test) is often positive. Specific leukocyte functional defects are not apparent.

Jordan's anomaly is a familial abnormality in which leukocytes, especially phagocytic cells, contain many large to fine vacuoles. The vacuoles are filled with lipids and they can be seen in marrow precursors, except for blast cells and megakaryocytes. Although specific functional defects have not been identified, patients exhibiting this abnormality had other pathological conditions, such as muscular dystrophy and icthyosis.

Pelger-Huët anomaly is a benign morphological abnormality of leukocytes that is characterized by condensed nuclear chromatin and the presence of nucleoli in otherwise mature cells. The nucleus of granulocytes, however, shows a decreased tendency toward segmentation. It is an autosomal dominant pattern, present in about 1 in 5000 people and it is not confined to any race or geographical area. Homozygous patients are relatively rare; most of the neutrophils contain a single, oval lobe with condensed chromatin. Examination of the marrow in homozygous patients shows normal granulocytic maturation up to the myelocyte stage. The cytoplasm appears normal at all stages, but as development continues the nucleus fails to lobulate. Heterozygous individuals have 70% to 90% neutrophils with a symmetrical bilobed nucleus (dumbbell or pince-nez appearance). The cells appear to be functionally normal and the incidence of infection is not increased.

An acquired form off Pelger-Huët anomaly (pseudo Pelger-Huët) is seen in many patients with myeloproliferative and myelodysplastic disorders. This is most likely to occur following toxic chemotherapy for acute leukemia, manifested by the presence of peripheral blood neutrophils with a single nuclear lobe. Pseudo Pelger-Huët is also sometimes seen in patients with malaria, myxedema, myeloid metaplasia, Fanconi's anemia, and infectious mononucleosis.

LEUKOCYTE RESPONSES TO INFLAMMATION AND INFECTION

Leukocytosis is an increase in white blood cells in the peripheral blood. **Neutrophilia** specifies a condition of increased peripheral blood neutrophils (greater than 7500 per μL). This occurs in a number of stressful situations, such as vigorous exercise, stimulation of catecholamine secretion, administration of certain drugs (especially steroids), and response to infections. A **leukmoid reaction** is a marked neutrophilic response, superficially resembling leukemia in that the number of granulocytes increases (50,000 to 100,000 per μL) and a degree of relative immaturity is evidenced as a "shift to the left" (see Chapter

8). Most of these changes are transient, reflecting the movement of PMNs between marrow storage, circulating, and tissue compartments. Quantitative criteria for defining increased (philic) and decreased (penic) concentrations of peripheral blood leukocytes are included in Table 21-3.

A staphylococcus infection stimulates a chemotactic response by circulating neutrophils (Fig. 21-3). Initially, neutrophil counts in the peripheral blood increase as cells demarginate from the vascular lining and move toward the focus of inflammation. The rate of increase is rapid but the response is transient, as neutrophils emigrate from the blood stream and enter the extravascular tissues. Additional or continuing chemotactic signals will stimulate the release of neutrophils from the bone marrow storage compartment. Depending on the strength of the signal and the rate of PMN depletion from the peripheral blood, neutrophils released from the marrow may be restricted to relatively mature segmented forms or they may include band and metamyelocytic forms (shift to the left). Thus, both numbers (concentration) and stages (degree of immaturity) are roughly proportional to the severity of the infection.

Bacterial sepsis can result in a leukmoid reaction, involving white cell counts of 100,000 per μL, the presence of myelocytes, and the appearance of **toxic granulation** in the cytoplasm of neutrophils (Fig. 21-4). Some evidence indicates that the toxic granules may contain immune complexes, consisting of microbial antigens and reactive immunoglobulins.

Obviously, it is important to distinguish white cell responses to inflammatory and infectious processes from those that are primary disorders, such as leukemic neoplasms. The bone marrow is usually definitive, since leukemic cells exhibit features (Auer rods, chromosome abnormalities, enzyme and cell membrane markers) that the normal precursors of a leukmoid reaction lack. A nonevasive procedure measures **leukocyte alkaline phosphatase (LAP)** activity in band and segmented neutrophils, using either a qualitative histochemical method or a quantitative enzyme assay. In the histochemical technique, the amount of LAP is visually observed in 100 cells and scored on a scale of 0 to 4 Kaplow units. Patients with chronic myelogenous leukemia usually have scores of less than 20 whereas leukmoid reactions often yield scores greater than 150. Other myeloproliferative disorders may produce higher or lower than normal values (normal is about 25 to 125 for males and 30 to 150 for females), but the distinction between

Table 21-3. Quantitative changes in leukocytes

Cell	Cytophilia	Cytopenia	Note
Neutrophil	> 7500 per μL	< 1500 per μL	< 500 per μL = agranulocytosis
Lymphocyte			
Adult	> 4000 per μL	< 1500 per μL	
Children	> 7000 per μL	< 2500 per μL	values for children < 3 years old
Monocyte	> 800 per μL	< 100 per μL	
Eosinophil	> 450 per μL	< 50 per μL	> 1500 per μL = hypereosinophilia
Basophil	> 100 per μL		or > 2% of total WBC count

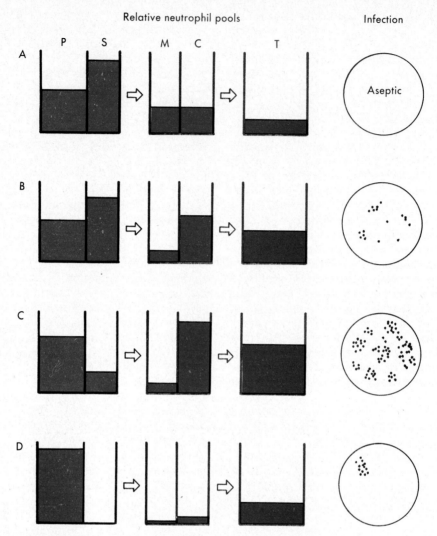

Relative neutrophil pools   Infection

Fig. 21-3.   Responses of neutrophils to severe bacterial sepsis.
A, Baseline state when no infection is present. **B,** Early stages of infection and response by circulating neutrophils. **C,** Continued infection results in release of marrow cells, including immature granulocytes. **D,** Exhaustion of marrow stores and peripheral blood neutropenia as infection overwhelms host defense. *P,* production pool; *S,* storage pool; *M,* marginal pool; *C,* circulating pool; *T,* tissue pool.

a marked leukmoid reaction and CML can be made without a bone marrow. It should be noted that the LAP score may increase in CML during a blast crisis (Chapter 20).

LYMPHOCYTIC RESPONSES

Lymphocytosis is an absolute lymphocyte concentration in the peripheral blood that exceeds 4000 per µL (adults) to 7000 per µL (children, depending on age). Abso-

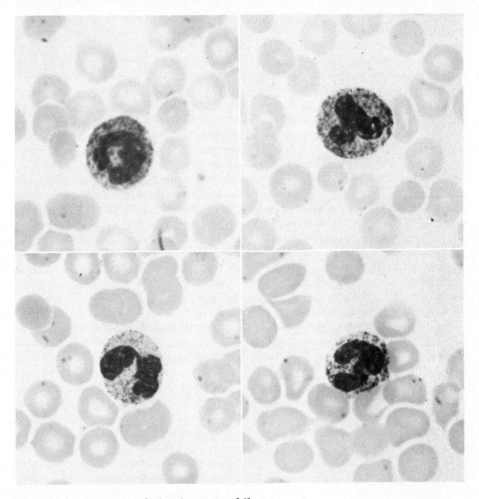

Fig. 21-4.   Toxic granulation in neutrophils
(From Miale, JB: Laboratory medicine: Hematology, ed 6, St Louis, 1982, The CV Mosby Co.)

lute lymphocytosis must be distinguished from a relative lymphocytosis due to a decrease in granulocytes. Benign lymphocyte increases can be divided into those that are dominated by small, mature lymphocytes and those that include a significant number (greater than 10%) of **reactive lymphocytes,** large cells with increased cytoplasm and "monocytoid" and/or immature features (Plate 7, *B* and *C*). These cells have been referred to as Downey cells (three types were described), virocytes, "atypical" lymphocytes, and other terms in association with specific conditions. The association between reactive lymphocytes and virus infections has long been recognized, but it wasn't until lymphocytic transformations were related to immunological responses that the basis for the "atypical" morphology was fully appreciated. The immature features are indeed indications of blast transformation, an event that heralds a response to antigen, usually by a B cell prior to immunoglobulin production as a plasma cell.

Increases in mature lymphocytes are particularly evident in children with whooping cough (pertussis); absolute lymphocyte counts can range from over 10,000 per μL to 50,000 per μL. The increase is self-limiting, abating as the infection resolves. Mature lymphocytes typically increase in adults that have disseminated forms of tuberculosis or brucellosis, both involving intracellular infections. Acute infectious lymphocytosis (AIL) is an enigmatic condition, primarily seen in children, that is not associated with a known infectious agent nor does it involve an acute illness other than diarrhea. This condition can be distinguished from infectious mononucleosis (IM) clinically because AIL has an absence of hepatosplenomegaly and adenopathy, both of which are usually present in patients with IM. Adults less often contract AIL, but they may also present with a moderate increase in mature cells. Hyperthyroidism may also be accompanied by lymphocytosis. In these conditions, as well as CLL (Chapter 20), the heterogeneity of lymphocyte morphology tends to increase as the cell count increases.

INFECTIOUS MONONUCLEOSIS

Reactive lymphocytoses are seen in many virus infections. The classic example of a moderate to marked increase in reactive cells occurs in patients, especially those who are immunocompromised, with EBV, CMV, and HIV infections. **Infectious mononucleosis (IM)** is caused by the Epstein-Barr virus, a DNA herpes-type virus that infects B lymphocytes. Patients display mild to severe adenopathy, hepatosplenomegaly in some, fever, malaise, pharyngitis, and a characteristic blood picture dominated by reactive lymphocytes. The latter comprise more than 10% of the total differential WBC count and lymphocytes comprise more than 50% of the white cell count (Fig. 21-5). Fortunately, the disease is most likely to strike healthy adolescents and young adults as the so-called "kissing dis-

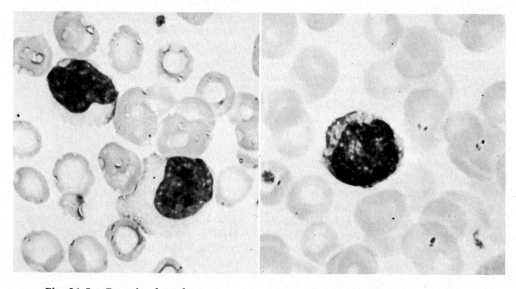

Fig. 21-5.　Reactive lymphocytes.
(From Bauer, JD: Clinical laboratory methods, ed. 9, St. Louis, 1982, The CV Mosby Co.)

LYMPHOCYTOSIS

Mature Cells Dominate

Mild

    Early chronic lym-
      phocytic leuke-
      mia

    Hyperthyroidism

Moderate to Marked

    Advanced chronic
      lymphocytic leu-
      kemia

    Acute infectious
      lymphocytosis
      (children)

    Pertussis (children)

    Disseminated tu-
      berculosis
      (adults)

Reactive Cells Dominate

    Upper respiratory
      infections

    Inflammatory pro-
      cesses

    Viral hepatitis

    Mumps, measles,
      chickenpox

    Epstein-Barr virus
      (infectious
      mononucleosis)

    Cytomegalovirus
      infections (CMV)

    Toxoplasma infec-
      tions

    Human immuno-
      deficiency virus
      (HIV)

ease" that is prevalent in high schools and colleges, and in most cases the condition is self-limiting.

The virus is transmitted primarily by infected saliva and evidence has accumulated that either the oropharyngeal epithelial cells or the salivary duct cells are the primary target for EBV. Many infections are probably transmitted by healthy carriers that are now immune to the disease, many of which acquired EBV in a milder form as young children. Keeling, in Thorup (1987), provides an interesting commentary on the reciprocal relationship between this early exposure to EBV and immunity to infectious mononucleosis. Almost all of the children in parts of Africa have been exposed to EBV by the time they are 2 years old, as evidenced by assays for antibody to EBV, and IM is extremely rare among their adult counterparts. Conditions in America restrict early exposure to EBV and IM is quite common. Unfortunately, the virus is not as benign in all cases. EBV has also been implicated in genital lesions of young women, in nasopharyngeal carcinoma, and in Burkitt's lymphoma. IM can also be fatal in some patients, involving systemic dysfunction and compromising immune function. Many of the cells that are infected will die, but some may be transformed and immortalized as memory cells containing the EBV genome.

Normally, NK and T cells limit the extent of infection. About 2 weeks after introduction into an immune-competent host, T cells are activated to counteract the infected B cells. The counterattack is usually optimal at 4 to 8 weeks and the disease is often resolved by 12 to 14 weeks. It is the activated T cells that comprise the majority of "atypical" or reactive lymphocytes in the peripheral blood. A few are B cells that contain EBV.

Other B cells also are involved in the defense, producing a variety of immunoglobulins (polyclonal) against determinants on the virus. Other antibodies are directed against determinants that have been identified in other animals. These are referred to as **heterophile antibodies** and they typically occur in IM as IgM antibodies with titers of 1:112 or more. Other conditions, such as myeloproliferative disorders and connective tissue diseases, also exhibit heterophile antibodies, but a differential test can distinguish IM on the basis of its absorption by beef red blood cells but not by guinea pig kidney. These can be performed with commercially available spot tests that are rapid and easy to interpret, providing an additional noninvasive method for discriminating between IM and monocytic leukemia.

IM may also be associated with a mild to severe hemolytic anemia due to the production of anti-i antibodies against host red cells. The i antigen is present on almost all fetal red cells, but most of the antigen converts to I after birth. Residual i antigen remains, however, and infection by EBV apparently uncovers the fetal determinant or stimulates production of immunoglobulin that can react with it, producing a cold hemolytic anemia (see Chapter 19). In most cases, hemolysis is extravascular and minor, but complement activation by an IgM antibody can produce intravascular destruction in a few patients. The resulting anemia can be severe (hemoglobin < 4 g per dL, reticulocyte count 30% to 40%). A mild thrombocytopenia, possibly also mediated by autoantibodies, may develop and result in some bleeding tendencies, especially if hepatic involvement is also extensive. The disease is relatively rare in elderly persons, but when it does occur it is often more severe. Treatment is typically supportive, as it is with many viral infections.

LYMPHOCYTE DEFICIENCY DISORDERS

A number of congenital disorders affecting lymphocytes have been described. Deficiencies range from absence of organs (thymus, spleen, lymph nodes) to impaired immunoglobulin synthesis. The deficiency can involve B cells, T cells, or both.

As might be expected, patients with B cell deficiencies are unable or only partially successful in humorally mediated defenses against microbes. The disorder may be evident from infancy due to recurrent infections; additional evidence includes decreased Ig production and failure to achieve immunization with vaccines. Radiographs and biopsies may reveal little or no lymphatic tissue. Semiquantitative immunoglobulin patterns can be verified by immunoelectrophoresis (IEP) and the concentrations by radial immunodiffusion (RID) in agar gels.

DiGeorge's syndrome is a congenital absence of thymic tissue, thus the maturation organ for T lymphocyte development is missing. The parathyroid glands are also absent or partially missing, disrupting calcium metabolism. Cell mediated immunity

LYMPHOCYTE DEFICIENCIES	
B cell deficiency	
Sex-linked agammaglobulinemia (Bruton's)	Absence of B cell production and tissue
Common variable hypogammaglobulinemia	Deficiency of immunoglobulin production
Selective IgA deficiency	Deficiency of IgA production
T cell deficiency	
Congenital thymic hypoplasia (DiGeorge's)	Absence of thymus, T cell production
B and T cell deficiency	
Severe combined immunodeficiency (SCID)	Several types: decreased or absent B and T cell production

(type IV hypersensitivity) is impaired, as evidenced by lack of response to skin tests for tuberculin and mycological antigens. Whereas B cell deficient patients are susceptible to many bacterial infections, T cell deficient patients have problems primarily with viral and fungal infections. Combined B and T cell deficiencies result in severe recurrent infections, usually proving fatal in infancy or early childhood unless a bone marrow transplant is successful.

In addition to congenital deficiencies of lymphocytes, acquired immunodeficiency can occur as a result of chemotherapy, radiation exposure, and viral infections. The most notorious example of the latter is **acquired immunodeficiency syndrome (AIDS)**, brought about by infection of T lymphocytes with **human immunodeficiency virus (HIV)**. As a result of the infection, AIDS patients are susceptible to many microorganisms that are usually classified as low grade or opportunistic pathogens (e.g., *Pneumocystis carinii*).

DISORDERS INVOLVING RESPONSES OF EOSINOPHILS

Eosinophil concentrations in the peripheral blood respond rapidly to stress and the presence of steroid hormones. Increased eosinophil counts (> 400 to 500 per μL) are most often associated with allergic reactions, particularly asthma, and the presence of parasites. A determination of **eosinophilia** is best based on sequential counts in a patient because considerable variation exists between individuals and within the same person at different times of day.

Eosinophil counts that exceed 1500 per μL in the absence of allergies or parasitic infections constitute a state of hypereosinophilia, indicative of systemic dysfunction, such as polyarteritis nodosa and Löffler's syndrome. **Eosinopenia** is less easy to define since a decrease in eosinophils on a blood smear is not apparent unless observations are directed to that purpose. Peripheral blood concentrations decrease in the presence of glucocorticoids, as in hyperadrenalism. The response is so sensitive that eosinophil counts, if done accurately, can be used as a bioassay to monitor changes in glucocorticoid steroid concentrations.

DISORDERS INVOLVING RESPONSES OF OTHER LEUKOCYTES

Monocytosis can be defined as concentrations of peripheral blood monocytes that exceed 800 per μL. Increases are most often associated with tuberculosis, syphillis, and connective tissue diseases. Interpretation of monocytosis on blood smears treated with Wright's stain must be done with caution because of the variety of reactive lymphocytes that are commonly encountered in other diseases. Decreased monocyte counts, like those of eosinophils, are less apparent because of the relative reference values (3% to 11%) usually cited. Decreases are seen in patients with hairy cell leukemia and in those receiving azathioprine or some steroids.

Basophilia is defined as basophil counts of more than 100/μL or greater than 2% of the differential count. If the latter criterion is used, at least 200 cells should be counted. Increases are most often associated with chronic myelogenous leukemia and decreases occur after the degranulation of anaphylactic shock (type I hypersensitivity).

SOME CAUSES OF EOSINOPHILIA

Parasites
Pneumocystis
Malaria
Cryptosporidium
Amebiasis
Giardia
Schistosoma
Ascaris
Strongyloides
Trichinosis

Drug hypersensitivity
Nitrofurantoin

Allergies
Allergic rhinitis
Asthma

Association with diseases
Terminal Hodgkin's disease
Cutaneous T cell lymphoma
Wiskott-Aldrich syndrome
Chronic hepatitis
Ulcerative colitis
Eosinophilic gastroenteritis
Chronic myelogenous leukemia
Some metastatic carcinomas (especially lung)

Case History

CONGENITAL PELGER-HUËT ANOMALY

The patient is a 20-year-old laboratory assistant who presented to her pathologist because of concern over a "significant shift to the left of my granulocytes." The pathologist obtained a bone marrow biopsy and aspirate and referred the patient for hematologic evaluation. The patient had no complaints other than intermittent fatigue. Physical examination was entirely normal.

Laboratory evaluation revealed a biochemical screening survey to be normal. The total WBC was 4,500/μL and the differential count was in-

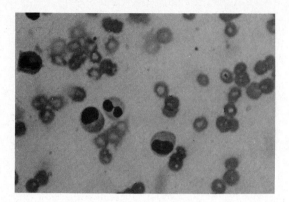

Fig. 21-6. Pelger-Huët anomaly, peripheral blood.

terpreted as 28% segmented neutrophils, 48% bands, 23% lymphocytes, and 1% monocytes. The hemoglobin was 13.0 g/dL, the hematocrit was 42.7%, and the platelet count was 250,000/μL.

Fig. 21-6 reveals peripheral blood neutrophils and demonstrates a typical Pelger-Huët cell. A CBC and peripheral smear from the sister revealed similar findings. The patient was told she was a heterozygote for the Pelger-Huët anomaly and was reassured regarding the benign nature of this defect, which is inherited as a simple autosomal dominant trait.

SUMMARY

- Lipid storage diseases of macrophages include Gaucher's disease (an accumulation of glucocerebrosides) and Niemann-Pick disease (an accumulation of sphingomyelinase). Both are hereditary deficiencies of specific lysosomal enzymes.
- Histiocytosis is one of a heterogeneous group of systemic disorders, probably congenital, characterized by proliferation and infiltration of macrophages into tissues. Examples are Letter-Siwe disease, Hand-Schüller-Christian disease, and eosinophilic granuloma.
- Compromised phagocytic function can occur from defects in enzymes that produce lethal oxides (chronic granuloma-tous disease), from defects of lysosomal fusion or granule contents (Chédiak-Higashi syndrome), or defects in chemotaxis and mobility (diabetes, lazy leukocyte syndrome).
- Other anomalies may be primarily observed as morphological aberrations but without direct functional defects: Alder-Reilly anomaly (large granules, seen in patients with other genetic defects), May-Hegglin anomaly (Döhle-like inclusions, giant platelets), Jordan's anomaly (cells contain many vacuoles), and Pelger-Huët anomaly (condensed nucleus with 1 or 2 lobes).
- Leukocytosis is any increase in total peripheral blood white blood cell concentration; neutrophilia is defined as >7500 per μL and neutropenia as <1500 per μL. A leukmoid reaction is a marked increase in neutrophils accompanied by a shift to the left, resembling leukemia. Leukmoid reactions can be differentiated from CML by bone marrow examination and by an increased leukocyte alkaline phosphatase score.
- Neutrophil responses to serious infection include rapid mobilization of the marginated cells and release of bands and segmented forms from the marrow storage pool. Increased demand can result in the release of progressively more immature forms, eventually resulting in depletion and neutropenia. Toxic granulation is often seen in neutrophils during septic conditions.
- Increased lymphocyte counts are seen in a variety of viral infections, especially in children and in patients with infectious mononucleosis. The lymphocytosis of IM is usually accompanied by the presence of reactive lymphocytes, larger than normal forms associated with the immune response.
- Infectious mononucleosis is an infection of oropharyngeal epithelial cells and B lymphocytes by Epstein-Barr virus; the re-

active cells are mainly T lymphocytes. Clinical signs include adenopathy, fever, and malaise. Laboratory diagnosis is usually confirmed with a heterophile antibody test.

- Eosinophilia is most commonly related to allergic reactions, particularly asthma, and parasites, particularly helminth worms. Monocytosis is most often seen in tuberculosis, syphilis, and connective tissue disorders.

22

Bleeding Disorders

OVERVIEW

Recognition of bleeding disorders predates by centuries an understanding of coagulation and the existence of hemostatic mechanisms. For example, it states in the second century Talmud to avoid circumcision in a male whose brothers had bled to death during the ritual surgery. Many other references appear in the writings of prerenaissance Arabic physicians. The first description of hemophilia in western medical literature appeared in 1793 and it was recognized as a sex-linked disorder by Otto in 1803. During the 1800s, several male members of European and Russian royal families fell victim. Queen Victoria of England (1819-1901) was one of the prolific carriers, passing it through two of her five daughters to the royalty of Spain (both uncles of King Carlos), Germany, and Russia (Alexis, brother of Anastasia). As investigations during the late nineteenth and early twentieth centuries revealed the clotting mechanism's intricacies and the role of platelets in hemostasis, a host of new disorders were described.

Classifications of bleeding and coagulation disorders can be initially organized to correspond with the four major components of hemostasis: the vascular tissue, platelets, coagulation proteins, and fibrinolytic system. Even with these simple categories, classification of a specific disease may be arbitrary. Interactions between hemostatic components may produce multiple defects (e.g., dysfunctional platelets may result in ineffective plug formation, an incomplete coagulation cascade, and reduced mainte-

nance of vascular tissue). Disorders may be hereditary, acquired, or undetermined in origin. They may be primary or secondary to other pathological processes. A defect may be morphological, functional, or a combination of both.

Successful diagnoses of bleeding disorders requires accurate medical histories, physical examinations, and appropriate laboratory tests (Fig. 22-1). The following terms describe bleeding manifestations (commonly used plural forms are given in parentheses).

Ecchymosis (ecchymoses): large, irregular areas of blue-black to brown-yellow discoloration caused by bleeding into skin or mucous membranes.

Epistaxis: bleeding from the nose or nasal sinuses.

Hemarthrosis: bleeding into the space surrounding a joint.

Hematemesis: vomiting of blood, originating from the gastrointestinal tract (blood is usually dark) or from the pharyngeal tract (blood is usually bright red).

Hematoma: bleeding into tissue around a vessel, resulting in a darkened swelling.

Hematorrhea: severe, profuse bleeding.

Hematuria: blood present in urine.

Hemoptysis: bleeding from the oral cavity, originating in the larynx, trachea, bronchi, or lungs.

Petechiae: small, flattened red spots on skin and mucosal surfaces caused by bleeding from capillaries.

Purpura: large area of bleeding into skin, mucous membranes, tissues, or organs and changing in color from red to purple to brown to yellow.

Definitions used to describe clinical conditions or hemostatic processes are:

Embolus (emboli): a thrombus (thrombi) or clot that has been dislodged from the site of formation and is moving through the blood stream.

Hemangiectasis: dilatation of the blood vessels.

Hemangioma (hemangiomata): benign tumor of blood vessels, usually appearing as a cluster of twisted capillaries.

Hemophilia: hereditary deficiency of coagulation factor VIII, IX, or XI.

Thrombosis: formation of a clot within the blood vessels; normal process to stop hemorrhage but pathological if occlusion of the vessel results.

Vasculitis: inflammation and damage to a blood or lymph vessel, involving loss of endothelium.

DISORDERS OF VASCULAR TISSUE

Bleeding problems caused by abnormalities of vascular tissue may be due to defects in the endothelial cell lining of the blood vessels or the supporting connective tissue around the vessels. They can also be a result of defective platelets and the products they secrete to maintain vessel walls. Usual clinical signs are the tendency to bruise easily or to bleed spontaneously, especially from mucosal surfaces. Diagnosis depends on obtaining a good family history, record of drug administration, history of past or present infections, and exclusion of primary platelet disorders. The latter is especially important since a wide variety of diseases and agents can produce bleeding manifestations. However, platelet deficiencies, either in number or quality, remain the most common causes of bleeding problems.

Hereditary hemorrhagic telangiectasia (Rendu-Osler-Weber Syndrome)

Hereditary hemorrhagic telangiectasia (HHT) is the most common *vascular* disor-

BLEEDING DISORDERS

Disorders of vascular tissue (Chapter 22)

1. Hereditary defects of vessel structure
   a. Hereditary hemorrhagic telangiectasia (HHT; Rendu-Osler-Weber syndrome)
   b. Hemangioma-thrombocytopenia syndrome (Kasabach-Merritt syndrome)
   c. Connective tissue dysplasias
2. Acquired defects
   a. Allergic purpura (Henoch-Schönlein syndrome)
   b. Senile purpura
   c. Secondary to systemic diseases
3. Other causes, undetermined
   a. Easy bruisability (purpura simplex)
   b. Psychogenic and other idiopathic purpuras

Disorders of platelets (Chapter 23)

1. Quantitative disorders
   a. Thrombocytopenias
   b. Thrombocytoses and thromocythemias
2. Qualitative disorders
   a. Abnormal interaction with vessel walls
   b. Abnormal adhesion
   c. Abnormal aggregation
   d. Abnormal procoagulant activity

Disorders of the coagulation cascade (Chapter 24)

1. Factor deficiencies
   a. Decreased or defective fibrinogen
   b. Hemophilias (decreased factor VIII, IX, or XI)
   c. von Willebrand's disease
   d. Other factor deficiencies
2. Abnormalities of circulating inhibitors
3. Presence of abnormal (pathological) inhibitors

Thrombotic disorders (Chapter 24)

1. Deficiencies of plasminogen system
2. Disseminated intravascular coagulation (DIC)

der associated with bleeding manifestations (Table 22-1). The disorder is inherited as an autosomal dominant trait. Nosebleeds are the major problem in early childhood, but

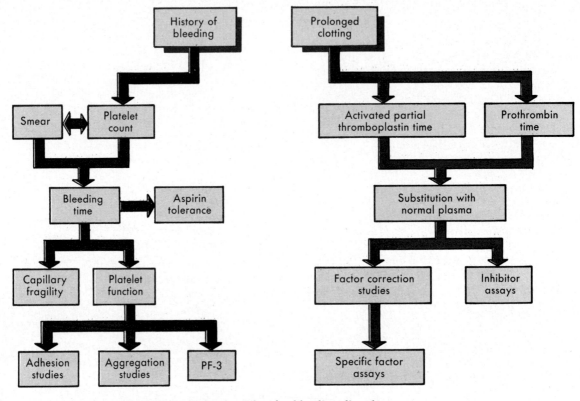

Fig. 22-1. Laboratory study algorithm for bleeding disorders.
Suggested flow chart of laboratory procedures in the investigation of bleeding problems, starting with screening tests and leading to specialized studies. Medical history and physical examination precede laboratory tests. Platelet count, prothrombin time, and partial thromboplastin time are usually ordered concurrently as a hemostasis-coagulation profile.

these usually decrease with increasing age. Small skin lesions, about 1 to 3 mm in diameter, appear in adults. These are reddish to purple and they blanch (lose color) when pressure is applied. This can be easily demonstrated with a glass microscope slide, pressing it over the lesion. The lesions are due to decreased content of elastic fibers in the vascular walls, resulting in coiled capillaries that are dilated with blood. These lie close to the surface of the skin and mucous membranes, especially on the hand and fingers, tongue and lips, and nasal surfaces. Bleeding can occur from these sites, as well as lesions in the gastrointestinal and geni-

tourinary tracts. Additional complications occur in patients with liver involvement and about one fifth of the patients exhibit small aneuryisms or arteriovenous fistulas in the lungs.

Laboratory results depend on the extent and severity of bleeding problems. Bleeding time is usually normal and the tourniquet test may be either normal or demonstrate increased capillary fragility. Platelet function tests are variable, being abnormal in some patients (decreased adhesion and aggregation). Iron deficiency anemia may result from chronic blood loss, especially if GI or GU hemorrhage is severe. Serum iron,

Table 22-1. Laboratory results in vascular disorders

Disease	Platelet count	Bleeding time	Tourniquet test	Bleeding problem	Other lab findings
Hereditary hemor-rhagic telangiecta-sia	Normal	Normal	Positive	Mucosal, purpura	DIC, IDA
Kasabach-Merritt syndrome	Decreased	Prolonged	Positive	Purpura	DIC
Marfan's syndrome	Normal	Normal	Normal	Absent to mild	Giant platelet, abnormal platelet functional study
Pseudoxanthoma elasticum	Normal	Normal	Normal or positive	Severe hemorrhage	Thrombosis
Osteogenesis imperfecta	Normal	Prolonged	Positive	Mucosal, purpura	Abnormal platelet functional study
Allergic purpura	Normal	Normal	Normal	Purpura	Increased ESR, Ig
Senile purpura	Normal	Normal	Normal	Purpura	
Scurvy	Normal	Normal or prolonged	Positive	Petichae, purpura	Decreased vitamin C
Drug toxicity	Normal	Normal	Positive	Purpura	DIC may be present

NOTES: Laboratory findings are the most typical for each disease, but considerable variation exists. Coagulation parameters will be abnormal when DIC is present. *DIC*, disseminated intravascular coagulation; *ESR*, erythrocyte sedimentation rate; *IDA*, iron deficiency anemia; *Ig*, immunoglobulin level.

transferrin, and RBC indices may reflect iron loss in these patients (see Chapter 18). More serious is a state of chronic disseminated intravascular coagulation (DIC) that may exist in some patients. At times, the DIC can become acute, resulting in platelet and coagulation factor consumption coupled with thrombotic problems (see Chapter 24). Treatment is largely symptomatic: iron therapy and transfusions to counteract severe blood loss, measures to control localized bleeding, and heparin to regulate the extent of DIC.

Hemangioma-thrombocytopenia syndrome

A hereditary basis for Kasabach-Merritt syndrome (giant cavernous hemangioma or hemangioma-thrombocytopenia syndrome) has not been established, but the condition is present at birth. The vascular tumor may be solitary and large. It usually occurs in the extremities, but in some cases it is present in an internal organ. Laboratory features include a low platelet count (10,000 to 40,000 per μL is common) and red cells that exhibit traumatic damage associated with thrombotic blood vessels. Signs of DIC may be present, affecting coagulation parameters. Fibrinogen levels may be very low. External hemangiomas may become engorged with blood and resemble hematomas. Treatment is usually accomplished with high dose, localized radiation. Thrombocytopenia is corrected with tumor regression.

Connective tissue dysplasias

Hereditary disorders that involve connective tissue may produce bleeding manifestations due to the lack of vascular tissue support. Most of these conditions are rare, but many of them are autosomal dominant in nature. Patients exhibit a tendency to bruise readily following minimal trauma or contact. The degree of bleeding varies from absent or minimal in Marfan's syndrome to severe in pseudoxanthoma elasticum. Abnormalities in collagen structure, elastic fibers, and fibronectin crosslinks of connective tissue have been documented for specific diseases.

Ehlers-Danlos syndrome is an autosomal dominant disorder that occurs in several clinical forms varying in severity of bleeding problems from easy bruisability to arterial rupture. There also may be an abnormality in platelet factor 3. Pseudoxanthoma elasticum is an autosomal recessive disorder often characterized by severe hemorrhage from the GI tract and from blood vessels in the brain, eyes, kidneys, bladder, and uterus. Bleeding is caused by multiple hemangiomas located in the vessels serving these organs. Other dysplasias include Marfan's syndrome and osteogenesis imperfecta, both autosomal dominant, and homocystinuria, an autosomal recessive disorder resulting in hydroxylysine-deficient collagen.

Allergic purpura (Henoch-Schönlein purpura)

Allergic purpura (anaphylactoid purpura) results from an autoantibody directed against the vascular endothelium. This disorder usually occurs in children following infection by rickettsial, viral, bacterial, or mycoplasmal agents. The organism may damage the endothelial lining of blood vessels, resulting in vasculitis. Antibodies or immune complexes (IgA is increased in half of the patients in one study) directed against the damaged vessels produce a symmetrically diffuse rash of petechiae or purpural spots, most often on the lower limbs and buttocks area. The appearance may be very rapid, accompanied by itching. Allergic origination has also been attributed to insect bite, certain foods, and various drugs and vaccinations. Joint pain and other signs of systemic autoimmune involvement (glomerulonephritis, myocardial necrosis, and neurological disturbance) may be present. Remission of the rash may be spontaneous and then reoccur one or more times.

Laboratory findings are not specific: bleeding time, tourniquet test, and coagulation test results are usually normal. Nonspecific indicators of inflammation, such as elevation of red cell sedimentation rate and peripheral blood neutrophilia and eosinophilia, are often present. Proteinuria and hematuria occur with renal involvement, but this is usually transitory. Treatment is generally supportive but largely ineffective.

Senile purpura

Onset occurs in older adults due to decreased elasticity of the connective tissues surrounding and supporting the superficial blood vessels. As a result, the skin, particularly on the backs of hands and extensor surfaces of the forearms, becomes thin, loose, and mobile. Sun exposure may also contribute to the decrease in subdermal connective tissue elasticity, accounting for superficial distribution of the purpura on the body. Blood vessels are exposed to additional stress and blood seeps into the surrounding tissue, forming red to purple ecchymoses. These dark blotches are flattened, about 1 to 10 mm in diameter, do not blanch with pressure, and resorb slowly. Similar lesions appear in patients treated with large amounts of corticosteroids and patients with Cushing's syndrome. Laboratory tests are normal and no other bleeding manifestations are present. This form of purpura should be ruled out if an elderly patient is worked up for a bleeding disorder.

Purpuras associated with systemic diseases

Purpuras are commonly seen in a number of other diseases. Paraproteinemias often involve the circulation and deposit of IgG-immune complexes that fix complement to vascular endothelial cells, resulting in vasculitis and bleeding. Deposition of abnormal lipids in vessel walls occurs in some patients with amyloidosis. The vessels are so fragile that mere contact with the skin can result in marked bruising ("touch purpura"). Hypothyroidism, diabetes mellitis, and malignant hypertension are other conditions that often result in purpura formation.

Other acquired purpuras

Drug toxicity. A number of commonly prescribed drugs can cause vasculitis or exacerbate vessel inflammation due to other causes. Aspirin, iodine compounds, digoxin, some antibiotics (chloramphenicol, sulfonamides), methyldopa, and estrogen compounds are among those implicated. Nictoine is an aggravating agent associated with heavy smokers. Coumadin (warfarin), the oral anticoagulant widely used to prevent thrombotic sequelae in myocardial patients, may be of particular interest and concern for the coagulation laboratory. Symptoms can be severe, leading to necrosis and gangrene. Surgical intervention may be necessary.

Tourniquet test results are often positive, but bleeding time, platelet count, and coagulation tests are normal unless DIC is present.

Vitamin C deficiency (scurvy). Insufficient dietary input of vitamin C (ascorbic acid) results in decreased synthesis of collagen and weakening of capillary walls. Epistaxis, petechial rashes, and purpural lesions occur with increasing vitamin deficiency. Petechiae are especially prominent around hair follicles, particularly on the thighs and upper buttocks area. Bleeding time is often prolonged and the tourniquet test usually indicates increased capillary fragility. Administration of ascorbic acid results in full recovery.

Infections. Bacterial, viral, and other microbial organisms can produce vascular damage directly, by their toxins, or by the immune complexes that result from inflammatory responses. Meningoccal, streptococcal and rickettsial infections are often associated with petechial or purpural symptoms.

Purpuras of unknown origin

Purpura simplex (easy bruisability). A diagnosis of simple vascular purpura or vascular fragility is made when other causes or conditions are not indicated. The ecchymoses are superficial, bleeding is usually mild, and laboratory results are most often normal. Bleeding time may be increased, especially after administration of aspirin or antiinflammatory steroids. Some patients may have platelets with slightly decreased retention on glass beads. The tourniquet test may be normal or positive and this may vary in the same patient at different times. Vascular purpura most commonly occurs in women and younger children; thighs and arms are the most frequent sites of bruising. Easy bruisability may be related to the lipid content of tissue around blood vessels, which is higher in women. Other studies have indicated a possible relationship to hypothyroidism. At least one form, not attributable to other conditions, is familial but it also occurs mainly in females.

Psychogenic purpura. Cutaneous bleeding and bruising through intact skin has been observed in patients in which no vascular defects or platelet disorders can be diagnosed. The patients are most often women with emotional problems and the bruising is often accompanied by nausea, vomiting, or fever. The sites of bleeding may be painful; burning or stinging may precede appearance of the purpura. Evidence for a psychosomatic origin has been equivocal: psychotherapy does not resolve many of the cases, but hypnotic suggestion can induce the lesions in some patients. Laboratory results are invariably normal. However, the lesions can be produced in some patients by intradermal injection of autologous red blood cells or RBC stroma (*autoerythrocyte sensi-*

tization). Similar results have been obtained with autologous DNA and some red cell components.

Some investigators have noted the similarity of psychogenic purpuras to the appearance of religious and supernatural stigmata, superficial marks occurring in some individuals undergoing exaggerated emotional stress. Other lesions may be a result of self-inflicted injury *(factitial purpura)*, which is also more likely to occur in individuals under emotional duress.

SUMMARY

- Bleeding disorders can be categorized in relation to the major hemostatic components: defects of the vascular system, platelet disorders, disorders of the coagulation cascade, and deficiencies of the fibrinolytic system.
- Vascular tissue disorders may be caused by hereditary or acquired defects in the endothelial cell lining of vessel walls, the connective tissue supporting blood vessels, or to platelet disorders that affect maintenance of the vascular lining.
- Hereditary hemorrhagic telangiectasia is the most common vascular disorder associated with bleeding problems. It is an autosomal dominant trait characterized by coiled thin-walled capillaries and purpural lesions of the skin, mucosa, and internal organs.
- Allergic purpura is most common in children, occurring as an autoimmune response to infections, some drugs, or other agents.
- Purpuras can also occur with aging (senile purpura), vitamin C deficiency (scurvy), in association with connective tissue dysplasias, various systemic diseases, as a result of psychological disturbance, unknown autoimmune mechanisms, and as simple lesions of unknown cause (purpura simplex).
- Laboratory tests of value include platelet count and function tests to rule out platelet disorders, tourniquet test for capillary fragility, and coagulation screening tests to rule out clotting disorders.
- Vascular disorders are often diagnosed on the basis of medical history and by excluding other sources of bleeding disorders.

23

Platelet Disorders

Platelet disorders are diverse and complex, reflecting the heterogeneous functional roles of these biochemical packets. Pathological changes in hemostasis or coagulation can result from decreased (**thrombocytopenia**) or increased (**thrombocytosis**) numbers of circulating platelets, dysfunction of platelets that are present in normal concentration (**thrombocytopathy**), or a combination of quantitative and qualitative changes. The defects can be primary, that is, inherent to platelet structure or metabolism, or they can result from other disease processes that secondarily affect platelet production, survival, or function. These disorders are classified below. The list includes conditions in which normal platelets interact with defective plasma components or vascular tissues, resulting in a bleeding disorder requiring platelet evaluation (an example is von Willebrand's disease, in which platelets fail to adhere to vascular subendothelial surfaces because a component of coagulation factor VIII is deficient).

Laboratory procedures for bleeding disorders caused by platelet problems may begin with screening tests, such as bleeding time and capillary fragility (tourniquet) tests. Tests of platelet function, such as aggregation profiles, are now routine in most hematology laboratories. More specialized procedures, such as platelet survival time, platelet antibody studies, and tests for abnormal adherence, require more advanced facilities. A typical sequence or algorithm for platelet disorders is presented in Fig. 23-1.

QUANTITATIVE DISORDERS: THROMBOCYTOPENIAS

Decreases in the numbers of circulating platelets account for the majority of platelet disorders. Although changes in platelet number are relatively easy to document by laboratory methods, the underlying causes can be difficult to evaluate. As with the disorders of other blood cells, thrombocytopenias can be etiologically classified into changes associated with decreased marrow production, increased destruction, and abnormal distribution.

In most normal individuals, platelet concentrations range from 130,000 to 370,000 per μL (mean of 250,000 per μL $\pm$ 2 standard deviations) and thrombocytopenia is defined as a platelet count of less than 100,000 per μL. Above this level, normally functioning platelets are adequate for participation in hemostatic plug formation and coagulation, so that excessive bleeding from trauma or surgery is not expected in an otherwise normal patient. Even at concentrations between 50,000 to 100,000 per μL, bleeding tendencies are usually not clinically evident, although the bleeding time results may be prolonged. Preoperative preparations may be necessary for counts of less than 50,000 per μL; counts of less than 10,000 per μL often result in sustained hemorrhage and should be considered life threatening.

Correlation between platelet count and bleeding time is approximately linear at concentrations of 10,000 to 100,000 per μL, if the thrombocytopenia is not complicated

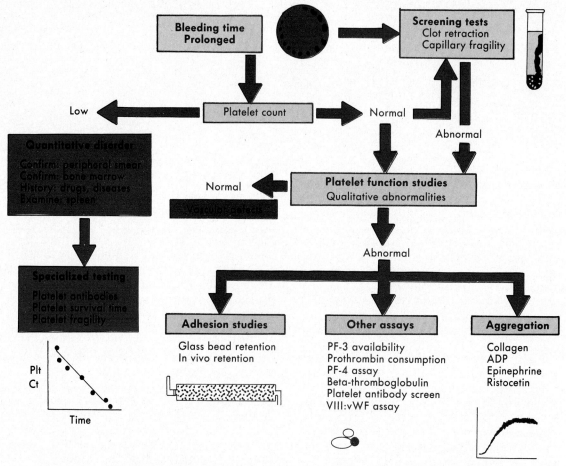

Fig. 23-1.   Algorithm for laboratory studies of platelets to diagnose bleeding disorders.
See Fig. 22-1 for algorithms of hemostasis and Fig. 24-1 for coagulation studies.

by qualitative changes (Fig. 23-2). Based on a normal bleeding time of 5 ± 1.5 minutes, this relationship is defined by the formula:

$$BT\ (mins) = \frac{30 - PLT\ CT\ per\ \mu L}{4000}$$

Thus a platelet count of 50,000 per μL would be expected to correlate with a carefully performed bleeding time of 17 to 18 minutes. Bleeding time results that are longer than expected imply functional impairment (e.g., the Wiskott-Aldrich and Bernard-Soulier syndromes in Fig. 23-2). Bleeding times that are shorter than expected may be associated with increased platelet competence which is a partial compensation exhibited by younger platelets that are released prematurely during destructive disorders (e.g., idiopathic thrombocytopenic purpura, ITP).

The importance of accurately determining platelet concentration, especially while trying to stabilize patients with bleeding disorders and coagulopathies, cannot be

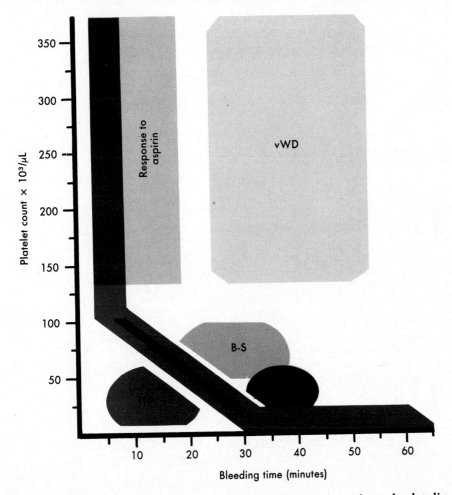

Fig. 23-2.   Correlation of bleeding time and platelet count in various platelet disorders.

Relationship between bleeding time and platelet count in patients that are normal, normal patients after aspirin ingestion, and patients with von Willebrand's disease *(vWD)*, Bernard-Soulier syndrome *(BS)*, Wiskott-Aldrich syndrome *(WA)*, and idiopathic thrombocytopenic purpura *(ITP)*. The linear relationship of thrombocytopenia to increased bleeding time *(T)* is indicated by the heavy line. (Adapted from Malpass and Harker, 1980, with supplemental data added).

overemphasized. Advances in automated hematology instrumentation have made it possible to obtain rapid, accurate platelet counts as a routine part of the complete blood count. However, some instruments do not provide optimal results in cases of severe thrombocytopenia. Very low counts are usually assessed by other methods, including manual counting techniques and correlation with morphology and density on stained blood smears (Chapter 26).

CLASSIFICATION OF PLATELET DISORDERS

Quantitative abnormalities: Changes in platelet numbers

A. Thrombocytopenia: decrease in circulating platelets
   1. Impaired or decreased production of platelets
      a. Resulting from damage to marrow cells by acquired agents
      b. Resulting from marrow replacement by other cells
      c. Resulting from congenital conditions
         1. Fanconi's syndrome with megakaryocyte hypoplasia
         2. Intrauterine exposure to drugs or infections
         3. Wiskott-Aldrich syndrome
         4. Thrombocytopenia with absent radii (TAR baby syndrome)
      d. Resulting from ineffective thrombopoiesis
         1. Defective DNA synthesis associated with megaloblastic anemia
         2. Thrombopoietin deficiency
   2. Increased destruction of circulating platelets
      a. Resulting from immunological mechanisms
         1. Drug induced: protein-drug-platelet complexes
         2. Idiopathic (autoimmune) thrombocytopenic purpura (ITP)
         3. Neonatal isoimmune thrombocytopenia
         4. Secondary autoimmune thrombocytopenia
         5. Posttransfusion purpura
      b. Resulting from increased platelet use or damage
         1. Thrombotic thrombocytopenic purpura (TTP)
         2. Disseminated intravascular coagulation (DIC)
         3. Interaction with nonendothelial surfaces (e.g., artificial heart valve)
         4. Hemolytic-uremic syndrome (HUS)
   3. Disorders related to distribution or dilution:
      a. Resulting from increased splenic sequestration accompanying splenomegaly
      b. Resulting from hepatic sequestration during hypothermia
      c. Resulting from dilution after massive transfusion with stored blood
B. Thrombocytosis and thrombocythemia: increase in circulating platelets
   1. Reactive thrombocytosis: secondary to other conditions
      a. In association with iron deficiency
      b. In association with inflammation, especially chronic diseases
      c. In association with certain malignancies
      d. Following splenectomy
      e. As a transient response to epinephrine, some drugs
      f. As a transient rebound after thrombocytopenia
   2. Thrombocytosis associated with myeloproliferative disorders
      a. Increased megakaryocyte mass associated with polycythemia vera and myeloid metaplasia
      b. Increased megakaryocyte number (decreased volume) associated with chronic myelogenous leukemia
   3. Thrombocythemia: essential or autonomous thrombocytosis

CLASSIFICATION OF PLATELET DISORDERS—cont'd

Qualitative abnormalities: Changes in platelet function (thromocytopathy)

A. Abnormalities involving platelet interaction with vascular tissue (Chapter 22)
  1. Ehlers-Danlos syndrome
  2. Hereditary hemorrhagic telangiectasia
  3. Acquired defects
    a. scurvy (vitamin C or ascorbic acid deficiency)
    b. amyloidosis
B. Abnormalities involving platelet adhesion
  1. Bernard-Soulier syndrome: vWF receptors (GP I) deficient
  2. von Willebrand's disease: various hereditary forms of factor VIII deficiency
  3. Acquired defects
    a. Autoimmune form of von Willebrand's disease (antibodies to VII:vWF)
    b. Uremia, metabolite accumulation
    c. Drug induced (especially, antithrombotic drugs)
C. Abnormalities involving primary aggregation
  1. Glanzmann's thrombasthenia: impaired binding of fibrinogen
  2. Acquired defects
    a. Resulting from increased fibrin degradation products
    b. Resulting from dysproteinemias
    c. Drug induced (especially synthetic penicillins and dextran)
D. Abnormalities involving secondary aggregation (release reaction)
  1. Storage pool deficiencies
    a. Gray platelet syndrome: absence of alpha granules
    b. Hereditary dense granule deficiencies
    c. Anomalies associated with other abnormalities
      1. Hermansky-Pudlak syndrome: albinism, ceroid deposits
      2. Chédiak-Steinbrinck-Higashi syndrome: albinism, abnormal WBC granules
      3. Wiskott-Aldrich syndrome: abnormal glycolysis, infections, eczema
      4. Thrombocytopenia with absent radii (TAR baby syndrome)
  2. Prostaglandin pathway deficiencies: "aspirin-like defects"
    a. Cyclooxygenase deficiency
    b. Thromboxane synthetase deficiency
  3. Defects in nucleotide metabolism
    a. Glycogen storage disease
    b. Fructose-1,6-diphosphate deficiency
  4. Acquired defects
    a. Viral infections
    b. Drug induced
      1. Aspirin
      2. Other nonsteroidal inflammatory drugs
    c. Ethyl alcohol, especially acute bouts of consumption
    d. Primary bone marrow disease (dyspoiesis) and myeloproliferative disorders
    e. Autoimmune diseases (e.g., AIHA, SLE)
    f. During open heart surgery: alpha granule depletion
E. Abnormalities involving coagulation factor receptors (procoagulant activity)
  1. Congenital deficiency of platelet factor 3 (factor V_m receptor)
  2. PF-3 nonavailability, secondary to defects in aggregation and release reaction

ABNORMALITIES OF PRODUCTION AND MATURATION

Damage to stem cells and megakaryocytes

Several of the physical, chemical, and biological agents known to interfere with production of red and white cells also affect megakaryocyte maturation and platelet production. Thrombocytopenia may be an early sign of general marrow damage or infiltration by other cellular elements. Causative agents may be acquired during postnatal life or by intrauterine exposure. In the latter case, a thorough maternal history is needed to distinguish hereditary neonatal thrombocytopenia from forms that are congenitally acquired.

Physical agents. Platelet precursors are slightly less sensitive to ionizing radiation than are other blood cell precursors. Mature platelets are relatively unaffected.

Chemical agents

1. Myelosuppressive drugs, used in cancer therapy, produce general bone marrow suppression (e.g., busulfan, 6-mercaptopurine, and methotrexate).

2. Thiazide diuretics, used in pregnant women and others to control water-related weight gain, can produce a mild to moderate chronic toxicity to megakaryocytes in sensitive individuals. In some cases this may be an immunological response.

3. Ethanol or its acetaldehyde metabolites produce disruptive effects in the absence or presence of vitamin deficiencies and liver dysfunction. The effects are more severe in acute toxicity (sporadic, heavy drinking binges) than in chronic abuse. Platelet counts can drop as low as 10,000 per μL, increasing bleeding tendencies and vascular abnormalities associated with alcoholism, although platelet numbers rapidly return to normal or higher (rebound phenomena) following alcohol withdrawal. Direct interference with platelet production and survival by ethanol or its metabolites has been postulated but not conclusively established.

4. Antibiotics, such as chloramphenicol (Chloromycetin), are especially toxic to marrow cells, producing reversible hypoplasia in most cases, but irreversible aplasia in a few patients. Immunological sensitization may also be involved in marrow cell destruction.

5. Estrogens may produce reversible suppression of platelet production, which is possibly the cause for an observed monthly cycle of platelet count fluctuations, known as **tidal thrombocytopenia.**

Biological agents

1. Viruses can infect megakaryocytes directly, resulting in vacuolation, nuclear degeneration, and decreasing platelet counts. Thrombocytopenia often accompanies influenza, infectious mononucleosis, hepatitis, rubella, rubeola, and other viral diseases. Some of this response may also be due to peripheral platelet destruction.

2. Disseminated tuberculosis, due to infections by species of *Mycobacterium*, can result in destructive lesions of the myeloid tissue.

Displacement by other cells

Infiltration of the marrow by neoplasms or by other invading cells results in generalized displacement of normal myeloid tissue, but thrombocytopenia is often an earlier and pronounced consequence due to the relative size and number of megakaryocytes among marrow elements. Pathological conditions that often, but not invariably, result in decreased platelet production include acute and chronic leukemias, Hodgkin's disease, various lymphomas, metastatic carcinomas, myelofibrosis, juvenile osteopetrosis, and multiple myeloma.

Congenital conditions

Fanconi's syndrome. Megakaryocyte hypoplasia is one of several congenital abnormalities seen in **Fanconi's syndrome,** which can also include hypoplastic anemia, dwarfism, mental and sexual retardation, and various abnormalities of skin, skeleton, spleen, and renal tract. The condition is evident during the first decade of life and appears to be inherited as a recessive trait, accompanied by random chromosome breaks. A variety of other congenital diseases associated with decreased marrow megakaryocytes, but without the visceral abnormalities, are also known.

Wiskott-Aldrich syndrome. A sex-linked condition known as **Wiskott-Aldrich syndrome** is characterized by bloody diarrhea, recurrent bacterial and viral infections, and chronic eczema. Bleeding usually occurs during the first year of life, but it becomes less severe thereafter. Platelet counts typically range from 10,000 to 75,000 per μL; platelet volume, in one study (Ochs et al., 1980), ranged from 3.8 to 4.6 fL (normal = 7.1 to 10.5 fL). Thus marked increases in bleeding time (30 minutes and more) correspond to decreases in both platelet number and size. Other platelet abnormalities include a shortened survival time (3.8 to 6.7 days) and a calculated turnover rate that is only 30% of normal. In addition, qualitative changes in platelets have also been reported.

Thrombocytopenia with absent radii. A severe decrease in marrow megakaryocytes is associated with a bilateral aplasia of the forearm bones (radii) and cardiac abnormalities, Some cases have been related to intrauterine exposure to rubella or tolbutamide at 6 to 8 weeks gestation. Intracranial hemorrhage is a leading cause of death, usually within the first 8 months of life. The associated abnormalities of thrombocytopenia and absent radii, termed **TAR baby syndrome,** are probably caused by concurrent developmental events at a time in which the fetal tissues may be particularly sensitive to chemical and biological agents.

May-Hegglin anomaly. Giant platelets (up to 20 μm in length) and large basophilic inclusions in leukocytes, resembling Döhle bodies (Fig. 23-3), characterize the rare disorder known as **May-Hegglin anomaly.** Thrombocytopenia may be absent to severe or intermittent. Most patients are clinically asymptomatic, but cases of se-

vere hemorrhage are known. Most studies of platelet and megakaryocyte structure have reported normal results for this disorder, although exceptions occur (Bellucci et al., 1983).

Intrauterine exposure. As noted previously, exposure to thiazide diuretics, rubella, and other agents can result in neonatal thrombocytopenia that is occasionally severe or fatal.

Other congenital disorders. In addition to those already listed, there are a number of cases of congenital thrombocytopenia which may be variants of other disorders or which are rare and poorly understood.

1. **Hereditary hypogranular thrombocytopenia,** inherited as an autosomal dominant trait, may be a form of storage pool disease.
2. **Familial thrombocytopenia** is characterized by neonatal or infant onset of bleeding, but without other obvious abnormalities or platelet dysfunction. Cases of autosomal dominant and recessive inheritance patterns have been described.

Ineffective thrombopoiesis

Although the existence of one or more substances that regulate platelet production has not been conclusively established (Chapter 12), a patient with a congenital deficiency of thrombopoietic hormone was followed over an interval of several years (Abildgaard and Simone, 1967). Far more common are cases resulting from vitamin B_{12} or folate deficiency in association with megaloblastic anemia and the interruption of DNA synthesis that affects all blood cells. Megakaryocytes may be decreased in number and show changes in lobulation or number of nuclei. Similar changes are seen with the myelodysplastic syndromes (Chapter 20). Platelet survival time is usually decreased. Results of hemostasis tests, such as bleeding time and capillary fragility, are often normal and bleeding manifestations are usually minimal or absent.

358

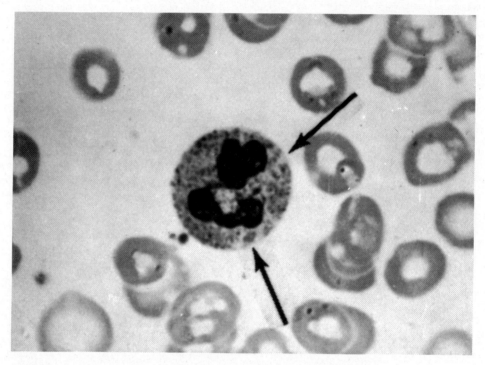

Fig. 23-3.   Peripheral blood cell morphology in May-Hegglin anomaly.
Leukocytes contain "Döhle-like" inclusions of basophilic material. Platelets vary greatly in size
and shape. (From Bauer, JD: Clinical laboratory methods, ed 9, St Louis, 1982, The CV Mosby
Co.)

DISORDERS OF DESTRUCTION AND CONSUMPTION

Thrombocytopenias due to platelet destruction can be separated into disorders resulting from mechanical damage and consumption (nonimmunological) and those caused by immunological responses. Mechanical damage occurs as platelets pass through damaged blood vessels and encounter thrombi or nonendothelial surfaces. Increased platelet consumption occurs during abnormal activation of the coagulation cascade, such as during disseminated intravascular coagulation. Regardless of the process, increased production is necessary to compensate for the accelerated loss of platelets. As in anemia, examination of the bone marrow can assess the response capacity and rule out production disorders. The presence of large (young?) platelets and a short platelet survival time, in the absence of an enlarged spleen, characterizes peripheral destruction or consumption disorders.

Destruction by immunological mechanisms

Drug-induced immune thrombocytopenia. The most common cause of immune-related platelet destruction is that caused by drugs or their metabolites, which combine with albumin or other plasma proteins to form antigens. The patient produces antibodies to the drug-protein complex and this adsorbs onto platelet surfaces. Subsequent recognition and removal of the coated platelets occurs by cells of the mononuclear-phagocytic system of the spleen and liver. If IgM, IgG1, or IgG3 is involved in the immune response, complement may also be activated and affixed to the platelet surface, resulting in intravascular lysis of the platelets (Fig. 23-4). Once the offending drug is discontinued, persistence of thrombocytopenia is dependent on the clearance rate of the drug-protein complex from the body and on compensating platelet production by the marrow. Despite the continued presence of antibodies to the drug (sometimes these can be demonstrated for years following an episode), platelet transfusions can restore hemostatic competence if the drug-protein complex is no longer present. A return to normal platelet concentrations may require days to months. Once sensitized, however, a second exposure to the offending drug can produce marked thrombocytopenia and bleeding in less than 24 hours.

Drugs often implicated include quinine, quinidine, digitoxin, gold salts, rifampicin, sulfonamide derivatives, alpha-methyldopa (Aldomet), morphine, and heroin. Heparin is also suspect. It may combine with a specific antibody, adsorb to the platelet surface and generate thromboxane A_2, resulting in granule release and aggregation.

Idiopathic (autoimmune) immune thrombocytopenia (ITP). In the absence of drugs, transfusions, or other conditions known to produce an immune thrombocytopenia, an autonomous process may be suspected.

Acute idiopathic thrombocytopenia (ITP). This form occurs most often in children between 2 and 6 years of age, in which it is often preceded by a virus infection 7 to 10 days before the onset of the thrombocytopenia and associated purpura. Platelet survival is extremely short, measured in hours instead of days. Remission is usually spontaneous, occurring 1 week to 6 months after onset (an interval of 4 to 6 weeks of thrombocytopenia is usual). Although reoccurrence is a problem for less than 10% of the childhood cases, more than 90% of the adults with acute ITP develop a chronic or recurrent form. A mortality rate of about 1% is cited by Thompson and Harker (1983). Compare this with allergic purpura (Chapter 22) in which thrombocytopenia is rarely present and the major consequence of infection appears to be an immune-related vasculitis and subsequent purpura.

Although the specific immune mechanisms of destruction are not well defined, it appears that a virus-viral antibody complex

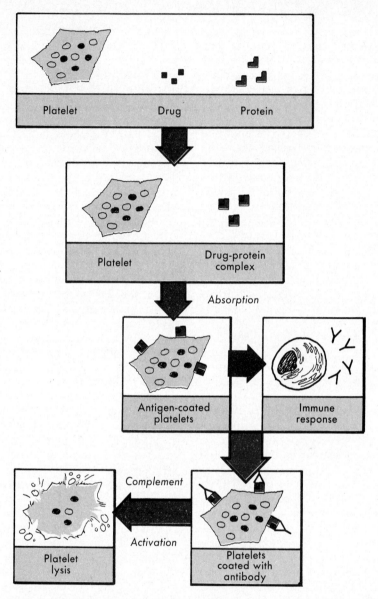

Fig. 23-4.   Platelet destruction by drug-induced immune thrombocytopenia.

attaches to the platelets. Complement is either activated, resulting in platelet lysis, or the cells are removed by splenic and hepatic macrophages (Fig. 23-5). It is also possible that immune responses are initiated directly by viral-induced changes in the platelet membrane antigens or by interference with suppressor T-lymphocyte function, thus the designation of this disorder as an autonomous entity.

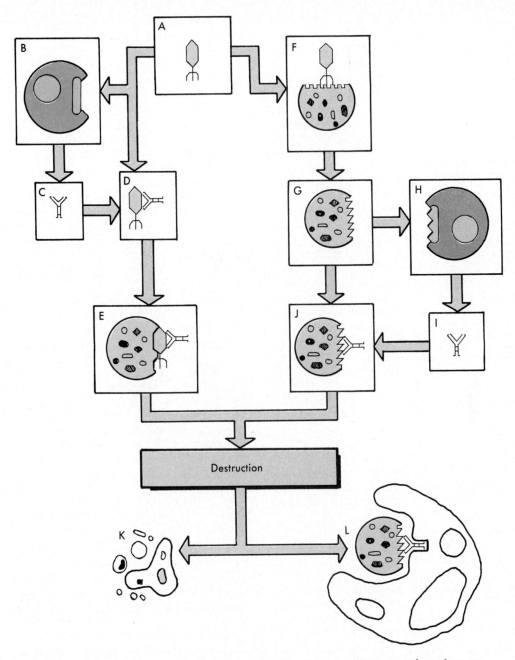

Fig. 23-5. Platelet destruction by idiopathic (autoimmune) immune thrombocytopenia.

Chronic ITP. This form occurs primarily in young and middle-aged adults, with a female to male ratio of about 3 to 1. The onset is gradual with mild bleeding in the form of purpura and menorrhagia being most common. Platelet destruction is not as rapid as in acute ITP; survival times range from 1 to 3 days. Unfortunately, chronic ITP rarely remits spontaneously. Furthermore, continuous production of antiplatelet antibodies and destruction of platelets in the spleen affects both the patient's (autologous) platelets and those obtained from donors, so that platelet transfusions are generally futile except as a desperate and transient effort to promote hemostasis. Platelet counts usually drop to levels of 20,000 to 80,000 per μL, although counts of less than 10,000 may be encountered. Bleeding is less severe than that of comparable thrombocytopenias due to the presence of young "supercompetent" platelets (Fig. 23-2). Platelet size averages 1.6 times normal; a threefold increase in megakaryocyte number has also been reported (Karpatkin, 1980).

Initial therapy often consists of glucocorticoids which interfere with splenic and hepatic macrophages to increase platelet survival time. However, the resultant immunosuppression and toxicity usually require splenectomy. A recurrent form of chronic ITP is also known in which episodes of purpura alternate with complete remissions (Owen et al., 1975).

Neonatal isoimmune thrombocytopenia

Neonatal isoimmune thrombocytopenia. This condition is analogous to hemolytic disease of the newborn (HDN or erythroblastosis fetalis) in that platelet antigens (usually Pl^{A1}) inherited from the father evoke maternal production of antibodies. These cross the placenta and destroy fetal platelets, a transient condition that ceases with delivery. A mortality rate of about 14% is reported (Pearson et al., 1964), but the severity, as in cases of HDN, increases with additional gestational stimulation of maternal response. The diagnosis is made by demonstrating maternal *isoantibodies* against infant or paternal platelet antigens. This form of the disease must be distinguished from transplacental ITP, in which maternal *autoantibody* crosses the placenta and destroys infant platelets that carry the corresponding antigen.

Secondary autoimmune thrombocytopenia. Autoimmune platelet destruction is observed in association with a number of diseases, including chronic lymphocytic leukemia, lymphocytic lymphoma, and various collagen diseases (particularly systemic lupus erythematosis). The clinical picture is similar to that of chronic ITP but the principal disease determines the specific manifestations, such as changes in megakaryocyte density.

Posttransfusion purpura. These patients display a dramatic purpura with severe thrombocytopenia about 7 to 10 days after receiving one or more units of blood. Most cases involve individuals, many of them women stimulated by previous pregnancies, that lack Pl^{A1} antigen, which is present on the platelets of 98% of random donor bloods. Although the disease is self-limiting, the ensuing hemorrhage may be life threatening and it can last for months. Exchange transfusion or plasmapheresis to dilute the offending donor antigens are therapeutic options.

Destruction due to mechanical damage or consumption

A variety of diseases, variously referred to as thrombotic thrombocytopenic purpura (TTP), platelet thrombosis syndrome, and hemolytic-uremic syndrome (HUS), are characterized by changes of the vascular endothelium and the formation of microthrombi in various organs.

Thrombotic thrombocytopenic purpura. A diagnosis of **thrombotic thrombocytopenic purpura (TTP)** is based on a syndrome of fever, renal abnormalities, microangiopathic hemolytic anemia, neurologic changes, and thrombocytopenia. The latter changes are the most common: intermittent neurologic signs and bleeding due to platelet counts as low as 8000 per μL. A moderate anemia and reticulocytosis with persistent red cell fragmentation are evident on blood smears, pointing to the microangiopathic association. Typically, hyaline thrombi occlude small arterioles and capillaries in most tissues examined.

Several studies have noted a greater frequency of occurrence in women than in men (about 3:2) with young to middle-aged adults comprising the majority of cases. Many cases of TTP are secondary to other conditions, such as pregnancy or immediately postpartum, in neoplastic and connective tissue disorders (especially SLE), following viral infections, bacterial endocarditis, and following administration of penicillin and some other drugs. Idiopathic manifestations include acute, chronic, and recurrent forms, and rare cases of congenital onset. The etiological basis of TTP is controversial, but a defect in endothelial prostacyclin has been postulated, resulting in poor maintenance of blood vessel linings.

Hemolytic-uremic syndrome. Although clinically similar to TTP, **hemolytic-uremic syndrome (HUS)** occurs primarily in children, has a high degree of association with viral infections, and results in pathological changes involving the glomerulus and renal arterioles, with resultant hypertension and renal failure. Sporadic adult cases of HUS may be particularly difficult to distinguish from TTP: the absence of neurologic symptoms and the prevalence of renal manifestations are considered diagnostic. With supportative therapy in the form of transfusions and hemodialysis, the prognosis for patients with HUS is relatively good.

Disseminated intravascular coagulation. The most common cause of destructive thrombocytopenia is activation of the coagulation cascade by a variety of agents or conditions, resulting in a consumptive coagulopathy that entraps platelets in intravascular fibrin meshes (Chapter 24).

Problems involving distribution and dilution

Decreased peripheral platelet concentrations may result from abnormal distribution in the body or from dilution following massive blood transfusion.

Sequestration. Normally, the spleen contains 20% to 30% of the circulating platelet mass, but this can increase to 90% in the presence of significant splenomegaly associated with disorders such as Gaucher's disease, various lymphomas, and portal hypertension with congestive splenomegaly. Because of compensating platelet production, blood levels usually remain above 50,000 per μL and survival time is essentially normal. Platelet kinetic studies reveal that less than 30% of a radio-labeled dose of platelets is recovered in cases of marked splenomegaly, compared to a normal value of about 65% (Thompson and Harker, 1983). Therapy is directed at the primary disease responsible for the splenomegaly. Hypothermia induced during open heart surgery also produces a transient platelet dysfunction and thrombocytopenia due to sequestration by the liver. Normal platelet circulation is restored to baseline levels during return to normal body temperature.

Dilutional thrombocytopenia. Rapid transfusion of more than 8 to 10 units of stored blood results in a progressive dilution of the patient's platelets with platelet-poor donor blood (survival time of platelets is dramatically reduced with routine blood collection and storage techniques). Platelet counts should be used to routinely monitor patients receiving massive transfusions and platelet components can be added to maintain hemostasis.

Increases in platelet density

Thrombocytosis is a secondary increase in circulating platelet concentration caused by an increase of production in association with another clinical condition. These platelets have normal functional attributes. **Thrombocythemia,** on the other hand, is an autonomous state of uncontrolled production in which many platelet functions may be abnormal. The following classification is modified from that of Thompson and Harker (1983).

Reactive thrombocytosis. Examination of the bone marrow reveals an increased number of megakaryocytes, each with a smaller cell volume, producing an increased, but controlled, peripheral platelet mass.

1. Following splenectomy, counts of 1,000,000 per μL or greater may persist for months.
2. Drugs such as epinephrine, antifungal agents, and *Vinca* alkaloids produce reversible elevated counts.
3. Rebound thrombocytosis may occur after resolution of thrombocytopenia due to cytotoxic drugs, alcohol abuse, surgery, or vitamin deficiencies associated with megaloblastic anemia. This is probably due to a slow rate of peripheral feedback regulation on marrow platelet production.
4. Association with iron deficiency states, particularly those due to blood loss, and with some sideroblastic anemias, indicating a possible involvement of iron in thrombopoiesis.
5. Association with chronic inflammatory diseases.
6. Association with Hodgkin's disease and malignancies, particularly with tumors of the lung, breast, stomach, or ovary.

Thrombocythemia. Autonomous increases in platelet production, defined as **essential thrombocythemia,** are characterized by increased numbers and volumes of megakaryocytes. Platelet concentrations in the peripheral blood may exceed 10,000,000 per μL! The relationship of this disease with other myeloproliferative disorders (myeloid metaplasia, chronic myelogenous leukemia,

and polycythemia vera) is discussed in Chapter 20.

There is often a paradoxical combination of thromboembolic (clotting) and hemorrhagic episodes associated with this condition. The bleeding manifestations are related to the many qualitative abnormalities found in these platelets, including deficiencies in epinephrine receptors and ultrastructural defects in granules, mitochondria, and microfilaments. Aggregation is thus absent in response to epinephrine, decreased with ADP, but normal with collagen. Platelet adhesion is probably decreased and thromboplastin activity is subnormal. The platelets may be notably clumped on blood smears, exhibiting marked variation in size and shape (Fig. 23-6). Neutrophilia and increases in other blood cells are indications of a generalized disorder of myelopoiesis. The hematocrit may be slightly elevated or a microcytic hypochromic anemia may be present as a result of iron deficiency due to blood loss. Therapy is directed at avoiding thrombotic episodes and reducing the platelet count by use of alkylating agents and thrombocytopheresis.

Qualitative disorders: thrombocytopathies

Abnormalities involving platelet function can be classified by reference to the major

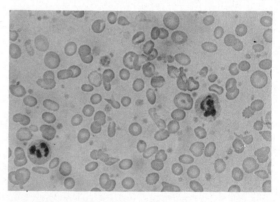

Fig. 23-6 Peripheral platelets in essential thrombocythemia.

Table 23-1. Laboratory findings in qualitative platelet disorders

Disorder	Bleeding time	Platelet count	Clot retraction	Adhesion	ADP release	Aggregation responses					
						ADP-1°	ADP-2°	Epinephrine	Collagen	Arachidonate	Ristocetin
Bernard-Soulier	Prolonged	Normal or decreased	Normal	Decreased	Normal	Normal	Normal	Normal	Normal	Normal	Absent
von Willebrand's	Prolonged	Normal	Normal	Decreased	Decreased	Normal	Normal	Normal	Normal	Normal	Decreased
Glanzmann's thrombasthenia	Prolonged	Normal	Absent or poor	Decreased	Normal	Decreased	Decreased	Decreased	Decreased	Decreased	Normal
Storage pool diseases	Prolonged	Normal	Normal	Decreased	Normal or decreased	Normal	Decreased	Normal 1° decreased 2°	Decreased	Decreased	Normal
Aspirin-like defects	Prolonged	Normal	Normal	Normal	Decreased	Normal	Decreased	Normal 1° decreased 2°	Decreased	Decreased	Normal

activities of platelets. These are: (1) interaction with vascular tissue, (2) adhesion, (3) aggregation, (4) metabolic dysfunction associated with storage products and the release reaction, and (5) participation in coagulation (Table 23-1). Two points will be emphasized in this section. First, dysfunction will be compared often to normal mechanisms (Chapter 12) and the tests that reveal the problem (Chapter 28). Secondly, abnormalities involving a particular platelet structure or metabolic pathway may result in diverse effects on plug formation, coagulation, and vascular maintenance. Conversely, a specific disease or syndrome may be the result of various abnormalities, not all of which directly involve the platelet.

Whenever bleeding manifestations or results of screening tests for hemostasis (e.g., clot retraction, bleeding time) are disproportionately abnormal in relation to the observed platelet count, qualitative platelet abnormalities should be considered. Although many of the hereditary conditions presented in this chapter are rare, they illustrate the principle that anything in a complex system can malfunction. Many of these obscure disorders, in fact, provided the basis for understanding the normal mechanisms of platelet function. Acquired disorders, however, are far more common, especially those associated with drugs and chemical toxicity.

Defects of platelets involving interaction with vascular tissue

Maintenance of the endothelial lining of the blood vessels by platelets can be disrupted as a result of thrombocytopenia or caused by functional defects in the molecular products secreted by platelets. Submucosal bleeding and the presence of petechial hemorrhages are most often associated with these disorders. Patients report that they bruise easily with minimal trauma. This tendency can often be confirmed by performing a tourniquet test for capillary fragility. Specific disorders of the vascular tissue are presented in Chapter 22.

Defects of platelet adhesion

Formation of a hemostatic plug requires that platelets adhere to tissue surfaces, particularly after vessel trauma and exposure of underlying collagen. Deficiencies in specific platelet surface glycoproteins have been identified in several rare, inherited disorders (Fig. 23-7).

Bernard-Soulier syndrome (giant platelet syndrome). The first description of this disorder appeared in 1948. A girl born in 1944 suffered submucosal bleeding at 8 months of age and died when 31 months old. She had a prolonged bleeding time (35 minutes), normal clot retraction, and slightly increased Lee-White coagulation time. Her brother, born in 1947, showed signs of bleeding manifestations within 2 weeks after birth. Like his sister, he exhibited bleeding times ranging from 15 to 30 minutes with a slightly increased coagulation time (12 minutes). Although his platelet count was normal, the platelets appeared abnormal in size and shape on peripheral smears. The central chromomere was dense and surrounded by a very clear hyaline zone. The clot retraction test was normal but the capillary fragility (tourniquet) test was positive. One other sister and both parents showed no signs of the disorder. Platelet counts decreased gradually, to 20,000 per μL by adulthood. When aggregation testing became available, a decreased response to fibrinogen and a total lack of response to ristocetin was noted (response to ADP was normal, see Fig. 23-8, A).

These findings became characteristic of the disease and about 70 cases were reported from 1948 to 1982. Fifty nine of these, from 37 families, have been described in detail. The sex ratio is equal (30 males, 29 females) and the geographical distribution includes Europe, Asia, Africa, and North America. Of the 59 cases, 14 involve consanguinous ancestry and the disorder is

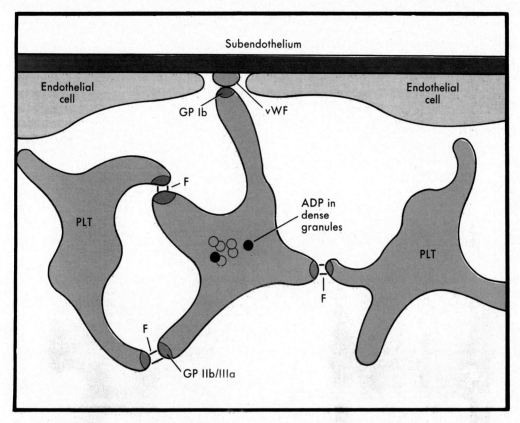

Fig. 23-7   Sites involved in disorders of hemostatic plug formation.
Sites of abnormalities that affect platelet adhesion and aggregation in vivo. *F,* Fibrinogen bridges linking platelets; *GP,* glycoprotein membrane receptors; *vWR,* collagen receptor site for von Willebrand's factor.

believed to be autosomal recessive. Ten deaths were reported from the case survey conducted by Bernard (1983), who termed the disorder "congenital hemorrhagic thrombocytopathic dystrophy".

Although most of the platelets (60% to 80%) appear larger than normal on smears, they may not be as enlarged while circulating in vivo. There is an in increase in the number of dense granules, as observed by electron microscopy. Functional testing shows that BSS platelets adhere normally to collagen substrates, but show decreased ad-

hesion with intact subendothelium and no response to microfibrils. Aggregation responses are essentially normal to all agents except the antibiotic, ristocetin. This lack of response is not corrected with factor VIII or normal plasma. Coagulation studies in BSS patients show decreased prothrombin consumption test times, decreased procoagulant fixation of factors V and VIII, and no fixation of factor XI, attesting to the complex nature of the deficiency. Measurements of platelet survival time indicate that the circulating lifespan is only 2 to 8

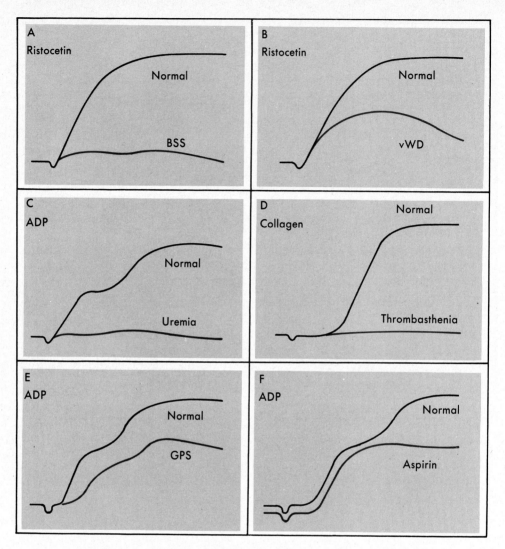

Fig. 23-8 Aggregation responses in qualitative platelet disorders.
A, Bernard-Soulier syndrome.
B, Von Willebrand's disease.
C, Uremia.
D, Glanzmann's thrombasthenia.
E, Gray platelet syndrome.
F, Cyclooxygenase deficiency; effects of aspirin ingestion.

days (normally, 8 to 12 days) and this may partly account for the observations of increased platelet size or volume.

Additional progress was made in the 1970s when specific glycoprotein deficiencies were observed. Glycoprotein Ib was quantitatively decreased and GP V was absent. GP I is a membrane complex that is required for ristocetin to produce an aggregation response and it also serves as an interacting site for adhesion to subendothelial microfibrils. In addition, this glycoprotein serves as the receptor site for platelet von Willebrand's factor. Furthermore, when an antibody to the GP Ib site is added to normal platelets, abnormal adhesion similar to that seen in BSS platelets results.

Diagnosis must distinguish BSS from von Willebrand's disease (vWD), usually on the basis of platelet morphology and failure to correct adhesion and ristocetin-induced aggregation with factor VIII or vWF. Intracranial, gastrointestinal, and menstrual hemorrhage may occur spontaneously and be life threatening. Therapy is largely symptomatic, replacing iron loss and providing supportive transfusions to correct anemia and thrombocytopenia. Note that normal plasma, used to correct the coagulation deficiency of vWD, is ineffective, as is treatment with steroids.

von Willebrand's disease (vWD). This disease is presented in this chapter in association with abnormal platelet function and it is reviewed in more detail as a coagulopathy related to the hemophilias (Chapter 24). Erik von Willebrand first described this disorder in 1926 in a family from the Aland Islands, located in the Gulf of Bothnia between Sweden and Finland. He catagorized it as a "pseudohemophilia" because of the hereditable bleeding manifestations that appeared early in life, but further studies revealed that in addition to a deficient clotting mechanism, the bleeding time was also prolonged.

Obviously, platelets were involved, but the defect did not appear to be intrinsic to the platelets. Platelet count and morphology are usually normal and clot retraction is also normal. Prothrombin time is normal, but the activated partial thromboplastin time is usually prolonged, if only slightly. As additional tests became available, the characteristic findings emerged: decreased retention on glass beads, deficiency of factor VIII procoagulant activity (VIII:C is usually less than 40%), and the aggregation response to ristocetin is greatly diminished. Responses to other agents are normal. This has been found to be correlated with a decrease in the large molecular weight component of factor VIII (VIIIR:Ag or VIII/vWF, see Chapter 13). The bleeding time is particularly sensitive to aspirin and subclinical cases can be demonstrated by means of the aspirin tolerance test, resulting in a marked but transient increase in bleeding time (Chapter 28).

Clinical manifestations and laboratory results vary greatly between affected patients of the same family and at different times in the same patient. Diagnosis can be difficult in milder forms of the disease and a repetitive series of tests may be necessary to demonstrate the deficiencies. Several types of vWD are now recognized, organized into the following broad catagories:

Congenital: often familial, usual onset at an early age
Autosomal dominant: the most common form
Type I: moderately severe with an absence or marked decrease in VIIIR:Ag
Type II: milder form, separated into subtypes based on differences in the distribution of the large and small molecular weight components of factor VIII (Chapter 24).
Autosomal recessive: rarer and more severe in manifestations
Acquired: sudden onset at any age, most commonly at middle age and later
Associated most often with lymphoproliferative and autoimmune disorders

and benign gammopathies. Most of these are associated with autoantibodies to factor VIII components which function as circulating inhibitors.

Since its discovery, vWD has been recognized as the most common genetic defect involving hemostasis. The deficiency in platelet function arises from the role that von Willebrand's factor (vWF) plays in binding platelets to the exposed subendothelium of injured blood vessels. An absence of the large multimers (VIIIR:Ag) prevents the adherent phase of hemostatic plug formation, accounting for the prolonged bleeding time and hemorrhagic manifestations. VIIIR:Ag is also the component that expresses ristocetin cofactor activity and the diminished aggregation response (Fig. 23-8, B) is correlated with a quantitative decrease in the immunologically-based measure. The prolonged coagulant activity is associated with a decrease in VIII:C, which is usually not as dramatic or abnormal as the platelet-dependent factor.

Acquired defects. Patients with uremia accumulate metabolites in their blood that inhibit platelet adhesion. The bleeding time can be greatly prolonged (30 minutes or more) and aggregation responses to ADP, collagen, and epinephrine can also be inhibited (Fig. 23-8, C). Normal function can be restored completely by peritoneal dialysis and partially by hemodialysis. A number of antithrombotic drugs (e.g., dipyridamole and prostacyclin) also inhibit platelet adhesion.

DEFECTS OF PLATELET AGGREGATION
Abnormalities of primary aggregation

Glanzmann's thrombasthenia. This severe bleeding disorder was first described in 1918, and about 200 cases have been reported since. Bleeding manifestations usually appear during infancy or early childhood and include submucosal bleeds (especially epistaxis) and easy bruisability. Hemorrhaging can be severe at times, involving the gastrointestinal tract (most often seen in infants), meningeal linings, and retina. Menorrhagia may be life threatening in postpubertal girls. Fortunately, the severity of bleeding appears to decrease with age, although a marked response to trauma or surgery should be anticipated at any age. Consanguinity has been noted in several cases and it is believed to be inherited as an autosomal recessive. Heterozygotes are either asymptomatic or exhibit very mild expressions of bleeding and laboratory abnormalities.

The first and most characteristic laboratory finding is a greatly diminished or totally absent clot retraction. The bleeding time is markedly prolonged, although this may be only moderately abnormal in some patients. The platelet count and coagulation tests are normal, although a slightly decreased platelet count has been reported in a few patients. Unlike the platelets seen in Bernard-Soulier syndrome, thrombasthenic platelets appear normal on peripheral smears, but they are isolated, showing no signs of clumping. The electron microscope may show some abnormalities of organelles. Aggregation studies (Fig. 23-8, D) show a complete absence of primary response to ADP, thrombin, epinephrine, collagen, and arachidonic acid, but a normal or slightly diminished response to ristocetin (just the opposite of the pattern seen in patients with BSS). Adherence to collagen and rabbit subendothelium is normal, as measured by the Baumgartner technique. Finally, because of the absence of aggregating capacity, thrombasthenic platelets show little or no retention on glass bead filters.

Despite the lack of primary aggregation to most agents, these platelets do change shape, release internal ADP and synthesize prostaglandins in the presence of these agents. Their inability to actually aggregate is due to the lack of the glycoprotein receptor complex, GP IIb/IIIa, which binds plasma fibrinogen to the platelet surface. This binding is necessary for the ADP-mediated interaction of calcium, thrombospondin, and fibronectin which forms bridges between platelets. Absence of the receptor explains why the platelet undergoes the internal responses to collagen, ADP, and thrombin without forming a hemostatic plug. Procoagulant activity is also diminished: PF-3 availability is decreased and factor XI and XII activation is limited, correlating with the severity of the bleeding manifestations. There may also be an absence of glycoproteins IVa, IVb, and VII. The PL^{A1} antigen, associated with GP IIIa, is either absent or defective and antigen Bak^a, associated with GP IIb, is also diminished.

Caen (1972) distinguished two types of thrombasthenia, both showing an absence of response to most aggregating agents. Type I is associated with an absence or marked defect in clot retraction, an absence of membrane GP IIb/IIIa, and a moderate decrease in platelet fibrinogen. Type II is associated with a moderate defect in clot retraction, a partial loss of GP IIb/IIIa, a slight decrease to low normal platelet fibrinogen, and a decreased platelet ATP content. The ultrastructural abnormalities in organelles are also more pronounced in type II GT: abnormal dense granules, an increase in large mitochondria, and clusters of small vesicles.

Acquired defects. Conditions resulting in increased fibrinolysis and the presence of circulating FDPs will inhibit primary aggregation. Patients with hepatic cirrhosis and other liver diseases often display increased plasminogen activation and subsequent clot lysis. Some forms of protein abnormalities, especially those involving increased concentrations of paraproteins, may inhibit aggregation responses by interferring with platelet membrane receptors. Similarly, dextran (a commonly used plasma volume expander), may interfere with either plasma components or the platelet membrane to inhibit aggregation and adhesion. Some antibiotics, particularly the artificial penicil-

lins (e.g., carbenicillin and ampicillin) stimulate formation of IgG antibodies which may attach to platelet membranes, either altering the receptor molecules or blocking them.

Abnormalities of secondary aggregation (release reaction)

A number of the hereditary disorders that affect the release reaction can be identified on the basis of morphological abnormalities demonstrated with the electron microscope. These have been collectively termed "storage pool deficiencies" since they are associated with an absence, decrease or abnormality of organelles containing products secreted from the platelet.

Gray platelet syndrome. This disorder was first described in an 11-year-old boy (Raccuglia, 1971) with thrombocytopenia that was corrected by splenectomy. The platelet cytoplasm appears gray on Wright's-stained smears and electron microscopy reveals that both the megakaryocytes and larger than normal platelets are highly vacuolized and agranular. This is caused by a decrease in the number of alpha granules. Other ultrastructural studies show an increase in elements of the dense tubular system.

Bleeding time is increased and clot retraction is prolonged, but these abnormalities are usually mild. A decrease in thrombospondin and fibrinogen associated with the decreased number of alpha granules may be responsible for the diminished aggregation response seen with ADP, collagen, and thrombin, although results of these tests vary (Fig. 23-8, *E*). One case of familial occurrence that includes affected female children has been reported, raising the possibility that this syndrome is inherited as an autosomal recessive trait.

Deficiencies of dense granules or contents. The primary deficiency involves decreased or absent stores of ADP and serotonin that would be released from the platelet. Autosomal dominant forms are most common, but other hereditable variations occur. The bleeding times are often very prolonged and aggregation responses may be markedly abnormal to collagen and the secondary response to ADP and epinephrine is absent. The ATP:ADP ratio is higher than normal and the uptake of granule-bound nucleotides is greatly diminished.

Acquired forms of dense granule deficiency can be associated with some diseases, such as leukemia and systemic lupus erythematosus, and with the toxic effects of acute alcoholism. Autoimmune diseases may produce antibodies that promote release of dense granule products, resulting in an ultrastructural appearance that resembles the inherited storage pool disorders.

Platelet anomalies associated with other abnormalities. Similar changes in platelet dense granules are seen in various systemic abnormalities. Most of these conditions are associated with prolonged bleeding times and mild to severe bleeding diatheses, but this is most likely related to the corresponding thrombocytopenia rather than the storage pool deficiency. Because of the accompaning thrombocytopenia, most of these disorders are also described in the section on quantitative disorders.

Hermansky-Pudlak syndrome. Hermansky-Pudlak syndrome (tyrosinase-positive oculocutaneous albinism) is an autosomal recessive disorder characterized by ceroid depositions in macrophages. The bleeding time is only moderately prolonged and bleeding problems are usually minor.

Chédiak-Steinbrinck-Higashi syndrome. This syndrome is also an autosomal recessive trait associated with abnormally large lysosomal granules in the leukocytes and megakaryocytes (Chapter 21). This disease also features oculocutaneous albinism, and recurrent fungal and pyogenic bacterial infections are prominent. The disorder progresses, involving episodes of thrombocytopenia, leukopenia, anemia, macrophage accumulations in tissues, and death at an early age. Bleeding varies from mild to moderate as platelet counts decrease.

Wiskott-Aldrich syndrome. This is a sex-linked trait characterized by severe eczema, recurrent infections, and life-threatening thrombocytopenia during the first years of life. Platelet glycolysis and oxidative phosphorylation are also abnormal.

TAR baby syndrome. This is another autosomal recessive trait that results in the absence of radial bones of the arm, a number of cardiac and skeletal abnormalities, and thrombocytopenia. The platelets show similar signs of ultrastructural defects in dense granules with corresponding abnormal aggregation responses. Marrow megakaryocytes may be decreased, immature, or normal.

DEFECTS OF METABOLIC PATHWAYS
The "aspirin-like defects"

Deficiencies involving the prostaglandin pathways produce functional defects similar to those acquired by administration of certain drugs, most notably acetylsalicylic acid (aspirin) and other nonsteroidal inflammatory agents. Aggregation depends on synthesis of thromboxane A_2 as a product of prostaglandin intermediates. An absence or decrease of an enzyme in this pathway inhibits this process. Since the bleeding diatheses associated with these enzyme defects are usually mild or moderate, the enzyme block is either partial or other pathways help mediate platelet release reactions and aggregation. The two most common deficiencies involve cyclooxygenase and thromboxane synthetase (Fig. 23-9).

Cyclooxygenase deficiency. An inherited deficiency in the enzyme that converts arachidonic acid to prostaglandin G_2 (PGG_2) can produce moderate bleeding symptoms. Laboratory results are characterized by a normal to prolonged bleeding time (depending on the severity of the deficiency), decreased retention of platelets on glass beads, decreased adhesion by the Baumgartner technique, and decreased secondary aggregation response to ADP, epinephrine, and collagen (Fig. 23-8, *F*). Aggregation with

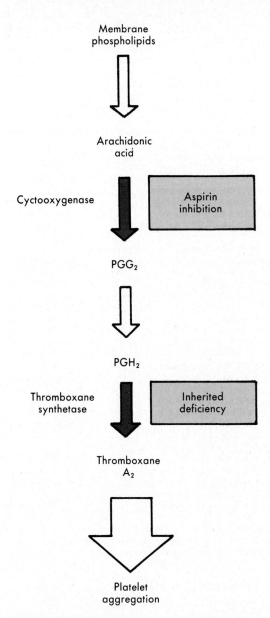

Membrane
phospholipids

Arachidonic
acid

Cyctooxygenase   Aspirin
                      inhibition

PGG_2

PGH_2

Thromboxane   Inherited
synthetase   deficiency

Thromboxane
A_2

Platelet
aggregation

Fig. 23-9 Deficiencies in the arachidonic acid-prostaglandin pathway.
Shaded areas indicate metabolic steps that are identified with hereditable or acquired defects resulting in impaired platelet function.

ristocetin is normal. PF-3 availability varies. To date, four cases of this defect have been described.

Aspirin administration results in specific and irreversible inhibition of cyclooxygenase for the lifespan of the circulating platelet. As a result, the release of endogenous ADP by the platelet is blocked, although the platelet can respond to exogenous ADP. A single 200 mg tablet of aspirin can acetylate 90% of platelet cyclooxygenase (Thompson and Harker, 1983). In spite of this, most patients do not suffer bleeding problems, again indicating that the arachidonic-prostaglandin pathway is not the primary or only mechanism for stimulating platelet responses. Patients undergoing evaluations for hemostasis should avoid aspirin ingestion for a minimum of 7 days prior to having a bleeding time determination, corresponding to the normal platelet turnover time. Platelet donors for single unit transfusions (mainly used for infants) should similarly avoid drugs known to impair platelet function.

Thromboxane synthetase deficiency. The inability to form thromboxane A_2 from endoperoxide intermediates also interferes with aggregation. Aggregation responses to arachidonic acid and PGG_2 are diminished, and the platelets are incapable of responding normally to ADP or epinephrine. The disorder is extremely rare, but it has been shown to be transmitted as an autosomal dominant trait.

Defects in nucleotide and energy metabolism

A number of metabolic deficiencies have been investigated to explain defective platelet release function, including glycogen storage disease (glucose-6 phosphatase deficiency), fructose-1,6-diphosphate deficiency, and deficiencies of adenylate cyclase with increased phosphodiesterase activity. The relationship between these disorders and impaired platelet aggregation remains unclear.

Miscellaneous acquired defects

Many divergent agents have been demonstrated to affect secondary aggregation. In addition to the effects of aspirin and other antiinflammatory drugs mentioned above, effects have been documented for eicosapentaenoic acid found in some seafoods, artificial penicillins (especially carbenicillin), the antimalarial drug hydroxychloroquine, acute or chronic ethyl alcohol ingestion, heparin administration, sympathetic blocking agents (phentolamine and dihydroergotamine), and exposure to some viral infections.

Patients with myeloproliferative and primary dyspoietic diseases of the marrow also exhibit abnormalities in dense granule components that can produce bleeding manifestations. Alpha granule depletion occurs as a result of platelet activation during open heart surgery while patients are on bypass blood oxygenators.

DEFECTS OF PLATELET MEMBRANE RECEPTORS AND PROCOAGULANT ACTIVITY

Platelet procoagulant activity, as measured by PF-3 availability, may be abnormal in a patient without corresponding anomalies in aggregation, adhesion, or release responses. The bleeding time in one such patient (Weiss et al., 1979) was normal, yet substantial bleeding occurred during surgical procedures. A deficiency of the factor V_m receptor site was discovered which affected binding of activated factor X to the platelet membrane. The reduction in number of binding sites (30% of normal) corresponded well to the reduction in PF-3 availability. As a result, the prothrombin consumption test result may be very low. Transfusion of normal platelets and prothrombin complex concentrates may be needed during surgical procedures. Two cases of this type have been reported to date. PF-3 associated abnormalities may be seen in other platelet disorders, since exposure of the receptor site depends on the release reaction. Therefore, the results of PF-3 availability tests should be evaluated in conjunction with aggregation and release function results.

SUMMARY

- Quantitative platelet disorders are defined as abnormal levels of circulating platelets; most are thrombocytopenias (<100,000 per μL). Clinically evident bleeding manifestations are usually not present until counts are well below 50,000 per μL.
- A linear relationship exists between the bleeding time determination and platelets count at concentrations between 10,000 and 100,000 per μL; bleeding time does not decrease above this density.
- Thrombocytopenias are the most common causes of platelet-mediated bleeding disorders. Low densities can result from production and maturation problems involving marrow megakaryocytes, increased destruction or consumption in the peripheral blood, or abnormal sequestration by the spleen.
- Increased platelet densities can occur as a secondary reaction to other conditions (thrombocytosis) or as a primary myeloproliferative disease (essential thrombocythemia).
- Increased bleeding times in association with normal platelet counts may imply a qualitative platelet defect (thrombocytopathy). Functional tests for clot retraction, adhesion, and aggregation in response to chemical agents provide the basis for defining many of the hereditary diseases and acquired defects that underlie bleeding disorders.
- Abnormalities include absences or defects in specific organelles (alpha granules, dense granules, membrane receptors for aggregating agents and procoagulant factors), deficiencies or inhibitions of critical enzymes (e.g., inhibition of cyclooxygenase by aspirin), and inability to synthesize normal amounts or types of proteins that interact with platelets (e.g., von Willebrand's factor, thrombospondin).

24

Congenital and Acquired Coagulation Protein Defects Associated with Hemorrhage or Thrombosis

Rodger L. Bick

CONGENITAL COAGULATION FACTOR DEFECTS AND VON WILLEBRAND'S SYNDROME

Coagulation factor disorders are characterized by deep tissue bleeding, including intraarticular bleeding with resultant crippling hemarthrosis, deep intramuscular bleeding with resultant compartmental compression syndromes, and, at times, intracranial bleeding. In addition, patients with single or multiple coagulation factor defects suffer moderate to severe mucosal membrane hemorrhage. Membranes affected may be gastrointestinal, genitourinary, intrapulmonary, and paranasal sinuses. It may also be manifest as diffuse, bilateral epistaxis. Patients tend to develop large ecchymoses but not petechiae and purpura except in von Willebrand's syndrome.

Most clinically significant coagulation protein disorders are detected by noting prolongation of global tests of coagulation, which are tests which depend on conversion of fibrinogen to fibrin for an end-point determination. These include such tests as the prothrombin time, activated partial thromboplastin time, thrombin time, Lee-White clotting time, activated clotting time, whole blood clotting time, and others.

One or a combination of them will usually be prolonged in clinically significant coagulation protein defects. The other screening tests of hemostasis are normal in patients with isolated coagulation protein problems, including the platelet count, peripheral blood smear, and template bleeding time. A definitive diagnosis of coagulation factor defects usually requires a specific quantitative factor assay after demonstrating prolongation of one or several of the global tests of coagulation.

Coagulation factor disorders are most easily thought of as being hereditary or acquired. The hereditary defects are almost always a single factor deficiency or dysfunction. Acquired defects usually involve multiple factor deficiencies, such as those seen in patients with acute or chronic liver disease, generalized intravascular proteolytic syndromes such as disseminated intravascular coagulation (DIC), or primary fibrinolytic syndromes (see box, p. 376).

The afibrinogenemias, hypofibrinogenemias, and dysfibrinogenemias are quite rare. However, dysfibrinogenemia may be more common than previously thought as only during the past 2 decades has awareness of this disorder initiated laboratory testing for its presence. Isolated deficiencies of factors II, V, VII, or X are extremely rare clinical oddities. Isolated factor XII deficiency, Fletcher factor deficiency, and Fitzgerald factor deficiency are also rare. Until more widespread screening is done as specific assays become available to most clinical laboratories, the incidence of these disorders remains undefined. The three hemophilias are not uncommon and account for about 1 in 8,000 to 10,000 male births in the United States, although differences are noted regionally and worldwide (see box below).

Fibrinogen (factor I) defects

Congenital abnormalities of fibrinogen consist of afibrinogenemia, hypofibrinogenemia, or dysfibrinogenemia. It is important to remember that most of the isolated coagulation factor disorders may occur in the "a" form (absence of protein) or the "dys" form (presence of a dysfunctional protein which has abnormal or absent biological coagulant activity).

Both defects are inherited as autosomal dominant traits. Quantitative defects are hypofibrinogenemia, representing the heterozygote, and afibrinogenemia, representing the homozygous patient. The hypofibrinogenemic patient will have about 50% normal fibrinogen levels. The afibrinogenemic patient has essentially no fibrinogen. The qualitative defects of fibrinogen consist of the dysfibrinogenemias; these are also manifest in the homozygous or heterozygous state. If the patient is homozygous, all fibrinogen is dysfunctional. If, however, the patient is heterozygous, 50% of circulating fibrinogen will be dysfunctional, and 50% will function normally.

Hypofibrinogenemic patients rarely suffer severe bleeding. Some have a mild tendency, but most bleed significantly only following surgical or traumatic stress. Afibrinogenemic patients have occasional spontaneous hemorrhage. This may be manifest as gastrointestinal blood loss in the form of melena, hematochezia, or hematemesis. Patients may develop large hematomata, massive hematuria, or hypermenorrhea. They often have umbilical stump bleeding, gingival bleeding with tooth brushing, and other mucosal membrane bleeding. In addition,

---

COAGULATION FACTOR DISORDERS

Hereditary defects (usually monofactorial deficiency/dysfunction)
Hemophilias
von Willebrand's syndrome
Deficiencies of II, VII, IX, or X (rare)
Fibrinogen defects
Other single factor defects (factors V, XI, XIII)
Contact activation defects
Kininogen defects

Acquired defects (usually multifactorial deficiency/dysfunction)
Disseminated intravascular coagulation
Syndromes
Primary fibrinolytic syndromes
Liver disease
Circulating anticoagulants
Drug induced

HEREDITARY COAGULATION FACTOR DEFECTS

A/hypo/dysfibrinogenemia
Factor II defects
Factor V defects
Factor VII defects
Factor VIII:C defects (hemophilia A)
Factor VIII:vW defects (von Willebrand's)
Factor IX defects (hemophilia B)
Factor X defects
Factor XI defects
Factor XII defects (Hageman trait)
Factor XIII defects
Passovoy defect
Prekallikrein defects (Fletcher trait)
Kininogen defects (Williams, Fitzgerald, Reid, Flaujeac, Fujiwara traits)
Fibrinolytic system defects

intraarticular bleeding with resultant hemarthroses and occasional intracranial bleeding occurs.

Global tests of coagulation (whole blood clotting time, recalcification time, activated partial thromboplastin time, prothrombin time, or reptilase time) will be prolonged in the hypofibrinogenemic (heterozygous) patient. However, the same global tests of coagulation (dependent upon the conversion of fibrinogen to fibrin) will be markedly prolonged or infinite in the afibrinogenemic (homozygous) patient. When measuring fibrinogen concentration by coagulation, protein precipitation, or immunological techniques, hypofibrinogenemic patients (heterozygotes) will have fibrinogen levels about 50% of normal. However, afibrinogenemic patients (homozygotes) will demonstrate no detectable fibrinogen by these techniques. Some afibrinogenemic patients will have trace amounts of fibrinogen by sensitive immunological techniques. This may represent cross-reactivity with nonfibrinogen material, possibly fibronectin. Patients with congenital dysfibrinogenemia often display no hemorrhagic diathesis. However, some do have a mild bleeding tendency with easy and spontaneous bruising. Patients with dysfibrinogenemia may have profuse and prolonged bleeding following trauma or surgery and females may suffer excessive menstrual flow. These findings are most commonly seen in homozygous patients where all fibrinogen is dysfunctional; heterozygous patients have one half normal functioning fibrinogen and one half dysfunctional fibrinogen and are often asymptomatic. Several congenital dysfibrinogenemias have been associated with a thrombotic tendency. These are fibrinogens Baltimore, Chapel Hill, Charlottesville, Copenhagen, Marburg, Naples, New York, Oslo I, Paris II, and Wiesbaden. Dysfibrinogenemias are named after the city in which the patient lives.

Global coagulation tests will be normal or moderately prolonged in the heterozygous dysfibrinogenemic patient, as these patients have about one half normal functioning fibrinogen and one half dysfunctional fibrinogens. In general, 100 mg/dL functional fibrinogen will render a normal clotting time with global coagulation tests. However, the homozygous dysfibrinogenemic patient has all dysfunctional fibrinogen and infinite clotting times will be noted. When measuring fibrinogen concentration by clot-based techniques, the heterozygous dysfibrinogenemic patient will have reduced levels, but the homozygous dysfibrinogenemic patient has no detectable fibrinogen by clotting technique. Protein precipitation or immunological methods for fibrinogen determination reveal both the heterozygous or homozygous dysfibrinogenemic patient to have normal fibrinogen levels.

In most instances of congenital dysfibrinogenemia, the defect accounting for defective function of the fibrinogen molecule is not known. Most have crucial amino acid substitutions, defects of fibrinopeptide A or B release, or abnormal carbohydrate constituents. About 90 forms of congenital dysfibrinogenemia have been described.

The therapy of afibrinogenemia, hypofibrinogenemia, and dysfibrinogenemia is component replacement therapy when significant bleeding occurs or when extensive surgery is planned that is likely to severely compromise hemostasis. Whole blood or plasma can be used. However, the best therapeutic component is cryoprecipitate. Bleeding is usually controlled easily by infusing enough cryoprecipitate or other fibrinogen-containing components to render a clottable (functional) fibrinogen level of 75-100 mg/dL.

Factor II defects

Congenital factor II (prothrombin) defects are extremely rare with less than 40 families being described. Prothrombin defects are inherited as autosomal recessive. Both quantitative and qualitative (dysfunctional) types have been described. The quantitative defects are hypoprothrombinemias and aprothrombinemias. Patients are cross-reacting material negative (CRM−) if they have an absence of factor II or are cross-reacting material positive (CRM+) if they have a dysfunctional form of factor II. This terminology is commonly used to distinguish quantitative and qualitative defects of coagulation factors. Qualitative defects of factor II are the dysprothrombinemias. Quantitative defects are more common than qualitative defects. Results of functional and immunological assays will be concordant in patients with quantitative defects. However, in the dysprothrombinemias, functional (clot-based) assays will show decreased or absent prothrombin levels, but immunological assays will reveal normal levels (discordant results). Several of the dysprothrombinemias have also been associated with a moderate quantitative defect (dysprothrombinemias Havana, Houston, Metz, Molise, and Quick). Like the dysfibrinogenemias and other qualitative coagulation protein defects, the dysprothrombinemias are named after the city in which the family lives.

Homozygous patients can have severe spontaneous bleeding consisting of large hematomata and ecchymoses, and life-threatening mucosal membrane hemorrhage. Heterozygous patients can suffer similar bleeding and may suffer severe bleeding with surgery or trauma. Once the diagnosis of a congenital factor II defect is made, an immunological assay of factor II should be performed to differentiate between a qualitative or quantitative defect. Patients with congenital factor II defects demonstrate a prolonged prothrombin time and activated partial thromboplastin time. The diagnosis is usually made after a specific factor II assay is performed.

Management of congenitally defective factor II patients is required when clinically significant hemorrhage occurs or surgery is contemplated. Prothrombin complex concentrates are the therapy of choice; however, plasma may also be used. The level of functional factor II should be raised to about 50% of normal to stop hemorrhage or to afford surgical hemostasis in presurgical patients. The half-life of factor II is about 3 days, so infusions need not be frequent.

Factor V defects

Factor V deficiency was first described by Owren and is extremely rare, with about 30 cases being reported. The defect is inherited as an autosomal recessive trait. Factor V deficiency has also been referred to as parahemophilia. There have been some cases of combined congenital factor VIII and V deficiency and combined factor V deficiency associated with von Willebrand's syndrome. It has been suggested that combined factor V and factor VIII deficiency may represent a congenital protein C inhibitor deficiency. Most patients studied have an absence of factor V. Recently, however, several cases of dysfunctional factor V have been described. The clinical features include moderate to severe mucosal membrane bleeding, large hematomata, and large ecchymoses. Bleeding with surgery can be particularly severe and spontaneous intraarticular bleeding episodes have been described. Heterozygous patients rarely have spontaneous bleeding, but propensity to hemorrhage correlates very poorly with levels of circulating factor V.

The laboratory diagnosis is suggested by noting prolongation of prothrombin time and partial thromboplastin time. A specific diagnosis depends upon a quantitative factor V assay. There are no factor V concentrates available and patients are managed with infusions of fresh frozen plasma at about 10 cc per kg/body weight or with cryoprecipitate. The factor V levels should be kept above 30% for hemostasis; since the half-life of factor V is around 24 hours, infusions need only be daily.

Factor VII defects

Factor VII deficiency is extremely rare and is inherited as an autosomal recessive.

Less than 150 cases of factor VII deficiency have been reported. Both the absence (CRM−) form and dysfunctional (CRM+) form of the disease exist. The absence of factor VII appears more common than dysfunctional factor VII defects. The clinical features are similar to other congenital single-factor defects. Patients may suffer significant life-threatening hemorrhage with surgery or trauma. Umbilical stump bleeding is also common. Spontaneous bleeding rarely occurs in heterozygous patients unless trauma or surgery is experienced. The laboratory diagnosis depends upon noting a prolonged prothrombin time and a normal PTT. When this combination of abnormalities is noted, a factor VII assay should be performed. The Stypven time (prothrombin time with Russell's viper venom) is normal. The management of homozygous patients, when clinically significant hemorrhage occurs, is with prothrombin complex concentrates or plasma. It should be noted that several of the commercially available prothrombin complex concentrates contain minimal or no factor VII. Thus, if treating a factor VII deficiency patient, the characteristics of concentrates must be known. Factor VII levels should be maintained at 30% of normal; infusions need to be frequent in bleeding or surgical patients, as the plasma half-life of factor VII is 4 to 6 hours.

Factor VIII:C defects

The hemophilias are more common congenital coagulation defects than those previously discussed. The incidence of hemophilia is around 1 in 10,000 male births, although regional differences are observed.

Hemophilia A, referred to as classical hemophilia, is inherited as a sex-linked recessive and is a deficiency or defect of factor VIII:C. About 90% of patients have a deficiency of both factor VIII:C and factor VIII:CAg and are, thus, truly deficient (CRM−), or factor VIII:C−. The remaining 10% of patients are missing factor VIII:C activity but have normal factor VIII:CAg;

these patients have, therefore, dysfunctional factor VIII:C. They are referred to as CRM+ or factor VIII:C+ patients. A positive family history is elicited in 70% of hemophilic patients, and in about 30% of patients the gene appears to arise spontaneously.

Factor VIII:C− and factor VIII:C+ patients suffer similar clinical courses. Hemophilic patients typically experience hemorrhage, primarily manifest as deep tissue bleeding. The types of bleeding are usually deep intramuscular bleeding, intraarticular bleeding with resultant joint fibrosis (hemarthroses), and potentially fatal intracranial bleeding. Patients commonly suffer hematuria. Particularly severe and potentially crippling bleeding can occur when hemorrhage into one of the closed muscular compartments of the extremities occurs. The severity of bleeding in hemophilia A closely parallels the level of circulating factor VIII:C. Severe bleeders are those who have 5% or less of circulating factor VIII:C or who have circulating inhibitors to factor VIII:C. Moderate hemophiliacs are those who have 5% to 10% circulating factor VIII:C levels. These patients have minimal to moderate numbers of spontaneous bleeding episodes, but bleed profusely when subjected to surgery or trauma. Mild hemophiliacs are those who have 10% to 40% circulating factor VIII:C. Patients with mild hemophilia rarely have spontaneous bleeding, but may have severe life-threatening bleeding with surgical or traumatic stress.

It is important to realize that severe hemophilia is usually clinically obvious and, in general, these patients are identified early in life due to frequent bleeding. However, mild hemophiliacs may not be identified until a major surgical or traumatic bleed occurs. For this reason, a sensitive activated partial thromboplastin time and reliable associated reagents are of paramount importance when using this test as a presurgical screening procedure or when using it to evaluate a bleeding patient for potential hemophilia.

The key to a rapid diagnosis of hemophilia A is to note a prolonged PTT in the face of a normal prothrombin time in a (usually) male child who has a positive bleeding history or a positive family history. In this setting, there is an 85% likelihood that the child will have factor VIII:C deficiency and, thus, would dictate a quantitative factor VIII assay to be performed. If factor VIII is negative, a factor IX:C and, if warranted, a factor XI:C assay would be in order.

About 10% of hemophilia A patients develop anti-VIII:C antibodies. These are most commonly IgG_4 kappa. The anti-VIII:C antibody is long acting, and may require a long incubation in the PTT system for demonstration. Thus, it is wise to incubate the activated partial thromboplastin time system for 15, 30, 45, and 60 minutes when seeking the factor VIII:C antibody.

The therapy of hemophilia A is dependent upon the site and severity of hemorrhage. Mild bleeding can often be controlled with cold compresses, topical thrombin when necessary, and other supportive measures. Serious bleeding episodes, including intraarticular bleeding, should be treated with factor VIII concentrates. In general, infusion of 25 units per kg will render a 50% increase in activity in a hemophilia A patient; a level of 50% normal activity should readily achieve hemostasis in most instances. High titers of antibodies are treated with "activated" prothrombin complex concentrates and the response is generally, but not consistently, good. Anti-VIII antibodies in hemophilic patients are generally not responsive to immunosuppressive therapy. Methods of detecting carriers of hemophilia A and B approach 90% accuracy.

Factor IX defects

Factor IX deficiency is also known as hemophilia B, Christmas disease, or PTC deficiency. This disorder is also inherited as a sex-linked recessive. The clinical features are identical to those of hemophilia A. The disease can be clinically divided into patients who are mild, moderate, or severe. Correlation between factor IX:C and severity of the disease is the same as that noted with factor VIII deficiency. Most patients, 70% to 90%, are truly deficient in factor IX:C and are CRM−. However, 10% to 30% are CRM+. As an added variable, some CRM+ patients have prolonged ox brain thromboplastin times and others are normal; thus, at least four variants of hemophilia B exist. An additional variant is hemophilia B Leyden, in which the factor IX:C levels increase with age. Additional variants are factor IX Chapel Hill and factor IX Alabama. Variants of hemophilia B are summarized in Table 24-1.

About 60% to 70% of patients have a positive family history. Patients will characteristically have a prolonged activated partial thromboplastin time and a normal prothrombin time. The diagnosis is usually made when a patient with an appropriate history, family history, or appropriate bleeding history presents with a prolonged activated partial thromboplastin time, a normal prothrombin time, and a normal factor VIII:C assay. In this circumstance the next assay to be performed would be a factor IX assay. Management, like that for hemophilia A, depends on the clinical signifi-

Table 24-1. Variants of hemophilia B

Factor IX protein	Ox brain thromboplastin time	Term used
CRM+	Normal	Hemophilia B+
CRM+	Long	Hemophilia B+$_M$
CRM−	Normal	Hemophilia B−
CRM−	Long	Hemophilia B−$_M$

Others: factor IX Chapel Hill (CRM+); factor IX Alabama (CRM+); Hemophilia B Leyden (IX levels increase with age).

cance of hemorrhage. Severe bleeding or preparation for surgery is managed with factor IX-containing prothrombin complex concentrates. The hazards of these concentrates are hepatitis and thrombus formation, including initiation of DIC-type syndromes. About 5% to 7% of patients with factor IX deficiency develop anti-IX antibodies. The only therapy for this complication is to neutralize the antibody with prothrombin complex concentrate, followed by raising the factor IX:C level to achieve hemostasis.

Factor X defects

Factor X deficiency is an extremely rare disorder with about 50 families described. The disorder is inherited as an autosomal recessive; homozygous patients have very low factor X:C levels and heterozygotes have around 50% of normal factor X:C activity. Both the absent form, factor X:C− and dysfunctional form, factor X:C+, are known. Clinical features are similar for both. Factor X deficient patients are more prone to have severe mucosal membrane and skin hemorrhages and fewer deep tissue hemorrhages than those seen in the hemophilias. Mucosal membrane hemorrhages can be from any site, and is often quite severe in homozygous patients. Umbilical stump bleeding is a particularly common early manifestation of factor X deficiency.

The activated partial thromboplastin time and prothrombin time are markedly prolonged in homozygous patients and mildly prolonged or, at times, normal in heterozygous patients. In addition, since Russell's viper venom will activate factor X in vitro, this test is also prolonged. Russell's viper venom time, however, may be normal in some factor X:C+ patients. These findings should prompt a quantitative factor X:C assay for definitive diagnosis. Since hemostasis can be achieved with 15% to 20% levels of factor X, management can often be achieved with plasma infusions. Serious

bleeding can be controlled or higher levels for surgery can be achieved with prothrombin complex concentrates.

Factor XI defects

Factor XI deficiency is also referred to as plasma thromboplastin antecedent (PTA) deficiency, Rosenthal's disease, or hemophilia "C". The latter term should probably be abandoned. The disorder was first described by Rosenthal and coworkers in 1953. Factor XI deficiency was initially thought to be inherited as an autosomal dominant. However, more recent studies have revealed it to be inherited as an incomplete autosomal recessive trait. Homozygous patients have about 1% factor X while heterozygotes have about 50% of normal factor X levels. A high incidence occurs in Jewish patients of Russian descent (Ashkenazic Jews), and in this population homozygotes comprise about 0.2% of the population and heterozygotes comprise as much as 11%. Many other races are also affected. All patients studied appear to have a true impaired factor XI synthesis defect, as no dysfunctional forms have been described.

The clinical features are quite variable and confusing. Homozygous patients have spontaneous bleeding from mucosal membranes which may be serious. However, deep tissue bleeding, including intraarticular bleeding, is extremely rare. Up to 50% of homozygous patients may experience serious and life-threatening bleeding with surgery or trauma. Bleeding from the oral mucosal or the genitourinary tract is a particular problem and has been ascribed to the enhanced fibrinolytic activity which may occur in these areas. Most heterozygous patients have no bleeding. However, a few may suffer spontaneous mucosal membrane hemorrhages, especially epistaxis, and some will have minor bleeding with surgery or trauma. Homozygous patients may have no bleeding, minimal bleeding, or profuse bleeding. The severity of bleeding does not correlate with levels of circulating factor XI.

Patients with factor XI deficiency will demonstrate a prolonged activated partial thromboplastin time and normal prothrombin time. Unless the patient is female, in which case a factor XI level should be considered immediately, the diagnosis is usually made by noting a typical personal or family history or significant bleeding and a prolonged PTT, a normal prothrombin time, a normal factor VIII and factor IX level, and a subsequent decreased level of factor XI. Management is primarily use of fresh frozen plasma infused at 10 cc per kg per day for significant bleeding episodes or in preparation for surgery. The factor XI levels should be raised to 30% to 40% of normal to achieve hemostasis.

Factor XII defects

Congenital factor XII deficiency was first described by Ratnoff and Colopy in 1955. Several hundred cases have been reported since then. The name of the first patient studied by Ratnoff and Colopy was John Hageman, and the disorder is commonly called the Hageman trait. The disorder is usually inherited as an autosomal recessive, but instances of autosomal dominant inheritance have been described. Homozygous patients of the autosomal recessive variety have very low levels of factor XII. Heterozygotes can be quite variable, but tend to have around 50% of normal factor XII activity. The disorder is known to exist in the absence form, factor XII:C− and the dysfunctional form, factor XII:C+ (CRM+). However, the absence form appears much more often.

In many instances, factor XII deficiency is found by chance when a screening PTT is performed and noted to be markedly prolonged, often in a routine presurgical patient. Since this is the manner in which many patients present it is assumed and often taught incorrectly that patients with factor XII deficiency have no bleeding diathesis. In fact, some patients do have a mild bleeding tendency and life-threatening bleeding can occur, although rarely. Of particular interest, patients with factor XII deficiency have defective surface-mediated activation of fibrinolysis and many patients dying with factor XII deficiency have died of thrombosis or thromboembolism. John Hageman, a railroad worker, died from a pulmonary embolus following a traumatic hip fracture.

The diagnosis is most often made by noting a markedly prolonged PTT and normal prothrombin time in an asymptomatic patient or a patient with a mild hemorrhagic diathesis. A definitive diagnosis requires specific quantitative factor XII assay by clot-based or synthetic substrate-based techniques. Since hemorrhage is rare or nonexistent, replacement therapy is generally not required. In those exceptionally rare patients with significant hemorrhage, replacement should be with fresh frozen plasma.

Prekallikrein defects

Prekallikrein deficiency was first noted by Hathaway in 1965. The defect was noted to correct with factor XII deficient plasma and the new disorder was referred to as Fletcher trait, after the surname of the family first studied. The mode of inheritance is unclear or variable. Some have described autosomal recessive characteristics while others have noted autosomal dominance. Although most patients studied have a true deficiency (CRM−), several instances of a dysfunctional form (CRM+) have also been described. Patients with prekallikrein deficiency have no bleeding tendency, but like those with factor XII deficiency, they also have defective activation of the fibrinolytic system. The diagnosis is suggested when noting a markedly prolonged PTT and a normal prothrombin time in an asymptomatic individual, usually during presurgical screening. The diagnosis is made by performing a specific prekallikrein assay by clot-based or synthetic substrate-based techniques. A characteristic of prekallikrein deficiency is correction of the partial thromboplastin time when incubating the PTT system for 10 minutes with kaolin, celite, silica, or ellagic acid. This test should *not be used* for a diagnosis since the same phenomena can be noted with Passovoy deficiency. An erroneous interpretation could lead to a missed diagnosis of Passavoy defect and a potential bleeding problem.

Kininogen defects

High molecular weight kininogen (HMWK) deficiency is known by a variety of surnames, including the most common, Fitzgerald trait. It is also known as Williams, Flaujeac, Fujiwara, and Reid traits. The disorder is inherited as an autosomal recessive. Patients do not have a hemorrhagic tendency, but do have abnormal surface-mediated activation of fibrinolysis. All patients studied have a true deficiency of HMWK. Fitzgerald and Reid traits represent a deficiency of high molecular weight kininogen. However, Williams, Fleaujac, and Fujiwara traits represent a deficiency of both high molecular weight and low molecular weight kininogen. These last three forms of deficiency are also deficient in prekallikrein. The diagnosis is suspected by noting a prolonged partial thromboplastin time and a normal prothrombin time and noncorrecting of the PTT with prolonged incubation in an asymptomatic individual, usually during a routine preoperative screening work-up. A definitive diagnosis is made by immunological assay for HMWK.

Passovoy defect

Passovoy deficiency was first described by Hougie in 1975. It appears to be inherited as an autosomal dominant. The molecular characteristics are unknown. Patients typically have a moderate bleeding tendency characterized by mucosal membrane bleeding (including epistaxis), easy and spontaneous bruising, and excessive menstrual flow. Intraarticular bleeds are uncommon. Severe bleeding may occur with trauma or surgery. The PTT is moderately prolonged and the prothrombin time is normal. The partial thromboplastin time will shorten with incubation, so the disorder can be erroneously confused with prekallikrein deficiency. Plasma infusions are used for traumatic or surgical hemorrhage.

Alpha-2-antiplasmin defects

Alpha-2-antiplasmin deficiency is inherited as an autosomal recessive. Alpha-2-antiplasmin levels are less than 10% in homozygous patients and around 50% in heterozygous individuals. No dysfunctional forms have been noted and all patients studied have parallel levels of biological and immunological alpha-2-antiplasmin. Bleeding can be severe in homozygous patients and typically consists of mucosal membrane bleeding (with hematuria predominating), large subcutaneous hematomas, spontaneous bruising, and severe bleeding with trauma. Intraarticular bleeding may also occur. Laboratory tests are generally normal except for low to nonexistant levels of alpha-2-antiplasmin by biological or synthetic substrate assay. Occasionally, elevated fibrin(ogen) degradation products may be seen. The therapy of choice is epsilon aminocaproic acid given as 10 mg per kg t.i.d., orally or intravenously. Tranexamic acid (cyclokaprone) can be used as an alternate.

Factor XIII defects

Congenital factor XIII deficiency has been described in over 100 families and is inherited as an autosomal recessive, although originally thought to be sex linked. A high incidence of consanguinity has been noted. Homozygous patients are missing the alpha chain, which contains the site at which thrombin activates factor XIII. Homozygotes may also have decreased levels of the beta chain, but patients have been described who have absent or normal beta chains. Heterozygotes generally have decreased alpha and beta chains. Thus, if immunological techniques are used to assay factor XIII, anti-alpha chain and anti-beta chain antibodies must be used.

The clinical manifestations of factor XIII deficiency are characteristic and the bleeding diathesis only occurs in homozygotes, as only 10% of normal factor XIII levels are necessary for normal fibrin monomer cross linking to occur. Ninety percent of patients demonstrate delayed umbilical stump bleeding at childbirth. Patients with homozygous factor XIII deficiency also usually suffer significant deep tissue hemorrhages, especially into muscle and muscle compartments. These commonly develop several days after minor trauma but may occur spontaneously. Many patients develop subsequent destruction of bone and pseudotumors. They are especially prominent in the thigh and gluteal areas. The most common cause of death is intracranial hemorrhage, which occurs in factor XIII deficiency more commonly than in any of the other congenital coagulation protein defects. These bleeds are also commonly preceded by minor trauma occuring several days previously. Most homozygous males are sterile and a high incidence of spontaneous abortion is seen in homozygous females.

A screening test for factor XIII consists of observing for clot solubility in 5 molar urea or 1% monochloroacetic acid. These are two agents that will disrupt hydrophobic bonds, but not the gammaglutamyl-lysine bonds created by factor XIIIa. These solubility tests are, however, poor screening techniques as they are insensitive to levels slightly more than 1% normal activity and potential deficient bleeders can be missed. More specific techniques are available including assays for gamma-gamma dimer (cross-linked by factor XIIIa), radioactive amine incorporation tests, latex agglutination inhibition tests, or radioimmunoassay. Therapy for factor XIII deficiency consists of infusion of fresh frozen plasma at 10 cc per kg every 7 to 10 days. Cryoprecipitate can be used. Adequate levels of factor XIII are also rendered to the surgical patient who may have received several units of whole blood.

von Willebrand's disease

von Willebrand's syndrome was reported by Eric von Willebrand in 1926. This bleeding disorder was first noted in families living on the Aland Island off the coast of Sweden. The islands have since been renamed Ahvenanmaa. The patients had a severe bleeding disorder which was autosomally inherited. In addition, a prolonged bleeding time, normal clot retraction, normal platelet counts, and a normal coagulation time were characteristic. This original group, labeled as "pseudohemophiliacs," was restudied by use of a capillary "thrombometer" several years later by von Willebrand and Jurgens. This closer evaluation revealed prolonged thrombometer times and patients were then labeled as having "constitutional thrombopathy." The criteria for a diagnosis became (1) a bleeding tendency, (2) autosomal inheritance, (3) a normal platelet count, (4) a long bleeding time, and (5) a normal whole blood clotting time. In 1953 Ben Alexander, Armand Quick, and Professor Larrieu simultaneously discovered a new characteristic of von Willebrand's syndrome, that of low factor VIII:C levels. This important discovery was a catalyst to launch investigations which have lead to a more complete understanding of the factor VIII macromolecular complex, classical hemophilia, and von Willebrand's disease. In 1971, Zimmerman, Ratnoff, and Powel developed an antibody to factor VIII and demonstrated that the presence of an antigen (factor VIII:RAg) existed in normal and hemophiliac plasma, but not in von Willebrand's plasma. This initiated the era of molecular biology of hemophilia, von Willebrand's disease, and factor VIII moieties. It also provided a tool for the discovery and defining of von Willebrand types as well as the separately-recognized portions/activities of the factor VIII macromolecular complex. The bleeding in von Willebrand's disease is reminiscent of a platelet-vascular problem and consists of purpura, easy and spontaneous bruising, increased menstrual bleeding, mucosal membrane bleeding (including gastrointestinal and genitourinary hemorrhage), and bilateral epistaxis. Bleeding, often in the form of bilateral epistaxis, and easy, spontaneous bruising typically begins in early childhood. These findings should prompt early suspicion of von Willebrand's disease. Deep tissue bleeding and intraarticular bleeding are far less common than mucosal membrane bleeding. Hemorrhage, however, can be profuse with surgery or trauma. Table 24-2 compares hemophilia A and von Willebrand's disease.

There are four subtypes of von Willebrand's syndrome:

Homozygous von Willebrand's disease is characterized by severe bleeding of the sites and a high incidence of consanguinity. The bleeding time is usually markedly prolonged. Ristocetin cofactor activity is markedly abnormal or absent and factor VIII:RAg

Table 24-2. Comparison of von Willebrand's syndrome and hemophilia A

	von Willebrand's	Hemophilia A
Inheritance	Autosomal dominant	Sex-linked recessive
Bleeding time	Long	Normal
Factor VIII:C	Moderate decrease	Marked decrease
Factor VIII:RAg	Decreased	Normal
Factor VIII:vW	Decreased	Normal
Platelet adhesion	Abnormal	Normal
Clinical features	Mucosal bleeds Petechiae Purpura	Deep tissue bleeding

and factor vW are markedly reduced or absent. Factor VIII:C and factor VIII:CAg are reduced but not as profoundly as factor VIII:vW and factor VIII:RAg. This variant is also referred to as type III.

Heterozygous von Willebrand's type I is inherited as an autosomal dominant and is characterized by concordant decreases in factor VIII:C, factor VIII:CAg, factor VIII:RCo (factor VIII:vW), and factor VIII:RAg. This type, thus, is a quantitative defect in the entire factor VIII macromolecular complex.

Heterozygous von Willebrand's type II is subdivided into two forms. Heterozygous von Willebrand's type IIA is also inherited as an autosomal dominant and appears to represent a dysfunction of factor VIII:vW (factor VIII:RCo). There is absent or almost nonexistant factor VIII:vW (factor VIII:RCo) activity and discordance with levels of factor VIII:C, factor VIII:CAg, and factor VIII:RAg, all of which are usually much higher than levels of factor VIII:vW (factor VIII:RCo). This suggests a dysfunction of the complex rather than a quantitative defect. In this form of disease it appears that there is depolymerization of the macromolecular complex, with many monomeric forms circulating. This type may, therefore, represent an abnormality of polymerization ability of the complex.

Heterozygous von Willebrand's type IIB is also inherited as an autosomal dominant and has the same discordant findings as seen in type IIA. There are normal or near normal factor VIII:C, factor VIII:CAg, and moderately reduced levels of factor VIII:RAg in this type. There are two major differences from type IIA. The first is enhanced platelet aggregability to ristocetin (enhanced factor VIII:RCo activity). The second, although this form also appears to be associated with a defect in polymerization, is fewer of the monomeric forms and more of the polymerized forms circulating than are typically seen in type IIA.

Laboratory diagnosis of von Willebrand's

disease can be complex. This complexity is further enhanced by the variability of laboratory parameters in a patient as well as the unreliability of two tests which were popular for diagnosing von Willebrand's disease but are no longer recommended for use. These tests are ristocetin-induced platelet aggregation and the platelet adhesion technique using glass bead columns. The ristocetin cofactor assay has replaced ristocetin-induced aggregation and is a reasonably sensitive test. However, primary laboratory tests are the factor VIII:C, factor VIII:RAg, and template bleeding time used in conjunction with factor VIII:RCo assay.

The therapy for von Willebrand's syndrome is cryoprecipitate, which contains abundant levels of factor VIII:R. The amount used is variable according to the amount of factor VIII:R. The response, by monitoring correction of the bleeding time, is also quite variable. However, a rough guideline is to give 1 to 3 units of cryoprecipitate per day per 10 kg/body weight. The presurgical patient should receive three units per 10 kg the morning of the day of surgery.

Other rare defects

Congenital protein C inhibitor deficiency has been reported in patients who were deficient in factors V and VIII:C. In one report all patients studied who had only an isolated singular factor V or isolated factor VIII:C deficiency had normal protein C inhibitor activity. Because of these findings it has been suggested that many previously-reported cases of combined factor V and factor VIII:C deficiency may be found to represent congenital protein C inhibitor deficiency.

DISSEMINATED INTRAVASCULAR COAGULATION

Disseminated intravascular coagulation (DIC) is not an independent disease but rather an intermediary mechanism of disease that is usually seen in association with well-defined clinical entities. In addition, the pathophysiology of DIC serves as an intermediary mechanism of disease in many localized disease processes which, in many instances, remain organ specific. This catastrophic syndrome spans all areas of medicine and presents a wide clinical spectrum that remains confusing.

Most consider DIC to be a systemic hemorrhagic syndrome. However, this is only because hemorrhage is obvious and often impressive. However, what is less commonly appreciated is the significant amount of microvascular thrombosis and, in some instances, large vessel thrombosis. In fact, the hemorrhage is often easy to contend with in patients with fulminant DIC and it is the small vessel and large vessel thrombosis with impairment of blood flow, ischemia, and associated end-organ damage which usually leads to irreversible morbidity and mortality of the patient. In this section, acute disseminated intravascular coagulation versus chronic disseminated intravascular coagulation and the attendant differences in clinical manifestations, laboratory findings, and treatment will be discussed. However, it should be realized that these are often pure and theoretical clinical spectrums of a disease continuum. Patients may present anywhere in it and may lapse from one end to the other.

Etiology

Acute DIC is usually seen in association with well-defined clinical entities (see box page 387). Obstetrical accidents are common events leading to DIC. In DIC associated with the retained fetus syndrome, its incidence approaches 50% if the woman retains a dead fetus in utero for more than 5 weeks.

Intravascular hemolysis of any etiology is a common triggering event for DIC. A frank hemolytic transfusion reaction is certainly a triggering event. However, hemolysis of any etiology, even of minimal degree, may provide a trigger. Septicemia is often associ-

CONDITIONS ASSOCIATED WITH ACUTE DISSEMINATED INTRAVASCULAR COAGULATION

Obstetrical accidents
Amniotic fluid embolism
Placental abruption
Retained fetus syndrome
Eclampsia

Intravascular hemolysis
Hemolytic transfusion reactions
Minor hemolysis
Massive transfusions

Bacteremia
Gram negative (endotoxin)
Gram positive (mucopolysaccharides)

Viremias
Cytomegalovirus
Hepatitis
Varicella

Disseminated malignancy
Leukemia
Acute promyelocytic
Acute myelomonocytic
Many others

Burns
Crush injuries and tissue necrosis
Liver disease
Obstructive jaundice
Acute hepatic failure

Prosthetic devices
(LeVeen shunting and aortic balloon)

Vascular disorders

ated with DIC, especially by meningococcus and other gram negative organisms. The triggering mechanisms have been well described and consist of the initiation of coagulation by endotoxin: bacterial coat lipopolysaccharide. Following this, many gram-positive organisms were also noted to be associated with DIC and are also aptly described. Bacterial coat mucopolysaccharides may demonstrate the same activity as endotoxin. Many viremias are associated with DIC and the most common are varicella, hepatitis, or cytomegalovirus infections.

Malignancy is often associated with DIC. Most individuals with disseminated solid malignancy will at least have laboratory evidence of DIC which may or may not become clinically manifest. Patients with leukemias of acute or chronic types are also subject to DIC. The most common acute leukemia associated with DIC is acute hypergranular promyelocytic leukemia (see Chapter 20). Other malignancies commonly associated with DIC are gastrointestinal, pancreatic, prostatic, ovarian, melanomas, lung neoplasms, myelomas, and myeloproliferative syndromes.

Acidosis and, less commonly, alkalosis may also provide triggers for DIC. Patients with extensive burns are also candidates and several mechanisms may be operative. Any patient with a large degree of crush injury and attendant tissue necrosis may develop DIC by the release of tissue enzymes and/or phospholipoprotein-like material into the systemic circulation.

Selected vascular disorders and a number of other disorders may be associated with acute DIC. However, these are more commonly associated with chronic DIC. Up to 25% of patients with giant cavernous hemangiomata will develop a chronic low grade "compensated" DIC which may or may not progress into an acute DIC, the so called Kasabach-Merritt syndrome. About 50% of patients with hereditary hemorrhagic telangiectasia will also have a chronic DIC syndrome and many may develop an acute DIC for unexplained reasons. Individuals with small vessel disease, such as vasospastic phenomena (including Raynaud's syndrome or severe diabetic angiopathy) or angiopathy associated with autoimmune disorders, may also develop chronic DIC which may or may not become acute.

Many chronic inflammatory disorders, including sarcoidosis, Crohn's disease, and ulcerative colitis, may also be associated with compensated DIC. Selected prosthetic devices may provide a triggering event for DIC. LeVeen (Denver) valves for peritoneovenous shunting has become a common palliative procedure for treatment of intractable ascites. A generalized DIC-type syndrome is common with the use of these shunts. It has been noted that removal of ascitic fluid at the time of valve implantation, as well as selected anticoagulants, may forestall DIC in these patients.

Chronic DIC is a compensated event and again represents the pure end of a clinical spectrum which may not always represent reality. Conditions most commonly associated with a chronic DIC-type process are listed in the accompanying box.

Fig. 24-1 shows how a variety of seemingly unrelated pathophysiological insults can give rise to the common result of DIC. There are many disorders which can cause endothelial damage, including circulating antigen-antibody complex, endotoxemia, tissue damage of any type (with resultant release of tissue procoagulant materials or tissue procoagulant enzymes), platelet damage and subsequent release, or red cell damage. When one of these insults occurs, there is a wide range of potential activation pathways which may eventually give rise to systemically-circulating plasmin plus systemically-circulating thrombin. DIC is usually the result.

Pathophysiology

The pathophysiology of DIC, once a triggering event has been provided, is highly complex (Fig. 24-2). After the coagulation system has been activated and both thrombin and plasmin circulate systemically, the pathophysiology of DIC is relatively constant in all disorders. When thrombin and plasmin circulate systemically, they behave

CONDITIONS ASSOCIATED WITH CHRONIC DISSEMINATED INTRAVASCULAR COAGULATION

Obstetrical accidents
Eclampsia
Retained fetus syndrome
Saline-induced abortion

Cardiovascular diseases
Acute myocardial infarction
Peripheral vascular disease
Leriche's syndrome

Metastatic malignancy
Hematologic diseases
Paroxysmal nocturnal hemoglobinuria
Polycythemia vera
Agnogenic myeloid metaplasia

Collagen vascular disorders (especially if a microvascular component)
Renal disorders
Glomerulonephritis
Renal microangiopathies
Hemolytic-uremic syndrome

Miscellaneous disorders
Allergic vasculitis
Sarcoidosis
Amyloidosis
Chronic inflammatory disorders
Diabetes mellitus
Hyperlipoproteinemias

as they would locally, forming clinically recognized FDPs (the X, Y, D, and E fragments). The consequences of thrombin circulation are primarily thrombosis, with deposition of fibrin monomer and polymerized fibrin in the microcirculation and, at times, large vessels. The systemic plasmin circulation primarily accounts for the hemorrhage seen in DIC because of the creation of fibrin(ogen) degradation products and their interference with fibrin monomer polymerization and induction of platelet dysfunction. Plasmin-induced lysis of many

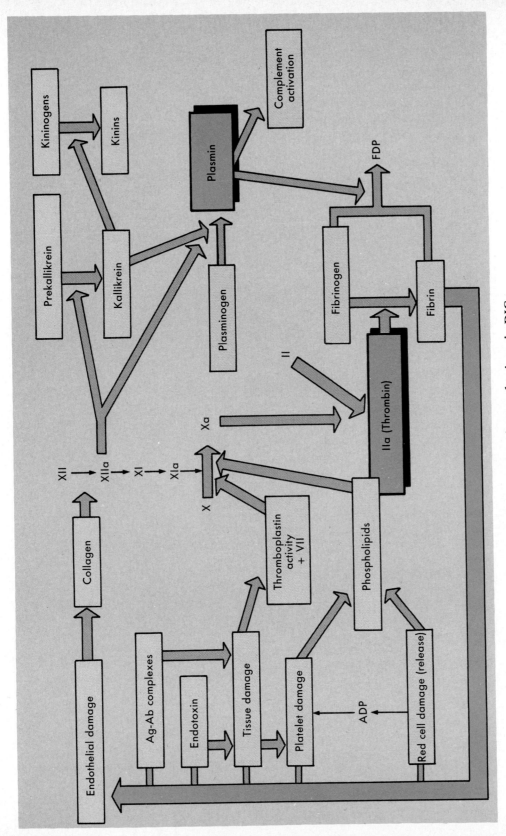

Fig. 24-1. Triggering mechanisms in DIC.

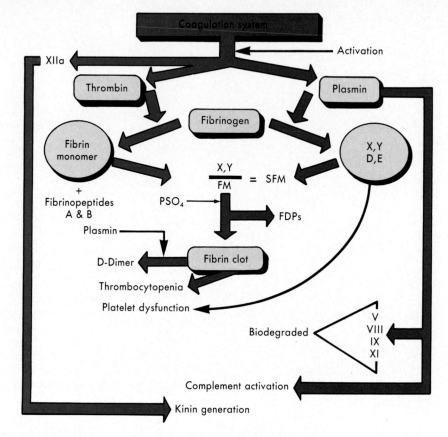

Fig. 24-2. Pathophysiology of DIC.

clotting factors also leads to hemorrhage. By appreciating this circular type of pathophysiology it is easy to understand why most patients with DIC are sustaining *hemorrhage plus thrombosis.*

Clinical findings of acute DIC

The signs and symptoms of DIC can be highly variable. They generally consist of fever, hypotension, acidosis, proteinuria, and hypoxia. These findings are rather general and are not particularly helpful in diagnosis. However, more specific signs are found and should raise the possibility of DIC in the appropriate clinical settings. They consist of petechiae and purpura (found in most patients with DIC), hemorrhagic bullae, cyanosis and, at times, frank gangrene. Wound bleeding, especially oozing from a surgical or traumatic wound, venipuncture site, or intraarterial line, is common in patients with DIC who have undergone surgery or sustained trauma.

The patient usually bleeds from at least three unrelated sites. Bleeding may occur in deep tissues, including intracranial bleeds and compartmental compression syndromes. Any combination of types of bleeding sites can be seen. A significant amount of microvascular thrombosis and, at times, large vessel thrombosis may also occur and may not be clinically obvious.

Clinical findings of chronic DIC

The clinical findings of chronic DIC are usually significantly different from those of acute DIC. Patients with chronic DIC more often have bothersome bleeding and diffuse thromboses rather than acute fulminant life-threatening hemorrhage. These patients have been appropriately described as having a "compensated DIC". In this instance there is usually an increased turnover and decreased survival of many components of the hemostasis system. Because of this, most coagulation laboratory parameters are near normal or normal. However, patients with chronic DIC almost uniformly have elevated fibrin(ogen) degradation products leading to impairment of fibrin monomer polymerization. In addition, they will have a platelet function defect resulting from the coating of platelet membranes by FDP. Thus, patients with chronic DIC often present with findings of gingival bleeding, easy and spontaneous bruising, large cutaneous ecchymoses, and mild to moderate mucosal membrane bleeding (often manifest as genitourinary or gastrointestinal hemorrhage). However, patients may also present with diffuse or singular thromboses.

Morphological findings in DIC

Morphological findings in DIC consist of characteristic but not pathognomonic peripheral smear findings as well as hemorrhage in any organ or combination of organs. It is again emphasized that any organ may be associated with rather severe hemorrhage in patients with acute or chronic DIC. Peripheral smear alterations typically seen in DIC include schistocytes and red cell fragments, including atypical "Heilmeyer helmet cells" (seen in about 50% of individuals with acute DIC). Most patients with acute DIC also present with a mild reticulocytosis and a mild leukocytosis usually associated with a mild to moderate shift to immature forms. The degree of thrombocytopenia is often obvious by examination of the peripheral blood smear.

In addition, many "large bizarre platelets" representing young platelets are usually seen on the peripheral smear in patients with DIC. This finding likely represents simply an increased population of young platelets caused by increased platelet turnover and decreased survival. Fig. 24-3 reveals a typical peripheral smear from a patient with acute DIC.

Laboratory abnormalities in DIC

With the complex pathophysiology described, laboratory findings of DIC may be highly variable, complex, and difficult to interpret. Likewise, evaluation of patients with DIC, especially with respect to significant laboratory tests useful for aiding in a diagnosis and monitoring therapy, remain confusing and sometimes controversial. The prothrombin time is prolonged in about 75% of patients with acute DIC, and in 25% the prothrombin time is normal or shortened. The activated partial thromboplastin time is prolonged in 50% to 60% of patients with acute DIC for many reasons. The thrombin time and reptilase time are also usually prolonged. They may be normal or shortened, however, in isolated cases.

The platelet count is usually significantly decreased in patients with acute DIC. However, the range may be as low as 2,000-3,000 per μL or greater than 100,000 per μL. In most patients the degree of thrombocytopenia is usually obvious by examination of a peripheral smear and averages around 60,000 per μL. Virtually all tests of platelet function will be abnormal in patients with DIC, but coagulation factor assays provide little, if any, information. Most patients with acute DIC have systemically circulating activated clotting factor, often factors Xa, IXa, or thrombin. Thus, coagulation factor assays done by the standard APTT-derived or prothrombin time-derived laboratory techniques using deficient substrates will render uninterpretable and meaningless results. Fibrin(ogen) degradation products are elevated in 85% to 100% of these

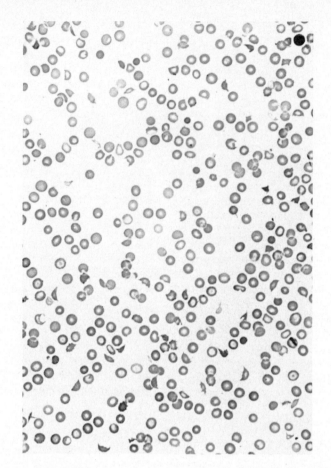

Fig. 24-3. Peripheral blood from a patient with DIC. Note the many red cell fragments.

patients. The protamine sulfate test or ethanol gelation test for circulating soluble fibrin monomer is positive in 80% to 85% of patients with acute and chronic DIC. Both elevated FDPs and circulating soluble fibrin monomer can be noted in other clinical situations as well, including women using oral contraceptives, patients with pulmonary emboli, some patients with myocardial infarction, patients with some renal diseases, and those with arterial, venous thrombotic, or thromboembolic events.

The antithrombin III test has become a key for diagnosis and monitoring of ther-

apy. In DIC there is an overwhelming generation of activated clotting factors (serine proteases) during activation (triggering), as well as during the ongoing intravascular coagulation event. When this occurs, there is an irreversible complexing of some circulating activating clotting factor with antithrombin III, thus leading to significant decreases of functional AT-III. Immunological assays for AT-III should not be used.

Increased platelet turnover and decreased platelet survival will usually be seen in these patients. Platelet factor 4 levels and beta thromboglobulin levels are newer assays that are markers of overall platelet reactivity and release. Either one may be highly useful in diagnosing DIC, as well as monitoring therapy. Both platelet factor 4 and beta thromboglobulin are elevated in most instances. However, it should be readily appreciated that neither of these modalities are diagnostic of DIC as they may be elevated in a wide variety of intravascular coagulation disorders, including pulmonary emboli, acute myocardial infarction, deep venous thrombosis, and in disorders associated with microvascular disease.

Fibrinopeptide A is commonly elevated in patients with DIC and is an overall assessment of hemostasis, much like platelet factor 4 and beta thromboglobulin. Fibrinopeptide A determinations may aid in assessing therapy. A newer modality, also available by radioimmunoassay, is that of B-beta 15-42 and related peptide determinations. Elevated levels of B-beta 15-42 and related peptides may, when performed in conjunction with fibrinopeptide A levels, add greatly to the differential diagnosis of DIC versus primary lysis.

Fibrinolytic system assays typically reveal decreased plasminogen levels and circulating plasmin. The degree of fibrinolytic activation can be assessed by measuring plasminogen and plasmin levels by synthetic substrate techniques. Measurement of fibrinolytic inhibitors, including fast-acting alpha-2-antiplasmin and slow-acting alpha-2-macroglobulin, may also help assess the overall fibrinolytic system in DIC patients. Recently, assays for tissue (endothelial) plasminogen activator (TPA) and TPA-inhibitor (TPA-I) have become available. These determinations may become useful in DIC patients.

A newer assay of major importance in DIC is the D-dimer assay. Recently, monoclonal antibodies have been harvested against D-dimer and a simple latex agglutination test is available for D-dimer detection. D-dimer signifies the presence of plasmin plus thrombin. It requires plasmin to create the D fragment, and thrombin is required to activate factor XIII to factor XIIIa to cross link the D fragments. Thus, the D-dimer assay is fibrin specific, unlike the FDP assay which measures fibrinogen and/or fibrin degradation products. This test may replace both the FDP assay and the protamine sulfate (or ethanol gelation) tests in diagnosing DIC. The D-dimer assay, being fibrin-degradation product specific and requiring thrombin for its formation, will be negative in instances of primary fibrino-(geno)lysis.

By understanding the pathophysiology of DIC it is clear that most tests of hemostasis will be highly altered and thus most common laboratory tests will be significantly abnormal. Useful tests are listed in Table 24-3. In general, this author does not indulge in "DIC panels" and prefers to let the clinical situation, in conjunction with

Table 24-3. Laboratory modalities available for evaluation of disseminated intravascular coagulation

Old methods (manual)	New methods (automated)
Prothrombin Time	AT-III*
Activated PTT	Plasminogen*
Thrombin time	Plasminogen activator*
Reptilase time	Plasmin*
Platelet count	Alpha-2-antiplasmin*
Fibrinogen level	Fibrinogen†
Soluble fibrin monomer (protamine/ETOH)	Fibrinopeptide A‡
	Fibrinopeptide B‡
	B-beta 15-42 peptides‡
FDP titer	Fibronectin†
Blood smear	Platelet survival
	Platelet factor‡
	Beta thromboglobulin‡
	Prostaglandin derivitives‡
	D-dimer assay†

*Synthetic substrate
†Immuno/ELISA
‡RIA

Table 24-4. Laboratory evaluation of chronic disseminated intravascular coagulation

Procedure	Typical findings
Platelet count	Usually normal/borderline
Fibrinogen	Normal or elevated
Factor VIII:C	Normal or elevated
Prothrombin time	Normal or fast
Activated PTT	Normal or fast
Schistocytes	Present in 90% of patients
Fibrin(ogen) degradation products	Usually elevated
Protamine sulfate	Usually positive
Fibrinopeptide A	Usually elevated
Plasminogen	Usually decreased
Plasmin	Usually present

Table 24-5. Reliability of laboratory tests in all types of disseminated intravascular coagulation

Procedure*	Pretherapy (% abnormal)	Posttherapy (% abnormal)
Elevated FDP	100	31
Decreased AT-III	89	8
Low platelets	89	18
Positive protamine test	89	10
Long prothrombin time	82	47
Long thrombin time	76	18
Low fibrinogen	71	5
Long reptilase time	66	58
Long activated PTT	63	21

*(Descending order of reliability)

judgement dictate which laboratory tests are to be obtained both initially and subsequent to therapy. None of these tests are diagnostic of DIC and, as in all areas of clinical medicine, laboratory modalities must be evaluated in the *appropriate clinical setting.* In addition, most of these laboratory tests are not specific. Typical laboratory findings of chronic DIC are significantly different from those seen in acute DIC. Many usual tests of hemostasis are normal or near normal and typical findings in chronic DIC are shown in Table 24-4.

Table 24-5 shows the probability of pretreatment and posttreatment coagulation abnormalities in all forms of DIC. Noting elevated fibrin(ogen) degradation products, elevated D-dimer, a depressed AT-III level, thrombocytopenia and a positive protamine sulfate test or ethanol gelation test appear to be the most reliable laboratory indices for confirming DIC and to help determine success of therapy. Traditional global tests, including the prothrombin time, thrombin time, fibrinogen level, reptilase time, and partial thromboplastin time, are less reliable. Molecular marker profiling for DIC is

Table 24-6. Molecular markers for the differential diagnosis of DIC versus primary lysis

Marker	DIC	Primary lysis
Fibrinopeptide A	Elevated	Normal
Fibrinopeptide B	Elevated	Normal
B-beta 15-42 peptide	Elevated	Normal
B-beta 1-42 peptide	Elevated	Elevated
B-beta 1-118 peptide	Elevated	Elevated
Platelet factor 4	Elevated	Normal
Beta-thromboglobulin	Elevated	Normal

now available and is automatable. These molecular markers are not only useful for diagnosing DIC, but are also useful for providing a differential diagnosis of DIC versus primary fibrinolysis or DIC versus TTP (Tables 24-6 and 24-7).

Therapy of disseminated intravascular coagulation

Acute disseminated intravascular coagulation. My approach to therapy in acute DIC

Table 24-7. Molecular markers for differential diagnosis of DIC versus TTP

Marker	DIC	TTP
6-keto-PGF-1-alpha	Normal	Decreased
Thromboxanes	Increased	Increased
Platelet factor 4	Increased	Increased
Beta-thromboglobulin	Increased	Increased
Plasminogen activator	Normal/ increased	Decreased
B-beta 15-42 peptide	Increased	Normal
Fibrinopeptide A	Increased	Normal
Fibrinopeptide B	Increased	Normal

SEQUENTIAL THERAPY OF ACUTE DISSEMINATED INTRAVASCULAR COAGULATION

Treat or remove the triggering process
Evacuate uterus
Antibiotics
Control shock
Volume replacement
Maintain blood pressure
Steroids ?
Antineoplastic therapy
Other indicated therapy

Stop intravascular clotting process
Subcutaneous heparin
Intravenous heparin ?
Antiplatelet agents
AT-III concentrate therapy

Component therapy as indicated
Platelet concentrates
Packed red cells (washed)
AT-III concentrate
Fresh frozen plasma
Cryoprecipitate (fibrinogen)
Prothrombin complex

Inhibit residual fibrino(geno)lysis
Aminocaproic acid

is somewhat vigorous and is summarized in the box at right. Although aggressive, it is associated with a high survival rate (76%) and low morbidity in patients with classical acute DIC. The most important therapy is treatment of the triggering disease process which is thought to be responsible for DIC.

In many instances removal of the triggering pathophysiology will stop the disease process and the classical example is an obstetrical accident. Anticoagulant therapy, especially heparin, is rarely (if ever) indicated in obstetrical accidents of any type. Simply evacuating the uterus or, in rare instances, hysterectomy will usually rapidly stop the intravascular clotting process. In septicemia, therapies include antibiotics, alleviation of shock, volume replacement, possibly steroids, and others to maintain hemodynamics. These will often cause significant blunting of the intravascular clotting process and may actually stop the DIC process. Each case must, of course, be evaluated on its merit depending upon the clinical situation and the dominant triggering event.

Most patients, except those suffering from DIC secondary to obstetrical accidents or massive liver failure, will often require anticoagulant therapy. Subcutaneous low-dose heparin has been this author's choice for the last 9 years. Anticoagulant therapy is indicated if the patient continues to bleed or clot significantly for about 4 hours after initiation of therapy. This time period depends upon the sites and severity of bleeding. With continued bleeding the patient is given subcutaneous calcium heparin at 80 to 100 units per kg every 4 to 6 hours as the clinical situation, site, severity of bleeding and thrombosis, and patient size dictates. With this approach one often notes cessation of antithrombin III consumption, lowering of FDP, and increases in fibrinogen levels. In addition, there will usually be slow or rapid correction of other abnormal laboratory modalities of acute DIC in 3 to 4 hours, followed shortly thereafter by blunting or cessation of clinically-significant hemorrhage and thrombosis.

Other anticoagulants available, depending upon the clinicians experience, are intravenous heparin, combination antiplatelet agents, or antithrombin III concentrates. Combination antiplatelet agents are far less effective in acute DIC, but may be called for as discussed later under chronic DIC. Acute DIC has been successfully treated with investigational antithrombin III concentrates in small groups of patients by several investigators.

Chronic disseminated intravascular coagulation. Therapy for chronic DIC is approached much differently than acute DIC. Most patients with chronic DIC do not suffer life-threatening hemorrhage. Instead, they have bothersome hemorrhage often associated with diffuse superficial or deep venous thrombosis and thromboembolus. Therapy for the underlying disease process is most important. In many instances, this will cease the intravascular clotting process and alleviate hemorrhage and thrombosis. Even if treatment for the triggering disease process responsible for intravascular coagulation does not stop the event, it will often blunt it so that bleeding or thrombosis ceases to be a clinical problem. If this first step is vigorously attempted and any combination of hemorrhage, thrombosis, and thromboembolus continues, anticoagulant therapy is indicated. Vigorous therapy may be contraindicated, as in some instances of malignancy, especially intracranial metastases. Combination antiplatelet therapy is often successful in stopping chronic DIC, provided attempts to treat the triggering pathophysiology are also used. Replacement therapy is not indicated unless the patient demonstrates significant component depletion. Inhibition of the fibrinolytic system with epsilon aminocaproic acid is also rarely, if ever, indicated.

LIVER DISEASE

Patients with acute and chronic liver disease have significant hemorrhage. This is a major challenge in clinical care, taxes the laboratory and local blood bank facilities, and is often the patient's terminal event. Alterations of hemostasis are complex and multifaceted. It has been taught that hemorrhage in chronic liver disease is caused by defective hepatocyte synthesis of the vitamin K-dependent prothrombin complex factors. These are factors II, VII, IX, and X. However, many other alterations of hemostasis, including primary hyperfibrinolysis, platelet function defects, and thrombocytopenia, must also be considered. DIC may play a role as chronic liver disease becomes terminal, however, it is more often significant in acute hepatic failure and biliary stasis.

The most common sequence of events in patients with chronic liver disease is development of a localized bleed, usually from a ruptured esophageal varix, peptic ulcer disease, or hemorrhagic gastritis. These bleeds tend to cascade into massive hemorrhage which is poorly responsive to usual therapies of massive transfusions with whole blood, fresh frozen plasma, plasma expanders, and vasopressin infusion. While many hemostasis defects are corrected (primarily defects in the prothrombin complex factors), many others are left unattended and effective hemostasis cannot be achieved (see box page 397).

Coagulation protein changes (impaired synthesis)

The hepatocyte is responsible for synthesizing factors I, II, V, VII, VIII:C, IX, X, XI, XII, and XIII; prekallikrein (Fletcher factor); high molecular weight kininogen (Fitzgerald, Flaujeac, Williams, Reid, and Fujiwara factors); as well as antithrombin III, alpha-2-macroglobulin, alpha-2-antiplasmin, and plasminogen. In addition, patients with chronic liver disease demonstrate abnor-

ALTERATIONS OF HEMOSTASIS IN LIVER DISEASE (IN DESCENDING ORDER OF PROBABILITY)

Acute

Defective (PIVKA) synthesis
Disseminated intravascular coagulation
Thrombocytopenia
Platelet dysfunction
Decreased factor synthesis

Chronic

Defective synthesis
Primary fibrino(geno)lysis
Thrombocytopenia
Platelet function defects
Vascular defects (poorly defined)
Disseminated intravascular coagulation
(terminal stages)

---

mal carboxylation leading to synthesis of PIVKAs (proteins induced by vitamin K absence/antagonists) or abnormal factors II, VII, IX, and X. The decrease in factor VII best correlates with the prothrombin time determination. However, decreases in factors IX and X best correlate with predisposition to clinical hemorrhage.

Patients with chronic liver disease may also synthesize defective fibrinogen, leading to pseudodysfibrinogenemia. As liver disease becomes "end-stage" there may also be decreased synthesis of factors V and VIII:C. Alternatively, these factors may be decreased simply due to significant activation of the fibrinolytic system and circulating plasminemia. Patients with acute hepatic failure of any etiology, especially viral, drug, or toxin/chemical induced, may develop a DIC-type syndrome. In addition, patients developing long term intrahepatic or extraheptic cholestasis by biliary obstruction often develop decreased synthesis of the vitamin K-dependent factors due to the inability of vitamin K to be used. Vitamin K is lipid soluble and thus may be malabsorbed in these obstructive syndromes. Thus, these patients will often demonstrate abnormal synthesis (PIVKA synthesis) of factors II, VII, IX, and X.

Enhanced destruction (primary fibrinolysis)

The manifestation of primary fibrino(geno)lysis is hemorrhage. Thromboses do not occur if this is an isolated hemostatic defect. The precise mechanisms of pathological activation of the fibrinolytic system in liver disease are unclear. Decreased inhibitors of the fibrinolytic system, primarily alpha-2-antiplasmin and alpha-2-macroglobulin may lead to pathological activation. This may be partially responsible for primary activation processes in liver disease and failure. Increased plasminogen activators may cause pathological activation. This mechanism, by way of poor hepatic clearance of activators, appears to be operative in hepatic cirrhosis. The end result of fibrinolysis in liver disease is biodegradation of many coagulation factors by plasmin and creation of fibrinogen/fibrin degradation products, which have serious deleterious effects on already compromised hemostasis.

Biological effects of fibrinogen/fibrin degradation products

The biological effects as fibrin(ogen) degradation products are formed from the plasmin-induced lysis of fibrinogen and fibrin are: (1) inhibition of the hemostasis system by interference with fibrin monomer polymerization, (2) an antithrombin effect, and (3) interference with platelet function. These fragments may also induce hyperpyrexia.

Laboratory manifestations of primary fibrinolysis

The consequences of circulating plasmin are elevated fibrinogen/fibrin degradation products. In association with these products are severe platelet dysfunction, plasmin-induced degradation of clotting factors, and elevation of B-beta 15-42 related peptides.

It is extremely important to recall that primary activation of the fibrinolytic system occurs in many instances of chronic liver disease. This defect in hemostasis must, like other defects, be recalled in the patient with liver disease and hemorrhage assessed from the laboratory standpoint.

Platelet defects

Thrombocytopenia. Thrombocytopenia is seen in up to 35% of patients with chronic liver disease (cirrhosis). The most common cause is portal hypertension with resultant congestive splenomegaly and hypersplenism. However, hypersplenism (increased splenic sequestration of platelets and other cellular elements) need not always be associated with significant splenomegaly. In most patients with chronic liver disease the degree of thrombocytopenia correlates with the degree of splenomegaly. In addition, the degree of splenomegaly correlates with the severity of hepatic damage. Hypersplenism results in decreased platelet survival; marrow megakaryocytes are usually normal to increased in number. Portacaval shunts will correct the thrombocytopenia of hypersplenism secondary to portal hypertension in about 30% of patients.

Thrombocytopenia may occur in patients with cirrhosis, secondary to folate deficiency, as a consequence of DIC in patients with chronic liver disease and in acute liver failure of viral-, drug-, or chemical etiology. The thrombocytopenia of acute viral hepatitis and hepatitis seen with mononucleosis or cytomegalovirus may be multifactorial. In these instances there may be an element of DIC contributing to or accounting for thrombocytopenia. There may also be selective suppression of megakaryopoiesis, or the thrombocytopenia may be part of a pancytopenia associated with marrow aplasia which occasionally occurs in patients with acute hepatic failure. In acute hepatic failure of viral, drug, or chemical etiology, thrombocytopenia may also result from development of antiplatelet antibodies or circulating immune complexes. In clinical practice, the thrombocytopenia of chronic or acute liver diseases usually is a summary of several or all mechanisms.

If the patient with chronic liver disease is also an alcoholic, additional mechanisms for development of thrombocytopenia may be operative. Thrombocytopenia is seen in up to 25% of ill patients who are actively drinking. One half of these will have concomitant cirrhosis. Persistent thrombocytopenia is usually caused by portal hypertension, splenomegaly, and associated hypersplenism. However, if it is primarily caused by acute ethanol intoxication rather than splenic sequestration, the thrombocytopenia will usually abate within 1 to 3 weeks after abstinence. A rebound thrombocytosis is seen in up to 30% of patients, and in some instances may be responsible for thrombotic episodes.

The degree that thrombocytopenia contributes to hemorrhage in the patient with liver disease is unclear. Not only are the causes of thrombocytopenia multifaceted, but thrombocytopenia is only one of many alterations of hemostasis in patients with acute or chronic liver disease. Thus, thrombocytopenia should be thought of as being part of a summation of events when hemorrhage is present.

Platelet function defects. Significant platelet dysfunction also occurs in patients with liver disease and hemorrhage, although this hemostatic defect is less appreciated and often goes unrecognized. As with thrombocytopenia, causes of platelet dysfunction in these patients may be multifactorial. Most patients with chronic liver disease have primary activation of the fibrinolytic system and resultant elevated circulating fibrin(ogen) degradation products (FDPs). These circulating FDPs may severely compromise platelet function. Patients with both acute and chronic liver disease often demonstrate secondary aggregation defects or storage pool-type aggregation defects. These are manifested as blunted aggregation to collagen, thrombin, and ristocetin, and absent secondary aggregation waves after aggregation with ADP and epinephrine. In addition, platelet factor 3 release is commonly impaired. Platelet dysfunction in liver disease may be the effects of altered platelet membrane palmitate and/or stearate metabolism, the result from coating of platelet membranes by fibrin(ogen) degradation products, or a combination of these defects. They may also be a manifestation of undefined alterations in platelet metabolic pathways.

Laboratory findings

Liver disease will cause most tests of hemostasis, including global screening tests, to be markedly abnormal. Laboratory alterations will be a summation of not only the underlying defect (for example, acute liver disease, chronic liver disease, or cholestatic liver disease), but will also be a manifestation of all defects that are present singularly or in combination (see accompanying box).

The mainstay laboratory test for assessing function of prothrombin complex factors is the prothrombin time. In significantly decreased or dysfunctional synthesis of factors II, VII, IX, and X, the prothrombin time will be significantly prolonged. Whether the degree of prolongation is related to clinical hemorrhage is controversial. The decrease in factor VII closely correlates with prolongation of the prothrombin time. However, decreased/dysfunctional synthesis of factors IX and X more closely correlate with clinical hemorrhage. The activated partial thromboplastin time is likewise prolonged in a patient with acute or chronic liver disease.

Tests for fibrinolysis will be abnormal in greater than 75% of patients with chronic liver disease, and may be abnormal in patients with acute hepatic failure or cholestasis if DIC and secondary fibrinolysis are

---

LABORATORY MODALITIES FOR ASSESSING HEMOSTASIS IN LIVER DISEASE

Impaired factor synthesis

Prothrombin time
Partial thromboplastin time
Thrombin time

Primary fibrino(geno)lysis

FDPs
Plasminogen
Plasmin

Thrombocytopenia

Platelet count

Platelet dysfunction

Template bleeding time
Platelet aggregation

Vascular dysfunction

Template bleeding time

---

present. Circulating plasmin and elevated FDP will be found in conjunction with decreased levels of plasminogen due to activation of the fibrinolytic system and plasminogen depletion. Good differential diagnostic tools for noting whether DIC is operative or whether low levels of clotting factors are present because of primary lysis are the B-beta 15-42 and related peptide determinations, FDP and D-dimer levels in conjunction with fibrinopeptide A, the platelet release proteins (platelet factor 4, and beta thromboglobulin) and a positive or negative paracoagulation reaction.

Tests of platelet function will likewise be abnormal. Prolongation of the template bleeding time may be caused by a combination of platelet function defects previously discussed. Other causes may include thrombocytopenia and/or defects in vasculature of patients with acute or chronic liver disease.

A thrombin time and/or reptilase time will offer an indication of the degree of dysfibrinogenemia or hypofibrinogenemia. However, both will also be prolonged in the face of FDPs, making the results difficult to interpret. Most tests of hemostasis will be markedly abnormal in patients with chronic or acute liver disease or cholestasis. Only a well-chosen hemostatic profile can assess each component of hemostasis in conjunction with knowing what liver disease is present and the defect or combination of defects identified.

Summary

Hemorrhage in the patient with chronic liver disease can no longer be contributed to a simple decrease in synthesis of factors II, VII, IX, and X. Many defects may occur and when significant or life-threatening hemorrhage develops, it may be caused by any combination of them. In the patient with hemorrhage in chronic liver disease, it is a major clinical and clinical laboratory challenge to define defects most likely at fault and deliver effective therapy. If primary hyperfibrino(geno)lysis is the major cause of hemorrhage, as it often is, the appropriate therapy is antifibrinolytic therapy. Fresh frozen plasma may be used to correct hemorrhage associated with decreased/dysfunctional synthesis of factors II, VII, IX, and X. If significant thrombocytopenia or platelet dysfunction is present, infusion of platelet concentrates is indicated. Thus, one must recall all defects and document the presence or absence of DIC when designing therapy.

ACQUIRED CIRCULATING ANTICOAGULANTS

Acquired circulating anticoagulants (inhibitors) directed against single or several factors are interesting but extremely rare causes of clinical hemorrhage. Acquired circulating anticoagulants are commonly associated with reasonably well-defined disease entities, drugs, or other clinical situations and may occur in otherwise normal individuals. Any coagulation factor may be af-

fected. This section is concerned with acquired circulating anticoagulants in otherwise hemostatically healthy individuals and will not discuss circulating anticoagulants as complications in patients with congenital coagulation factor defects.

Clearly the most common circulating anticoagulants of clinical significance are fibrin(ogen) degradation products. The next most common is that of malignant paraprotein. In addition, when suspecting circulating anticoagulants one must also consider Munchausen syndrome, the deliberate self-administration of warfarin-type drugs or heparin. In hospitalized patients one must recall the potentially unrecorded use of heparin to keep intravenous lines open.

Acquired inhibitors occurring in noncongenitally deficient patients are divided into two types. The first includes inhibitors which inactivate individual coagulation factors, often in a progressive, usually irreversible, time-dependent manner. Most are immunoglobulins (specific antifactor antibodies) and comprise most of this section. Subtyping of these reveal most of the immunoglobulins to be IgG and the most common subtype is IgG_4. Kappa light chains are more common than lambda light chains in circulating IgG anticoagulants.

The second type of circulating inhibitor is characterized by being reversible (or partially reversible), immediate in action, representing a strictly protein-protein interaction (complex formation) with either a specific coagulation factor or group of factors. These anticoagulants often do not destroy the coagulation factor and its biological activity may be recovered if the complex can be dissociated. These are most often seen in malignant or benign paraprotein disorders with the interaction being between paraprotein and a specific clotting factor or group of factors. Circulating anticoagulants should be strongly suspected when an otherwise healthy individual develops unexplained bleeding or when coagulation testing gives contradictory or confusing results.

Acquired inhibitors to specific coagulation factors

Fibrinogen (factor I) inhibitors. Less than 10 cases of acquired inhibitors to fibrinogen have been reported. Of these, two have occurred in transfused afibrinogenemic patients. In noncongenital deficient patients, the anticoagulant has been associated with autoimmune disorders (two cases of systemic lupus), chronic inflammatory disorders (chronic active hepatitis) and in a patient with Down's syndrome. In addition, one case was reported in a multiple transfused patient who most likely had DIC. In cases studied the antibody was identified as an IgG, and in one case the antibody was found to interfere with release of fibrinopeptide A. In some patients a mild hemorrhagic tendency has been present, but in others no abnormal clinical hemostasis defects were encountered.

Factor II inhibitors

Antiprothrombin (factor II) antibodies in cases of noncongenital factor II deficiency are extremely rare and have only been seen in patients with systemic lupus erythematosus. In this instance a clear-cut distinction from a specific anti-II antibody versus a lupus anticoagulant has remained unclear.

Factor V inhibitors

Acquired antibody to factor V has occurred in at least 16 patients. In almost 70% of patients developing an anti-factor V antibody, development of the antibody was preceded by a surgical procedure. To further complicate etiological mechanisms, 50% of the surgical patients reported had ingested streptomycin as part of their operative course. An anti-factor V antibody has also been associated with the use of streptomycin in several nonsurgical patients. Most patients have had a mild bleeding problem, but bleeding has been severe or fatal in a few cases. Both IgG and IgM immunoglobulins have been incriminated. Therapy, when necessary, is generally limited to fresh frozen plasma. However, one patient was treated successfully with platelet concentrates.

Factor VII inhibitors

Anti-factor VII antibodies have only been reported once and this was in association with a case of probable carcinoma of the lung. The antibody was determined to be an IgG. Surgery was not performed because of abnormal hemostasis studies. Thus, the diagnosis was not confirmed and the cell type remains unknown.

Factor VIII:C inhibitors

Anti-VIII antibodies occur in 8% to 10% of patients with hemophilia A. These were previously discussed. Anti-VIII antibodies are one of the more common circulating anticoagulants occurring in otherwise healthy individuals and in selected clinical situations. Therefore, they should be suspected in healthy individuals who suddenly develop an unexplained hemorrhagic diathesis. In addition, an anti-VIII antibody is the most likely circulating anticoagulant in the nonlupus patient who develops a circulating anticoagulant in the absence of malignant paraprotein or elevated fibrin(ogen) degradation products. A survey of 215 nonhemophiliac patients with inhibitors to factor VIII found that more than 46% had no underlying disease condition, 8% had developed an anti-VIII antibody in association with rheumatoid arthritis, more than 7% developed an anti-VIII antibody in the course of a normal postpartum state, almost 7% were associated with a disseminated malignancy, slightly more than 5% were associated with drug ingestion, an equal number were associated with systemic lupus, more than 4% were associated with less common autoimmune disorders, an equal number were associated with dermatological disorders, and about 10% were thought to be caused by other rare clinical disorders. The peak incidence was in individuals 50 to 80 years of age and this group contained more than 65% of patients in this survey who developed an anti-VIII antibody.

This survey also indicated that patients developing a circulating anticoagulant in association with an autoimmune disorder fared rather poorly and persistence of the antibody and/or death occurred in 36% of patients. The rest survived with the use of immunosuppressive therapy. When evaluating the cases in this large survey, 56% survived development of an antiplatelet antibody and 44% died from a hemorrhagic complication of the circulating anti-VIII antibody. Of those surviving, most received immunosuppressive therapy. Of those not surviving, 62% received no immunosuppressive therapy. This large survey confirms the suggestions of others that the use of immunosuppressive therapy in nonhemophilic patients who develop an anti-VIII antibody is clearly warranted. Interestingly, nonhemophilic patients who develop an acquired anti-VIII antibody do not usually suffer the types of bleeding usually associated with hemophilia A. Therefore, they rarely have intraarticular bleeding, deep intramuscular bleeding, or intracranial bleeding. They more commonly have large subcutaneous ecchymoses.

von Willebrand (factor VIII:vW) inhibitors

Acquired von Willebrand's disease, or development of an acquired anticoagulant to the von Willebrand portion of the factor VIII macromolecular complex, has been reported in over 20 individuals. Most have had an autoimmune disorder, lymphoma, myeloproliferative/myelodysplastic syndrome, or a malignant paraprotein disorder. One individual developed an anti-von Willebrand Factor antibody after pesticide exposure and one was noted to develop in a patient with Wilms' tumor. In the patient with Wilms' tumor the antibody improved with surgical resection of the malignancy. In most instances, the bleeding has not been severe and has been compatible with a mild acquired von Willebrand's-type syndrome. Therapy has been that of immunosuppression, cryoprecipitate, and other measures to control the underlying disease process whether it be myeloma, other paraprotein disorders, or autoimmunity.

Factor IX inhibitors

Anti-IX antibodies only rarely occur in patients with rheumatic fever and nonhemophilia B. The most common clinical situation in which they occur are postpartum females and patients with systemic lupus. Like anti-VIII antibodies in the nonhemophilic patient, the anti-IX antibody often abates with immunosuppressive therapy in the form of prednisone, azathioprine, or cyclophosphamide.

Factor X inhibitors

Only two cases of an anti-X antibody have been reported. Both occurred in patients with leprosy. One patient was ingesting dapsone. However, the patient was untreated at the time of developing the antibody and thus leprosy, rather than drug ingestion, appeared to be the common denominator. Neither patient had a clinically-significant bleeding diathesis. Of more clinical relevance is the association of a selective factor X deficiency associated with systemic amyloidosis. Although an anti-X antibody has not clearly been found in the circulation, it is thought that amyloid fibrils may selectively bind with factor X and remove it from the circulation. Thus, although a "circulating anticoagulant" can not be demonstrated, it appears that amyloid may represent an extra circulatory factor X inhibitor through interaction of factor X and amyloid fibrils.

Factor XI inhibitors

Anti-XI antibodies in noncongenital patients have occurred in only 11 individuals. Ten have had an autoimmune disorder and one suffered pneumonia thought to be caused by an adenovirus.

Factor XII inhibitors

Anti-factor XII antibody has only been reported in systemic lupus, in Waldenström's macroglobulinemia, and in a patient with glomerulonephritis. A severe deficiency of factor XII has been found in association with angioimmunoblastic lymphadenopathy, but a circulating anticoagulant has not been demonstrated.

Factor XIII inhibitors

Acquired anti-XIII antibody has occurred in at least eight otherwise hemostatically normal individuals. Most had received isoniazid therapy and one developed an anti-XIII antibody in the face of a drug-induced systemic lupus-type syndrome. It is thought that the inhibitor either reacts with the thrombin activation site on the alpha chain of factor XIII or prevents fibrin cross-linking by reacting with sites on fibrinogen. Some individuals developing an anti-XIII antibody have had associated profuse bleeding.

Lupus inhibitors

The lupus anticoagulant has long been described. Several reviews have shed light on the nature of this elusive "anticoagulant". Lupus anticoagulants have been defined as immunoglobulins interfering with phospholipid dependent tests of coagulation. Unlike the other factors previously discussed, lupus anticoagulants do not inhibit activity of specific coagulation factors; these may occur in up to 10% of patients with systemic lupus erythematosus (SLE).

The frequency of bleeding due to the lupus anticoagulant is clearly less than 1% of patients developing it. Of interest, almost one fourth of the patients with SLE plus the lupus anticoagulant will have a concomitant significant prothrombin deficiency and over 40% will have significant associated thrombocytopenia. In this regard, bleeding in association with the lupus anticoagulant almost always occurs in patients with associated hypoprothrombinemia and/or thrombocytopenia and there is no reported increase in surgical hemorrhage in patients with the lupus anticoagulant alone.

Another unclear feature is that isolated prothrombin deficiency may occur in patients with SLE who do not have the lupus anticoagulant. In this instance the mechanism(s) remain unknown. Infusions of plasma have failed to correct the isolated factor II deficiency in lupus patients, suggesting the presence of an anti-factor II antibody as previously discussed.

A laboratory characteristic of lupus anticoagulants is that all phospholipid-dependent coagulation tests are prolonged, including the prothrombin time, activated partial thromboplastin time, and Russell's viper venom time. Of these tests, the activated PTT appears to be the most sensitive. When studying lupus it is important to recognize that if the prothrombin time is significantly prolonged (defined as a prothrombin ratio of greater than 2.0), hypoprothrombinemia rather than the lupus anticoagulant should be suspected. It has also been clearly shown that sensitivity of the activated PTT to the lupus anticoagulant is highly dependent upon the reagents used. It has been noted that platelet-poor plasma enhances the sensitivity of the phospholipid dependent tests to the presence of the lupus anticoagulant. Also, platelet rich plasma may diminish the test's sensitivity to lupus anticoagulants and may mask their presence.

Two lupus anticoagulant assays are popular. The first is a prothrombin time in which the thromboplastin is diluted. The thromboplastin is diluted to give a normal time of 60 seconds. When noting a time of 65 seconds or longer, a lupus anticoagulant is considered present. A problem with this test is that it may miss IgM lupus anticoagulants.

It has been suggested that a superior test is a modified Russell's viper venom time in which the venom is diluted to give a normal time of 23 to 27 seconds. The phospholipid is then diluted to a minimal level which will continue to support this range. A prolongation of this system will not correct with a mixture of patient and normal plasma. In addition, the advantage of this system is that both IgG and IgM lupus anticoagulants are thought to be detected. It is interesting to note that biological false-positive tests for syphilis are seen in up to 40% of patients with systemic lupus. However, biological false tests for syphilis are seen in more than 50% and up to 90% of patients with systemic lupus plus the lupus anticoagulant. In addition, it should be recognized that almost 40% of patients with biological false-positive tests for syphilis will have a lupus anticoagulant and in this clinical setting the lupus anticoagulant should be sought.

Thromboembolism occurs in about 10% of patients with systemic lupus. However, if a patient with SLE also has the lupus anticoagulant, thromboembolism is a complication in 25% to 50% of cases.

Lupus anticoagulants may occur in normal individuals and in other disease states and may occur in association with drug ingestion. The most commonly cited drugs are chlorpromazine or procainamide hydrochloride.

Summary

This section has summarized rare clinical instances of acquired circulating anticoagulants in noncongenitally deficient patients. Although these circulating anticoagulants are interesting and may, on rare occasion, give rise to clinically significant or fatal hemorrhage, it should be kept in mind that they are extremely rare. Circulating fibrin-(ogen) degradation products and malignant paraprotein acting as circulating anticoagulants are far more common causes of clinically significant hemorrhage. The circulating anticoagulants in the absence of circulating fibrin(ogen) degradation products or paraprotein most likely to be found are an anti-factor VIII antibody or the lupus anticoagulant.

BLOOD PROTEIN DEFECTS ASSOCIATED WITH HYPERCOAGULABILITY AND THROMBOSIS

Hypercoagulability and thrombosis remain poorly understood. In at least half of patients undergoing thrombotic or thromboembolic events, a definitive etiological reason is not identifiable. The discovery of new inhibitor systems and congenital deficiencies may allow definition of the etiology in many patients experiencing arterial or venous thrombotic events. We are just beginning to understand etiological aspects and develop diagnostic tools for assessment of hypercoagulable and thrombotic disorders. In general, as described over 100 years ago, there are only three primary factors in thrombus formation. These are: (1) changes in the blood flow, (2) changes in the circulating blood, and (3) changes in the vessel wall. Factors associated with an increased risk of arterial or venous thrombotic or thromboembolic events are listed in the box on page 405. This section will be limited to a discussion of hereditary and acquired blood protein defects associated with thrombosis and thromboembolus, as listed in the box on page 405.

Antithrombin III defects

Antithrombin III is an alpha-2-globulin with a molecular weight of about 65,000 daltons. In the absence of heparin, antithrombin III appears to inactivate thrombin and other serine proteases in a progressive, irreversible manner. In addition, antithrombin III inactivates other serine proteases, including factors Xa, IXa, XIa, XIIa, and kallikrein, although with less efficiency than its inhibition of thrombin. In the presence of heparin, inactivation of thrombin and Xa by antithrombin III is markedly accelerated and almost instantaneous. The physiologic range of antithrombin III in normal human blood is quite narrow. Moderate decreases of antithrombin III are often of significant clinical relevance with re-

THROMBOSIS/THROMBOEMBOLUS RISK FACTORS

Arterial
Atherosclerosis
Male sex
Cigarette use
Hypertension
Diabetes mellitus
LDL Cholesterol
Hypertriglyceridemia
Family history
High hematocrit
Left ventricular hypertrophy
Oral contraceptive use
Venous
Obesity
Oral contraceptive use
Varicose veins
Infection
Trauma
Surgery
General anesthesia
Pregnancy
Malignancy
Immobility
Congestive heart failure
Nephrotic syndrome
Blood protein defects

BLOOD PROTEIN DEFECTS ASSOCIATED WITH HYPERCOAGULABILITY AND THROMBOSIS

Antithrombin III deficiency
Protein C deficiency
Protein S deficiency
Plasminogen deficiency
Dysfibrinogenemia
Tissue plasminogen activator (t-P.A.) deficiency
Heparin cofactor II deficiency
Cystathionine beta synthetase deficiency
Factor XII deficiency
Lupus anticoagulant
Anticardiolipin antibodies

spect to thrombus formation or thromboembolus.

Infants have about half of normal adult antithrombin III levels; however, the adult level is reached at an early age. The mechanisms by which a potential deficiency of antithrombin III may occur are: (1) a defect in synthesis which may occur in the congenital form, as well as in several acquired forms such as liver disease, (2) increased consumption of antithrombin III resulting from generation of pathological levels of serine proteases as might be expected to occur in DIC-type syndromes, extensive deep venous thrombosis, massive pulmonary embolization, and diffuse small and large venous and arterial thrombo-occlusive events, (3) loss of antithrombin III from the

intracellular compartment as may occur with selected renal diseases, and (4) increased protein catabolism.

Hereditary Defects of Antithrombin III. Hereditary thrombophilia or congenital deficiency of antithrombin III is usually inherited as an autosomal dominant disease. However, variant inheritance has also been described. In most patients with classic hereditary deficiency of antithrombin III there appears to be a reduced synthesis of a biologically normal antithrombin III molecule. However, hereditary deficiency of antithrombin III may also be associated with a dysfunctional antithrombin III molecule as well. Thus, the absence and dysfunctional forms exist. The incidence appears to be between 1 and 2,000 to 5,000.

Patients with classical hereditary deficiency of antithrombin III have an increased risk of venous thrombotic events and pulmonary embolism. These events typically appear in mid to late teenagers. The most common sites of thrombosis are deep venous structures of the lower extremities. However, an additional characteristic site of thrombosis is the mesenteric veins. The classical presentation is that of recurrent deep venous thrombosis with or without pulmonary embolization. From the family studies reported, it appears that the deficiency of antithrombin III need not be especially severe for thrombotic events to occur. Some individuals have deep venous thrombosis and pulmonary emboli at between 50% and 70% biological activity whereas others with low antithrombin III levels may not suffer thrombosis at all. Thus, heterozygotes are certainly also at an increased risk for severe venous thrombotic and thromboembolic events. Many patients with hereditary thrombophilia treated with oral anticoagulants have an increase in antithrombin III levels after the initiation of therapy. However, some patients are reported to be unresponsive to oral anticoagulant therapy and demonstrate no significant increases in antithrombin III levels. Very potent antithrombin III concentrates for treating hereditary antithrombin III deficiency are recently available.

Acquired defects of antithrombin III. Acquired AT-III deficiency may be seen in patients with extensive deep venous thrombosis or extensive thromboembolic disease. In addition, AT-III deficiency is commonly seen in patients with DIC and in patients with severe liver disease and impaired protein synthesis. Some women using oral contraceptives, especially estrogen containing preparations, may demonstrate decreased AT-III levels. However, the significance remains unclear. Patients with nephrotic syndrome and significant proteinuria often have marked decreases of AT-III through urinary loss. The nephrotic syndrome is commonly associated with increased risk of thrombotic and thromboembolic disease.

Antithrombin III determinations

Patient populations considered candidates for antithrombin III are determined by: (1) a history of deep venous thrombosis or pulmonary embolus, (2) active deep venous thrombosis or pulmonary embolus, (3) recurrent thrombotic event during heparin therapy, (4) preoperative patients with a family history of deep venous thrombosis or pulmonary embolus, (5) DIC or related syndrome, (6) significant proteinuria, (7) family history of deep venous thrombosis or pulmonary embolus, (8) inadequate prolongation of an activated partial thromboplastin time or other global clotting tests while on intravenous heparin, (9) patients receiving subcutaneous or intrapulmonary heparin, and (10) possibly, patients who are considering taking oral contraceptives, but indications are not clearly established.

Heparin cofactor II deficiency

Heparin cofactor II is a protein of molecular weight 66,000 daltons. Like AT-III, heparin cofactor II inhibitory activity is markedly accelerated by addition of heparin. However, the dose at which acceleratory activity occurs is much higher than necessary for AT-III. Heparin cofactor II is a more limited serine protease inhibitor than AT-III and only demonstrates inhibitory activity against thrombin and chymotrypsin. There appears to be no inhibitory activity against factors Xa, IXa or XIa. The first case of congenital deficiency was described in 1985 and since then subsequent congenitally deficient patients with thrombosis have been reported. However, many heterozygous patients with HC-II deficiency have now been found that have not yet suffered thrombotic or thromboembolic events. Thus, the actual incidence of thrombosis associated with this deficiency is yet to be determined.

Protein C defects

Protein C is a newly rediscovered vitamin K-dependent protein which also appears to be a major inhibitor of the procoagulant system and may actually exceed the importance of antithrombin III. Protein C was first discovered in 1960 by Mammen, Thomas, and Seegers. These investigators also noted the inhibitory nature of protein C.

Protein C was rediscovered in 1976 by Stenflo. Seegers and coworkers, in 1976, quickly demonstrated that their initial protein C, originally called autoprothrombin II-A, and Stenflo's rediscovered protein C were the same inhibitory protein. Protein C is synthesized in the hepatocyte and has a molecular weight of about 56,000 daltons. It exerts its primary inhibitory activity by inactivating factors V and VIII:C. To perform this inactivation, protein C must first be activated by thrombin. Thrombin which activates protein C to protein Ca (activated form) must first be bound to endothelial thrombomodulin. Following binding to endothelial thrombomodulin thrombin acquires its ability to activate protein C. The inhibitory activity of protein C in degrading factors V and VIII:C is markedly enhanced by protein S, another vitamin K-dependent factor. This factor was discovered in 1977 by DiSchipio in Seattle, hence the designation protein S. The mechanisms by which protein S accentuate activated protein C in degrading factors V and VIII:C, which must occur in the presence of phospholipid, remains unclear.

Congenital deficiency of protein C. Congenital deficiency of protein C is inherited as an autosomal dominant trait, and the clinical characteristics are amazingly similar to congenital antithrombin III deficiency. Recurrent deep venous thrombosis and pulmonary embolus begins to typically occur in the late teenage years. Two forms of the disease exist. Patients may have an absence of the protein (CRM− form) or may have a dysfunctional protein (CRM+ form). Absence of the protein appears to be more common. In addition, like antithrombin III deficiency, venous thrombi and thromboemboli (especially pulmonary emboli) commonly occur in heterozygous patients as well as homozygous patients. Most homozygous patients have succumbed to thrombi and thromboemboli during early infancy. One homozygous infant is surviving with the prophylactic use of a protein C-containing prothrombin complex concentrate. It has recently been noted that many patients with protein C deficiency develop skin necrosis with warfarin-type drugs.

Congenital protein C deficiency may be a more common cause of thrombosis or thromboembolus than antithrombin III deficiency. The incidence of congenital protein C deficiency will only become known when assays become more available. It should be noted, however, that many protein C assays, some fully automated, are available for the clinical laboratory. It is known that congenital antithrombin III deficiency accounts for about 4% of patients presenting with deep venous thrombosis or pulmonary embolus. However, preliminary estimations suggest that congenital protein C deficiency may account for up to 10% of patients presenting with venous thrombosis or pulmonary embolus.

Acquired protein C deficiency. Acquired protein C deficiency is commonly seen in patients with acute DIC, extensive deep venous thrombosis, and severe liver disease. In addition, protein C levels may be decreased in postoperative patients, but the role of this decrease in contributing to or causing postoperative deep venous thrombosis remains unclear. Assays for protein C biological and immunological activity are available and in most instances can be readily automated by synthetic substrate technique for biological reactivity or immunological activity.

Protein S defects

Although the incidence of congenital protein S deficiency remains to be determined, it appears to be a more common defect than congenital AT-III deficiency. It appears to be inherited as an autosomal dominant, since heterozygotes and homozygotes suffer increased predisposition to venous thrombosis and thromboembolism. The clinical characteristics appear to be similar to those of congenital AT-III or protein C deficiency.

Acquired protein S deficiency occurs in women using oral contraceptives, during pregnancy, in patients with nephrotic syndrome, in type I diabetes mellitus, and in patients with deep venous thrombosis. Of course both protein S and C are decreased in patients taking warfarin drugs.

Congenital plasminogen deficiency

Congenital plasminogen deficiency is rare. However, this deficiency may be found to be much more common than previously suspected with the availability of reliable and simple plasminogen assays by synthetic substrate methodology. The disorder is inherited as an autosomal recessive trait. Both the absence form (CRM−) and the dysfunctional form (CRM+) have been described, although the dysfunctional form appears to be more common. Patients clinically demonstrate similarities to congenital antithrombin III deficiency and congenital protein C deficiency. Congenital deficient plasminogen patients begin to experience thrombotic events in their late teenage years. The most common thrombotic events are deep venous thrombosis and pulmonary embolization, occurring when the plasminogen level is less than 40% of normal biological activity.

Both homozygous and heterozygous patients can be identified by synthetic substrate assays for biological activity of plasminogen. Additionally, a comparison of biological activity with immunological levels may be used to identify patients with dysfunctional plasminogen versus those with quantitative hypoplasminogenemia (heterozygotes) or aplasminogenemia (homozygotes). Usual global tests of coagulation, including the platelet count, prothrombin time, partial thromboplastin time, thrombin time, and bleeding time, are normal and the diagnosis depends on specific plasminogen assays for biological activity performed by synthetic substrate methods. Successful therapy has included heparin,

warfarin-type drugs, antiplatelet agents, and, interestingly, urokinase.

Acquired plasminogen deficiency

Acquired plasminogen deficiency is seen in patients with severe liver disease and in those with DIC. In addition, decreased plasminogen levels are noted postoperatively and in patients with extensive thrombotic or thromboembolic disorders. It is also found in some infants and adults with respiratory distress syndrome (hyaline membrane diseases.)

Congenital dysfibrinogenemia

Most congenital dysfibrinogenemias are associated with hemorrhage. However, several are associated with a thrombotic tendency. Those associated with thrombosis are fibrinogens Baltimore, Chapel Hill, Charlottesville, Copenhagen, Marburg, Naples, New York, Oslo I, Paris II, and Wiesbaden. None of the acquired dysfibrinogenemias have yet been associated with a thrombotic tendency.

Lupus anticoagulants and thrombosis

Lupus anticoagulants are not associated with a hemorrhagic tendency. However, patients with the lupus anticoagulant are at increased risk of thrombosis or thromboembolic disease. The lupus anticoagulant was discussed previously.

Antiphospholipid syndromes and thrombosis

Patients with anticardiolipin antibodies are at increased risk of both arterial and venous thrombotic and thromboembolic disease. This risk is seen with IgG, IgA or IgM anticardiolipin antibodies. Three clinical syndromes appear to exist with these antiphospholipid antibodies: (1) deep venous thrombosis and pulmonary embolus, (2) cerebrovascular and retinal arterial occlusive disease, and (3) cardiac and large arterial occlusive disease, including coronary artery occlusion and thrombo-occlusive disease of the aorta and other great vessels.

Tissue (endothelial) plasminogen activator (t-P.A.) defects

Hereditary deficiency of t-P.A. or t-P.A. release appears to be very rare. The congenital form was first reported in 1978 and is inherited as an autosomal dominant trait. The clinical manifestations are similar to those noted with AT-III, protein C and protein S deficiency and primarily consist of venous thrombotic disease. From the few reports available, it seems that a high probability of venous thrombosis exists if an individual has the defect.

Case History

CASE 1: HEMOPHILIA A

The patient is a 29-year-old black female referred after a prehysterectomy evaluation revealed an activated PTT of 63.0 seconds and a normal prothrombin time (11.5 seconds). Historically, the patient related that her son was a "bleeder" and two brothers, living outside of the area, were also "bleeders". However, she did not know their diagnoses. Further history revealed that she did not take medications and had never received a blood transfusion. Past medical history was positive for both gonorrhea and syphilis, both successfully treated. Her only past bleeding had been associated with childbirth, but did not require transfusion therapy. She denied a history of easy or spontaneous bruising, petechiae, purpura, epistaxis, hemoptysis, gingival bleeding, or hematuria. She also denied excessive menstrual flow until 2 months ago and denied intramenstrual bleeding or spotting.

Physical examination was unremarkable.

Initial laboratory evaluation:
Prothrombin time = 12.0 sec.
APTT = 59.5 sec.
Template bleeding time = 4.0 min.
White Blood Cell Count = 5,700/μL
Hemoglobin = 11.1 gm/dL
Hematocrit = 35.4%

Indices are normal
Platelet count = 331,000/μL

Additional laboratory studies:
Factor VIII:C = 26%
Factor VIII: vW = 118%
Factor VIII:RAg = 80%

Diagnosis: This patient is a carrier of hemophilia A. Although it is unusual for these individuals to bleed, if the factor VIII:C level is low enough, carriers may bleed, especially if subjected to surgery or trauma.

Treatment for abdominal hysterectomy: Patient was given DDAVP (desmopressin), 0.3 micrograms per kg (=22 micrograms) IV in 50 mL. D5/water over 20 minutes, given 30 minutes before surgery, in conjunction with EACA (5 gm/ IV over 15 minutes, *preceding* the DDAVP). Factor VIII:C level was 128% after DDAVP administration and the patient tolerated the surgical procedure well.

CASE 2: DISSEMINATED INTRAVASCULAR COAGULATIONS

The patient was a 55-year-old white female initially complaining to her physician of left hip pain and a 3 month history of easy and spontaneous bruising, lethargy and fatigue. Four days after her original complaints, she suddenly developed more severe hip pain and the inability to ambulate. At the same time she spontaneously developed a large ecchymosis of the left hip which, in a few hours, had extravasated up into the left lateral chest wall approaching the axilla. At this time, she presented to an emergency room.

Physical examination revealed the patient to be pale, to have numerous petechiae and purpura, and to demonstrate the large ecchymosis.

Initial laboratory evaluation in the emergency room revealed a hemoglobin of 9.7 gm/dL, a total white cell count of 165,000/μL, a platelet count of 112,000/μL, a prothrombin time of 13.9 seconds and a partial thromboplastin time of 43.0 seconds. A peripheral blood smear was reviewed and is shown in Fig. 24-4. Based on this information the patient was admitted.

More detailed laboratory evaluation after admission revealed an elevated uric acid, elevated LDH, and elevated GGT, SGOT, and alkaline phosphatase. In addition the AT-III was

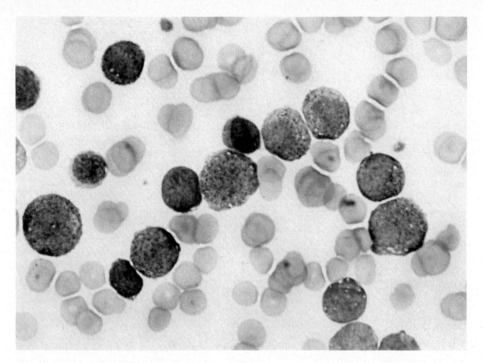

Fig. 24-4.   Peripheral blood from a patient with acute promyelocytic leukemia and DIC.

52%, FDP were > 80 mg/dL, the fibrinogen was 65 mg/dL, the protamine sulfate test was positive and both the thrombin time (19 seconds) and reptilase time (32 seconds) were prolonged.

Diagnosis: Based on these findings, a diagnosis was made of (1) acute promyelocytic leukemia (FAB-M3) and (2) disseminated intravascular coagulation secondary to acute promyelocytic leukemia.

Subsequent course: The patient was started on subcutaneous calcium heparin at a dose of 100 units per kg every 6 hours. After 24 hours, her laboratory parameters of DIC were near normal and no new bleeding occurred. Following this the patient was continued on subcutaneous heparin and started on the TAD (thioguanine, Ara-C, and daunomycin) protocol and achieved complete remission. After 13 months she relapsed and a second remission was not achieved. However, she did not develop subsequent episodes of DIC.

CASE 3: CONGENITAL PROTEIN S DEFICIENCY

The patient is a 16-year-old white female high school student who was sitting in her chair in class and experienced sudden onset of pain in the right calf and popliteal fossa (behind the knee). Shortly after this, she developed dyspnea and chest pain and was immediately taken to an emergency room.

On evaluation in the emergency room she was found to have a positive thromboscintigram of the right leg and a positive lung scan. She was then admitted to the hospital. Historically, the patient denied significant medical problems and specifically denied oral contraceptive use, cigarette smoking, or any type of thrombotic or thromboembolic disease. In addition, she denied trauma or strenuous physical activity preceding this event.

Interestingly, the father had suffered a deep vein thrombosis and pulmonary embolus at age 42; this followed a cholecystectomy and gastric stapling. In addition, he had an acute myocardial infarction 5 days after his pulmonary embolus. The mother had experienced a deep vein thrombosis of the left calf at age 12, following an appendectomy and subsequent peritonitis. Three siblings had suffered no thrombotic or thromboembolic episodes.

What diagnoses should be considered and what work-up would be justified?

Diagnosis: The AT-III level was 103% of normal, the protein C level was 72% of normal, the plasminogen level was normal at 3.0 CTAU/dL and a lupus anticoagulant was not found. However, her protein S level was 12%; this was confirmed by repeat measurement. When this was found, both the mother and father were studied and the father was 78% of normal and the mother was 12.5% of normal. Thus, a diagnosis of congenital protein S deficiency was made.

Subsequent course: After initial heparinization, the patient was placed on warfarin, aiming for a prothrombin ratio of 1.2 to 1.5; she has now been followed for 2 years without a repeat thrombotic event.

SUMMARY

- Hereditary defects of coagulation pathway proteins may result in bleeding from mucosal membranes and deep body tissues. The bleeds are characteristically manifested by ecchymoses, in contrast to the petechial hemorrhages of capillary and platelet disorders.
- Most clinically-significant coagulopathies are detected by one or more abnormal test results of total coagulation. These include prothrombin time (PT), partial thromboplastin time (PTT), thrombin time, and clotting times.
- Disorders of coagulation proteins may be quantitative (decrease or absence) or qualitative (a dysfunctional form of the molecule) or both. Severity of a hereditary disorder depends on how the trait is transmitted (sex-linked or autosomal, dominant or recessive) and whether the patient is homozygous or heterozygous.
- The most common disorders involve factor VIII. Hemophilia A (classical) is a

sex-linked recessive deficiency of factor VIII:C, the coagulant component. The PTT is prolonged and the PT is normal.
- Hemophilia B (Christmas disease) is a sex-linked recessive deficiency of factor IX. The clinical symptoms are identical to factor VIII deficiency. The PTT is prolonged and the PT test is normal.
- Fibrinogen disorders include quantitative deficiencies and almost 100 different dysfibrinogenemias, some associated with thrombotic tendencies.
- von Willebrand's disease is an autosomal defect of factor VIII:Ag (VIII:vW), the component responsible for platelet adhesion to endothelial cells. Several subtypes of this disorder, with different inheritance patterns and clinical symptoms, are known. Diagnosis is made by assays for factor VIII components (ristocetin cofactor and factor VIII:Ag).
- Most defects of other factors are rare or have less severe clinical manifestations.
- Disseminated intravascular coagulation (DIC) is a syndrome of bleeding and hypercoagulability that results in consumption of platelets and several coagulation factors. Common triggering stimuli include intravascular hemolysis, retention of a dead fetus, gram-negative bacterial endotoxins, viral infections, certain malignancies, and severe burns.
- Significant laboratory findings in D/C include decreased platelet count and fibrinogen concentration, increased fibrin(ogen) degradation products (FDPs) and decreased antithrombin-III activity. PT and PTT results are often prolonged, but they are not reliable indicators.
- Most coagulation system proteins are synthesized in the liver. Liver disease adversely affects coagulation at many points, thus laboratory findings are complex and treatment is complicated. Hyperfibrinolysis is a major cause of hemorrhage that must be distinguished from other hemostatic defects, such as de-

creases in factors II, VII, IX and X (the vitamin K-dependent proteins).

- Acquired disorders may be caused by circulating anticoagulants that act as inhibitors to specific components of the coagulation cascade. Increased FDPs and paraproteins are the most common inhibitors; hemophiliacs may develop antibodies to the factors that are deficient. Lupus anticoagulants interfere with coagulation tests dependent on phospholipid activity (PT and PTT).

SUGGESTED READINGS—SECTION V

Barnhart MI, Henry RL, and Lusher JM: Sickle cell, ed 3, Kalamazoo, Mich, 1979, Upjohn Co.

Barrett JT: Textbook of immunology: an introduction to immunochemistry and immunology, ed 5, St Louis, 1988, Times Mirror/Mosby College Publishing.

Behrens JA and Kidd PG: Adult acute leukemia, J Med Technol 4:12, 1987.

Bellucci S, Tobelem G, and Caen JP: Inherited platelet disorders, Prog Hematol 13:223, 1982.

Bennett JM, Catovsky D, Daniel M-T et al.: Proposals for the classification of the myelodysplastic syndromes, Br J Haematol 51:189, 1982.

Bennett JM, Catovsky D, Daniel M-T et al.: Criteria for the diagnosis of acute leukemia of megakaryocytic lineage (M7). A report of the French-American-British Cooperative Group, Ann Intern Med 103:460, 1985.

Bennett JM, Catovsky D, Daniel M-T et al.: Proposed revised criteria for the classification of acute myeloid leukemia. A report of the French-American-British Cooperative Group, Ann Intern Med 103:626, 1985.

Bernard J: History of congenital hemorrhagic thrombocytopathic dystrophy, Blood Cells 9:179, 1983.

Bertina RM: Hereditary protein S deficiency, Haemostasis 15:241, 1985.

Bick RL: Disorders of hemostasis and thrombosis: principles of clinical practice, New York, 1985, Thieme, Inc.

Bick RL: Hemostasis defects associated with cardiac surgery, prosthetic devices, and other extracorporeal circuits, Semin Thromb Hemost 11:249, 1985.

Bick RL: Disseminated intravascular coagulation: a clinical review, Semin Thromb Hemost 14:299, 1988.

Block AJ, Boysen PC, Wynne, JW et al.: Sleep apnea, hypopnea, and oxygen desaturation in normal subjects: a strong male predominance, N Engl J Med 300:513, 1979.

Booth WJ and Berndt MC: Thrombospondin in clinical disease states, Semin Thromb Hemost 13:298, 1987.

Broekmans AW: Hereditary protein C deficiency, Haemostasis 13:233, 1985.

Browman GP, Neame PB, and Soamboonsrup P: The contribution of cytochemistry and immunophenotyping to the reproducibility of the FAB classification in acute leukemia, Blood 68:900, 1986.

Caen JP: Glanzmann thrombasthenia, Clin Haematol 1:383, 1972.

Caen JP, Nurden AT, Jeanneau C et al.: Bernard-Soulier syndrome: a new platelet glycoprotein abnormality. Its relationship with platelet adhesion to subendothelium and with the factor VIII von Willebrand protein, J Lab Clin Med 87:586, 1976.

Chessells JM: Acute lymphoblastic leukemia, Semin Hematol 19:155, 1982.

Comp PC: Hereditary disorders predisposing to thrombosis, Prog Hemost Thromb 8:71, 1986.

Cowan DH: Effect of alcoholism on hemostasis, Semin Hematol 17:137, 1980.

Desnick RJ, Gatt S, and Grabowski GA (editors): Gaucher disease: a century of delineation and research, New York, 1982, Alan R Liss, Inc.

Deutsch E: The liver and blood clotting, Semin Thromb Hemost 4:1, 1977.

Dutcher TF: Cytochemistry of acute leukemias and hairy cell leukemia, Chicago, 1982, American Society of Clinical Pathologists.

Gan TE, Sawers RJ, and Koutts J: Pathogenesis of antibody-induced acquired von Willebrand syndrome, Am J Hematol 9:363, 1980.

Gehan EA, Smith TL, Freireich EJ et al.: Prognostic factors in acute leukemia, Semin Oncol 3:271, 1976.

Golde DW, Jacobs AD, Glaspy JA et al.: Hairy-cell leukemia: biology and treatment, Semin Hematol 23:3, 1986.

Hemker HC and Frank HLL: The mechanism of action of oral anticoagulants and its consequences for the practice of oral anticoagulation, Haemostasis 15:263, 1985.

Huang AT (editor): Hairy cell and chronic lymphocytic leukemia. Thirty years of progress, New York, 1985, Elsevier Science Publishing Co, Inc.

Kaplow LS: The relationship of myeloperoxidase activity to neutrophil maturity and other hematologic indicators of infection, Blood 12:153, 1986.

Karpatkin S: Autoimmune thrombocytopenic purpura, Blood 56:329, 1980.

Kauffman RH, Herrmann WA, Meyer CJ et al.: Circulating IgA-immune complexes in Henoch-Schönlein purpura, Am J Med 69:859, 1980.

King DJ and Kelton JG: Heparin-associated thrombocytopenia, Ann Intern Med 100:535, 1984.

Kitchens CS: Concept of hypercoagulability: a review of its development, clinical application, and recent progress, Semin Thromb Hemost 11:293, 1985.

Koike T: Megakaryoblastic leukemia: the characterization and identification of megakaryoblasts, Blood 64:683, 1984.

Lahey ME: Histiocytosis. In: Spivak JL (editor), Fundamentals of clinical hematology, ed 2, Philadelphia, 1984, Harper & Row Publishers, Inc.

LeBeau MM: Chromosomal fragile sites and cancer-specific rearrangements, Blood 67:849, 1986.

Lee SL, Kopel S, and Glidewell O: Cytomorphological determinants of prognosis in acute lymphoblastic leukemia of children, Semin Oncol 3:209, 1976.

LeMaistre A, Powers CN, and Reuben JM: Monoclonal antibodies and flowcytometry in characterization of acute leukemias, Clin Lab Sci 1:29, 1988.

Malpas TW and Harker LA: Acquired disorders of platelet function, Semin Hematol 17:242, 1980.

Mammen EF: Congenital coagulation defects, Semin Thromb Hemost 9:1, 1983.

Marchesi SL, Knowles WJ, Morrow JS et al.: Abnormal spectrin in hereditary elliptocytosis, Blood 67:141, 1986.

McCusick VA: Multiple forms of the Ehlers-Danlos syndrome, Arch Surg 109:475, 1974.

Miale JB: Laboratory medicine: hematology, ed 6, St. Louis, 1982, CV Mosby Co.

Moake JL and Funicella T: Common bleeding problems, Clin Symp 35:1, 1983.

Nydegger UE and Miescher UE: Bleeding due to vascular disorders, Semin Hematol 17:178, 1980.

Ochs HD, Slichter JS, Harker LA et al.: The Wiskott-Aldrich syndrome: studies of lymphocytes, granulocytes, and platelets, Blood 55:243, 1980.

Osserman EF, Merlini G, and Butler VP Jr: Multiple myeloma and related plasma cell dyscrasias, JAMA 258:2930, 1987.

Pedraza MA, Doslu FA, Marsh RA et al.: Acute leukemias: ultrastructural, cytochemical, and immunologic diagnostic approaches, Lab Med 14:45, 1983.

Raccuglia G: Gray platelet syndrome: a variety of qualitative platelet disorders, Am J Med 51:818, 1971.

Ratnoff OD: The psychogenic purpuras: a review of autoerythrocyte sensitization, autosensitization to DNA, "hysterical" and factitial bleeding, and the religious stigmata, Semin Hematol 17:192, 1980.

Rodgers GM and Shuman MA: Congenital thrombotic disorders, Am J Hematol 21:419, 1986.

Rose N, Frieman H, and Fahey J (editors). Manual of clinical immunology, ed 3, Washington, D.C., American Society for Microbiology.

Rosse WF: Brief review: the control of complement activation by the blood cells in paroxysmal nocturnal hemoglobinuria, Blood 67:268, 1986.

Rosse WF and Parker CJ: Paroxysmal nocturnal hemoglobinuria, Clin Haematol 14:105, 1985.

Roth EF Jr: Red cell polymorphisms and the malaria hypothesis, Diagn Med 8:29, 1985.

Rowe JM: Clinical and laboratory features of the myeloid and lymphocytic leukemias, Amer J Med Technol 49:103, 1983.

Ruggeri ZM and Zimmerman TS: Platelets and von Willebrand disease, Semin Hematol 22:203, 1985.

Sandberg AA: The chromosomes in human leukemia, Semin Hematol 23:201, 1986.

Shapiro SS and Thiagarajan P: Lupus anticoagulants, Prog Thromb Hemost 6:263, 1982.

Silverstein MN and Ellefson RD: The syndrome of the sea-blue histiocytes, Semin Hematol 9:299, 1972.

Stewart JG, Ahlquist DAA, McGill DB et al.: Gastrointestinal blood loss and anemia in runners, Ann Intern Med 100:843, 1984.

Sun T, Li C-Y, and Yam LT: Atlas of cytochemistry and immunochemistry of hematologic neoplasms, Chicago, 1985, American Society of Clinical Pathologists Press.

Thorup OA Jr: Leavell and Thorup's fundamentals of clinical hematology, ed 5, Philadelphia, 1987, WB Saunders Co.

Weatherall DJ: The thalassemias. In: Williams WJ et al. (editors): Hematology, ed 3, New York, 1983, McGraw-Hill, Inc.

Weiss HJ: Congenital disorders of platelet function, Semin Hematol 17:228, 1980.

Whelby MS: Disorders of iron metabolism. In: Thorup OA Jr (editor): Fundamentals of clinical hematology, ed 5, Philadelphia, 1987, WB Saunders Co.

White JG: Ultrastructural studies of the gray platelet syndromes, Am J Pathol 95:445, 1979.

Williams WJ, Beutler E, Ersler AJ et al. (editors): Hematology, ed 3, New York, 1983, McGraw-Hill, Inc.

Wu KK, Minkoff IM, Rossi EC et al.: Hereditary bleeding disorder due to a primary defect in platelet release reaction, Br J Haematol 47:241, 1981.

Zaino EC: Paleontologic thalassemia, Ann NY Acad Sci 119:402, 1964.

SECTION VI
Technical Hematology

25

Collection of Blood and Marrow Samples

Susan Aycock and Lawrence Powers

SAMPLE COLLECTION

Collection of a blood sample is one of the most critical phases of obtaining accurate laboratory test results. Although a detailed presentation of patient and specimen processing is beyond the intention of this book, some discussion is warranted on blood collection technique, errors associated with improper sampling, differences between venous and capillary blood, uses of anticoagulants, and other factors that have an impact on hematological results. Specialized textbooks in techniques of blood collection are available (e.g., Stockbower and Blumenfeld, 1983), but none can substitute for experience. The following discussion assumes some experience with blood collection.

BLOOD COLLECTION EQUIPMENT

Syringes. In the past, syringes were the only practical way blood could be collected. They were made of glass and after each use they were placed in paper bags or cloth wraps and sterilized for reuse. Although glass syringes are still available, they have been largely replaced by plastic, disposable syringes. These, in turn, have given way to the evacuated tube and needle-holder systems used for most routine blood collecting needs (Fig. 25-1). Syringes are still used for

collecting some types of samples, such as arterial blood gases, blood cultures, and various body fluids. Syringes may also be the best choice for patients with small veins, veins that easily collapse when exposed to the negative pressure of the evacuated tubes. They may also be the best choice when other collecting or administering devices are used, such as butterfly infusion sets. Two advantages of syringes are:

1. Blood usually appears in the hub of the syringe as a vein is entered, which is helpful for novice phlebotomists and when collecting blood from arms with fragile, deep, or mobile veins.
2. Blood flow rate and withdrawal pressure is easily controlled by the phlebotomist, so that "collapse" of thin-walled veins can be avoided. Large amounts of blood (20 to 30 mL) can be withdrawn from a small vein, using a small-gauge needle, by a steady but gradual pull on the plunger.

Evacuated systems. The most common blood collecting systems use a disposable needle, a needle holder, and an evacuated tube (Fig. 25-1). The needle screws into the holder and each end of the needle is pointed—one to enter the vein, the other to puncture a collecting tube. The vein is entered first, then any number of collecting

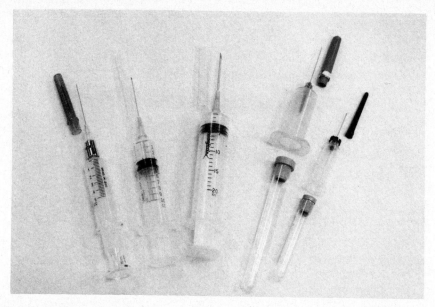

Fig. 25-1. Phlebotomy equipment: syringe, needles, and evacuation system.
Left to right: glass syringe with Luer-lock needle, disposable plastic syringes and needles. Vacutainer evacuation systems.

tubes can be added to the other end. Each tube is punctured through a rubber cap and blood flows into it due to the partial vacuum. One drawback to this system is gradual loss of vacuum from tubes that have been on the shelf a few years.

Collecting tubes are available in many sizes and the tube walls are made of soda lime glass (this may release trace elements such as calcium or magnesium into the blood sample) or borosilicate glass (widely used). Some tubes also employ a special material that separates serum from the blood clot, facilitating rapid processing. Last, but not least, the collecting tubes may contain additives such as anticoagulants and preservatives, which are usually denoted by a stopper color code. Many tubes are also coated with silicon to minimize clotting and hemolysis. Advantages of evacuation systems include:

1. One needle holder can replace many bulky syringes, saving space on phlebotomy trays.

2. A number of collecting tubes, with various additives, can be used sequentially. Some patients experience anxiety at the sight of a 30 mL syringe being filled with their blood, whereas five or six small tubes may not seem as threatening.

3. Blood enters each tube and mixes rapidly with a specific anticoagulant, whereas blood in a syringe must either forego anticoagulation until the phlebotomy is complete, or the syringe must be coated with the anticoagulant, thus limiting the variety of additives used.

4. Blood collection is faster with evacuated tubes than with a syringe, especially if several tubes are to be filled.

Anticoagulants. Most procedures used in hematology require whole blood or plasma.

Anticoagulants prevent blood clotting by enhancing the action of natural inhibitors (heparin potentiates antithrombin-III) or by removing calcium from the plasma (most other anticoagulants). Selection of an anticoagulant depends on requirements of the procedure (Table 25-1). Some anticoagulants used in hematological procedures include:

Table 25-1. Anticoagulant requirements of hematological procedures

Procedure	Anticoagulant
Complete blood count, most routine hematology procedures	EDTA
Studies of cell morphology	None (P); EDTA (A)
Platelet counts, some function studies	EDTA
Platelet aggregation studies	Heparin
Osmotic fragility	Heparin
Prothrombin time, partial thromboplastin time, most coagulation procedures	Sodium citrate
Erythrocyte sedimentation rate	Sodium citrate (P); EDTA (A)
Abnormal hemoglobin pigments	EDTA
Heinz body formation	Heparin
Sugar-water or test for PNH	Sodium oxalate (P); Sodium citrate (A)
Sickle cell screening tests and electrophoresis	EDTA
LE cell preparation, glass bead method	1% Heparin
Leukocyte alkaline phosphatase stain	Heparin (do not use EDTA)
Myeloperoxidase stain	EDTA or heparin

A, acceptable; *P*, preferred.

Heparin. Heparin is a mucositin polysulfonic acid, available as sodium, potassium, and ammonium salts. Its action as an antithrombin prevents transformation of prothrombin to thrombin (Chapter 13). About 20 units of heparin are required to anticoagulate 1 mL of blood.

Advantages	Disadvantages
Minimum interference in most tests	Relatively expensive
Available as a liquid or powder	Produces blue background on Wright-stained smears
Can be used in tests for phosphorus	Inhibits acid phosphatase activity

Ethylenediaminetetraacetic acid (EDTA). EDTA is used as a disodium or dipotassium salt that prevents coagulation by chelating or binding calcium in the plasma. Calcium is required in several steps of the coagulation cascade. About 1 to 2 mg of EDTA is needed for each milliliter of blood. EDTA is the most common anticoagulant used in routine hematological studies.

Advantages	Disadvantages
Preserves cellular morphology	Inhibits alkaline phosphatase activity
Little effect on most chemistry tests	Not useful for calcium and iron studies

Sodium citrate. This is the anticoagulant of choice for studies of coagulation. A concentration of 3.4 to 3.8 g/dL is used, mixing 1 part of anticoagulant to 9 parts of whole blood. Calcium is chelated, a result that is easily reversed by addition of ionized calcium.

Advantages	Disadvantages
Anticoagulation easily reversed	Not suitable for many chemistry studies
	Inhibits alkaline phosphatase

Oxalates. Sodium, potassium, ammonium, and lithium oxalates inhibit coagulation by forming an insoluble complex with plasma calcium ions. Concentrations of 1

to 2 mg per mL are used; potassium oxalate is the salt most widely used. There is little use of oxalates in hematology.

Advantages	Disadvantages
None	Na and Li oxalates draw water from RBCs, results in crenation, 10% decrease in hematocrit
	Inhibits alkaline phosphatase

Other anticoagulants are available for blood collection, but these are used only for chemistry studies. **Sodium fluoride** is a weak anticoagulant that inhibits a glycolytic enzyme. Therefore, it acts as a preservative and it is the anticoagulant of choice for blood glucose determinations. **Sodium iodoacetate** is also an antiglycolytic agent (it can substitute for sodium fluoride) which can be used for glucose and blood urea nitrogen (BUN) studies.

Needles. The gauge (diameter) and length of the needle used on a syringe or evacuated system depends on the amount of blood to be drawn, type of analysis to be performed, and condition of potential phlebotomy sites in the patient. The bore size, or diameter, of a needle is indicated by gauge: high numbers (e.g., 24 gauge or 26 gauge) indicate small needle lumens and low numbers (e.g., 16 gauge or 18 gauge) indicate needles with large lumens (Fig. 25-2). Most blood samples are collected with needles of 19 to 21 gauge. Patients with very small veins or with veins that collapse easily when negative pressure is applied during blood withdrawal may require a small needle, used with a syringe. On the other hand, blood donors providing a unit (450 mL) of plasma or whole blood are usually drawn with a 16 gauge needle. Collection of large single

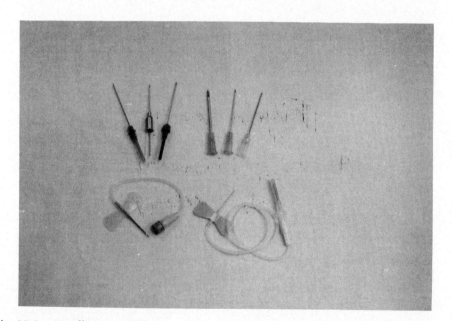

Fig. 25-2.   Needle types and sizes.
Top left: needles for evacuation systems; top right: disposable needles for syringes; bottom: disposable butterfly needle sets.

sample volumes (25 to 50 mL) can be facilitated with a butterfly set (Fig. 25-2). This consists of a needle and long flexible tube attached to a syringe. The tube can be taped to the patient's arm to withdraw a large sample over a longer interval of time than would occur with an evacuated system or syringe alone. This may be necessary in elderly or critically ill patients with delicate or badly scarred veins. Anticoagulants are sometimes used in the tubing or syringe to insure adequate blood flow and prevent clotting if sample collection is prolonged.

The effect of needle size on the blood sample is controversial. Both large bore and small bore needles have been implicated as potential sources of red cell damage and hemolysis. Large bore (low gauge) needles facilitate rapid passage of the blood and cells are swirled against the needle wall because of turbulance and high fluid pressure. Small bore (high gauge) needles have a large surface area compared to intraluminal volume, again facilitating cell contact with the needle wall. The rate of blood withdrawal, therefore, should be adjusted to the needle diameter. When a smaller needle (22 gauge or higher) is used with small veins, blood withdrawal should be slower to prevent hemolysis and venous collapse. Most modern needles are lubricated with a silicon-containing compound which minimizes trauma from wall contact during red cell passage.

The length of the needle is usually either one inch or 1½ inches. The choice of length depends on characteristics of the phlebotomy site (depth of vein, scar tissue, etc.) and on the phlebotomist's preference. All needles in routine use today are disposable and sterile, so that blunt, barbed, or contaminated needles should not be a factor. Visual examination of the tip prior to venipuncture is a good practice, however.

Drawing order. Some tests require that the blood sample be exposed to minimal coagulation and hemostatic activity, such as assessments of platelet function and most coagulation studies. Therefore, blood for these analyses should be mixed with an appropriate anticoagulant as soon as possible. Anticoagulants can interfere with assessment of blood morphology on smears, so these should be made from blood "fresh from the source" when microscopic examination is critical. When an evacuated system of tubes is used, collection of multiple samples for diverse analyses becomes important. One study (Caalm and Cooper, 1982) recommends that prepared sample tubes be collected in the following order: (1) sterile blood culture tubes, (2) tubes without additives (serum studies), (3) coagulation study tubes (usually sodium citrate or heparin), and (4) tubes with other additives (EDTA, then oxalates and fluorides). Some transfer of additives from tube to tube is a possibility, especially if blood withdrawal is difficult. For example, if the EDTA tube is collected prior to a heparinized tube for electrolyte analysis, the potassium salt of EDTA may falsely elevate the potassium determination. Since EDTA is a calcium chelator, EDTA contamination can elevate plasma or serum calcium results if the heparin or nonadditive tubes are drawn after the EDTA tube. Oxalates can interfere with some enzyme determinations and produce membrane alterations that affect red cell morphology.

PHLEBOTOMY

Phlebotomists develop variations of techniques and successful approaches based on individual experiences and special requirements for certain patients and situations. Drawing blood from children, mental patients, and critically ill individuals may require ingenuity and the ability to adapt to these circumstances. Some guidelines can be identified, however, that form the basis for an acceptable blood collection protocol. They are:

1. Patient identification; note isolation and dietary restrictions
2. Reassure and position the patient
3. Assemble required supplies

4. Apply the tourniquet and select phlebotomy site
5. Cleanse phlebotomy site
6. Perform venipuncture and collect required sample
7. Release tourniquet and remove needle
8. Place gauze over site and apply pressure
9. Fill tubes and mix (syringe) or mix (evacuation system)
10. Dispose of needle in appropriate container
11. Label sample tubes, slides; sign request slips or logbooks; other documentation
12. Examine patient's arm, apply bandage if needed; recheck identification
13. Transport samples to laboratory

The venipuncture procedure (Figs. 25-3 through 25-7)

1. *Identify the patient.* Perhaps the most important consideration in quality patient care is to assure that correct samples are obtained from the intended individual. Test results posted to the wrong records could have adverse effects on the diagnosis, treatment, and medical condition of a patient.

   a. If possible, the patient should state his or her name when asked by the phlebotomist.

   b. The phlebotomist should compare identification data on the test request slip with that provided by the patient (bed or door labels and wrist identification bands for inpatients).

   c. Compare request slip data with data of labels to be placed on collecting tubes.

2. *Reassure the patient.* Some patients, particularly children, may be uneasy about blood collection. The phlebotomist should gain the patient's confidence by proceeding in a professional, confident manner. Explain the procedure and assure them that any discomfort will be minor and of a short dura-

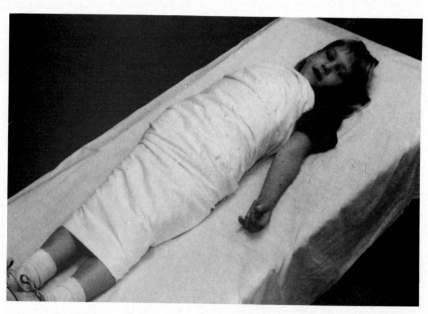

Fig. 25-3. Child wrapped in a sheet for immobilization.

tion. Do not tell a patient that "it won't hurt" or that "you won't feel a thing."

3. *Position the patient* (Fig. 25-3). A successful venipuncture is much more probable if the patient is immobilized and the phlebotomist is comfortable. Seated patients should sit comfortably with arm extended, below shoulder level, on an armrest or supporting surface. Placement of their other hand beneath their elbow may provide added support. A reclining patient should lie on his or her back with an arm extended either outward (distally) from the body or along side the body. A rolled towel or pillow can provide additional support near the elbow.

4. *Assemble the required supplies (Fig. 25-4).* All items needed during the procedure, including a few spares, should be close at hand. For a routine venipuncture, supplies include:

    a. tourniquet: several types are available; a blood pressure cuff may also be used.

    b. alcohol preps or swabs.

    c. dry gauze pads, to dry the alcohol and place over the site after the needle is removed.

    d. collection tubes, as needed, with appropriate additives for requested tests.

    e. needle holder or syringe.

    f. needles, usually 20 or 21 gauge, either for evacuated tube system or syringe.

    g. adhesive bandages or tape and gauze pads to protect site after procedure.

5. *Select venipuncture site.* In most cases, blood will be drawn from an arm vein, since these vessels are usually large, close to the skin surface, and easy to penetrate. On occasion, an alternate site must be selected because of burns, amputation, presence of a cast, or other medical considerations. Alternate sites include the back of the hand, the ankle, or foot. A few special considerations should be noted:

    a. Avoid using skin areas marked by

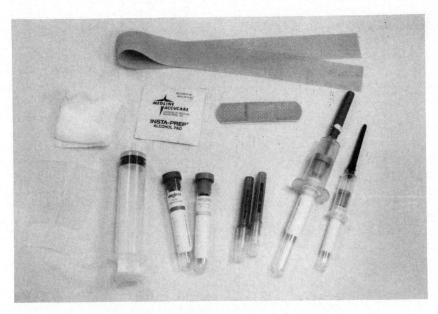

Fig. 25-4.   Assembled phlebotomy supplies.

excessive scarring or containing large hematomas.

b. Do not draw from an arm in which an intravenous line is inserted, since dilution of the blood sample may occur. If the IV needle is inserted high in the arm (proximal to the body), it is possible to draw blood from a lower (more distal) site of the same arm. If intravenous therapy is occurring in both arms, a nurse can usually discontinue fluid administration for 5 minutes. Blood is drawn from the IV connector. The first 5 mL is discarded to avoid IV fluid contamination and the sample is drawn as usual. This should be noted by the phlebotomist in case discrepancies arise when sequential test results are compared.

c. Women who have undergone a recent unilateral mastectomy will experience lymphostasis on that side of the body. This change in lymphatic drainage alters composition of the blood, so that a phlebotomy should be performed on the opposite arm.

6. *Apply the tourniquet.* A latex band, velcro strap, or rubber-tubing tourniquet should be placed 8 to 10 cm above the proposed venipuncture site. This produces filling and swelling of the veins distal to the tourniquet. The patient can further facilitate vein selection by making a fist, which firms the lower arm muscles and helps display the veins. The phlebotomist palpates the veins with an index finger to test for a pliable, "spongy" vessel. Hard, wire-like or "knotty" vessels should be avoided. Vessels that contain extensive scarred tissue may be difficult to penetrate. The tourniquet should be applied no more than 1 to 2 minutes, since the resulting venous stasis changes the cellular composition of the blood.

7. *Select a vein (Fig. 25-5).* Most venipunctures are made in an arm vein at, or just below, the bend of the elbow. The median cubital vein is most often used since it is large, superficial, and lies in a site that is relatively insensitive to pain. The cephalic and basilic veins may also be used, but they are more likely to roll and bruise. During this inspection, the choices of syringe versus evacuated system and needle size are made.

8. *Clean the venipuncture site.* Routine phlebotomy sites are cleaned with an alcohol pad (commercially prepackaged) or a cotton swab soaked in 70% isopropyl alcohol. The alcohol should be applied in a circular motion, working from the center of the site outward. Allow the skin to dry since residual alcohol could result in some hemolysis of the sample. Do not touch the clean site again until after the venipuncture. If repalpation is needed, the site should also be recleaned before a needle enters the skin. This step is often combined with number seven since selecting a vein and cleaning the site should take no more than 30 seconds. In some patients, however, vein selection may be prolonged or interrupted. If the tourniquet is removed to prevent excessive stasis, reapply the tourniquet just prior to venipuncture. The needle, collecting tubes and syringe or needle holder should be at hand and ready to use. Depending on vein quality, it may be desirable for the patient to open and close the fist several times to increase vein distension.

9. *Perform the venipuncture (Fig. 25-6).*

a. Remove the protective cap from the needle and visually inspect the needle point for damage. If the needle is attached to a syringe, slide the plunger back and forth one or two times to assure smooth motion. Hold the syringe or holder so that the needle bevel faces upward.

b. With the opposite hand, place the index finger or thumb about 3 cm below the puncture site and draw the skin taut. This helps immobi-

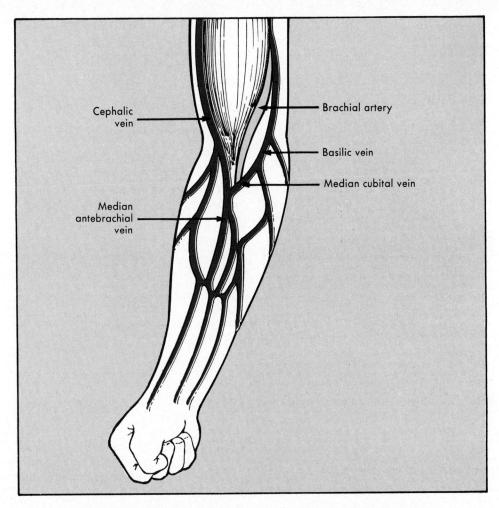

Cephalic vein

Brachial artery

Basilic vein

Median cubital vein

Median antebrachial vein

Fig. 25-5.   Blood vessels and related structures of the forearm.

lize the vein (prevents "rolling") and steadies the patients arm. The patient should maintain a fist.

c. Align the needle with the arm and insert the needle under the skin and into the vein at a 15 to 20 degree angle. The hand holding the syringe or holder can rest on the patient's forearm, providing further stability.

Evacuated system: One hand grasps the holder while the other hand pushes the col-lecting tube into the needle. If the needle is situated properly in the vein, blood should enter and fill the tube within a few seconds. When additional tubes of blood are re-quired, filled tubes are replaced by empty ones. Modern needles prevent blood leakage during tube exchange.

Syringe: One hand grasps the barrel and the other hand is free to pull back on the plunger. If the needle is properly located in the vein, blood should enter the hub of the

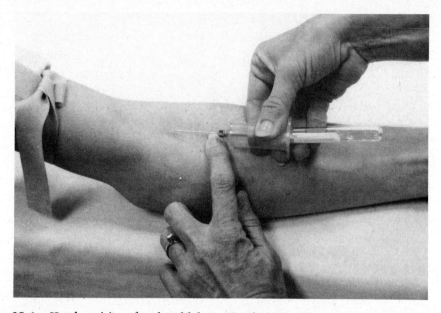

Fig. 25-6.   Hand positions for the phlebotomist during collection.
The phlebotomist pulls the skin taut with one hand while inserting the needle with the other hand.

syringe. Pull back slowly on the plunger until the desired volume of blood has been obtained.

10. *Remove the needle from the arm.* After the desired amount of blood has been obtained, the patient should open the fist. Remove the tourniquet. Place a dry gauze over the needle and puncture site and withdraw the needle in a swift, smooth backward motion, pulling the needle out without vertical or horizontal motion. If a syringe is used, remove the needle and transfer the blood to appropriate containers.

11. *Apply pressure (Fig. 25-7).* The patient should press the gauze firmly over the puncture site. The common practice of simply bending the elbow to hold the gauze in place should be discouraged since it may not provide enough pressure to prevent formation of a hematoma. The arm should be extended horizontally and pressure applied at the site for about 3 minutes. When bleeding or oozing at the puncture site has ceased, an adhesive bandage can be applied to the wound.

Sample tube processing. While the patient applies pressure to the puncture site, the phlebotomist should tilt tubes containing anticoagulants to assure mixing. Label all sample tubes with information appropriate to the collecting and processing facility. In most hospitals, a label might consist of: (a) patient's full name, (b) patient's hospital case or record number, (c) patient's room or ward number, (d) the date and time that the sample was drawn, and (e) the initials or code number of the phlebotomist. Outpatient samples are also usually numbered with a case or referral number. Alternately, an address, social security number, or other positive means of identification can be used. Labels should be legible (anyone should be able to read the information); they can be preprinted or written with nonsmearable ink. All labeling on the sample tubes should be affixed *after* the sample is

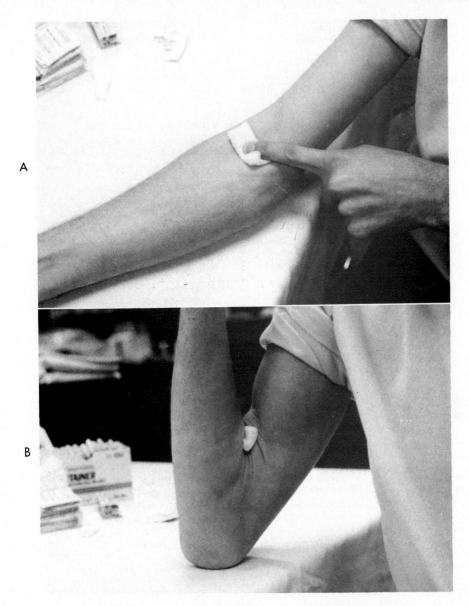

Fig. 25-7.   Application of pressure following phlebotomy.
A, Right method; **B,** wrong method.

collected and *before* the phlebotomist leaves the patient's bedside. Review the request slips since some tests require special sample handling, such as immediate icing or incubation at 37° C.

Documentation procedures for phlebotomy vary widely. In some institutions, blood collectors are also required to sign and note collection time on the request slip as well as the sample tube label. Other requirements may include logging the sample collection in a record book or on the patient's hospital chart.

Finally, transport the blood samples to the laboratory under conditions appropriate for the test procedures to be performed. Transport time should be minimized since delays can affect test results for some procedures.

Sources of error

Errors that can be made while doing a venipuncture include the following.

1. The patient is not properly identified by the phlebotomist. Information on request forms should agree with the patient's wristband (inpatients) or verbal responses (outpatients).

2. Isolation and/or dietary restrictions are not followed so that the sample is inappropriate for the analysis requested. This is more of a problem for chemistry tests than for hematology procedures.

3. The tourniquet remains on the arm for a prolonged period before venipuncture, resulting in stasis and hemoconcentration of the blood. Cellular concentrations and hemoglobin values will be increased.

4. The phlebotomy site is not adequate to assure a satisfactory venipuncture. Difficulty in obtaining blood may be characterized by formation of clots before mixing with anticoagulants can occur, resulting in activation of platelet responses and the coagulation cascade. Hemolysis of red blood cells can occur in traumatic phlebotomies, resulting in a reduced red cell count and hematocrit.

5. Withdrawal of blood downstream from infusion of intravenous fluids, resulting in hemodilution and lowered cell counts. Infusion of heparin near the sampling site interferes with some coagulation studies.

6. The phlebotomy site is not adequately dried before insertion of the needle. Alcohol contamination is obviously a major error if a blood alcohol determination is the requested test. Besides, alcohol burns when it is introduced into a cut or puncture.

7. Position of the needle is incorrect (Fig. 25-8). The needle bevel must be up and it must be intraluminal in the vein. Too shallow or too deep a puncture will result in failure to obtain blood and the possibility of hematoma formation in the adjacent tissue.

8. The tubes are not properly filled, resulting in an inappropriate ratio of blood to anticoagulant. An excess of EDTA or heparin can adversely affect red cell morphology as well as dilute the blood sample. For coagulation studies, the ratio of sodium citrate to blood must not vary greatly from the recommended 1:9 ratio (see Chapter 28).

9. Postcollection handling is inappropriate. This includes delays in processing (such as mixing anticoagulant and blood or removing plasma from blood cells for coagulation studies), exposure to excess temperatures (high or low), and failure to label the sample tubes correctly. Excessive shaking or bumping can cause mechanical hemolysis of red cells and activate platelets.

10. Failure to release the tourniquet before withdrawal of the needle or insufficient application of pressure to the venipuncture site may result in the formation of a hematoma.

Since the results of a blood test are only as good as the sample collected and processed, careful attention to these and other sources of error is important. The following are some collecting errors that can result in red cell lysis:

a. Needle bore too small for blood volume drawn
b. Too much draw force applied to plunger of syringe
c. Expelling blood at high force through syringe needle into sample tubes
d. Expelling blood through a needle after clotting has begun
e. Vigorous shaking of tube instead of gentle inversion to mix blood with anticoagulant
f. Venipuncture made through wet alcohol area, carried on needle to mix with blood

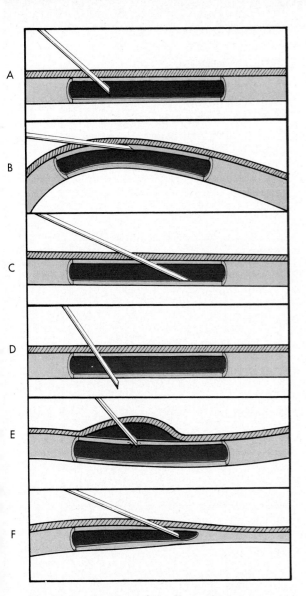

Fig. 25-8.   Position of needle in the vein.
A, Correct insertion, blood flows into the needle. **B,** Bevel is on upper wall of vein, blood does not flow into needle. **C,** Bevel is on the lower wall of the vein and bevel is down, blood does not flow into needle. **D,** Needle penetrates vein completely, blood may infiltrate surrounding tissue, little blood is collected in needle. **E,** Needle is partially inserted into vein wall, allowing blood to leak into surrounding tissue; hematoma results. **F,** Vein collapses around needle.

g. Blood drawn from a hematoma or other area of infiltration

h. Difficult or prolonged venipuncture

i. Exposing blood to water at any phase of collecting or processing

CAPILLARY PUNCTURE

When only a small amount of blood is required or when a venipuncture is too difficult or impractical, a skin puncture of the finger, heel, earlobe, or toe may provide an alternate collection site. The majority of capillary puncture methods are performed on children (usually by fingerstick) or newborn infants (heel stick). Unfortunately, this method of blood collection is also more painful than venipuncture and additional reassurance may be necessary for the child who has had prior experience with a fingerstick. Capillary collection is indicated in adults when the patient is severely burned or extremely obese. It is also indicated when accessible veins are few, damaged, or they must be preserved for intravenous fluid administration. Capillary collection, however, is time consuming and imposes obvious restrictions on the volume of blood that can be obtained. There is also a greater risk from infection from skin puncture, a consideration of particular importance to patients already immunocompromised by disease or some forms of therapy.

Puncture and collection devices

A number of instruments are available for puncturing the skin to collect capillary blood (Fig. 25-9). These include:

1. sterile disposable lancets, such as the Monolet (Monoject) and Microlance (Becton-Dickinson)

2. spring activated devices, such as Autolet, Hemalet, and Monojector, which have a lancet held in place by a cocking lever. When the blade is released, it penetrates the skin to a depth of 2 millimeters. Similar instruments have been designed to standardize bleeding time determinations, such as the Surg-

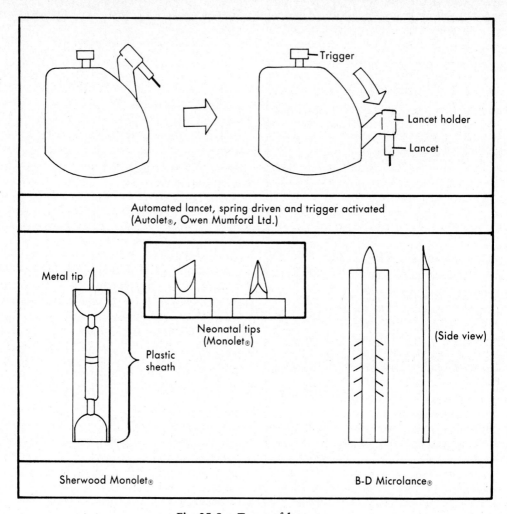

Fig. 25-9.   Types of lancets.

icutt (International Teledyne) and Sim-plate (General Diagnostics).

After the skin puncture, the capillary blood may be collected in a variety of containers. Heparinized and plain microhematocrit capillary tubes can be used for general purposes. When EDTA or other additives are required, various commercial microsamplers and containers can be used (Fig. 25-10). Most microcontainers have the disadvantage of blood drops collecting near the mouth of the tube and unless the blood

is mixed periodically with the anticoagulant in the bottom of the tube, the blood clots. This can be accomplished by a flicking motion of the wrist of the hand holding the tube while waiting for the next drop of blood to well up from the puncture site.

Capillary puncture procedure (Figs. 25-11 through 25-13)

Procedures for patient identification are identical to those for the phlebotomy proto-

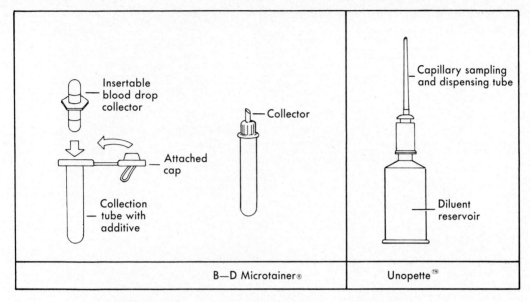

Fig. 25-10.   **Types of microsample tubes and devices.**

col. Positioning of the patient and technologist are different, however, depending on the age and condition of the patient and the skin puncture site. An ambulatory adult or older child should sit comfortably with the arm extended, below shoulder level, to a supporting surface, such as an arm rest or table top. Some blood collectors prefer to face the patient, others sit alongside with arms extended in the same direction (Fig. 25-11). A young child can be held in the lap of an adult, which serves as reassurance as well as providing support and immobilization (Fig. 25-12). When another adult is unavailable, a child can be effectively supported but immobilized in the collector's lap during a fingerstick. In either case, keep all materials well out of the reach of thrashing hands and feet! A very agitated or uncooperative patient can be wrapped in a blanket or sheet, but this should be avoided if a reassuring approach can gain the child's confidence. Sometimes this means requesting that the parent step out of the room so that the technologist can interact with the child in a one-on-one manner. Experience

will dictate the approach to be used for each child.

As with a venipuncture, assembly of collection materials is essential. Extra slides, capillary tubes, gauze pads, and collection devices should be within reach. Check the request forms carefully to be sure that the appropriate devices are available and that capillary blood will suffice for the tests ordered. A typical skin puncture assembly consists of:

a. Lancets
b. Alcohol preps or swabs
c. Dry gauze pads, usually 2 in. × 2 in. or 4 in. × 4 in.
d. Microsample containers and/or capillary tubes
e. Sealing clay, if microhematocrit tubes are used
f. Adhesive bandages or tape and gauze to protect the site after collection.

A bandage is often not necessary for adults, but it can make the difference between tears and smiles for a young child.

1. Select a puncture site. In adults and children older than 18 months, Blumenfeld

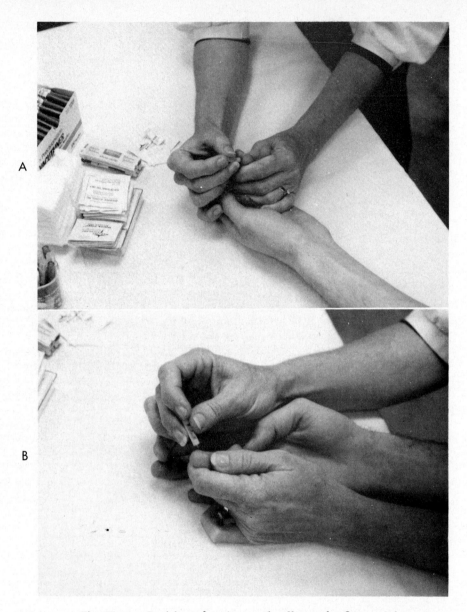

Fig. 25-11.   Position of patient and collector for fingerstick.
A, Facing patient; **B,** parallel to patient.

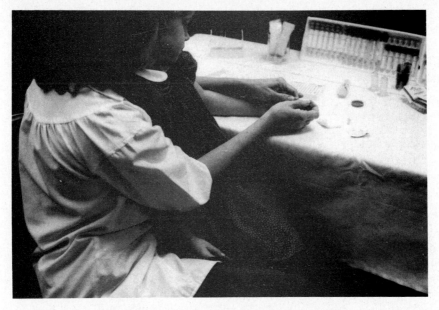

Fig. 25-12.   Supporting and holding a child during capillary puncture.

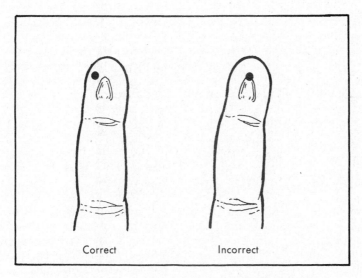

Fig. 25-13.   Sites for capillary puncture: fingerstick.

(1983) recommends the palmar surface of the distal portion of the second, third, or fourth finger (Fig. 25-13). Avoid the sides or tip of the finger (near the nail) because tissue thickness in these areas is only about half that of the fleshy center portion, but displace the puncture from the mid-line. Do not use old puncture sites or areas with obvious callouses.

2. *If necessary, warm the puncture site.* Patients with impaired circulation or those that have been outside and exposed to cold temperatures will have poor capillary blood flow. One can simply hold or rub the patient's hands; a moist towelette warmed to body temperature placed on the site for about 3 minutes is usually effective.

3. *Cleanse the puncture area* with isopropyl alcohol and dry it with a clean gauze. Residual alcohol can cause hemolysis of red cells as they flow from the wound. Iodine is not recommended as a site preparation for routine blood sampling and it may interfere with various chemical analyses.

4. *Grasp the finger firmly* but not too tightly with one hand and use the other hand to hold the lancet and perform the puncture. Use a quick, decisive motion to cut across fingerprint ridges. The puncture should not be brutal, but a timid or hesitant motion will usually require a second attempt. This can be unnerving for patient and collector alike. Maximum puncture depth should not exceed 3.1 mm. Discard the lancet immediately into a biohazards container. Never use the same lancet twice, even on the same patient at the same site.

5. *Wipe the first drop that wells up* from the wound with a clean gauze. This drop contains a large amount of tissue fluid that may dilute the blood and interfere with some coagulation studies.

6. *Collect subsequent blood drops* into the appropriate containers, tilting or flicking the tubes periodically to mix the blood with the anticoagulants. Capillary tubes and many of the microcontainers permit the drops to flow into them by capillary ac-tion. Blood should flow freely from the puncture site with a minimum amount of pressure on the finger. Gentle massaging or milking of the finger can promote blood flow without forcing tissue fluids to contaminate the sample. The site can be wiped from time to time to remove platelet clumps and facilitate additional blood flow.

7. *Cap containers and seal capillary tubes* with plugs or clay. Some collectors tape capillary tubes to a card or request slip to permit identification and prevent the tubes from rolling around during transport.

8. *Apply pressure to the puncture site* with a clean gauze or cotton ball until bleeding has stopped. A bandage may be used with adults and older children. Do *not* place a bandage on the hands or fingers of infants or very young children because they could ingest it and suffocate.

9. *Transport the labeled samples promptly* to the laboratory. The small sample volumes are more sensitive to environmental factors, such as temperature, than the larger volumes obtained by venipuncture.

Heelsticks in newborn infants

The heel is usually used for capillary blood collection in children younger than 1 year old. Most comments on fingersticks also apply to heel punctures. Choice of puncture site is restricted to the lateral and medial edges of the plantar surface (sole) of the foot (Fig. 25-14). The central portion and posterior curvature of the heel are *not* to be used because bone lies close to the surface; bone puncture can result in osteochondritis. Maximum puncture depth should be 2.4 mm. Previous punctures sites and edematous areas should not be used to avoid tissue fluid contamination of the blood sample. Since commercial blood lancets are available in a number of shapes and lengths, selection of the right type is critical. A lancet with a maximum tip length of 2.5 mm should be used for routine sticks, but a shorter tip should be used for small or premature infants. Scapel blades without

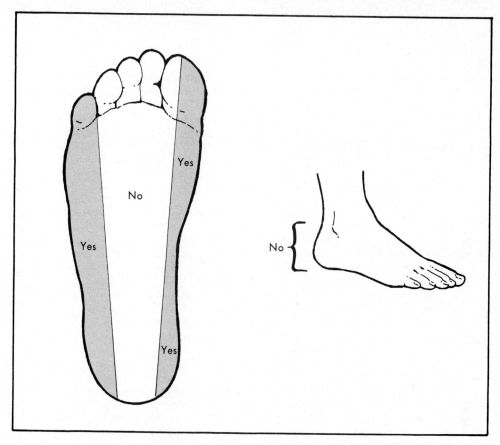

Fig. 25-14.   Sites for capillary puncture: heelstick in infants.

depth control guards should never be used for capillary punctures in infants.

1. Examine the site and warm the heel with a moist warm towel, if necessary. Clean with alcohol and dry.

2. Grasp the heel firmly, placing the index finger at the arch of the foot and the thumb proximal to the puncture site, around the ankle (Fig. 25-15). The puncture should be made with a continuous, deliberate motion at an angle slightly rotated from perpendicular.

3. The heel should be held downward and a gentle but continuous pressure applied to promote blood flow. The first drop should be discarded. Subsequent drops are collected in appropriate containers.

4. After collection is completed, elevate the infant's foot and apply a sterile gauze pad to the site with pressure. When bleeding has stopped, the gauze is removed. Most hospitals discourage the use of bandages on active infants because of the danger of ingestion and suffocation.

Collection from other sites

Ear lobes are an additional source of capillary blood in children and adults. Nerve endings are few at the lobe tip and so it is an almost painless site for a skin puncture.

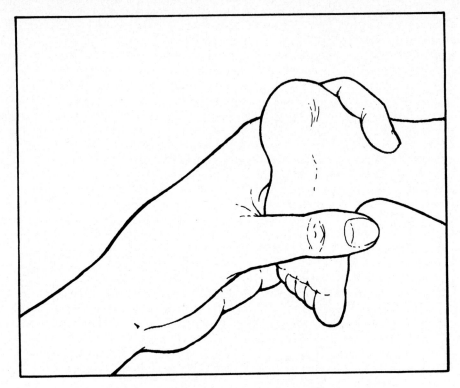

Fig. 25-15.   Holding an infant's heel for capillary puncture.

Badly burned hands and feet may require blood collection from this site, but blood pooling in the lobes produces slightly different cell counts and other values that are sensitive to hemoconcentration. The big toe is an alternate site to the heel in older infants (generally, 6 months to 1 year). Follow the same guidelines as for a fingerstick.

Venous blood can also be obtained from the umbilical cord of a neonate by a physician. This is often the first blood sample received by a laboratory after the birth of a critially-ill infant. In some patients with bad burns or missing limbs, the jugular vein can be used by a physician as a source of blood. Femoral artery punctures can also be done by physicians when other limb veins are unsuitable. Any use of a nonroutine col-

lection site should be noted on laboratory request forms.

BONE MARROW ASPIRATION AND BIOPSY

Examination of the marrow is routinely requested for evaluating hematological conditions in which hematopoietic processes must be examined. Since many blood diseases are characterized by pathological changes in proliferation, maturation, and release from the marrow, direct observation of cell morphology and tissue structure is essential for diagnosis and treatment. Collection is performed by a physician, usually in a clinic or hospital-room setting. In some special instances such as collection for research purposes or when working with immunocompromised patients, the marrow

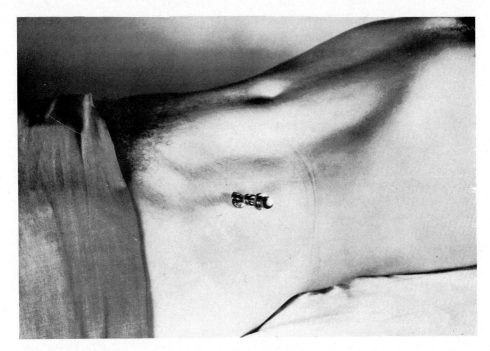

Fig. 25-16. Bone marrow collection: anterior iliac crest.
(From Miale, JB: Laboratory medicine hematology, ed 6, St Louis, 1982, The CV Mosby Co.)

collection may be done in an operating room. Collection of large amounts of marrow for transplantation requires excision in a sterile environment.

Collection sites and techniques

Routine marrow collection is done by aspiration, trephine (needle) biopsy, or a combination of both. Collection sites depend on the pathological condition being investigated, the age of the patient, other medical indications, and the preference and experience of the physician doing the puncture.

Aspiration is the technique most widely used. After penetration into the marrow cavity, a syringe is attached to the needle and the semiliquid marrow is withdrawn by forced, negative pressure. Unfortunately, this disrupts the normal architecture of the marrow and destroys relationships between cellular and noncellular elements. As the

sinusoidal membranes rupture, bleeding dilutes the marrow elements with circulating cells. Aspiration does, however, yield a quantity of individual cells that can be easily smeared for staining. The morphology of abnormal cells is well preserved and identification of cells for differential counts is made with aspirated material.

Needle biopsy uses a needle that cuts a core or plug of tissue from the marrow. It is extracted and preserved so that the marrow structure is intact. Estimates of cellularity (cell to fat and fibrous tissue ratio) are facilitated and the clustering of abnormal cell elements can be evaluated more accurately. Touch preps can also be made from the surface of the marrow plug and these are smeared to provide some cellular detail. Biopsies may also be required in some conditions in which aspiration yields no marrow (a "dry tap"). Dry aspirations can occur because of poor sampling technique, in aplastic marrows, or in conditions in which normal marrow tissue is replaced by infiltrating elements such as lymphosarcomas, granulomatous processes, sclerotic and fibrotic replacement (e.g., myelofibrosis), and some infactions (e.g., miliary tuberculosis). Dry aspirations can also occur for no apparent reason. Aspiration and biopsy can be obtained from the same puncture site by using an instrument such as the Jamshidi needle. Aspiration is done first, followed by biopsy (the iliac crest must be used for a combination collection).

The site of puncture is determined by the physician. The anterior iliac crest is the preferred site in infants and young children (Fig. 25-16), although the medial aspect of the head of the tibia can also be used in young infants (less than 18 months old). The posterior iliac crest is often used in adults, especially in those that may be apprehensive about the procedure (Fig. 25-17). The mid-sternum, adjacent to the second intercostal space, is another traditional site of collection (Fig. 25-18). This site is contraindicated in infants because their sternums are cartilaginous and excess penetration could risk cardiac damage. Apprehensive patients may prefer to have the procedure done to their backsides, out of view. Other possible sites include the spinous processes of the lumbar vertebrae (L2, L3, and L4) and the ribs. The sternal and spinal sites are less likely to be diluted by sinusoidal blood during aspiration, but the iliac

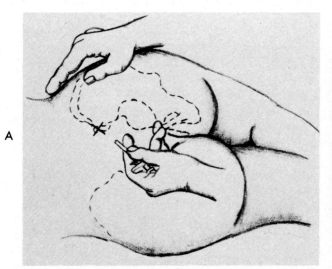
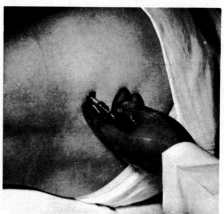

Fig. 25-17.   Bone marrow aspiration: posterior iliac crest.
A, Drawing of anatomical site. **B,** Photograph of aspiration technique. (**A** From Miale, JB: Laboratory medicine hematology, ed 6, St Louis, 1982, The CV Mosby Co; **B** From Bauer, JD: Clinical laboratory methods, ed 9, St Louis, 1982, The CV Mosby Co.)

crest offers multiple sites when a single collection is unsuccessful or likely to be unrepresentative of the pathological process. Considerable heterogeneity of sites exists with regard to the cellular material obtained, especially in the early stages of some myeloproliferative and metastatic diseases. Thus, it is possible to obtain marrow material that is essentially normal from one puncture yet discover pathological cells in a separate aspirate or biopsy only a few millimeters away.

General procedural guidelines

The techniques of collection and methods used to examine marrow vary greatly from institution to institution, but the following are widely-used procedures (see Bauer, 1982, for details of preparing fixatives and processing specimens).

1. The patient is made comfortable, preferably in a quiet examining room or other isolated area. Positioning depends on the collection site to be used: supine (face up) for sternal and anterior iliac puncture, prone (face down) for posterior iliac puncture, and sitting bent forward for vertebral puncture.

2. All required materials, including duplicate items, should be collected and placed in an accessible location prior to the procedure. Once collection starts there will be no time to gather slides, coverslips, or other items. Slides should be cleaned and solutions ready to use. Bone marrow trays containing the surgical instruments may be reusable and autoclavable or they may be disposable.

3. The puncture site is examined, shaved

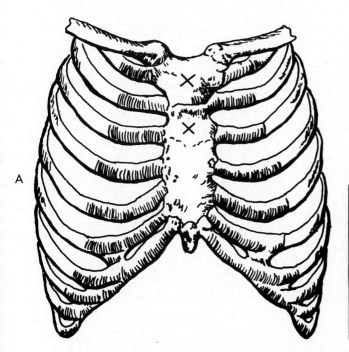
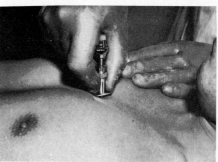

Fig. 25-18. Bone marrow aspiration: sternal puncture.
A, drawing of anatomical site; **B,** photograph of aspiration technique. (**A,** from Miale, JB: Laboratory medicine hematology, ed 6, St Louis, 1982, The CV Mosby Co; **B,** from Bauer, JD: Clinical laboratory methods, ed 9, St Louis, 1982, The CV Mosby Co.)

(if necessary) and thoroughly cleaned with a surgical soap. An antiseptic solution is then applied.

4. The site is numbed with a topical solution, such as 1% procaine hydrochloride (Novocain) or 2% lidocaine, by first infiltrating the skin and then the periosteum covering the bone.

5. The puncture instrument is grasped firmly by the physician and penetration into the marrow cavity is achieved (Fig. 25-19). The stylet is removed and a 10 mL syringe is attached for aspiration. If only a biopsy is performed, the cutting needle is inserted into the outer needle. Aspiration is achieved by pulling the plunger back forceably. The sudden negative pressure sucks a small amount of the marrow into the syringe, producing a sharp pain at the collection site. Children and apprehensive adults need to be carefully restrained and reassured during this step.

6. A small amount of marrow (0.2 mL or less) should be obtained at this point and expressed into a watchglass or onto a clean slide to be examined for marrow particles or spicules. They resemle grains of sand, whitish to yellowish in color. Thin smears should be made from this initial sample for routine stains. The slides can be smeared in the manner of peripheral blood smears. Individual particles can also be placed between cover slips and crushed by pulling the coverslips in opposite directions. A properly-prepared smear will have one or more yellowish-white smudges among the blood.

7. Additional marrow (up to 1.0 mL) can be obtained with a second syringe for more smears and for sectioning. Some protocols permit the additional aspirate to clot in Zenker's solution or in acrolein, whereas others use heparin or EDTA to process the specimen (Fig. 25-20). The anticoagulated aspirate can be separated into particulate matter for additional crush smears and the liquid portion centrifuged in a Wintrobe or capillary tube to obtain layers of lipid,

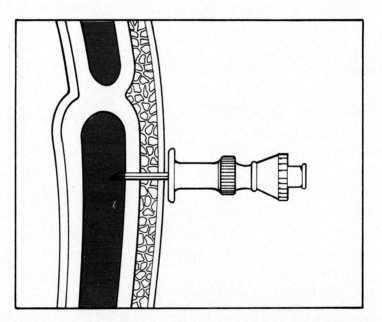

Fig. 25-19. **Bone marrow aspiration: penetration into marrow cavity.**

plasma, nucleated cells, and erythrocytes. The nucleated cell layer is used to prepare a buffy coat smear that is especially useful for detecting and identifying abnormal cells that may occur infrequently.

8. Biopsy cores are also expressed into a watchglass or petri dish. Touch preps are made by lightly pressing a coverslip or slide to the surface of the core and allowing some cells to adhere. The plug is then placed into Zenker's solution or into acrolein for paraffin or methacrylate embedment and sectioning. Tissue for hematoxylin and eosin (H&E) histological staining

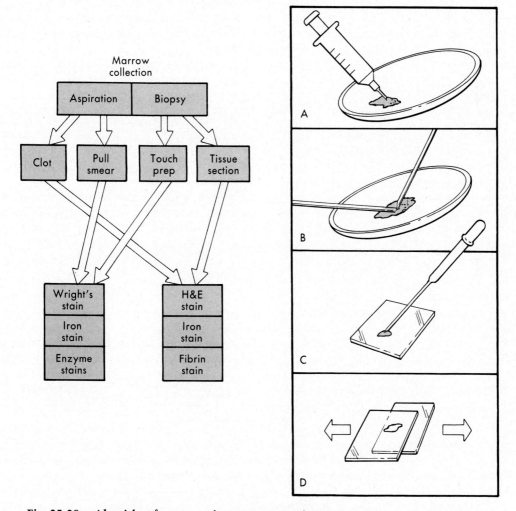

Fig. 25-20.   Algorithm for processing marrow specimens.
Smears are made by (**A**) placing some of the marrow aspirate in a watchglass or petri dish, (**B**) locating some of the gritty marrow particles and (**C**) transferring these to coverslips. A particle is crushed gently between two coverslips (**D**) and a smear made on both when they are pulled in opposite directions.

must be decalcified, a process requiring several days.

9. Combined aspiration and biopsy is done by tilting the needle in the marrow to an angle away from the initial aspiration site. The biopsy tool is inserted, the plug cut, and the needle withdrawn.

10. After the final sample is obtained, the outer needle is withdrawn and a dry, sterile compress is applied with pressure to the site for several minutes. After hemostasis is realized, a bandage is taped over the site and routine hygiene is observed for 1 or 2 days.

• • •

Special cytochemical stains are widely used for cellular identification, particularly to differentiate acute leukemias. The slides should be cleaned in 95% alcohol, fixed in acetone, and air dried. The slides can be stored at 1 to 6° C until used. Some techniques call for the marrow material to be fixed in specific solutions (formaldehyde and absolute ethyl alcohol for peroxidase, citrate buffered acetone for alkaline phosphatase, and citrate-acetone-methanol for esterases). In addition, cytogenetic studies require preservation of the aspirate in chromosome culture medium or into sterile Hank's solution with sodium heparin (Bauer, 1982, p. 269).

SUMMARY

- Routine phlebotomy is performed with a syringe and needle or with an evacuated-tube system. The advantage of the latter is rapid collection of multiple samples, employing a variety of anticoagulants for different analytical procedures.
- Anticoagulants are selected for the effects they produce on cellular morphology or for the manner in which they affect coagulation processes. EDTA is used for most routine tests, citrate for most coagulation studies.
- Blood collection is the first critical phase in processing and analysis of a blood sample. Positive identification of patient and sample is one of the most important steps in this phase. Proper collection technique requires practice and patience. Errors during collection and transport to the laboratory can adversely affect test results.
- Routine capillary punctures are done from the fingertip of adults and children or from the heel of infants. Standardized lancets assure proper puncture depth. Capillary puncture may be necessary in some patients with severe burns, poor veins, or other medical problems.
- Bone marrow collection is achieved by aspiration or biopsy through a needle into the sternum, anterior or posterior iliac crest, vertebrae of the lumbar spine, ribs, or head of the tibia. The site and technique depends on the age of patients, their medical condition and preferences of the physician performing the puncture.
- Marrow samples must contain spicules of material with hematopoietic tissue in order to evaluate proliferation and maturation processes.
- Aspiration destroys the marrow structure, resulting in dilution by sinusoidal blood. The morphology of individual cells is usually well preserved, facilitating identification of abnormal cells by routine and special stains.
- Biopsy results in a plug of intact marrow tissue that poorly reveals individual cells but preserves the structure and relationships of marrow elements.

26

Routine Blood Examination

PREPARING BLOOD FOR EXAMINATION

Most hematological studies are conducted either on blood cells or on coagulation components, using whole blood and plasma, respectively. Chapter 25 described techniques for collecting blood and the use of anticoagulants to prevent clotting. This chapter outlines preparation of blood smears for cell studies and the numerical evaluations that comprise the complete blood count (CBC) and other routine studies. These chapters are not intended to be procedure manuals or present sources of error. Several references are listed that provide expanded methodological information.

EXAMINATION OF WET PREPARATIONS

It is often advantageous to observe blood in its living state, free from the artifacts resulting from drying, fixation, and staining. White cell motility and phagocytosis is best observed in wet preparations, some inclusions are easily seen with polarized light or phase microscopy, and some poikilocytic forms (e.g., stomatocytosis and echinocytosis) can be evaluated for artifact versus in vivo occurrence.

A drop of blood placed between a glass microscope slide and a coverslip permits observations of single cells, with or without staining. Dilution of the blood with physiological saline facilitates dispersion of the cells for observations or photography. Since an unsealed coverslip is subject to desiccation (within minutes to an hour, depending on heat from the microscope stage and hu-

midity of the surrounding air), observations over an extended time require additional steps (Fig. 26-1).

1. *Humidity chamber.* A simple slide chamber to retard the rate of desiccation can be prepared from a petri dish. Toothpicks or applicator sticks are used as a platform to separate the glass slide from a damp gauze or tissue square. With petri dish cover in place, the chamber air is rapidly saturated and the coverslip preparation dries slowly.

2. *Coverslip sealed along edge.* The perimeter of the coverslip is ringed with a sealant, such as petroleum jelly. The drop of blood is placed in the center of the coverslip on the same side as the sealant, then the glass slide is lowered onto the coverslip and carefully pressed into place. The preparation is turned over for examination. With practice, the sealant will form a complete barrier around the liquid drop and only a small amount of air will be trapped. This technique can also be used to demonstrate crystal formation in red cells as oxygen decreases within the droplet.

3. *Slides with wells.* Special glass slides containing one or more depressions can also be used. The wells hold sufficient liquid volume so that desiccation is not an immediate problem. These slides can also be used with a sealant and coverslip for observations over an extended time. Because of the liquid depth, the blood may require additional dilution to facilitate observations.

PREPARATION OF BLOOD SMEARS

Smears can be made by a variety of staining methods. The essential step involves

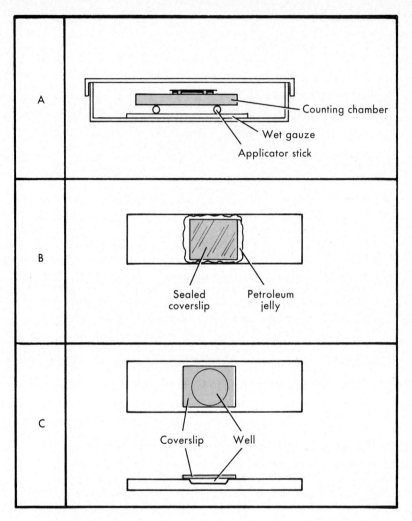

Fig. 26-1.   Wet preparations.
A, Humidity chamber made from a petri dish. A hemacytometer or slide and coverslip lies on applicator sticks. **B,** Sealed coverslip on glass slide. **C,** Slides with concave wells.

formation of a monolayer of cells with a minimum of distortion or artifact introduction.

   1. Coverslip preparation. The blood can be spread between two coverslips. When the slips are pulled apart, a thin layer of blood is left on each. This is a common technique for preparing marrow smears since only a small droplet is required for two coverslips. Each coverslip is then inverted on a rubber, stopper, stained, and placed face down on a glass slide.

   2. Wedge smear. A drop of blood placed on a glass slide can be spread by using a second slide held at an acute angle (Fig. 26-2). The drop is placed at one end of the slide and a second "spreader" slide is brought into contact with the drop. As the drop

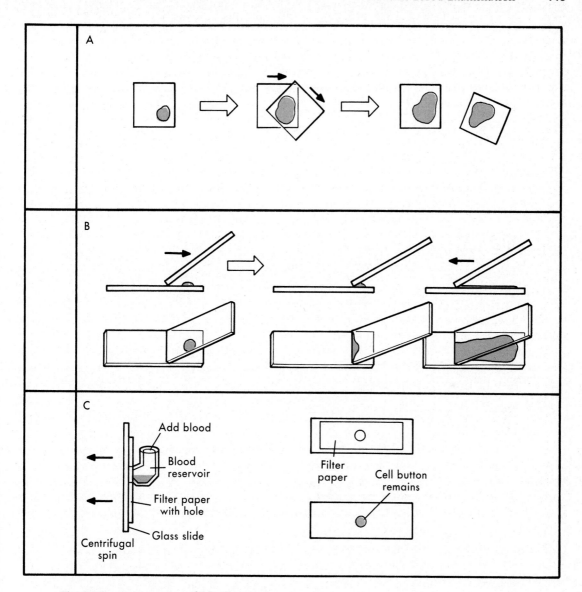

Fig. 26-2. Preparation of blood smears.

A, Coverslip preparation. A drop of blood or marrow is spread between two coverslips as they are pulled in opposite directions. **B,** Wedge smear. A drop of blood is pulled across the slide by another slide at an acute angle, creating a wedge-shaped smear with decreasing cell density. **C,** Centrifugal smear. A drop of blood is spun from a central point, creating an evenly dispersed monolayer of cells.

moves outward along the edge of the spreader, this second slide is moved along the surface of the first slide in a smooth motion. Diluted bloods or liquids of thin viscocity are spread quickly, whereas thicker bloods are moved at a slower rate. Some workers prefer to lay the first slide on a flat surface, others prefer to hold it at an angle with the other hand. The goal is to achieve a wedge-shaped smear with a thin, feathery edge. Observations of cell morphology are optimal adjacent to the edge.

3. Smears prepared by centrifugation. A monolayer of cells can be prepared by using cytological centrifuges. These instruments have high torque, low inertia motors that facilitate rapid spreading of the cells across a slide from a central point. This eliminates some of the artifacts and signs of cell destruction that are inevitable with the wedge technique. Only small volumes of liquid are needed, making this an ideal means of preparing smears from bone marrow, buffy coats, spinal fluid, and other body fluids. The cells are less distorted and more evenly distributed, presenting better conditions for critical morphological studies and photographic documentation.

ROUTINE STAINING TECHNIQUES

Routine morphological studies of bone marrow and blood smears use a Romanowsky stain, which contains oxidized methylene blue and eosin. A number of commercial preparations are available, but most are based on modifications of the Wright-Giemsa technique.

Wright-Giemsa blood stain

Principle. **Methylene blue** at alkaline pH forms a complex of basic azures, methylene blue, and methyl violet. The dye is dissolved in methyl alcohol, which also serves as a fixative for the blood cells. These basic blue dyes have an affinity for the acidic components of the nucleus (DNA) and cytoplasm (RNA). **Eosin** or derivatives of eosin are acidic components and they combine with basic elements of the cells, such as hemoglobin and eosinophilic granules. The dye also contains neutral components that stain other cell structures. The resulting polychrome dye produces a complex staining pattern to facilitate identification of most types of blood cells. The following directions are provided for a manual procedure, but automated staining instruments are available from several manufacturers.

Reagents

1. Wright-Giemsa stain consists of 9 g of powdered Wright stain and 1 g of powdered Giemsa stain, dissolved in 90 mL of glycerin and 2910 mL of absolute anhydrous methyl alcohol. The materials are mixed and left to stand in the dark for about 1 month at room temperature. The preparation can also be heated to 37°C, decreasing the incubation time to several days. The stain should be shaken daily for the first few days. Aliquots can be placed in small brown dropper bottles. Each working bottle should be filtered daily or before use.

2. Sodium phosphate buffer, pH 6.4

Procedure. Slides can be stained on horizontal racks; coverslips are stained on inverted rubber stoppers. The smear is either air dried or dipped in methyl alcohol. Stain is added to the slide, covering the surface without spilling over the side. The staining time, determined empirically, varies from 1 to 3 minutes, depending on the particular batch of stain and the thickness of the smear (bone marrows usually require longer times).

The phosphate buffer is added to the stain, again avoiding overflow. The diluted stain-buffer combination can be mixed by gently blowing across the slide surface and a bluish-green metallic sheen indicates active staining of the cellular material. The stain buffer is left for an additional 3 to 6 minutes, as determined empirically. Tap water or distilled water, which is slightly acidic, can be substituted for phosphate buffer.

The stain is washed off the slide by a gentle rinse with tap or distilled water. The back of the slide is wiped with gauze or paper towel to remove excess stain before the slide dries. After drying, the slide can be examined directly or permanently fixed under a coverslip with mounting medium.

Results. Macroscopically, a properly stained smear appears pinkish-gray. Microscopically, erythrocytes stain pink to orange, eosinophil granules stain a bright orange, neutrophil cytoplasm stains a light pink, and lymphocyte cytoplasm a light to medium blue. The nuclei of granulocytes and lymphocytes stain dark blue to purple. Improperly stained slides usually result from buffers that are overly acidic (too pink) or overly basic (too blue). Inappropriate ratios of stain time to buffer time is another cause of improper stains. Precipitated dye may appear if the slide dries during the staining process or if the slides (or coverslips) are not clean prior to making the smear. Slides can be cleansed with methyl alcohol and restained.

Vital staining

Some cellular components can only be stained while the blood cells are living. Some techniques kill the cells. Others permit observations of stained, living cells.

The vital dyes, **brilliant cresyl blue** or **new methylene blue,** precipitate the cytoplasmic organelles of living reticulocytes (mitochondria, ribosomes, and residual RNA) as a blue-green reticulofilamentous substance (Plate 8A). Mature erythrocytes do not display this precipitate. This permits enumeration of reticulocytes in the peripheral blood by counting the number of cells with intracellular precipitate as a percentage of total erythrocytes. An automated procedure uses **acridine orange,** a fluorescent dye when exposed to ultraviolet light, to achieve the same results but with more precision.

Other vital stains include either Janus green or pinacyanol in combination with neutral red for staining vacuoles and mitochondria. Methyl violet, new methylene blue, or brilliant cresyl blue demonstrate Heinz bodies in living erythrocytes.

These dyes are added to small amounts of blood in a ratio according to instructions of the manufacturer. A common technique is to fill a microhematocrit tube about 1/3 volume of blood and 1/3 of dye, then mix by tilting the tube back and forth several times so the dye and blood zones merge. The tube sits at room temperature for several minutes to permit dye uptake by the cells, then a drop or two of the mixture is expelled and discarded. The drops near the center of the mixture should be well stained and these are placed on a slide under a coverslip for direct observation, or the drop is smeared by the wedge technique and dried for extended observations or counting. Other staining techniques are described in the next chapter that use cytochemical and immunological reactions to identify cell types or to observe cell inclusions.

BLOOD CELL COUNTING TECHNIQUES
Manual counting procedures

Blood cell enumeration is a critical component of a hematological evaluation. Before the advent of automated instruments, blood cell counts were performed manually, using a counting chamber (**hemacytometer**). Blood was diluted with an appropriate solution, the diluted blood placed in the chamber under a coverslip, and the cells in a ruled area were counted. A formula was used to derive the blood cell count, based on the dilution factor and the area and volume of the chamber in which cells were counted. A typical diluting system (Unopette) is shown in Fig. 25-10, and the ruled area of a hemacytometer is shown in Fig. 26-3. Manual counting is still used for counting eosinophils, platelets in thrombocytopenic patients, and leukocytes in neutropenic patients.

Procedure
1. The pipette shield is used to open the diaphragm of the dilutant vial.
2. Blood is obtained from a venipuncture

or a capillary stick and drawn into the micropipette (capillary action ceases when the pipette is filled). Wipe excess blood carefully from the outside of the pipette.

3. Using one finger to cover the base of the pipette, insert the pipette (tip first) into the diluent vial while simultaneously squeezing the diluent container.

4. Release the reservoir and the end of the pipette at the same time. This will draw the blood sample into the diluent (some practice may be required). Blood is rinsed from the pipette by squeezing the diluent container several times, then cover the opening and invert several times to thoroughly mix the contents.

5. The base of the pipette can be reinserted into the vial for transportation and the outside of the container can be labelled. The pipette serves as the dispensing dropper to fill the hemacytometer chamber.

6. The hemacytometer is placed on a flat surface and a special coverslip is placed over the counting surface. One or two drops of diluted blood are expelled from the mixed vial; the next drop is touched to the groove protruding from under the coverslip and capillary action draws the drop across the counting surface. The entire chamber surface of each side should be filled, but no excess should spill over the sides of the counting surface.

7. Depending on the cells to be counted, the chamber should sit for up to several minutes in a covered, moist petri dish to prevent desiccation. This insures that the cells will lie along the same focal depth

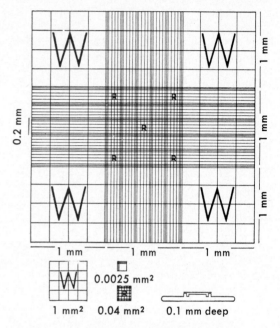

Fig. 26-3.   Hemacytometer counting grid.
Improved Neubauer ruling. R = red cell counting area; W = white cell counting area (from Bauer JD: Clinical laboratory methods, ed 9, St Louis, 1982, The CV Mosby Co).

Table 26-1. Manual cell counting data

Cells	Diluent	Area counted
Leukocytes	2% acetic acid or 1% hydrochloric acid (vol/vol)	4 large squares (4 mm²)
Erythrocytes	Gower's solution, Hayem's solution, or isotonic saline	5 small squares (0.2 mm²)
Platelets	1% ammonium oxalate	10-25 small squares (0.4-1.0 mm²)
Eosinophils	1% aqueous phloxine	18 large squares (18 mm²)
Basophils	Toluidine blue	18 large squares (18 mm²)

when viewed under the microscope. This is particularly critical for platelets.

8. The cells of interest in a portion of the ruled hemacytometer area are counted (Fig. 26-3) separately in each of the two chambers. The blood concentration is calculated on the basis of number of cells counted, depth of counting chamber (0.1 mm), total area of chamber in which cells are counted, and dilution factor (see Unopette vials and pipettes):

Cell concentration (per μL) = number of cells × dilution factor × volume factor (Table 26-1)

Additional information on sources of error, calculations, and counting methods can be found in the textbooks by Brown (1988), Pittiglio (1987), or Turgeon (1988). Other counting chamber designs are available that use larger volumes or different counting area patterns for specialized cell studies. Counting chambers can also be used to quantitate blood cells in body fluids, such as cerebral spinal fluid. Thoma blood cell pipettes have also been used to mix blood and diluents. The pipettes have volume calibration marks and a mixing bead. They require a mouthpiece, tube, and filter or a syringe attachment to draw blood into the pipette and a special shaker or wheel for mixing.

Automated cell counting

Two methods are most often used to enumerate blood cells in automated cell counters. These are the impedence method (Coulter principle) and optical methods using focused laser beams. Each of these have

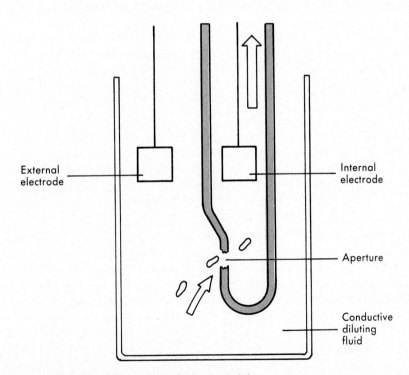

Fig. 26-4. Impedence counting (Coulter principle).
Cells flow through an aperture that separates two compartments. Electrical potential between electrodes changes as cells pass. Number of pulses translates to cell count and amplitude of pulse depends on cell volume that displaces conductive fluid.

been incorporated into an increasingly-sophisticated series of instruments that combine basic cell counting with identification and calculation procedures. These instruments make it possible to count thousands of cells in a few seconds, decreasing the coefficient of variation (see Chapter 29) and increasing the precision of such counts manyfold in comparison to manual methods.

Impedance counting was developed by Coulter in the late 1950s, thus this method is also referred to as the **Coulter principle.** Nonconductive cells or other solid particles displace a volume of a conducting diluent. When the particles flow through a small aperture, the change in this conducting volume can be sensed by disruption of electron flow (increased resistance or impedence) between electrodes placed on either side of the aperture (Fig. 26-4). The number of disruptions or pulses is expressed as the particle or cell count and the magnitude (amplitude) of the impedence change is correlated with the volume of the particle. Thousands of particles pass through the aperture in a few seconds and the integral data on each pulse can be collected, stored, and displayed as a histogram. Particle size discrimination can be made electronically by setting thresholds above and below which particles will be recognized or ignored. Thus, platelets can be enumerated at discrimination settings consistent with platelet volumes while red blood cells are counted simultaneously within their respective volume range (Fig. 26-5).

Optical detection

A thin stream of particles or cells passing through a focused beam of a **laser** can also be used for counting. The blood is diluted in isotonic saline and passed through the light beam as a stream of single cells. This is accomplished by focusing the blood cells with a second fluid, forming an outer sheath of liquid moving in the same direction. This is a principle known as **hydrody-**namic focusing. The resulting instrument is generically defined as a **flow cytometer.** As each cell passes through the beam, it scatters the light at angles proportional to structural features of the cell (Fig. 26-6). Most laser systems incorporate light sensors that detect forward scatter of the beam (180° from the light source) and right angle (90°) scatter. The former is correlated with cell volume or density, analogous to the impedence amplitude of the Coulter principle. Right angle deflection is a function of cell contents, primarily cytoplasmic granularity. Photodetectors convert the light signals to electrical signals that are processed by a computer. Data display routinely includes cell count and MCV, but simple cell differential counts can also be assigned (e.g., granulocytes versus nongranulocytes).

Cell identification can be enhanced by incorporating fluorochrome dyes in the cell suspension to be counted. The dye can be used directly to stain or "tag" certain cell components (e.g., a granule or an enzyme) or the dye can be attached to an immunological component (e.g., antibody to a lymphocyte surface antigen). Different types of fluorochromes can be excited by different wavelengths of light, thus a particular cell with a specific tag can be counted independently. A differential leukocyte count or an automated reticulocyte count is made by using two or more laser detection systems in sequence.

In addition to detection, the flow cytometry principle is used to separate cells for specialized testing. As each specified or labelled cell passes through the beam, the computer can direct a charging collar to apply a positive or negative electrical charge to the cell (Fig. 26-7). The charged cell is deflected or sorted into a unique stream and container, making it possible to obtain a sample of monocytes or T4 lymphocytes or any other cell subset that can be identified by specific cell markers. These **cell sorters** were initially reserved for the research laboratory, but recent diagnostic applications

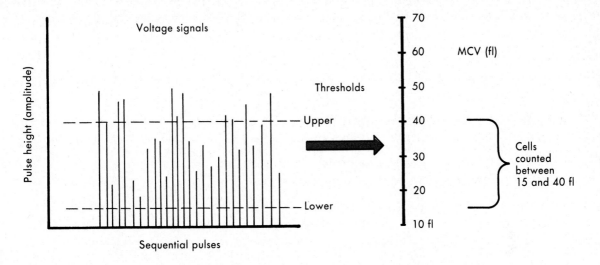

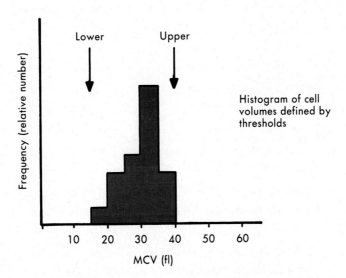

Fig. 26-5. Histogram of cell counts with limiting thresholds.

(e.g., T4/T8 ratios) have assured their use in large clinical laboratories as well.

RED BLOOD CELL EVALUATION
Hemoglobin

A quantitative determination of hemoglobin concentration provides essential information for diagnosis of anemia. The spec-trophotometric assay is simple. Lyse the erythrocytes (releasing the hemoglobin as a pigment), measure the pigment in a colorimeter or spectrophotometer as a function of light transmission or absorption, and compare these values with those of a standard solution of known hemoglobin concentration. Most clinical procedures mea-

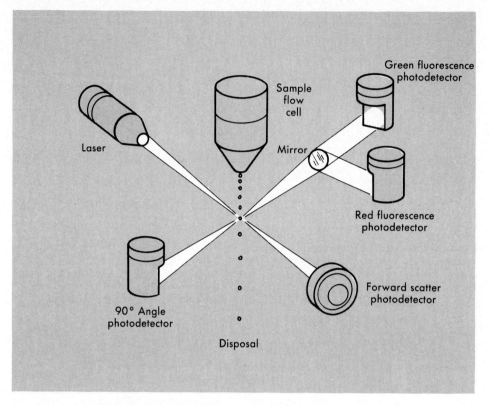

Fig. 26-6.   Optical detection of cells by a laser-based system.
Cells are focused by the laminar flow of a sheath fluid. Cells are counted and partly identified by differential light scatter of a laser beam.

sure hemoglobin as **cyanmethemoglobin,** a method that includes most forms of hemoglobin (including those that do not carry oxygen). The procedure involves oxidation of ferrous iron to the ferric state (formation of methemoglobin) by ferricyanide and subsequent conversion to cyanmethemoglobin by potassium cyanide. The cyanide containing reagent, Drabkin's solution, is widely used for both manual procedures and automated instruments and the reagent is relatively stable. This method does not measure sulfhemoglobin.

Procedure

1. Blood is collected by capillary puncture into heparinized tubes or, preferably, by phlebotomy into EDTA, heparin, or oxalate. The blood should be tested within 24 hours of collection, although nonhemolyzed specimens can be assayed up to 1 week later with good results.

2. For a manual method, a standard curve is prepared by diluting a commercially-prepared standard solution of hemoglobin (e.g., 80 mg per dL of cyanmethemoglobin, equiuvalent to 20 g per dL of hemoglobin in a blood sample) and plotting a standard curve of concentration against light transmission or absorbtion (optical density) at 540 nm. Test samples are processed in the same manner, except that 0.02 mL of blood is added to 5.0 mL of reagent, mixed, and

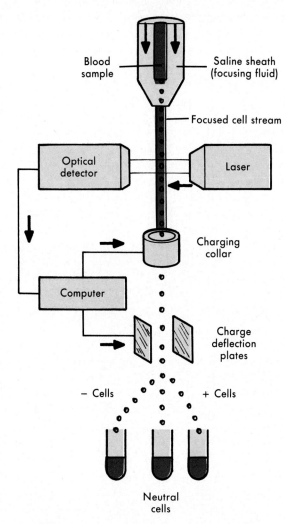

Fig. 26-7.   Flow cytometry: sorting cells.
A laser detection system is combined with a computer and a charging collar. Cells of a particular identity (carrying fluorescent tags that react to the laser) are charged and deflected to a collection contained.

with a modified Drabkin's solution and measurement of light absorbance at 540 nm.

Comments. Because hemoglobin is determined spectrophotometrically, dirty glassware (manual method) or contamination of the reagents can produce elevated results. Blood with a high plasma lipid content is also unsuitable, but the red blood cells can be washed several times in buffered saline and resuspended to their original volume, effectively removing the interferring plasma. In some leukemia patients, an exceptionally elevated leukocyte count may also interfere with the hemoglobin determination. After the cells are lysed, white cells can be centrifuged and the lysate (supernatant) used in the spectrophotometer. This method may also be applied to some lipemic bloods.

Reference range

Adult males: 13-17 g/dL	Newborn infants: 16-23 g/dL
Adult females: 12-16 g/dL	Infants at one year: 9-15 g/dL

Hematocrit

The packed cell volume (PCV) or hematocrit is the ratio of red blood cells to plasma, expressed as a percent of the whole blood volume. This can be written as either a percent (e.g., 36%) or a decimal (0.36). The hematocrit, like the red blood cell count and the hemoglobin, is a relative measure, varying as a function of both the cell or liquid component.

Procedure

1. Blood is placed in a capillary or microhematocrit tube, filling about 3/4 of the tube. The blood can be collected into heparinized tubes directly from a capillary puncture or added to nonheparinized tubes from an EDTA tube.

2. One end of the tube is sealed with clay or a commercial sealant. This must be done carefully to assure a good plug without breaking the tube. Avoid trapping air between the blood and plug.

3. The tubes are placed in a calibrated microhematocrit centrifuge, sealed ends out

allowed to sit for several minutes. Duplicate determinations should agree within 0.3 g per dL.

3. Automated instruments process the blood for cell counts and hemoglobin determination by a series of parallel dilutions, but the principle is the same: lysis of the sample

against a rubber ring. The lid is placed firmly over the centrifuge head, the cover closed and the timer set as determined by calibration with control samples. Most instruments require 3 to 5 minutes centrifugation time.

4. The tubes should be removed and read within a minute or two after the centrifuge has stopped to avoid redispersion of the cells into the plasma. Hemolysis of the plasma should be noted, since this may lower the hematocrit results in relation to the hemoglobin determination (the hematocrit is roughly three times the value of the hemoglobin if the cells are normocytic).

5. A variety of devices are available to determine the hematocrit value: lined cards, wheels, and optical instruments. All work by the same principle, measuring the height of the total plasma and cell column and the height of the red cell layer. If a buffy coat, consisting of white blood cells, is unusually large, this can also be noted (Fig. 26-8).

Comments. A poorly-calibrated centrifuge will provide erroneous results. Since the rotation speed is fixed (preset), calibration consists of noting the time required to compact a standard red cell sample (commercially available as preserved erythrocytes or other particles) to a predetermined value. If a blood sample is well mixed before each microhematocrit tube is filled, replicate readings should not vary by more than 1%. Some laboratories report values to the nearest whole number, others to the nearest half percent.

Automated instruments also report a hematocrit value, often to the nearest 0.1 or 0.2%, based on calculations from the MCV and red cell count:

Hematocrit = [red blood cell count (in millions/μL) × MCV (fL)] ÷ 10

This is the reciprocal of the formula for calculating MCV as a red cell indice. Because the cells are not physically packed by centrifugation, the calculated hematocrit may be slightly lower than one determined manually (a small amount of plasma is trapped between the cells during centrifugation, expanding the red cell layer).

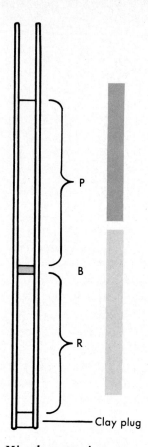

Fig. 26-8. Microhematocrit.
B, Buffy coat of leukocytes and platelets; *P*, plasma; *R*, red blood cells.

Reference values

Adult male: 38-50%	Newborn infant: 50-70%
Adult female: 36-46%	Infant at one year: 28-45%

Red blood cell count

Red cells are counted manually in hemacytometers or by automated instruments based on the principles described previously. Blood is diluted in an isotonic solution to facilitate enumeration, so all blood cells and platelets are present. For most samples, the contribution of leukocytes is negligible (e.g., 8000 per μL WBCs compared with an RBC count of 5,000,000 per μL is an inclusive error of 0.16%). However, a leukemia patient with a white cell count of 300,000 per μL and a red cell count of 3,000,000 per μL has a leukocyte contribution that equals 9.1% of the total cell count (excluding platelets). Discrimination thresholds and identification protocols must be used on automated instruments that distinguish red cells from white blood cells or the white cell count must be subtracted from the total blood cell count. Platelets, in most conditions, are small enough so that volume overlap does not interfere with the red cell determination. White cells are easily distinguished from red cells under the microscope when counting cells manually and the differences can be further enhanced by adding methylene blue or a similar dye to the diluting fluid.

A manual red cell count uses the central square of a Neubauer hemacytometer (Fig. 26-3). Red cells in five or more of the small squares are counted and the volume factor is calculated accordingly (each square equals 0.004 mm^3). Manual methods for RBC counts range from 5% to 30%, depending on technique, the red cell concentration, and the area counted. Severely anemic bloods may require less dilution than normal bloods and bloods of polychemia patients may require additional dilution. In clinical practice, automated red cell counting has all but replaced manual techniques.

Reference values

Adult male: 4.2-6.0 × 10^6/μL	Newborn infant: 4.8-7.0 × 10^6/μL
Adult female: 3.8-5.4 × 10^6/μL	Infant at one year: 4.0-5.5 × 10^6/μL

Red blood cell indices

Calculation of the red blood cell indices provides information to assess the size (volume) and hemoglobin content of erythrocytes when evaluating types of anemia. The indices are calculated from data on red cell numbers, hematocrit and hemoglobin.

Mean Corpuscular Volume (MCV) indicates the average volume of red blood cells, expressed in femtoliters (fL):

$$MCV\ (fL) = \frac{\text{hematocrit (\%)} \times 10}{\text{RBC count, in millions}}$$

Mean corpuscular hemoglobin (MCH) indicates the average amount (mass) of hemoglobin in red blood cells, expressed in picograms (pg):

$$MCH\ (pg) = \frac{\text{hemoglobin (g/dL)} \times 10}{\text{RBC count, in millions}}$$

Mean corpuscular hemoglobin concentration (MCHC) indicates the average concentration of hemoglobin in red blood cells, expressed in percent (%) or g per dL:

$$MCHC\ (\%) = \frac{\text{hemoglobin (g/dL)} \times 100}{\text{hematocrit (\%)}}$$

$$MCHC\ (g/dL) = \frac{\text{hemoglobin (g/dL)}}{\text{hematocrit (decimal)}}$$

Reference values
Mean corpuscular volume: 85 to 95 fL
Mean corpuscular hemoglobin: 27 to 31 pg
Mean corpuscular hemoglobin concentration: 32 to 36 g/dL or %

Red blood cell distribution width (RDW) is a quantitative measure of anisocytosis, the variability of red cell size, usually measured as mean cell volume. This parameter is derived by automated instruments that measure MCV directly. A histogram of red cell volumes is plotted and the RDW is defined as the coefficient of variation of the MCV:

$$RDW\ (\%) = \frac{\text{standard deviation of MCV}}{\text{mean MCV}} \times 100$$

Reference value. 11% to 14%.

RETICULOCYTE COUNT AND INDEX

Reticulocytes represent effective erythrocyte productivity, that is, erythroblastic replication, maturation, and release. Residual and ribosomal RNA content can be detected in reticulocytes, but not mature erythrocytes, by exposing the living cells to a supravital stain such as new methylene blue N or brilliant cresyl blue. The dye is absorbed and the RNA is precipitated as reticulofilamentous substance, visible on the dried slide as amorphous intracellular blue-green granules (Plate 8A). The smears can be counterstained with Wright's stain subsequently, facilitating comparisons to the degree of anisocytosis and polychromasia that accompany the appearance of immature red blood cells.

Procedure

1. Add anticoagulated blood to one third of the capacity of a nonheparinized microhematocrit tube. EDTA or heparin are the anticoagulants of choice.

2. Add filtered dye to the blood in the microhematocrit tube, bringing the total liquid volume in the tube to two thirds of capacity. The dye should be in direct contact with the blood, leaving about one third of the tube volume empty.

3. Tilt the tube back and forth, twirling it between the fingers, so that the blood and dye mix as each coats the inner surface of the tube.

4. Let the tube sit horizontally for 10 minutes to permit absorption of the dye and precipitation of the RNA.

5. Expel the first two or three drops at either end and prepare wedge or spun smears with the dye-blood mixture from the center of the tube. Dry the slides and examine with the oil immersion lens. The slides can also be counterstained at this time, if desired.

6. One thousand erythrocytes are counted and the number of reticulocytes detected are tabulated within the 1000 cell count. Example: 23 reticulocytes are observed during the 1000 red cell count (977 cells were mature red cells), yielding a reticulocyte count of 2.3%.

Comments. Protocols for enumerating the cells vary from laboratory to laboratory.

Turgeon (1988) suggests that 500 cells on each of two slides be counted and compared. If results vary by more than 20%, a third slide of 500 cells should be counted. Bauer (1982) indicates that 2000 cells should be enumerated for low reticulocyte counts. If two slides of 1000 cells each agree within 10%, the two values can be averaged and reported. The cells should be examined in areas of the slide where they do not overlap. An oil immersion field containing between 100 and 200 cells is optimal.

An automated procedure uses flow cytometry to count cells that have been stained with the fluorochrome dye, **acridine orange.** This dye preferentially stains RNA and it fluoresces when exposed to ultraviolet light. The instrument can count thousands of reticulocytes in a few seconds at accuracies of about 0.1%, compared to average values of 2 to 10% for manual methods.

The **absolute reticulocyte count** provides a comparable basis for following progression or treatment of anemia and this is now the preferred form of reporting values. The absolute value can be determined by multiplying the red cell count by the reticulocyte percent:

$$\text{Absolute reticulocyte count (per } \mu\text{L)}$$
$$= \frac{\text{Reticulocyte count (\%)}}{100}$$
$$\times \text{RBC count (per } \mu\text{L)}$$

The reticulocyte count can also be corrected for the degree of anemia present, since a decreased hematocrit and an increased reticulocyte ratio exaggerates the production response. The **corrected reticulocyte count** is based on normal hematocrit values of 42% for women and 45% for men:

$$\text{Corrected reticulocyte count (\%)}$$
$$= \frac{\text{patient hematocrit (\%)}}{\text{normal hematocrit (\%)}}$$
$$\times \text{reticulocyte count (\%)}$$

If the anemia is severe and the erythropoietic response includes release of marrow reticulocytes, the **reticulocyte index** compensates for the amount of time it takes for reticulocytes to mature in the peripheral blood. The additional correction simply divides the corrected reticulocyte index by 2, a number that represents the increased reticulocyte maturation time in the peripheral blood.

Reference values
  Newborn infants: 2.0% to 6.5%
  Children: 0.5% to 4.0%
  Adults: 0.5% to 1.5%
Reticulocyte counts are decreased in conditions that reflect decreased erythropoiesis: aplastic anemia, aplastic crises of hemolytic anemias, marrow replacement by tumor cells, and dyserythropoiesis. Increased reticulocyte counts are seen in response to hemorrhage (acute or chronic blood loss), hemolytic anemias, and during erythropoietic response to iron or cobalamin therapy.

WHITE BLOOD CELL EVALUATION
White blood cell count

When blood is diluted with a weak acid solution, the red blood cells are lysed, while white blood cells and platelets remain intact. The addition of a dye to the solution enhances visualization of the leukocytes for manual counts. The principles of enumeration are the same as for the red cell count. A large counting area of the hemacytometer is used for white cell counts, usually consisting of 4 square millimeters in each chamber (Fig. 26-3). Dilutions are not as large, usually on the order of 1:20 (Thoma pipettes) to 1:100 (Unopette system). Manual leukocyte counts are useful for patients with marked neutropenia (e.g., during the aplastic phase of marrow response to cancer chemotherapy) and in other conditions when the white cell count falls below 2000 per μL.

Nucleated red blood cells (NRBCs) will be counted as leukocytes by automated instruments nor will the cells be hemolyzed by the weak acid of the diluting fluid used in manual counting procedures. The white cell count can be corrected by examination of the blood smear and noting the number of NRBCs per 100 WBCs. Correct the count whenever the ratio of NRBCs to WBCs is greater than 20:1 (>5%) by the formula:

Corrected WBC count =
$$\frac{\text{uncorrected WBC count} \times 100}{100 + \text{number of NRBCs per 100 WBCs}}$$

Correction is most often required in patients with severe anemias, some types of blood dyscrasias, and neonates with large numbers of erythroblasts.

Differential count

Leukocytes are identified and enumerated from their morphological appearance on stained blood smears or by automated instruments that use a combination of optical characteristics and histochemical reactions. Blood smears are most often stained with Wright's stain, Giemsa stain or a modification of one of these methylene-based polychrome dyes.

The slide is examined with the high dry objective (40 to 44 ×) to observe cell distribution, red cell morphology, and to screen for infrequent, abnormal cells that might be missed during the differential count. A drop of oil is added to the slide and the oil immersion lens (95 to 100 ×) carefully lowered into focus. The count should be made in the "feathered edge" area of the smear, where the red cells are evenly dispersed with little overlap. A consistent search pattern should be used that permits examination of a representative portion of the optimal area of the smear, but without counting the same area twice (Fig. 26-9).

Absolute leukocyte counts are often reported along with or in place of percentages:

Absolute cell count/μL = total WBC count/μL
  × % of the cell on the differential

Manual differential counters are used to tabulate the results. Each major cell type is represented by a key and this is pushed as

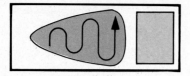

Fig. 26-9. Search pattern and area for differential counts on a blood smear.

the cell is located and identified. Most counters have eight keys and registers plus a register that records the total leukocytes counted. A bell rings each time 100 cells are registered. A routine differential count includes 100 cells, but unusual counts may require additional cells. Quantitative counts of bone marrow smears usually require a 200 cell tabulation (in practice, most routine marrow differentials are done by estimate). Unusual cells or cells not represented by a register (NRBCs, reactive lymphocytes, etc.) should be tabulated separately, using one miscellaneous register to enter them in the counter.

Automated differential counters have been designed using various principles. One system uses stained smears and performs the count the same way a human does a manual count: cells are located and the optical patterns of cell dimensions, shape, nucleus-to-cytoplasm ratio, chromatin density, granularity, and staining reactions are compared with information in a data bank. A cell identification is made on the basis of the characteristics stored in the instrument's memory (image analysis). Cells that don't match a particular set of identifiers are "flagged" for manual review and identification. The instrument contains a microscope and video display screen to facilitate review and data entry. The slides must be stained uniformly (a smear preparation and staining module is available). Although this type of instrument is no longer in production (Hematrak, made by Geometric Data Corporation), some laboratories may still have the system.

Another approach (Coulter S Plus, Coulter Electronics, Inc.) uses the Coulter principle to construct a size-distributed histogram of leukocytes. In most instruments, three subpopulations (modes) are identifiable, corresponding to lymphocytes, other mononuclear cells, and granulocytes. A computer calculates the number of particles in each area as a percent of the total WBC histogram. Abnormal histograms (e.g., a large number of blasts or other immature cells that creates overlap with the adjoining areas) are flagged for manual review. For routine screening, the calculated values are useful approximations of a three-part WBC differential count.

Cytochemical staining is used by the Technicon H6000 analyzer to produce full differential counts. Myeloperoxidase activity is used to separate lymphocytes from monocytes and granulocytes, which along with cell size produces a two dimensional scattergram. Very high peroxidase activity is characteristic of immature neutrophils. Monocytes are further identified by a non-specific esterase reaction (Chapter 27) and the heparin-containing granules of basophils are stained with alcian blue. Lymphocytes and blasts are unstained and the largest unstained cells (LUC) are counted as a distinct catagory (Fig. 26-10).

The EPICS system (Coulter Electronics, Inc.) is a cell sorter that uses laser technology. Blood cells are passed through a focused laser beam as a suspension surrounded by a laminar sheath fluid (see the previous discussion of automated counters). Fluorescent tags (fluorescein) on the cells interact with an argon ion laser and the scattered light is received as forward and right angle scatter. Cell identification, up to 10,000 cells per second, is made by comparing the light scattering characteristics and wavelengths with stored criteria. The flow cytometer sorts cells by differentially charging the cell droplets as they are identified. Data can be displayed as scattergrams, or as single and two parameter histograms.

A detailed description of automated hematology analyzers is beyond the scope of this

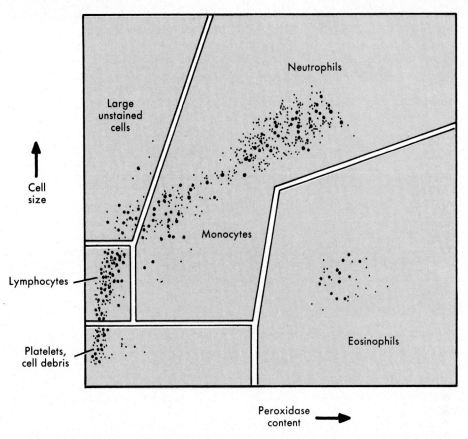

Cell size

Neutrophils

Large unstained cells

Monocytes

Lymphocytes

Platelets, cell debris

Eosinophils

Peroxidase content

Fig. 26-10.   Differential cell identification by peroxidase content and cell size.

book and continuing advances in commercial instruments would soon date any such presentation. Operating instructions and discussions of analytical results for some instruments can be found in the textbooks by Brown (1988) and Pittiglio (1987). The best sources for information, biased or not, are the manufacturers. Several references have been included in the reading list that provide comparative evaluations and discuss interpretive problems with different instruments.

PLATELET EVALUATION
Smear morphology and numerical estimate

The appearance of platelets on the peripheral blood smear is a useful indication of thrombocytopathology. Platelets that are unusually large are seen in some hemostatic disorders, such as Bernard-Soulier syndrome and idiopathic thrombocytopenic purpura (Chapter 23). Large numbers of platelets characterize thrombocythemia and decreased concentrations typify various thrombocytopenias. For an estimate of platelet concentration from a blood smear to be valid, the platelets must not be clumped. If the smear is made from a capillary stick, the blood should be spread on the slide immediately after the drop is collected (the first drop from the puncture is wiped with a gauze). Blood collected in an anticoagulant (EDTA) should be mixed as soon as possible to assure that platelet remain dispersed. Platelets should be observed in the same area of the smear in which differential counts are made. About 8 to 20 platelets per oil immersion field correspond to a normal platelet concentration. An estimate can also be calculated from the formula:

Platelets/µL = number of platelets/100 RBCs
× hematocrit in % × 100

Lack of azurophilic granularity, the occurrence of excess numbers of large platelets (more than 5% macrothrombocytes), or occurrence of platelet strands should be noted.

Manual platelet count

The enumeration methods, using diluting pipettes or Unopettes, are similar to those described for manual white cell counts. Diluting fluid contains 1.0% ammonium oxalate; red cells are hemolyzed while WBCs and platelets remain intact. The hemacytometer counting area consists of 10 to 25 small squares (0.04 mm^2) from the central square. The platelets should sit in the hemacytometer, placed in a humidity chamber, for at least 15 minutes so that they rest at the same focal plane. Counts are preferably made with a phase microscope to enhance refractiveness and facilitate differentiation from dust particles and other artifacts. Platelets appear as refractile round, oval, or comma-shaped structures, 2 to 4 µm in diameter.

Counts of 25 squares (1 mm^2) from each side of the hemacytometer should agree within 10%; they are average and the concentration is calculated from the general formula previously presented in the discussion of red cell counts. As with smear estimates, evidence of platelet clumping necessitates a redilution or, if persistent, collection of a new sample. The blood of some patients may display a phenomenon in which neutrophils are ringed by the platelets (satellite formation). This type of aggregation can be prevented by collecting blood in sodium citrate.

Platelet counts by automated analyzers are routinely available on instruments that perform complete blood counts. Some also provide histograms of platelet volumes, a mean platelet volume (MPV), and a platelet distribution width (PDW). In an instrument such as the Coulter S Plus, platelets are counted as particles in the 2 to 20 fL range. If the resulting histogram fits a lognormal distribution, the volume range is expanded to 70 fL and all particles within this range are tabulated as platelets. If red cell fragments or abnormal platelet volume distributions result in a different distribution, the reported platelet count is restricted to the original 2 to 20 fL range and the count is "flagged" for further review. Platelet counts of less than 20,000 per µL may be inaccurate on some instruments that are not specialized for platelet enumeration.

Reference values

Adults: 150 to 400 × 10^3 per µL
Neonates: 100 to 350 × 10^3 per µL

ERYTHROCYTE SEDIMENTATION RATE (ESR)

Anticoagulated whole blood in a cylinder or tube will separate into an upper plasma layer and a lower cell layer as a result of gravity interacting with the denser cells. The distance that cells fall within a specified time interval is the **erythrocyte sedimentation rate (ESR)**. The rate of fall, conventionally expressed as millimeters per hour (mm/hr), depends on:

1. The density and surface area (shape and size) of the red blood cells. Large cells settle faster than small cells and fewer cells settle faster than a high concentration of cells. Thus, ESRs are most increased in cases of macrocytic anemia, moderately increased in anemias associated with low red cell counts, and relatively slow to normal in patients with polycythemia. Variations in cell shape, such as those associated with

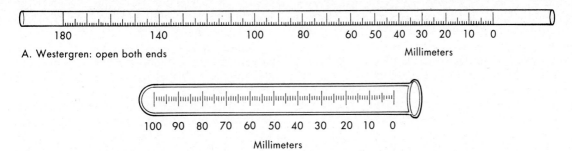

A. Westergren: open both ends

Millimeters

B. Wintrobe: open one end

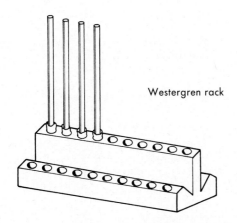

Westergren rack

C.

Fig. 26-11   Erythrocyte sedimentation rate.
A, Westergren tube. **B,** Wintrobe tube. **C,** Tubes in vertical rack.

sickle cell anemia, thalassemia, and sphero-cytosis, retard the sedimentation rate be-cause the cells are unable to aggregate in the stacks (rouleau formation) typical of discocytes.

2. Viscosity of the plasma also influences sedimentation rate. Increased concentra-tions of plasma proteins (inflammation, multiple myeloma, hyperfibrinogenemia) increase the amount of rouleaux and the ESR. Increased concentrations of albumin, however, reduces the ESR. The effect of in-creased plasma viscosity is the basis of us-ing the ESR as a screening test for inflam-mation (increased gamma globulins).

In addition, ESR is a function of the phys-ical environment: tube diameter, angle of tube sides to vertical, temperature, and the presence of vibrations. An increase in any of these produces an increase in ESR. Therefore, standardized tubes held at a specified angle (usually vertical) at room temperature for a specified time period (usually 1 hour) are used in the procedure.

Sedimentation occurs in three stages. First, the red cells form rouleaux (stacks of coins), depending on the shape of the eryth-rocytes and composition of the plasma. Sec-ond, the large aggregates of red cells settle rapidly, depending on the degree of rouleaux. The third stage is defined by the slow settling and compacting of red cells within the bottom layer.

Procedure (modified Westergren)

1. Whole blood (EDTA) at room temperature is well mixed and added in a 4:1 ratio to 0.85% saline (2.0 mL of blood and 0.5 mL of saline provides sufficient volume). Mix the solution well.

2. Fill a Westergren disposable sedimentation tube exactly to the 0 mark, without bubbles, and place in a vertical rack (Fig. 26-11). The rack must be vertical (a leveling bubble is provided on some types of racks).

3. Allow the tube to stand for exactly 60 minutes, then record the number of millimeters to which the red cells have settled.

Wintrobe and Landsberg procedure

1. Add well-mixed whole blood directly to a Wintrobe tube, filling without bubbles to the 0 mark.

2. Place the tube in a vertical rack and let the tube stand for 60 minutes. Record the number of millimeters to which the red cells have settled.

Reference values

	Westergren	Wintrobe
Adult males (mm/hr)	0 to 10	0 to 9
Adult females (mm/hr)	0 to 15	0 to 20

27

Special Procedures

Cheryl Lee Drennan and Lawrence Powers

SPECIAL STAINING PROCEDURES

Special stains include those histochemical techniques other than Wright-Glemsa that are used to locate specific blood cell components (granules, iron deposits, enzyme activity) and to identify immature and abnormal cells, such as those of the acute leukemias. Technically, the most common pitfalls in these procedures are similar to those for preparing routine slides. A well-made slide will result in a clear, easily-read stain.

Preparation of smears for cases of acute leukemias should include sets of bone marrow and peripheral blood slides, stained at the same time. If either the peripheral white cell count or the number of circulating blasts is low, buffy coat smears can be used to facilitate cell location and identification. Marrow smears should be representative and contain spicule material (see preparation of bone marrow smears, Chapter 25).

Development of commercial kits for most staining techniques has greatly reduced the inconsistencies associated with these procedures in the past. Fixatives for the stains have been improved, making the results cleaner and easier to interpret. Directions for blood collection, storage of reagents, and the staining procedure must be followed carefully, especially for those involving enzymatic reactions (dependent on time, pH, and temperature).

Stains used in classifications of acute leukemia

Assignment of a patient to one of the FAB types of acute leukemia depends on morphological features of the marrow and peripheral blood cells and the results of a battery of staining reactions (Table 27-1 and Chapter 20). Interpretation of these staining reactions can be easy or exceedingly difficult. The stains *do not* selectively define-malignant cells. In fact, many of the mature, normal cells stain positively with one or more of these histochemicals, providing a positive control for stain performance. In addition, comparison of the distribution, size, and other characteristics of the malignant cells should be made between Wright-stained smears and special-stained smears, facilitating location on slides on which the stains do not delineate the cells as well. This is particularly essential when malignant replacement of the marrow or peripheral elements is only partial, leaving normal elements that also react positively with the special stain. Localization and identification of abnormal cells requires frequent comparison between smears and interpretative experience with the technical procedure so that evaluation of the staining results is meaningful.

A typical staining battery for adult leukemias consists of: (1) **Sudan black B** and/or **myeloperoxidase,** (2) **periodic acid Schiff (PAS),** (3) **napthol AS-D chloroacetate es-**

Table 27-1. Special stains used to classify acute leukemias

Stain	Myel	Mono	Lymph	Eryth	Mega
Sudan black B	+	±	–	–	–
Myeloperoxidase	+	±	–	–	–
Periodic acid Schiff	–	–	(+)	+	±
Specific esterase	+	–	–	–	–
Nonspecific esterase	–	+	–	–	±

Myel, Granulocytic blasts; *Mono*, monocytic blasts; *Lymph*, lymphocytic blasts; *Eryth*, malignant erythroblasts; *Mega*, megakaryoblasts; ±, variable staining reaction; (+), positive 70% of cases of ALL.

terase, and (4) **alpha-naphthyl acetate esterase.** Currently, an **acid phosphatase stain** is done on smears from adult patients with acute lymphocytic leukemias (ALL), but this protocol is subject to change. In fact, pediatric oncology groups have discontinued use of the latter stain because no significant patterns or benefits were realized in children with ALL.

Most pediatric leukemias are acute lymphoblastic and their classification now relies heavily on the use of monoclonal antibodies to cell antigens. Therefore smears from these patients are evaluated with Sudan black B and alpha-napthyl acetate esterase to identify myeloid and monocytoid cell lines, respectively. For each of these stains, information is summarized on chemical reactions, expected positive and negative staining patterns for each cell line, and the manner in which the stain is used in assigning FAB designations.

Sudan black B

Sudan black B stains lipids in myeloid cells and it is probably the most reliable of all the stains used to classify adult leukemias. Staining reactions closely parallel the patterns observed with myeloperoxidase and only rarely do myeloid cells stain with either Sudan black or myeloperoxidase but not the other. Granulocytic blasts usually show a moderate to heavy staining pattern whereas monocytic blasts are either sparsely stained or negative. Lymphocytic and megakaryocytic blasts typically are not positive with these stains, although exceptions do occur. All mature granulocytes stain with Sudan black B. Normal mature granulocytes contain myeloperoxidase and should give a positive reaction (deficiencies of this enzyme are discussed in Chapter 21).

Periodic acid Schiff (PAS)

Periodic acid oxidizes glycols to aldehydes, which react with Schiff's reagent, a mixture of pararosaniline and sodium metabisulfite, to produce a pararosaniline adduct. The adduct stains the glycol-containing components in cells (Plate 8, *C* and *D*).

Once thought to be the definitive stain to identify lymphoblasts, PAS is now considered less important for this purpose. Lymphoblasts in 20% to 30% of cases of ALL do not stain with PAS. When the characteristic block-positive pattern of lymphoblasts does occur, confirmation is usually obtainable by monoclonal antibody testing. PAS is also used to identify erythroblastic leukemia. Although normal erythroblasts are PAS negative, malignant cells of this line show both cytoplasmic diffuse and block-positive staining. Mature granulocytes and lymphocytes stain with PAS and mature monocytes show a very light reaction. Monoblasts yield a negative reaction; megakaryoblasts are variable.

Naphthol AS-D chloroacetate esterase (NACE, specific esterase) and alpha-naphthyl acetate esterase (ANAE, nonspecific esterase)

Esterase enzymes, in the presence of a stable diazonium salt, hydrolyze ester linkages to free naphthol compounds; naphthols couple with the salt to form colored deposits in the blood cells. The specific esterase stains granulocytic blasts and the nonspecific esterase stains monocytic blasts (Plate 8, E and F). Each stain also reacts with the mature cells of the respective lineages. ANAE often produces a very light, speckled staining pattern in lymphocytes, but much less positive than that seen in monocytes. Megakaryoblasts often show a distinct localized pattern of deposits, unlike the diffuse staining reaction of monocytic cells. Although most granulocytic blasts are clearly indicated with Sudan black B, it is helpful to have a confirmatory stain in some questionable cases. Since monoblasts show variable reactions with Sudan black, ANAE serves as a definitive stain for these cells. Further definition of monocytic lineage can be accomplished by adding a **fluoride inhibition** procedure to the ANAE stain. Monocytic esterase is rendered inactive in the presence of fluoride.

Leukocyte acid phosphatase

Acid phosphatase can be demonstrated in all leukocytes; sites of enzyme concentration are delineated with naphthol AS-B1 phosphate and a diazonium salt which combine at acid pH. The procedure is run with and without tartrate to recognize tartrate-resistant lymphocytes that are characteristic of hairy cell leukemia (HCL). As stated earlier, this stain has also been use to diagnose ALL, but characteristic staining patterns have not been recognized and acid phosphatase is used less often for this.

Iron stain (Prussian Blue reaction)

A representative evaluation of a patient's iron status is possible by examination of bone marrow smears stained for iron (Plate 8,B). Two pertinent questions can be answered: (1) is storage iron present, and (2) are normal sideroblasts present? Storage iron appears as very round, dense, blue-black siderotic granules in the matrix of the marrow spicules. With experience, iron can be judged to be increased, normal, or decreased. Normally, 20% to 50% of the marrow nucleated red cells should contain from one to three siderotic granules each.

Storage iron is markedly decreased or absent in patients with iron deficiency anemia and few or no sideroblasts are present. Patients having anemia associated with chronic disease have normal amounts of storage iron, but no sideroblasts. In contrast, patients with erythroblastic leukemia and with some forms of myelodysplastic syndrome often show increased storage iron and ringed sideroblasts containing numerous siderotic granules.

Procedure

1. Dry marrow smears are fixed in absolute methanol for 15 minutes. Remove excess alcohol.
2. While slides are fixing, prepare fresh staining solution:
   Equal amounts of 2% potassium ferrocyanide are added to 0.1 N hydrochloric acid, enough for immediate use (the stain is not stable).
3. Stain the marrow smears for 20 minutes (a rack or Coplin jars may be used).
4. Rinse the slides in gentle wash of tap water for 20 minutes.
5. Counterstain with 0.5% safranin for 15 to 30 seconds.
6. Air dry and mount with a coverslip.

Leukocyte alkaline phosphatase (LAP)

The sites of alkaline phosphatase activity are identified by incubating fresh peripheral blood smears with naphthal AS-MX phosphate and a diazonium salt. One hundred mature neutrophils (band and segmented forms) are counted and graded for the presence of alkaline phosphatase positive granules (Fig. 27-1). Depending on the salt used, the granules stain a purplish blue or orange-red. Grading of the cells ranges from zero (no activity) to 4+ (maximum activity, obscures nucleus). The score for the 100 cells is totaled and reported as the LAP score.

The LAP score is usually decreased in chronic myelogenous leukemia, except during blast crisis. In contrast, LAP is elevated during leukmoid reactions due to infections, stress, polycythemia vera, and during the third trimester of pregnancy (obstetric patients are often used as an elevated LAP control for the procedure). The LAP is also decreased in cases of paroxysmal nocturnal hemoglobinuria and refractory sideroblastic anemia.

Since grading LAP activity is somewhat subjective, technologists in a laboratory should agree on grading criteria. The stain is not stable, so photographs of slides must be used to provide a permanent reference set.

Reference values. LAP Score: 40 to 150.

SPECIAL METHODS FOR RED BLOOD CELL EVALUATIONS

Osmotic fragility. The erythrocyte osmotic fragility test measures resistance of red blood cells to hypotonic saline solutions. Resistance is a function of membrane integrity, including cytoskeletal structure, ability to maintain an ionic gradient, and the shape and volume of the cell. Diagnostically, this test can be used to recognize certain anemias that are characterized by increased fragility (decreased resistance) or decreased fragility (increased resistance).

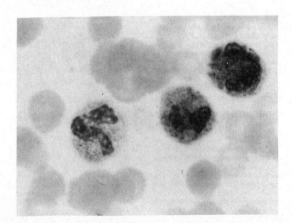

Fig. 27-1.   Leukocyte alkaline phosphatase (LAP) activity in neutrophils.
Neutrophils graded (from left to right) 2+, 3+, and 4+ for intensity of enzyme activity (from Bauer JD: Clinical laboratory methods, ed 9, St Louis, 1982, The CV Mosby Co.)

Increased fragility	Decreased fragility
Hereditary spherocytosis	Sickle cell anemia
Some acquired hemolytic anemias	Thalassemia
Pyruvate kinase deficiency*	Iron deficiency anemia
Hereditary elliptocytosis*	Leptocytosis of liver disease
In patients with severe burns	Polycythemia vera
Hemolytic disease of the newborn	Hemoglobin C disease

Spherocytes are particularly sensitive to hypotonic solutions, since the cell volume to surface area is already at a maximum. Additional water influx causes the cell to rupture. Red cells from patients with hereditary spherocytosis display increased fragility when placed in a series of saline dilutions, starting with 0.85%. Elliptocytes are also fragile in hypotonic solutions, but this is caused by the abnormal lipid composition of the membrane rather than the shape. Sickle cells, leptocytes, target cells, and other poikilocytes with large surface area-to-volume ratios are less fragile than normal cells.

The test consists of placing an aliquot of red cells in various dilutions of saline and recording the amount of hemolysis after a period of incubation. Results can be read visually or with a spectrophotometer.

Incubation for 24 hours at 37° C provides an additional level of sensitivity that can detect heterozygous individuals for hereditary spherocytosis. The incubated 24 hour test is more sensitive than the 30 minute test because the cells are also placed in hypoglycemic stress. Pyruvate kinase deficiencies, resulting in reduced ability to generate ATP, leads to increased sodium retention and less tolerance to osmotic stress.

Procedure

1. Saline solutions are prepared to obtain

---

*With incubation at 37° C for 24 hours.

final concentrations (%) of 1.00, 0.85, 0.75, 0.65, 0.60, 0.55, 0.50, 0.45, 0.40, 0.35, 0.30, 0.20, 0.10, and 0.00. These solutions can also be purchased as Unopettes (Becton-Dickinson, Inc.).

2. The manual procedure calls for a 1:100 blood to saline solution (e.g., 0.05 mL of heparinized blood + 5.0 mL of saline); the Unopette procedure uses $20/\mu L$ of blood for each 1.98 mL reservoir of saline (also a 1:100 dilution). Each tube or reservoir is mixed by gentle inversion. A control series (normal blood) should be run with each set of patients.

3. The tubes stand at room temperature for 30 minutes. Remix, then centrifuge at 1200 to 1500 g for 5 minutes. (Unopette solutions are spun at 2000 g for 5 minutes).

4. Read the absorbance of the supernatant fluid at 540 nm. The 0.85% saline solution should be clear in the normal control and this serves as a blank. Complete hemolysis should occur for both control and patient in the last dilution of the series (0.00%).

5. Calculate hemolysis of supernatant in each tube:

$$\% \text{ hemolysis} = \frac{\text{optical density of supernatant}}{\text{optical density of 0.00\% tube}} \times 100$$

6. Plot the results of the control and patient as percent hemolysis versus percent saline concentration (Fig. 27-2). The normal curve will be sigmoid, with a relatively linear middle segment.

Reference values. Nonincubated: hemolysis begins at 0.45% to 0.50% NaCl and is complete at 0.20% to 0.30%. Incubated (24 hours at 37° C): hemolysis begins at 0.55% to 0.65% and is complete at 0.30%.

Other tests for hemolytic anemias

The **ascorbate-cyanide screening test** is useful for detecting enzyme deficiencies of the hexose monophosphate shunt (HMS): glucose-6-phosphate dehydrogenase, gluta-

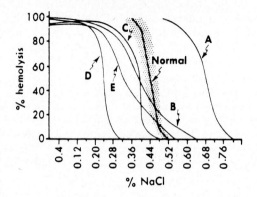

Fig. 27-2. Osmotic fragility curves.
A, Hereditary spherocytosis. **B,** Thalassemia major. **C,** Thalassemia minor. **D,** Hb E disease. **E,** Iron deficiency anemia (from Bauer JD: Clinical laboratory methods, ed 9, St Louis, 1982, The CV Mosby Co.)

thione peroxidase, and glutathione reductase. Hydrogen peroxide formation in the erythrocyte is normally inhibited or removed by catalase and by enzymes of the HMS so that hemoglobin is maintained in the reduced form. Sodium cyanide inhibits catalase, so that only the HMS can prevent accumulation of hydrogen peroxide. When red cells are incubated at 37° C for 2 to 4 hours in the presence of glucose and cyanide, deficient HMS enzymes result in the oxidation of hemoglobin to methemoglobin, turning the blood from bright red to reddish brown. The deficient red cells will also develop Heinz bodies that can be observed after staining with methyl violet.

A similar procedure is used to induce Heinz body formation. A fresh buffered solution of acetylphenylhydrazine is mixed with whole blood (collected in EDTA) and incubated for 2 hours at 37° C. The cell suspension is added to an equal volume of methyl violet, incubated for 10 minutes and placed under a coverslip. Patients with HMS enzyme deficiencies display multiple Heinz bodies in many of the red cells, characterized as large, irregular purple dots at the periphery of the cell. Normal controls will have only a single inclusion per red cell.

The **glucose-6-phosphate dehydrogenase fluorescence test** is another screening procedure for G-6-PD deficiency. In the presence of NADP and glucose-6-phosphate, normal red cells (with G-6-PD) convert the NADP to NADPH, a fluorescent molecule when exposed to ultraviolet light. The kit is available from Sigma Chemical Company, St. Louis, Mo. Blood is mixed with the substrate and a drop is placed on a filter paper at a prelabelled spot. The blood-substrate mixture is incubated at 37° C and an additional drop placed on the filter paper at 5 and 10 minutes elapsed time. A normal control and blank solution are also added to the paper. After the filter paper has dried, it is examined in a darkened room with an ultraviolet lamp. Little or no fluorescence should appear in the first spot (time 0) but should increase to maximum at the 10 minute spot. Patients with G-6-PD deficiency show less fluorescence, depending on the severity of the deficiency. Results should be confirmed with quantitative assays.

The **sugar water screening test** for paroxysmal nocturnal hemoglobinuria (PNH) is a simple procedure in which red cells, collected in sodium citrate, are incubated in a sucrose solution at room temperature for 30 minutes. An aliquot is added to cyanmethemoglobin ("total") and the remainder is centrifuged and the supernatant added to another tube of cyanmethemoglobin ("test"). A blank is prepared from sucrose solution and cyanmethemoglobin and all tubes stand for an additional 10 minutes. Absorbances are read at 540 nm and hemolysis is calculated as a ratio of test to total. Red blood cells from patients with PNH will bind complement under these conditions, resulting in hemolysis of more than 10%. Less than 5% is considered normal and between 5% and 10% is borderline abnormal.

The **acidified serum test (Ham test)** is an additional screening procedure for PNH. The patient's red cells are mixed with autologous serum and with normal serum (ABO group compatible with patient) and incubated in several tubes at 37° C. One set of tubes is incubated at 56° C to destroy complement and serve as a control. A weak acid (0.2N HCl) is added to some of the tubes and all of the tubes are incubated for 1 hour. The tubes are centrifuged and the supernatant observed for hemolysis. Normal bloods show no hemolysis, whereas patients with PNH show hemolysis in tubes in which complement is intact. Patients with HEMPAS (see Chapter 19) will have red cells that are lysed by other serums but not by their own.

Sickle cell screening tests

Two methods are used to detect sickle cell anemia or trait. The first places red blood cells in a hypoxic environment, created by a strong reducing agent (sodium metabisulfite). The cells sickle when the oxygen concentration is lowered sufficiently and this can be observed on a wet preparation under the microscope. The second method relies on the increased turbidity produced by Hb S crystals to a red cell lysate, whereas a lysate containing normal hemoglobin is relatively translucent.

Sodium metabisulfite test. Although heterozygous patients (trait) rarely demonstrate drepanocytes on peripheral smears, when the erythrocytes are deprived of oxygen they will undergo sickling. A drop of blood, collected in EDTA or heparin, is placed on a microscope slide. Two drops of 2% sodium metabisulfite or sodium bisulfite are added and mixed with the blood. One drop of reagent is sufficient if the hematocrit is very low. A coverslip is sealed over the blood solution with petroleum jelly, taking care to avoid air bubbles (see wet preparations, Chapter 26).

Examine the slide after 30 minutes incubation at room temperature or at 37° C (the latter produces maximal results). If sickle cells or holly leaf-shaped cells appear, the test is reported as positive. The cells must

have distinct points; elongated and crenated cells are not considered positive for this test. If negative, continue to incubate and examine periodically for up to 24 hours. Patients with sickle cell anemia (homozygous) will usually display sickling within a few minutes, but the actual amounts of Hb S must be confirmed by electrophoresis.

Dithionite solubility test. One mL of whole blood (EDTA, heparin, or sodium citrate) is centrifuged and the plasma and buffy coat are removed. Ten μL of the packed red cells are added to 2 mL of a freshly-prepared solution of sodium hydrosulfite containing saponin (available from commercial sources or prepared as per instructions in Brown, 1988). A normal control should be run with each set of patient bloods.

The solutions stand at room temperature for 5 to 10 minutes, forming a lysate. Then the normal and patient tubes are placed in front of a lined card. The dark lines on the card should be clearly visible if the blood is normal (negative), whereas Hb S (also Hb Bart's and Hb C_{Harlem}) forms a turbid solution that obscures the lines. Positive results should be confirmed by electrophoresis.

Hemoglobin electrophoresis

Identification of abnormal hemoglobins is crucial for diagnosis of many types of anemia. Hemoglobin electrophoresis is the definitive procedure, at this time, for quantitating hemoglobin variants. Electrophoresis uses differences in the charge distributions and molecular weights of various hemoglobin molecules to achieve separation. Hemoglobin is released from the erythrocytes as a lysate and placed on a medium, such as **cellulose acetate** at pH 8.4 to 8.5 or **citrate agar gel** at pH 6.0 to 6.2. The following is a brief synopsis of the procedure. Complete details can be obtained from manufacturers of the instruments and supplies (Helena Laboratories; Gelman Instruments; Corning Biomedical).

The hemolysate is prepared from anticoagulated blood (EDTA) by centrifugation of the red cells at high speed for 20 to 30 minutes. Some procedures call for washing the red cells in normal saline before rapid centrifugation. A hemolysing reagent is added to the packed red cells for a few minutes. If hemolysis is not complete, the cells can be frozen and thawed to complete the lysis. Normal bloods and abnormal controls are run with the patient samples.

The electrophoretic chamber is prepared and the power supply set according to the instructions of the manufacturer. Brown (1988) provides an excellent summary of the procedural steps involved in the Helena system, including pitfalls and sources of errors. The cellulose acetate electrophoretic strips are stained in Ponceau S and washed in glacial acetic acid and methanol. The strips are dried in an oven for a few minutes, and are then ready to be scanned with an optical densimeter. Citrate agar gels are stained with a reagent composed of orthotolidine, glacial acetic acid, sodium nitroferricyanide and hydrogen peroxide.

Most routine samples are separated on cellulose acetate, but some hemoglobins migrate at the same rate on this medium. These can usually be separated on citrate gel. Mobility patterns of major hemoglobin variants are shown in Fig. 27-3. For example, hemoglobins C, E, O and A_2 migrate very closely and hemoglobins S, D and G form another close group at alkaline pH on cellulose acetate. These are separated at pH 6.2 on citrate agar, but Hb S and C_{Harlem} migrate together. Detailed lists of mobility characteristics can be found in Williams et al. (1983) and Wintrobe (1981).

Reference values

	At birth	Adult
Hemoglobin F	60%-85%	0.0%-2.0%
Hemoglobin A	15%-40%	96%-99%
Hemoglobin A_2	0.2%-2.5%	0.3%-3.5%

SPECIAL METHODS FOR LEUKOCYTE EVALUATIONS

White blood cells can be concentrated in **buffy coat** preparations. Whole blood is spun at moderate speeds for 20 to 30 min-

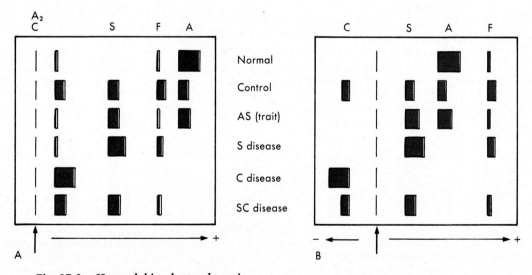

Fig. 27-3.   Hemoglobin electrophoresis.
The arrow indicates the point of application. **A,** Cellulose acetate at pH 8.5; **B,** citrate agar gel at pH 6.2.

utes and the cream-colored layer between the plasma and red cell layers is removed with a Pasteur pipette and transferred to another tube. This step can be repeated to remove additional red cells. Smears made with buffy coats will contain a high density of WBCs that permits screening for rare but abnormal cells. A cytocentrifugal slide preparation, resulting in an evenly-dispersed monolayer, further facilitates observations of the cells.

Separation of the leukocytes into granulocytes, monocytes, and lymphocytes can be achieved with the use of **ficoll density gradients** (Hypaque, Sigma Chemical Co.). Ficoll solutions of two different specific gravities are carefully layered in a centrifuge tube, the red cells are added on top, and the tubes are spun for 30 minutes at moderate speeds. Red cells settle to the bottom and the leukocytes are trapped in distinct layers (Fig. 27-4). These can be removed with a pipette for specific studies. The ficoll is poisonous to the cells, however, and should be removed if functional studies are to be made. This is done by washing the cells 2 to 3 times with normal saline.

Phagocytic activity in neutrophils can be evaluated with regards to chemotactic response, capability to migrate to a site of inflammation, ability to ingest microorganisms, the presence of key enzymes, and ability to generate oxygen radicals. Few of these tests are performed in the routine clinical laboratory, partly because the corresponding abnormalities are relatively rare and also because some of the tests are complex bioassays that are not conveniently packaged as commercial kits or procedures.

The Rebuck skin window and bipolar shape formation were described in Section III as qualitative techniques to evaluate gross responses of neutrophils to chemotactic stimuli. Attempts have been made to quantitate chemotaxis, using Boyden migration chambers and labelling the cells with radioisotopes to facilitate enumeration, but the procedures are tedious and the results are difficult to reproduce. Myeloperoxidase activity can be measured in cells with histochemical staining techniques and deficiencies of this enzyme can sometimes be observed in automated instruments that classify cells by peroxidase activity.

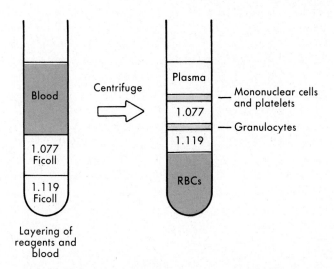

Fig. 27-4. **Ficoll density gradients for separating leukocytes.**

The **nitroblue tetrazolium test (NBT)** has been used to detect patients with chronic granulomatous disease (Chapter 21). Normal white blood cells are able to reduce nitroblue tetrazolium, a light yellow compound, to formazan, a bluish-black compound. Usually less than 10% of the neutrophils will show the colored aggregates if the cells are not undergoing active phagocytosis. NBT is primarily reduced by oxygen compounds formed during neutrophil stimulation (respiratory burst). When a microbial stimulant is presented at the same time, the reduction of NBT is greatly enhanced, occurring in 50% to 70% of normal neutrophils. Patients with CGD are unable to produce an oxidative burst and the amount of formazan deposition is zero. Female carriers of the sex-linked gene will display 50% normal neutrophils and 50% cells that are unable to reduce NBT. The test kit is available from Sigma Chemical Company, St. Louis, Mo.

28

Hemostasis and Coagulation Procedures

Laboratory tests for evaluation of hemostasis and coagulation are presented in the following order: hemostasis and platelet function, coagulation, and fibrinolysis. Only a few of the many types of procedures are presented. Others are listed with principles and applications. Many of these are available only from commercial sources and their instructions should be followed carefully. Because these tests are modified and updated frequently, technologists should periodically review the procedures for changes in technique, reagents used, and reference values reported.

PLATELET EVALUATION

These procedures can be separated into tests of gross capillary maintenance, functional assays of platelet aggregation and adherence, and assays of platelet factors or other components. Methods of platelet enumeration and microscopic morphology are presented in Chapter 26.

Capillary fragility test

This procedure is also known as the tourniquet test or the Rumpel-Leede test. It measures the ability of capillaries to withstand increased stress, reflecting the integrity of the vessel wall endothelium and the maintenance activities of platelets.

Principle. A blood pressure cuff is applied to the upper arm for a time interval and at a specified pressure. The appearance of petechiae is noted by comparing the arm before and after venous occlusion.

Procedure

1. Inspect the medial (inner) surface of the forearm for petechiae and circle any that are present. A circle, 5 cm in diameter, is drawn on the arm. Do not include, if possible, preexisting petechiae in this observation circle.

2. Determine the patient's blood pressure and inflate the cuff to a point halfway between the systolic and diastolic readings. Do not exceed 100 mm Hg, regardless of the readings.

3. After 5 minutes of inflation, remove the cuff and observe the arm for petechiae. Count any that appear in the 5 cm circle during the next 5 to 10 minutes.

Interpretation. Examination can be confined to the observation circle or it can include the entire forearm, from just below the elbow to just above the wrist and the back of the hand. A prescribed circle is recommended for patients in whom sequential comparisons may be required. Normally, less than 10 petechiae of less than 1 mm diameter will appear within 10 minutes. A semiquantitative scale may be assigned:

0-10 per circle	1+	normal
10-20 per circle	2+	borderline (doubtful)
20-50 per circle	3+	abnormal
>50 per circle	4+	positive, may indicate pathology

Discussion. Most people can withstand cuff pressures of 100 mm Hg for several minutes without capillary rupture. The procedure is not a comfortable one, however, and the patient should be advised of the time interval and be reassured that the discomfort is temporary. There is considerable variation between individuals as to capillary response. Women over 40 years of age are often positive at the 2+ to 3+ level without underlying vascular or hemostatic pathology. Abnormal (3+ to 4+) results are most often seen in thrombocytopenia, vascular purpura, and vitamin C deficiency (scurvy). Recent ingestion of aspirin can produce abnormal results in conjunction with adverse effects on platelet function and bleeding time determination.

Bleeding time

The time interval for bleeding to cease after a standardized capillary puncture is made provides a means of assessing platelet function and capillary-venular vasoconstriction. Various techniques have been used to produce wounds that constitute a standardized hemostatic challenge. Most procedures have the following elements in common:

1. The volar (inner) surface of the forearm is used as a site, avoiding superficial veins, areas of scar tissue, or other areas that might yield misleading results.
2. Mild venous stasis is achieved by placing a blood pressure cuff above the elbow on the arm selected as a puncture site. A pressure of 40 mm Hg is maintained during the timed interval, producing a constant stress to the hemostatic mechanism.
3. The wound or wounds are made by a lancet, freely held or enclosed in a triggered device to insure a standard incision.
4. The timer is activated when the incision is made, the first drop of blood is removed with a sterile gauze, leaving a clean, dry surface for subsequent drops.
5. The blood at the incision is carefully blotted (not wiped) with filter paper every 30 seconds, creating a sequence of spots along the outer perimeter of

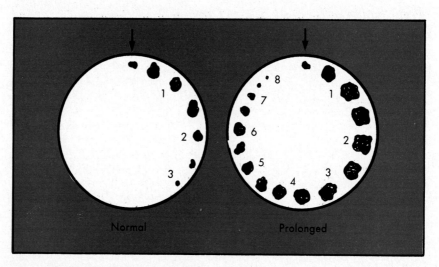

Fig. 28-1. Bleeding time determination.
Appearance of blood spots on filter paper from a patient with a normal bleeding time (left) and from a patient with a platelet defect (right).

the paper (Fig. 28-1). This provides both a record of elapsed time and the relative volume of bleeding.

6. The test is terminated when the incision ceases to bleed freely. Some patients, including some with normal hemostatic function, may ooze a blood-tinted fluid for several minutes more. Any discoloration or signs of hemorrhage into the tissue surrounding the wound should also be noted, as this may indicate problems of blood vessel integrity.

Duke earlobe bleeding time. The earlobe is cleaned with alcohol and dried. The ear should be warm (room temperature adjustment) for optimal blood flow. A disposable lancet is used to pierce the fleshy tip of the lobe and a timer is activated. Blot every 30 seconds until free bleeding ceases. Although the results are not as reproducible as other techniques, it is relatively painless, does not result in scarring, and it can be performed on small children (the manuevers are out of their sight).

Reference values. 1 to 3 minutes; 3 to 6 minutes is a borderline result that should be repeated, preferably by another method.

Ivy bleeding time. Two wounds are made in the forearm with a disposable capillary lancet, spaced 2 or 3 centimeters apart. Each incision should be about 3 mm in depth and the incision should be oriented perpendicular to the axis of the arm. The time for both wounds is recorded. If they agree within 1 minute, the results are averaged and reported. Because a standard incision is difficult to achieve with this method, considerable variation may exist in the times.

Reference values. 2 to 6 minutes; 6 to 10 minutes is considered borderline.

Template bleeding time. The procedure is similar to that of the Ivy method, except that the incision is 1 mm in depth and 10 mm in length. A spring-loaded blade is contained in a plastic housing; this is triggered by a button after the face of the device is placed firmly against the forearm surface. Single and double blade devices are available. The longer incision is believed to provide more consistent results, but a small scar usually results. This can be minimized by using a butterfly bandage to close the edges of the incision when the test is terminated.

Reference values. 3 to 10 minutes; 3 to 5 minutes in small children when 30 mm Hg pressure is used.

Aspirin tolerance test

The bleeding time is determined before and 1 hour after a dose of aspirin (5 to 10 grains) is given. This is a useful procedure for evaluating borderline normal results for von Willebrand's disease. Normal patients will often show a slightly longer time (2 to 5 minutes) and increased blood flow volume after aspirin ingestion, but patients with vWD have dramatically increased times (15 to 30 minutes) and may bleed profusely. This test should not be done if the initial test is grossly abnormal.

Clot retraction

Clot retraction represents the final stage of coagulation, corresponding to consolidation of the clot by the action of thrombosthenin. Patients with low platelet counts ($< 100,000$ per μL) or thrombasthenia display less clot retraction than normal. The clot should begin to retract, producing a distinct barrier between serum and red cell mass, within minutes after coagulation is complete. The clot is observed periodically while it incubates in a 37°C water bath. Retraction is complete by 4 hours in normal subjects but may be poor or absent 24 hours later in patients with inadequate thrombosthenin (Fig. 28-2).

A small amount of free red blood cells may be found at the bottom of the tube, but this "fallout" is increased in patients with hypo- or dysfibrinogenemia. Because the clot is composed primarily of erythrocytes, patients with polcythemia will show mini-

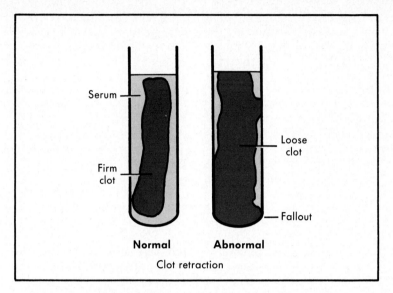

Fig. 28-2.   Clot retraction.
Normal and abnormal appearance of a clot after 24 hours' incubation.

mal clot retraction and patients with severe anemias will show marked retraction. If hyperfibrinolytic activity occurs, the clot may dissolve as it is formed, leading to increased red cells at the bottom of the tube and presence of a stringly, ill-formed clot. Other observations of the clot, including a technique for quantitating serum and cell components, is presented in Sirridge and Shannon (1983).

Platelet aggregation studies

Platelet activities during the hemostatic process includes a change in shape, increasing surface adhesiveness, and the tendency to aggregate with other platelets to form a plug (Chapter 12). These responses can be assayed in vitro to diagnose disorders of platelets. Aggregating agents (e.g., thrombin, adenosine diphosphate, collagen) are added to a suspension of platelets in plasma (**platelet rich plasma, PRP**) and the response is measured turbidimetrically as a change in light transmission (Fig. 28-3). A variety of commercial instruments (**aggre-**

gometers) are available to conduct these studies.

Principle. Platelet rich plasma (PRP) is placed in a tube or test well of an aggregometer and a baseline (dispersed) reading is obtained. An aggregating reagent is added to the PRP and the change in optical density is recorded as a function of time (moving strip chart recording). Increased platelet aggregation results in the transmission of additional light to a photodetector. The aggregation response (slope = rate; amplitude = maximum) of a patient is compared to a control subject.

Procedure (general)

1. The patient's PRP and platelet poor plasma (PPP) are prepared by centrifugation. The PRP should not contain red cells or other contaminants and the platelet count should be adjusted to a consistent concentration, as per the instrument manufacturer's instructions (usually between 200,000 and 500,000 per µL). The PPP can be used as a diluent.

2. Baseline values (0% and 100%) are set on the instrument with PRP and PPP re-

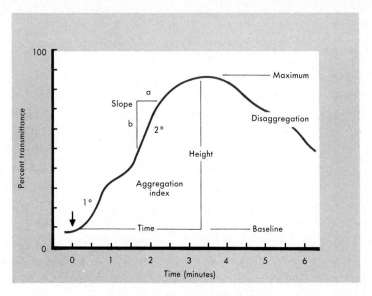

Fig. 28-3.   Features of a platelet aggregation curve.

spectively, the minimum and maximum transmission values.

3. Tests are conducted with PRP at 37°C. One volume of aggregating reagent is added per nine volumes of PRP. The strip chart recorder is activated with the addition of the reagent and the response curves are obtained. Most instruments also calculate slope parameters.

Results. A platelet response curve consists of distinct phases that vary with the type and concentration of aggregating agent used. Primary aggregation is the initial response of the platelets to the aggregating agent, seen as a rapid change in optical density due to change of shape (baseline oscillations cease as the platelets change from discs to spheres) and formation of clumps. A secondary phase of aggregation occurs with some reagents, caused by release of ADP from the aggregating platelets, producing further clumping.

1. Collagen (Fig. 28-4, A). A single phase of aggregation occurs after a brief lag time. If aspirin is given to the patient and the test

repeated, the secondary phase of ADP release is inhibited and only a small primary phase is seen.

2. Adenosine diphosphate (Fig. 28-4, B). A single or biphasic curve results, depending on the concentration of ADP used. Low concentrations produce a primary phase that is usually reversible (disaggregation is evidenced by a decrease in light transmission or deflection toward baseline). With higher concentrations of ADP, the primary and secondary waves are fused or evidenced by only a slight deflection in the curve. Change of shape is usually evident as a small downward deflection after addition of the reagent.

3. Epinephrine (Fig. 28-4, C). Epinephrine (adrenalin) also produces a biphasic response curve in most samples tested, but no evidence of platelet shape change is seen. Aspirin inhibits the second phase of aggregation.

4. Ristocetin (Fig. 28-4, D). A rapidly rising, single phase response curve is typical with ristocetin. The curve may show a

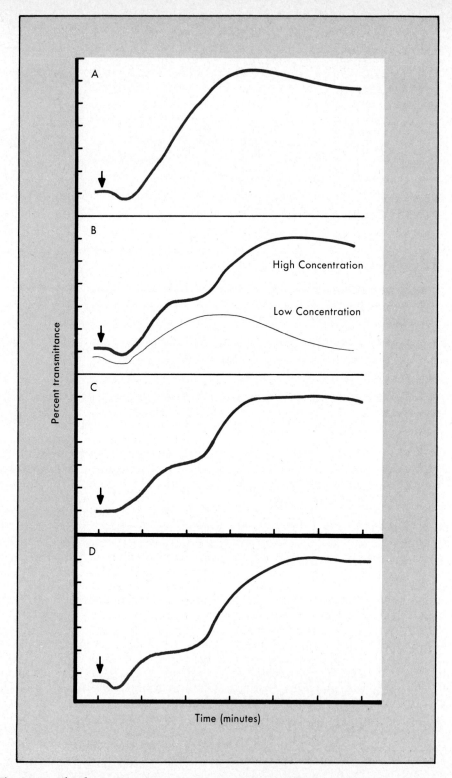

Fig. 28-4. Platelet aggregation curves in response to different agents.
A, Response to collagen. **B,** Response to ADP. **C,** Response to epinephrine. **D,** Response to risto-cetin.

broad trace because of the oscillations produced by the very large aggregates of platelets that are formed.

5. Arachidonic acid. The curve is similar to that produced by collagen, except that aspirin completely inhibits the aggregation response due to blockage of the arachidonic pathway (cyclooxygenase inhibition). For this reason, an absence of response to this agent should result in an investigation of the drug history of the patient before continuing with additional platelet function studies.

Table 28-1 compares aggregating agents with respect to findings in platelet disorders (also see Chapter 23). Patients refrain from aspirin ingestion for at least 8 days prior to aggregation testing. Other substances that may interfere with platelet aggregation include alcohol, some antihistamines, nonsteroid antiinflammatory drugs, and some antidepressants.

Reference values

60% to 90% of control values with each aggregating agent

Lag time for arachidonic acid: 15 to 30 seconds

Lag time for collagen: 45 to 60 seconds

Table 28-1. Aggregating agents with abnormal results in hemostatic disorders

Disorder	Agent
Bernard-Soulier syndrome	Ristocetin
Glanzmann's thrombasthenia	All agents except ristocetin
von Willebrand's disease	Ristocetin
Storage pool defects	Collagen, arachidonate
Release mechanism defects	Collagen, epinephrine, arachidonate, low ADP concentration
Aspirin or ethanol ingestion	All agents except ristocetin and high doses of ADP

Other platelet tests

Platelet factor 3 (PF-3) availability. PF-3 is an intrinsic platelet phospholipid that activates coagulation factors II and X of the common coagulation pathway. When the platelets in PRP are stimulated by kaolin or epinephrine, PF-3 response can be measured by plasma clotting time. Patients with thrombasthenia or thrombocytopenia have decreased amounts of PF-3 available, resulting in a prolonged clotting time. A patient sample is compared with a control sample (the platelet counts must also be adjusted to equal concentrations with PPP to obtain comparable results). Clotting times usually range from about 30 to 60 seconds. Abnormal patient samples should be at least 15 seconds longer than the control sample.

Platelet adhesion (retention). The Salzman glass bead method tests the ability of platelets to adhere to foreign substances. Whole blood is collected through a flexible tube containing glass beads into EDTA. A second sample is collected directly into EDTA. If the platelets are normal, the blood collected through the beads should contain 40% to 75% of the platelets observed in the direct sample. Each laboratory must establish its own normal values, based on the equipment and procedure followed. Since flow rate can affect platelet retention, a more precise method involves the use of a constant flow pump to draw the blood through the bead column. Blood is collected as a single sample in heparin, then an aliquot is drawn through the bead column with the pump. Percent adhesiveness (platelet retention) is calculated as the difference between platelet count without beads and with beads, divided by the count without beads, multiplied by 100 to express the result as a percentage.

EVALUATION OF COAGULATION

Assessing potential defects of the coagulation cascade is accomplished first by screening tests to determine what part of the cascade is abnormal (common, extrinsic, or intrinsic pathway), then performing differential or confirmatory assays to establish diagnosis and evaluate the disorder's quantitative extent. The major screening tests will be reviewed first.

Whole blood clotting times

The simplest technique to measure clotting ability is to merely collect a blood sample and observe the time it requires for a clot to form. Standardization of the results is improved when the amount of blood is consistent, the process occurs at a specified temperature, and clotting occurs in the same physical environment. The **Lee-White coagulation time** is a test of the intrinsic and common pathways, but the results are likely to be abnormal only when a major defect is present (e.g., factor concentrations of less than 1%). The test is not sufficiently sensitive to be used as a routine screening test for coagulopathies nor will it detect mild qualitative and quantitative factor deficiencies. Because the test requires continued monitoring for 15 to 20 minutes, it is also an impractical procedure for sequential monitoring (e.g., periodic testing during heparin administration) or for testing large numbers of patients.

Procedure

1. Blood is drawn, with minimal trauma, through a 20 gauge needle into a plastic syringe. The first few drops of blood are collected and the syringe is removed, to be replaced by a new syringe. About 5 mL of blood is drawn with the second syringe.

2. One mL of blood is placed into each of three 12 × 75 mm glass test tubes. A timer is started at the time blood is added to the third tube. The tubes are placed in a 37°C water bath or heat block. Blood should not be placed in the tube through the needle nor should the blood be ejected forcefully into the tube.

3. The first tube is tilted every 30 seconds until a clot forms; the blood doesn't flow even if the tube is completely inverted. The second and third tubes are tilted every minute until they clot; the Lee-White time is that at which the last tube clots.

The clot can be left in the water bath for observations of clot lysis. The clotting time will be prolonged if the volume of blood per tube or the diameter of the tube is increased, or if the temperature is decreased. The second tube usually clots within 1 to 3 minutes of the first and the third tube within 1 minute of the second.

Reference values. 5 to 15 minutes.

• • •

A more accurate whole blood clotting time uses diatomaceous earth to stimulate the clotting mechanism. The **activated clotting time** (ACT) uses a two tube technique (Vacutainer system, Becton-Dickinson) to draw the blood.

Procedure

1. A small amount of blood is drawn through the needle into a plain tube and this is removed from the needle holder and discarded. A second Vacutainer tube, containing 12 mg of diatomaceous earth (B-D no. 6522), is placed in the holder and blood is collected. A timer starts with the appearance of blood in the tube.

2. The filled tube is removed from the needle assembly and inverted a few times. The tube is placed in a 37°C water bath or heating block. At 1 minute elapsed time, tilt the tube to observe for clot then quickly return it to the water bath. Repeat this every 5 seconds until the blood clots.

This test is more reproducible than the Lee-White time and it takes considerably less time to perform. The heating block must be near the collection site and the phlebotomy must be completed quickly and cleanly for the results to be accurate. Alternatively, the test can be done with two syringes, in which case 2 mL of blood from the second syringe is transferred to the ACT tube.

Reference values. 70 to 105 seconds.

Screening tests based on plasma clotting time

The major screening test of intrinsic pathway function is the **partial thromboplastin time (PTT) or activated partial thromboplastin time (APTT).** When blood is collected into an anticoagulant, such as sodium citrate, calcium is removed from the plasma and it is therefore not available to participate in the key steps of factor complex formation (Chapter 13). The sample is centrifuged and most of the platelets are also discarded. Plasma clotting times are based on the readdition of calcium to the plasma (recalcification) plus a substitute for platelet activity that permits the coagulation process to proceed. If an intrinsic coagulation factor is deficient, clotting will be prolonged.

Procedure (APTT)

1. Draw blood carefully by evacuated system into 3.8% sodium citrate or add 4.5 mL of blood from a syringe to 0.5 mL of the anticoagulant.

2. The blood is centrifuged within 2 hours of collection (as soon as possible). High speed removes most of the platelets from the plasma (3000 rpm for 10 minutes in a table top model). Remove the plasma from the blood immediately and place it in a second tube. If a delay in testing of more than 15 minutes is inevitable, the plasma can be refrigerated.

3. Place calcium chloride (0.025 M) in a 37° C water bath or heating block (automated instruments have incubating wells for reagents). Plasmas and other reagents should also be incubated at 37° C for 1 or 2 minutes prior to testing.

4. Add 0.1 mL of activated thromboplastin reagent into tubes or instrument cups, one for each sample replicate.

5. Add 0.1 mL of plasma (patient or control) to a reagent tube/cup and incubate for 5 minutes. Automated instruments provide fixed intervals that sequence these steps at the appropriate times.

6. Add 0.1 mL of calcium chloride to the plasma-reagent mixture. If this is a manual procedure, a timer is activated as the $CaCl_2$ is added. After the tube sits for about 20 seconds, tilt it gently about once every 2 seconds, observing the side of the tube against a light or a dark background. Automated instruments use a mechanical agitator or an optical beam to measure clot formation. Clot formation is signified by the appearance of a fibrin mesh in the plasma and formation of a semisolid gel or lump. Unlike the whole blood clotting method, inversion of the tube will spill the clot. Whether by a manual or an automated method, each sample should be tested in duplicate and the results should agree within a few seconds.

Commercial reagents and control plasmas are reliable, but instructions of the manufacturer must be followed carefully. Data on control plasmas should be recorded and compared so that deviations in results due to temperature changes, different lots of reagents, or instrument malfunction can be monitored. Patient results are always reported with control values, typically in the range of 25 to 40 seconds. The major difference between the PTT and APTT is that the latter is activated by kaolin, which speeds up the slow contact phase of the cascade. The thromboplastin reagent contains the platelet phospholipids that form a complex with calcium and factors VIII and IX.

In addition to intrinsic factor and contact factor deficiencies, the APTT will be prolonged if circulating anticoagulants are present in the plasma. Thus, this test is used to monitor heparin concentration during intravenous administration and it can be used to detect circulating inhibitors, such as the lupus anticoagulant (see plasma recalcification time). The test is not sensitive to minor abnormalities in some of the common pathway factors, but it is useful for screening mild to moderate deficiencies of factors VIII and IX (the most common and potentially serious disorders!) and the contact factors. Abnormal results of a PTT or APTT determination should be followed by differential studies using adsorbed plasma and aged serum (below).

• • •

The **prothrombin time (PT)** measures functional activity of the extrinsic (and common) pathways. The procedure is similar to that of the APTT, except that it uses a tissue thromboplastin reagent combined with calcium chloride to provide a one step procedure for initiating plasma clotting. Tissue thromboplastin and factor VII activate factor X and the common pathway (X → V → II → I). The prothrombin time measures deficiencies in these factors to different degrees. It is least sensitive to disorders involving factor II (prothrombin). Based on observations cited in Sirridge and Shannon (1983), changes in PT times are associated with the indicated factor deficiencies:

Fibrinogen (I) < 80   →   prolonged PT
  mg/dL or dysfi-
  brinogenemia
Factors V, VII, and X →   longer than 70 sec-
  (homozygous state)   onds
Factors V, VII, and X →   prolonged by 1 to 3
  (heterozygous   seconds
  state)

The PT is especially useful in monitoring oral therapy with coumarin-type drugs (e.g., warfarin) since these interfere with production of the vitamin K-dependent factors (II, VII, IX and X). Intravenous heparin also prolongs the PT and this should be considered when evaluating a prolonged result in patients in intensive care units or recovering from surgery. Endogenous circulating anticoagulants also prolong the PT.

Procedure

1. Blood is collected in 3.8% sodium citrate, in the same manner as for the APTT. Centrifuge the sample to separate the plasma from red cells and platelets (3000 rpm for 10 minutes) and isolate the plasma in a clean tube as soon as possible.

2. Place 0.2 mL of thromboplastin reagent (contains calcium chloride) in a tube or cup and incubate at 37° C for a mini-

mum of 1 minute. Also incubate the plasma (patient and control) at 37° C prior to testing.

3. Add 0.1 ml of plasma to the reagent in the cup and start the timer. Automated instruments use mechanical agitation or an optical beam to measure clot formation. Manual methods rely on tilting and observation of a fibrin web. As with the APTT, each sample should be done in duplicate.

Reference values. 10 to 13 seconds, depending on instrument and commercial reagents used.

• • •

The **plasma recalcification time (PRT)** is a simple method for assessing activity of the intrinsic pathway in relation to platelet concentration which provides the phospholipid activating substrate. Depending on how the sample is centrifuged, a platelet rich plasma (PRP) or platelet poor plasma (PPP) is obtained. With PPP, all components of the intrinsic pathway are measured, including platelet factor 3. Since PF-3 is especially liable to inhibition by the lupus anticoagulant, the PPP-based PRT is a relatively sensitive method for detection of this circulating coagulation inhibitor. The APTT and PT, however, are more sensitive methods than the PRT for assessing coagulation factor deficiencies.

Procedure

1. Collect blood in 3.8% sodium citrate (4.5 mL blood + 0.5 mL of anticoagulant) and mix. The PRP method should use a two syringe or siliconized tube for collection.

2. Centrifuge the sample at 3000 rpm for 10 minutes to obtain PPP or at 1000 rpm for 10 minutes to obtain PRP. As with other clotting time tests, the sample should be run within 2 hours of collection.

3. Incubate calcium chloride (0.025 M) at 37° C in a water bath or heating block. Incubate the plasma samples, 0.2 mL per tube or cup, prior to testing.

4. Add 0.2 mL of calcium chloride to the plasma and activate a timer. After 60 seconds, tilt the tube once every 2 seconds (manual method) or use an automated in-

strument to mechanically agitate or optically monitor the plasma. Appearance of a fibrin web is the end point. Repeat each sample at least once.

Reference values. Platelet rich plasma: 120 to 160 seconds; Platelet poor plasma: 160 to 200 seconds

Differential testing for factor deficiencies

When a screening test (PT or APTT) is prolonged in the absence of anticoagulant therapy, a differential test is performed by mixing the patient plasma with normal plasma. If the prolonged result occurs because of a factor deficiency, the addition of normal plasma containing the missing or defective protein should "correct" the screening test to a normal time. If correction does not occur, the prolonged result is most likely caused by a circulating anticoagulant. Therefore, this procedure is often referred to as a **correction study.** The test is performed in the same manner as a regular PT or APTT, except that the patient plasma is added to normal plasma in a 4:1 ratio (20% of a coagulation factor is enough to correct either of these times to a normal or near normal value).

Identification of a likely factor deficiency can be made on plasma samples that are corrected with normal plasma. **Substitution**

studies are done in the same manner as correction studies, except that one of two reagents are combined with the patient plasma. Instead of normal plasma containing all of the coagulation factors, aged serum or adsorbed plasma is used, each containing some of the coagulation factors:

Absorbed plasma contains factors I, V, VIII, XI, and XII

Aged serum contains factors VII, IX, X, XI, and XII.

Adsorbed plasma is prepared by mixing normal plasma (pooled or single source) with aluminum hydroxide gel (use with sodium citrate anticoagulant) or with barium sulfate (use with oxalates). The salt absorbs factors II, VII, IX and X, leaving the others in solution. Aged serum is made by placing serum in a 37° C for 24 hours, destroying the heat labile factors. Directions for preparation are provided by Shannon and Sirridge (1983). Also, both reagents are available commercially.

When one of these reagents is used to correct the screening test time, it can only provide the factors present. In combination with the factors for which the PT and APTT test (extrinsic and intrinsic pathways, respectively), a differential result is obtained which is a presumptive factor identification (Table 28-2).

Table 28-2. Results of substitution studies for factor deficiencies

| APTT | PT | Adsorbed plasma | | Aged serum | | Probable deficiency |
		APTT	PT	APTT	PT	
A	N	N	—	N	—	Factor XI or XII
A	N	A	—	N	—	Factor IX
A	N	N	—	A	—	Factor VIII
N	A	—	A	—	N	Factor VII
A	A	A	A	N	N	Factor X
A	A	N	N	A	A	Factor V
A	A	A	A	A	A	Factor II
N	N	No further testing necessary				No apparent deficiency

N, Normal result; *A*, abnormal result; —, testing not required.

For example, a patient suffering from hemophilia B (factor IX deficiency) would have a normal PT result but a prolonged APTT. Absorbed plasma does not contain factor IX, so correction does not occur, whereas aged serum does contain the missing factor and the APTT result will be normal. It is not necessary to perform PT substitutions, since the initial PT result was normal. A factor V deficiency would result in an abnormal PT and APTT, since both tests also measure the function of the common pathway. Only adsorbed plasma contains factor V and either the PT or APTT (or both) should be corrected by this reagent but not by aged serum.

Both reagents contain factors XI and XII, so deficiencies of one of these factors in association with a prolonged APTT cannot be distinguished on the basis of a substitution study. Prekallikrein or high molecular weight kininogen (HMWK) deficiency is also a possibility. Clinical manifestations are most often associated with a deficiency of factor XI. A prolonged APTT result caused by a deficiency of prekallikrein usually can be detected by incubating the plasma with silica or kaolin for 10 minutes, which serves as an activator and corrects the time to normal.

Coagulation factor assays

The routine definitive test for a quantitative deficiency of a coagulation protein is the specific **factor assay,** in which the APTT or PT determines the factor's concentration in the patient plasma and in a control plasma. This semiquantitative test is performed on a sequence of dilutions of a factor deficient plasma (various types are commercially available) to which the patient's plasma is added. The amount of correction by the patient's plasma is compared with correction by normal plasma (arbitrarily defined as 100% activity). Results from the patient are expressed as a percent of the normal plasma, with reference ranges of 50% to 150% of normal. Factor deficient plasmas are expensive. Therefore the screening and substitution studies are completed first, providing a presumptive identification of the deficient factor.

General procedure

1. Blood is collected in 3.8% sodium citrate immediately prior to testing. Centrifuge the sample at high speed to separate platelets from the plasma and place the plasma in an ice bath.

2. Factor deficient plasma, corresponding to the suspected deficiency of the patient, is reconstituted and also placed in the ice bath. Reagent for a PT or APTT, depending on the factor deficiency, is incubated at 37° C.

3. Serial dilutions of the patient's plasma are made and 0.1 mL of each dilution is combined with 0.1 mL of the factor deficient plasma and incubated at 37° C. A parallel set of serial dilutions of normal plasma and factor deficient plasma is also incubated.

4. The results, averaged replicate test times at different dilutions, are plotted for patient and normal plasma on logarithmic (log-log) graph paper. A best-fit line drawn through the points from the normal plasma dilutions represents the normal activity curve, from about 1% to 100% activity.

5. Dilutions of patient plasma are compared to the normal activity curve to determine the amount of coagulation factor present in the patient's plasma. New normal activity curves are run for each set of assays. The procedure has a number of sources of error (incubation times and temperatures, processing times, reagent lots, etc.) and normal activity will vary each time.

6. Automated instruments have computers that calculate activity curves and patient results. Control data should be compared for assay to assay variation.

Prothrombin consumption test (PCT)

A prothrombin time performed on serum, instead of plasma, tests for prothrombin (factor II) after blood has clotted. If a factor deficiency related to the plasma thrombinase complex (platelet factor 3, factor VIII or IX) is present, conversion of prothrombin to thrombin will be incomplete and increased amounts of prothrombin will remain. On the other hand, if the patient has a factor II deficiency (the PT will be abnormal) or a deficiency in more than one factor, the PCT will most likely be normal. Thrombocytopenia or platelet disorders relating to PF-3 availability will also result in a decreased PCT time.

The PT is performed by adding fibrinogen reagent to thromboplastin reagent and calcium chloride. Reference times vary with the reagent system used, but normal PCT times are usually greater than 18 to 20 seconds.

Tests for fibrinogen activity

The **thrombin time test** is a method for evaluating the rate of formation of fibrin monomers from fibrinogen. A number of abnormalities will produce a prolonged test:
1. Plasma fibrinogen concentration of less than 100 mg/dL.
2. Presence of thrombin inhibitors, such as:
   a. Increased fibrin(ogen) degradation products (FDPs)
   b. Heparin or other circulating anticoagulants
   c. Increased amounts of immunoglobulins (e.g., associated with multiple myeloma)
3. Dysfunctional forms of fibrinogen

The test may also be prolonged in newborns. It is useful for evaluating prolonged PT and APTT results when other factor deficiencies have been ruled out. In cases of disseminated intravascular coagulation (DIC), the presence of increased FDPs and decreased fibrinogen produces a prolonged thrombin time and the test provides a means of monitoring the combined effect. Commercial kits, containing a thrombin reagent and calcium chloride, are available to

test plasma. A normal control plasma should always be run for comparison. A control time should fall between 10 and 15 seconds and a normal patient should be less than 20 seconds (most are less than 10).

Fibrinogen assays are quantitative techniques to measure fibrinogen present in the plasma. Different techniques have been developed to provide data in specific situations. In emergency situations involving hemorrhage (obstetric or surgical complications, DIC), a modification of the thrombin time is used (the Clauss method), employing dilutions of the plasma sample and a high concentration of thrombin to overcome the presence of heparin or other inhibitors. The test is rapid and simple to perform. Results are compared with a normal plasma of specified fibrinogen concentration and the results are plotted on log-log paper in the same manner as a factor assay (previously discussed). Normal results are read as concentration, in mg/dL, with reference values of about 160 to 400 mg/dL. Note that the procedure is a determination based on activity, but results are converted to concentration by comparison with control plasma results. The results can be misleading if the abnormality is dysfibrinogenemia rather than hypofibrinogenemia. As with other factor assays, the procedure can be run on automated coagulation instruments, reducing the time and increasing the precision of the test.

A direct measure of fibrinogen concentration can be done by weighing a clot and determining its protein content with a quantitative protein procedure (biuret or Folin-Ciocalieu technique). Immunological techniques have largely replaced this classic procedure, however. Monoclonal antibodies provide a means of identifying and quantitating the molecule specifically and without interference from circulating inhibitors. Nonspecific immunological techniques, such as radial immunodiffusion using nonspecific antibodies, may also be used to estimate concentration. However, increased amounts of FDPs may also be detected as fibrinogen, yielding falsely elevated results.

TESTS FOR FIBRINOLYSIS

Evaluations of the fibrinolytic system include screening tests to observe the gross breakdown of blood clots, determinations of soluble monomers and fibrinogen-fibrin degradation complexes, and direct measurements of the plasminogen system (see box).

Whole blood clot lysis time

Principle. Excessive fibrinolytic activity will result in premature lysis of a formed blood clot. Clots incubated at 37° C (optimal plasmin activity) and in the cold (control for low fibrinogen) are observed at various intervals for clot dissolution.

Procedure

1. By careful venipuncture with a 21 gauge or larger needle and plastic syringe,

---

FIBRINOLYSIS TESTS

Clot lysis
Whole blood clot lysis time
Diluted whole blood clot lysis time
Euglobulin clot lysis time

Soluble fibrin monomer complexes (SFMC)
Protamine sulfate serial dilution test
Plasma protamine paracoagulation test
Ethanol gelation test
Cryofibrinogen

Fibrinogen-fibrin degradation products (FDP)
Precipitation test for fibrin split products
Staphylococcal clumping test
Thrombo-Wellcotest
Neutrophil fluorescence test
Fibrin plate assay

Plasminogen and antiplasmin
Synthetic fluorogenic substrate assay for
    plasminogen
Synthetic chromogenic substrate assay for
    antiplasmin
Assay for protein C

---

draw slightly more than 6 ml of blood, avoiding prolonged venous stasis or irritation.

2. Add 2.0 mL of blood to each of 3 glass tubes (12 × 75 mm or 13 × 100 mm) and place these immediately into a 37° C water bath or heat block.

3. Observe the tubes periodically for clot formation, which should occur within 20 to 30 minutes. Note time and transfer one tube to a refrigerator (1 to 6°C).

4. Observe the remaining tubes in 37°C at intervals over 48 hours, noting any disintegration of the formed clot or fibrin "fallout" in the bottom of the tube. Typical observation times are: 1, 2, 3, 4, 24, and 48 hours.

5. Compare clot appearance with the refrigerated tube. Report lysis time as "no clot lysis at 48 hours" or "clot lysis observed at 4 hours." Report normal expected values, based on method or modification of method.

Interpretation. The clot should remain intact at either temperature for at least 48 hours. The formation of a small clot or no clot may be caused by hypofibrinogenemia. Pour the contents of a tube over filter paper to observe for clot fragments. If these are firm, low fibrinogen levels should be suspected. Rapid lysis of the clot at 37°C, but not in the cold, is indicative of increased fibrinolysin activity and this should be investigated with more sensitive and specific methods.

Discussion. Although slightly less sensitive, a widely used method is to use the clot formed during the clot retraction test. Because of the larger blood volume normally used, significant lysis is usually absent before 72 hours. Earlier methods for clot lysis usually permitted observations at room temperature (anything is possible), but plasmin activity would have to be very excessive to produce abnormal results.

Diluted whole blood clot lysis time

Principle. Circulating inhibitors of the fibrinolytic system extend the time required to observe increased plasmin activity and they decrease the sensitivity of the clot lysis method presented previously. This procedure uses refrigeration and dilution of the plasma to counteract inhibition of fibrinolysis.

Procedure

1. Place 1.7 mL of phosphate buffer and 0.1 mL of thrombin solution into each of 3 small glass tubes. Place all tubes in an ice bath. Add the thrombin just prior to collecting the blood sample.

> Phosphate buffer. Dissolve 9.47 g of Na_2HPO in one liter of distilled water. Add 3.02 g of KH_2PO_4 dissolved in 250 mL of distilled water, adjust pH to 7.4 and sterilize by heat. Store in refrigerator.

> Thrombin solution. Add 10.0 mL of 50% glycerol in barbital-buffered saline to 1000 units of bovine topical thrombin. Store in freezer as stock solution. For use, dilute 1:2 with barbital-buffered saline (working concentration = 50 U per mL).

2. Draw one mL of blood with minimal trauma into a syringe and transfer 0.2 mL to each of the three tubes. Gently tilt each tube once.

3. Transfer the tubes to a refrigerator for about 30 minutes to inactivate inhibitors.

4. Place two of the tubes in a 37° C water bath or heat block. After 10 minutes gently rotate the tubes to loosen the clots from the glass surfaces. Retraction will result in a small clot floating in the buffer solution.

5. Record the time of lysis, which first appears as a hazy blurring of the formed clot and leads to complete dissolution. As in the undiluted clot lysis time, the refrigerated tube serves as a control for the presence of fibrinogen.

Interpretation. In patients with normal fibrinolytic activity, clot lysis will occur at 2 to 12 hours (mean of about 5½ hours). Times are longer for samples drawn in the morning, so that time of collection should be consistent to establish normal values.

Euglobulin lysis time

Principle. A clot prepared from the euglobulin fraction of plasma, with antiplasmin and antiplasminogen activator absent, is observed for lysis, which occurs more rapidly than clots prepared from whole blood or plasma.

Procedure

1. Collect 4.5 mL of blood with minimal trauma and venous stasis and add it to 0.5 mL of sodium oxalate (0.1 M). Use plastic syringes and tubes.

2. Centrifuge rapidly (use refrigerated centrifuge, if available, at 2500 rpm) for 10 minutes to produce platelet-poor plasma (PPP) and separate from cells immediately. Keep plasma in an ice bath and test within 30 minutes of collection.

3. Add 0.5 mL of plasma to a large test tube (15-16 × 125 mm). Add 9.0 mL of cold distilled water and 0.1 mL of 1% acetic acid. The dilution and acidification steps separate the euglobulin proteins from others in the plasma, forming a white precipitate. Mix by inversion and centrifuge at 2500 rpm at 4° C for 30 minutes.

4. Pour off the supernatent and allow the inverted tube to drain onto filter paper for 2 minutes, removing the plasma portion containing antiplasmin. A cotton applicator can be used to wipe remaining liquid from the tube walls; do not disturb the precipitate.

5. Place the tube in a 37° C water bath and add 0.5 mL of sodium borate solution. Stir with a plastic rod until the precipitate is completely dissolved.

> Sodium borate solution. Dissolve 9.0 g of sodium chloride and 1.0 g of sodium borate in 100 mL of distilled water, adjust to pH 9.0.

6. Add 0.5 mL of calcium chloride (0.025 M) to the mixture and tilt the tube every few seconds until a clot forms. Record the time of clotting. Return tube to the 37° C water bath.

7. Check the clot periodically for lysis. If increased fibrinolytic activity is probable, check every 5 minutes for the first half

hour. When lysis begins, check every 5 minutes until completed and record the time. The results are reported as the elapsed time from clot formation to complete dissolution.

Interpretation. The euglobulin clot normally requires between 2 and 4 hours to lyse, but there are marked variations from day to day in the same patient. It is advisable to perform this test in parallel with a sample from a "normal" patient as a control. In the presence of normal fibrinogen levels, lysis times of less than 120 minutes are usually indicative of increased plasminogen activator activity.

Discussion. Times can also be shorter due to prolonged venous occlusion or as a result of vigorous arm rubbing, which results in increased activity of plasminogen activator. Prolonged lysis times can result from the antiplasmin activities of platelets, so PPP must be prepared soon after blood collection. Bacterial contamination of reagents, hypofibrinogenemia, or use of citrate as an anticoagulant will result in shortened lysis times. Optimal pH of the euglobulin precipitation reaction is 6.2, with longer times occurring as pH decreases.

Some procedures use a second sample drawn from the patient after venous occlusion with a blood pressure cuff (90 mm Hg for 5 minutes). The lysis time for this sample should be considerably shorter than the nonoccluded sample. If not, a decreased release of plasminogen activator is indicated. Euglobulin clotting is initiated by 0.5 mL of bovine thrombin (5 U per mL) in some procedures.

Protamine sulfate serial dilution test

Principle. Formation of fibrin monomers and early fibrin degradation products (FDPs) occurs in excess during some pathological processes, notably disseminated intravascular coagulation (DIC). These soluble complexes form fibrin strands or gelation in the presence of protamine sulfate and this result, paracoagulation, is indicative of secondary fibrinolysis.

Procedure

1. Draw blood with minimal trauma and add 9 parts blood to 1 part sodium citrate (3.8%).

2. Prepare platelet-poor plasma by centrifuging at 3000 rpm for 10 minutes and separating the plasma from the cells. The test should be performed within 2 hours of blood collection.

3. Add 0.05 mL of 1.0 M epsilon aminocaproic acid (EACA) to 1.0 mL of platelet-poor plasma. EACA inhibits fibrinolysis. EACA 1.0 M solution is made by diluting stock EACA (Lederle, 250 mg per mL) 1:2 with distilled water.

4. Prepare serial dilutions of protamine sulfate with normal saline to obtain 1:5, 1:10, 1:20, 1:40 and 1:80 dilutions, each in a labelled tube. 1% Protamine sulfate is supplied by Eli Lilly & Co. Adjust to pH 6.5 by adding a few drops of 0.5 N sulfuric acid.

5. Transfer 0.2 mL of each protamine sulfate dilution to a small test tube.

6. Add 0.2 mL of platelet-poor plasma to each tube and mix gently, resulting in protamine sulfate concentrations as follows:

Dilution	1:5	1:10	1:20	1:40	1:80
Concentration (μg/mL)	1000	500	250	125	62.5

7. Stopper each tube and incubate at 37° C. Observe the tubes against a dark background at 30 minutes and at 24 hours. Record results as gelation (G), fibrin strand (FS), or as amorphous precipitate (AP).

Interpretation. Fibrin monomer complexes (SFMC) usually polymerize earlier and can be detected at 30 minutes, if present. The tubes should be tilted gently during observations so that delicate fibrin threads are not destroyed. The presence of threads or a gelatinous button is positive for fibrin monomers or fibrin degradation products (fdp). The latter are more likely to be evident at the 24 hour reading. The presence of an amorphous, opalescent precipitate is negative for paracoagulation products.

Discussion. Many procedures use incubation at room temperature, but this is more likely to result in appearance of the amorphous precipitate. This test is less sensitive than some other paracoagulation procedures, but it is relatively specific for SFMC and fdp (specifically, $X°$), which are formed as a result of fibrinolysin acting on previously-formed clots. This is in contrast to primary fibrinolysis which acts on fibrinogen and results in fibrinogen degradation products (FDP), specifically X^{fp}, components not detected by this test.

Ethanol gelation test

Principle. Fibrin monomers in plasma are detected by precipitation with ethyl alcohol, resulting in strands or gel formation within a specified time period. Increased levels of fibrin monomers are observed in disseminated intravascular coagulation (DIC).

Procedure. (Breen and Tullis method, modified by Glueck.)

1. Collect blood in a plastic syringe with minimal venous stasis and add 9 parts of blood to 1 part of buffered sodium citrate. Collect blood from a normal patient and run in parallel as a control. (Buffered sodium citrate. Add 3 parts of 0.109 M sodium citrate to 2 parts of 0.1 M citric acid.)

2. Centrifuge the anticoagulated blood at 2500 rpm for 20 minutes to obtain platelet-poor plasma.

3. Place 9 drops of PPP into a 12 × 75 mm test tube; repeat for control plasma.

4. Add one drop of 0.1 N sodium hydroxide, mix well.

5. Carefully layer 0.15 mL of 50% ethyl alcohol over the PPP in each tube and allow to sit at room temperature for 1 minute.

6. Observe the interface between the layers of ethyl alcohol and PPP for a line of precipitation or presence of a gel, either of which denotes a positive test for fibrin monomers.

7. If the tubes are negative for precipitate or gel at 1 minute, observe again at 9 minutes. If a gel or precipitate is present at this time, add another drop of 0.1 N NaOH and gently shake the tube. The test is positive if the precipitate persists. If the precipitate dissolves, it is nonspecific and the test is considered negative.

Interpretation. The appearance of definite fibrin strand or gel constitutes a positive screening test for fibrin monomers, and this may support other indications of DIC. An amorphous flocculation, in the absence of a strand or gel, is not significant. Strands appearing after 10 minutes are also of doubtful significance.

Discussion. The buffered citrate is essential, since pH above 7.7 delays formation of strand or gel. Oxalate anticoagulants produce a pH that is too alkaline. The presence of heparin or slight red cell contamination does not interfere with this test. The test may be falsely positive if the fibrinogen level exceeds 400 mg/dL. Although the ethanol gelation test is not as specific as the protamine paracoagulation test, it is considered more sensitive.

Cryofibrinogen precipitation

Principle. Fibrin monomers precipitate from plasma when refrigerated for several hours.

Procedure

1. Place 1 ml of either oxalated or citrated plasma in each of two small test tubes.

2. Both tubes are stoppered and one is placed in a 1-6° C refrigerator and the other left at room temperature overnight.

3. Observe both tubes the next day.

Interpretation. The presence of a heavy precipitate, gel, or a few distinct strands in the refrigerated tube only, is positive for cryofibrinogen. This should disappear if the tube is warmed to 37° C.

Discussion. Cryoglobulins can also appear as a precipitate in refrigerated plasma, but these appear in serum as well. A refrigerated serum sample can be observed as an additional control.

Thrombo-Wellcotest for fibrinogen-fibrin degradation products (FDP)

Principle. Increased levels of FDP appear in the serum during primary fibrinogenolysis or as a result of secondary fibrinolysis. FDP is detected by a visible agglutination reaction with latex particles that have been sensitized with antibodies to purified FDP. Normal serum contains less than 8 μg per mL and the commercial latex test produces visible clumping at FDP concentrations of greater than 2 μg per mL. Serial dilutions of serum provide semiquantitative results.

Procedure

The following procedure is based on information supplied by the manufacturer, Wellcome Reagents Division of Burroughs Wellcome Company. Consult inserts or brochures for the other commercial kits.

1. Draw 2 mL of blood with minimum trauma. Either a syringe or evacuation system may be used with the sample collection tubes provided. These contain thrombin to ensure rapid clotting and a soybean enzyme (trypsin) inhibitor to prevent fibrin degradation in vitro.

2. Mix blood by inversion, place tube in 37° C incubator until clotting is complete, then centrifuge until a clear serum is obtained. If patient is receiving heparin and blood fails to clot, Reptilase-R can be added (see the following).

3. Prepare serum dilutions in two 10 × 75 mm test tubes, labelled 1:5 and 1:20. Using the graduated droppers supplied, add 0.75 mL of glycine saline buffer (pH 8.2) to each tube. Using the disposable dropper from the kit, add five drops of patient's serum to the tube marked 1:5 and one drop of serum to the tube marked 1:20; mix each tube.

4. Transfer one drop of each diluted serum to a separate, labelled ring on the reaction slide.

5. Add a drop of positive control and a drop of negative control serum to each of two separately marked rings on the reaction slide.

6. Mix the latex suspension by vigorous shaking, then add one drop of latex to each control and diluted serum. Stir the latex and serum with a clean, disposable stick or rod, filling the entire ring with the mixture.

7. Rock the slide gently for 2 minutes, observing for macroscopic agglutination of the latex against a dark background. A good light source, placed at an angle to the slide, will enhance particle visibility.

Interpretation. The negative and positive controls should be negative and positive for latex agglutination, respectively. Since the lower threshold of FDP detection is 2 μg per mL, the following results are reported:

Dilution	1:5	1:10	Report/Result
Test results	−	−	"Less than 10 μg per ml FDP"
	+	−	"10 to 40 μg per ml FDP"
	+	+	"Greater than 40 μg per ml FDP"

Agglutination should not be present in the 1:10 tube unless it is also present in the 1:5 tube. Other dilutions can be made and tested, as previously described, to follow a clinical course or response to therapy.

Discussion. This test, like many others for FDP, cannot distinguish between breakdown products of fibrinogen and fibrin. The serum sample may be refrigerated for up to 1 week or stored at −20° C for longer times before performing the test. Patients with serum positive for the rheumatoid factor may also give a false positive for FDP by this method.

Blood failing to clot because of heparin therapy can be treated with Reptilase-R (Abbott Laboratories). Add 1.0 mL of distilled water to reconstitute the vial. Use 0.1 mL of Reptilase-R for each 1.0 mL of blood. Mix well and incubate at 37° C; clotting should be complete within a few minutes.

A procedure is also available to detect FDP in urine, but correlation between serum and urine FDP is poor. See the package insert for procedure and interpretation.

Staphylococcal clumping test

The Neuman strain of *Staphylococcus aureus* contains clumping factors in the cell wall that reacts with either fibrinogen or fibrinogen degradation products (mainly fragments X and Y) and results in clumping of the bacteria. Lyophilized bacteria (Sigma Chemical Co, St. Louis, Mo.) are added to serial dilutions of serum produced by rapid clotting (EACA-thrombin solution). A serially diluted control of known fibrinogen concentration is run in parallel and the equivalent titer of clumped serum is expressed as "μg fibrinogen equivalents/mL". Normal values depend on the specific procedure used. Although fragments D and E are not detected directly by this method, they are detected when they combine with fibrinogen monomers to produce fibrin. Tube, slide, and microtiter methods are available. Procedures are available in Sirredge and Shannon (1983), Lenahan and Smith (1985), and Bauer (1982).

Tanned red cell hemagglutination inhibition

This immunoassay, using microtiter plates, is considered the reference and research method and it is sensitive to fragments X, Y, D and E at concentrations as low as 0.6 μg of fibrinogen equivalents per mL. The patient's serum is mixed with an antiserum to fibrinogen and then combined with sheep RBCs that are sensitized to fibrinogen. If FDPs are present, they combine with the antiserum and the RBCs fail to agglutinate. Less FDPs result in hemagglutination by the antiserum at a lower dilution. The procedure is commercially available from Wellcome Reagents as the FDP Kit. For most clinical purposes, this degree of sensitivity is not required. Correlation between the slide latex procedure and the TRCHI is good at concentrations greater than 2.0 μg FE per mL.

Neutrophil fluorescence for FDP phagocytosis

During DIC, neutrophils phagocytize FDP and fdp. The addition of a fluorescent antifibrinogen to peripheral blood will stain neutrophils containing the breakdown products. Since the products of secondary fibrinolysis are removed by reticuloendothelial macrophages before neutrophils can ingest them, this test has been suggested as a possible screening test to distinguish primary fibrinolysis from secondary fibrinolysis.

Plasminogen: fluorogenic substrate assay

Plasminogen in citrated plasma is converted to plasmin during incubation with streptokinase and reacted with a synthetic fluorogenic substrate. Plasmin enzymatically alters the substrate to a nonfluorogenic molecule and the change is measured kinetically in a fluorometer and compared to an assayed reference material. The reagents are supplied as a kit by Dade (Protopath Plasminogen Synthetic Substrate Assay Kit). A fluorometer suitable for this assay is also available from Dade. The procedure is summarized by Sirridge and Shannon, 1983. Values are expressed in CTA (Committee on Thrombolytic Agents) units per mL with a suggested normal range of 2.4 to 3.8 CTA U per mL.

29

Quantitation and Quality Assurance

Hematological studies provide much useful information about the health or pathological state of a patient. Some test results are descriptive and of a qualitative nature. Examples are presence or absence of iron deposits in the marrow, presence of various red cell inclusions, and positive results of screening tests for sickle cell hemoglobin and G6PD enzyme deficiency. Most laboratory data, however, are reported as discrete numerical values that are compared to a "normal" or reference range. Values higher or lower than the reference limits are regarded as indications of an abnormal physiological state. Extreme deviations may represent "crisis values" that initiate emergency medical intervention. But how reliable are the numbers generated by analytical procedures? To what extent do test results represent the patient's physiological status? How does the result of a particular procedure compare with that obtained by an alternate procedure? These questions are central to the operations and the objectives of the clinical laboratory as an integral component of the health care system.

DEFINING QUALITY ASSURANCE

Quality assurance or quality control (QC) is a *system* of procedures and evaluations used to monitor an output or product, such as manufactured materials. The concept can be applied to any process for which the detection, measurement, and documentation of output variables can assist in increasing product reliability and efficiency. Emphasis is placed on the word "system". Quality assurance is not a single test,

record of results, or statistical value. Rather, it is a continuous process for obtaining confidence in the methods used and for guaranteeing integrity of the final product.

In the laboratory environment, the final product is the analytical result of a test on a clinical specimen and quality assurance is the process of monitoring instruments, reagents, the test procedures, technologist performance, and the accuracy of the reported results. In modern laboratories, much of the QC data accumulation and analysis is performed automatically during sample testing by a computer component of the analytical instrument. Despite this, the responsibility for detection of procedural errors and interpretation of test reliability rests with the laboratory worker. Accomplishing this requires that the technologist or laboratory scientist have a full understanding of the test procedure and attributes of the clinical assay. Limitations of the test system must be considered, such as the levels of analyte that can be detected, substances and other variables that may interfere with the analysis, and reported values meeting health care requirements.

Samples and populations

Every laboratory analysis is an imperfect representation of the "real world" that it is assessing. Most laboratory tests are done in vitro on samples of body fluids that are imperfect representations of the physiological state of an individual. A blood sample, drawn from a specific site at a specific time, provides a single data point from which to extrapolate a patient's condition. That condition changes continuously as countless physiological mechanisms interact in every organ and cell of the body. One analogy to this situation is to predict the ending of a motion picture from an analysis of a few single frames taken at random. A knowledge of story plots, the film genre, and experience with similar films will aid the analyst. But, the probability for an accurate evaluation increases significantly if the number of frames to be analyzed increases and if they are chosen systematically, based on experience with other films and their characteristics. In this example, the entire film can be considered a *population* and the individual frames comprise one or more *samples.* By extension, a single film can also be a "sample" of other films of the same genre or representative of all films in general. The inclusive limits of sample and populations must be defined for each analytical situation.

Hematological samples also vary in their usefulness for predicting a patient's physiological state. A series of hemoglobin or leukocyte count values is more likely to provide a true picture of the patient than is a single determination. Likewise, a knowledge of the patient's clinical condition and the results of other diagnostic examinations provides a more reliable basis for interpretation of laboratory data and an assessment of its suitability for diagnosis. No amount of experience or analytical sophistication, however, can compensate for the fact that a blood specimen is only an incomplete and imperfect *sample* of a complex and dynamic *population* (the entire circulating blood supply of the patient).

The blood specimen also is a population from which a subsample is taken, represented by the amount consumed or processed during analysis. Assumptions must be made about the degree to which the analytical portion represents the total blood specimen and the patient's peripheral blood

population. Finally, the sample examined must be compared others that comprise various geographical groups, sexes, races, ages, and states of health (Fig. 29-1).

Fortunately, there are standards that establish a mathematical and practical basis for implementation and evaluation of analytical techniques so that a few microliters of blood can represent the physiological status of a patient. These protocols are the basis for quality assurance. They require that a level of *expected* performance be determined before testing and data accumulation begins. This expectation should, in turn, be based on a thorough knowledge of the procedures, instrument capabilities, and nature of the results that are achievable. These expectations and realizations can be expressed as two parameters of measurement: accuracy and precision.

Accuracy and precision

Accuracy is a measure of performance. It is the ability to reproduce or realize the true value of a population attribute. In target shooting, accuracy is defined by hitting the center of the bulls-eye (Fig. 29-2, *A*). To evaluate the accuracy of a measurement, one needs to know the "target" or true value. A standard hemoglobin solution, with a known assayed value expressed in g per dL, can assess the relative accuracy of a laboratory instrument and method. Deviation from the known value provides a means of comparing procedures, instruments, or laboratories. The amount of deviation is analagous to the distance from the target center (the rings might represent specific levels or *standard deviations*, see the following).

Methods of establishing the true value vary. The *definitive method*, establishes the value of an analyte by which all other methods are compared. In practice, any measurement is somewhat arbitrary. That is, results depend on the procedure used to obtain them. Therefore, a definitive method is selected on the basis of the consistency

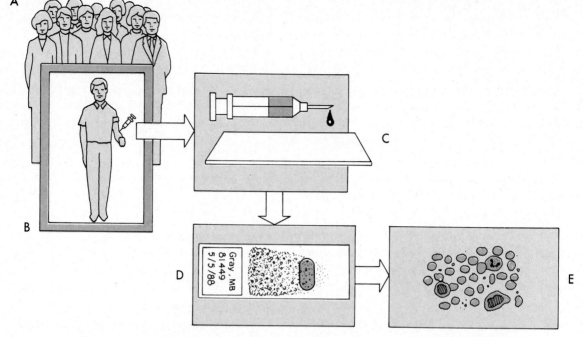

Fig. 29-1.   Samples of samples: the relationship between an analytical value and potential patient populations.

A, The population of individuals may represent different ages, sexes, races, and physiological states. A single individual (sample) may not be representative of either the total population or a particular subpopulation. **B,** A blood sample drawn from an individual may or may not be representative of the person's usual blood cell population. Time of day, medications, and physiological state can produce variations. **C,** A single drop of blood from the total sample is used to prepare a smear for a differential white count. Variation can occur because of clotting, hemolysis, or settling. **D,** The drop (population) is spread as a smear and a region (sample) selected for enumeration and identification. Some cells are carried to the edge and others are left behind. **E,** When 100 or 200 cells (sample) are counted manually, random and nonrandom variation can bias the interpretation of white cell responses.

by which the same results can be obtained and verified over a range of values. Often, the definitive method involves a physically-based measure (e.g., gravimetric, volume displacement, or mass determination) which may be too laborious for routine clinical use. A *reference method* is one that has been compared with the definitive method and displays little deviation (inaccuracy) from the definitive values. It is usually easier to perform than the definitive method and it may serve as a basis for stan-

dardizing reagents for commercial purposes. Thus, a hemoglobin solution supplied for instrument calibration may be analyzed by the manufacturer with a reference method. This value then permits the user to establish a standard for everyday use and calibration.

Accuracy has to be determined for each type of assay. Some measures might be expected to vary from the known value by only tenths of a percentage point, whereas other types of analyses may be much more

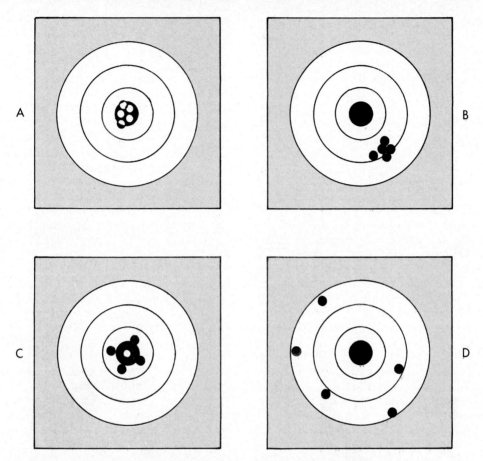

Fig. 29-2.   Accuracy and precision: the target analogy.
A, Accuracy is visualized as the ability to realize the center of the target. In this case, the aim was also precise, as evidenced by tight clustering about the bull's eye. **B,** Precision is seen as consistency of results, despite lack of accuracy of aim. **C,** The results are relatively accurate, scattered evenly about the center, but precision could be improved. **D,** Neither accuracy nor precision were achieved.

difficult to standardize. For example, a reaction product of interest may be unstable (e.g., some kinetic enzyme assays), so that the "target" value is a moving one. Repeated measurements may be required to obtain an average result that approximates the assayed value.

Precision is also a measure of performance. It is the ability to obtain the same results, time after time, on the same sample. Returning to the analogy of target shooting, precision is defined as the *consistency* of aim, producing a tight cluster of hits (Fig. 29-2, *B*). The degree of precision is easy to define by statistical methods: the amount of variation in any series of measurements of the same analyte. The series can consist of replicates made at the same time, at different times during the same testing interval, or extended to different testing sessions during any time interval in which the consistency of results needs to be evaluated. As with accuracy, acceptable levels of precision (or imprecision) need to be defined for each test on the basis of variations that are inherent to the procedure.

It should be obvious from the target analogy that accuracy and precision are somewhat independent properties. One can obtain results that are accurate when multiple determinations are averaged, as measured by the tendency to display little bias from the known standard value yet consist of individually variable values, indicating a low level of precision (Fig. 29-2, C). Conversely, results can be extremely precise (reproducible), yet display a consistent bias or deviation from the reference value (Fig. 29-2, B). The ideal situation, sometimes difficult to achieve, is to realize both accurate and precise results (Fig. 29-2, A). Unfortunately some results may be neither accurate or precise (Fig. 29-2, D).

Obtaining accuracy and precision in hematological testing requires a thorough understanding of the technical aspects of the procedure and the nature of the analyte. Cell counts, cell identifications, and quantifications of chemical substances, such as hemoglobin and serum iron, use different physical principles of analysis. Cell counts are usually determined as discrete events. Cells are counted individually, either as deflections of electric current, as interruptions of a laser beam, or as individual objects in a hemacytometer. Accuracy and precision of cell counts are functions of the number of particles enumerated and the amount of linearity that exists over the range of particle densities observed. For this reason, electronic cell counters, counting 10,000 or more cells, achieve *coefficients of variation* (see the following) that are at least an order of magnitude less than those obtained by manual methods that typically count 50 to 200 cells.

Differential counts are more difficult to standardize because of the inherent variability in cell morphology. Automated cell identification systems are programmed to classify cells types on the basis of defined criteria, such as size, nucleus to cytoplasm ratio, granularity of cytoplasm, and myeloperoxidase reaction. Many of these characteristics are qualitative rather than quantitative and some subjectivity is inherent to the program developed for the instrument. Abnormal and reactive cells may not fit standard schemes, requiring review and reclassification. The problem is likely to be one of accuracy, determining the true identity of the cell, rather than precision. Manual differential counts are subject to both sources of error. Lack of precision can result from inconsistency in identification by a single technologist or from lack of agreement as to identification criteria among several technologists (e.g., criteria for inclusions of cells as bands or segmented neutrophils, identity of reactive lymphocytes). Accuracy of identification is more difficult to evaluate because an individual hematologist must serve as the expert reference, and even experts, unfortunately, are apt to disagree. Survey slides can help redefine the criteria by which cells are classified, but each cell is a unique entity and some will defy identification regardless of criteria and expertise.

An indiscrete or continuous variable, such as hemoglobin concentration, can assume any value within the resolution limits of the instrument or method. The accuracy of the method should exceed, by an order of magnitude, the resolution required to be reported. Thus, a manual hematocrit can be read to 0.1% or 0.2%, but need be reported to only the nearest 0.5% or 1.0%. Hemoglobins can be determined to 0.01 g/dL, but it is clinically meaningless to report values that differ by less than 0.1 g/dL. In fact, clinical decisions require results that vary by greater amounts than this. The problem isn't one of laboratory precision, but of interpreting accuracy with regard to the physiological variation that occurs in the patient. Communication between practitioners of clinical medicine and laboratory medicine is needed to define the limits of precision and accuracy required for meaningful health care.

STANDARDIZATION OF TEST RESULTS

A quality assurance program is based on a continuous evaluation of accuracy and precision in obtaining analytical results. *Standardization* is the process of using materials of known values or properties to establish performance values of a procedure. Accuracy and precision are measured empirically, usually by several repetitions of tests at different times that represent normal operating conditions. Examples include dilutions of hemoglobin solutions to establish a spectrophometric concentration-response curve, particle or preserved cell suspensions to measure electronic responses of an automated counter, and standard normal plasmas to standardize coagulation factor assays.

Calibration is the process of comparing instrument responses to known physical properties, such as electronic signals (cell counters), radioisotope emissions (well scintillation counters), and light spectra (spectrophotometers). Calibration assures that the instrument is performing properly so that data output is predictably proportional to sample input. Calibration requirements vary with the instrument. Some require calibration with each sample run whereas others maintain stability for weeks at a time.

Controls are samples of known constituents and properties that are analyzed in sequence with the test samples. The controls may be preassayed, providing a target or reference value, or they may be unassayed so that values are established empirically. Controls can be obtained from commercial sources with constituents of normal and abnormal reference ranges, or they can be "homemade" by pooling plasmas or sera from patient or normal volunteer sources. Assayed commercial controls have the ad-

vantage of use as a check for both accuracy and precision, whereas unassayed materials are primarily used to evaluate precision. Commercial manufacturers, because of their proprietary interest in promoting quality assurance methods, are an excellent source of information. Booklets, wall charts, sample forms, and videotapes can be obtained from companies that sell instruments and reagents.

Monitoring test performance requires that decisions be made about the results achieved. Statistical treatment of the performance data is a means of standardizing the evaluation. Thus, different laboratory workers, in different laboratories, can compare analytical results with a common yardstick. Quality control statistics are simple and easy to apply. The following outline is intended to provide an informal summary of terms and concepts rather than a formal mathematical basis.

DESCRIPTIVE STATISTICS FOR MONITORING HEMATOLOGY LABORATORY PERFORMANCE

The central question for any laboratory analysis is, "Does the result reliably represent the state of the patient or contents of the sample"? There are many ways to answer this question, none of which are entirely satisfactory. As stated before, every analysis is a compromise. The "true value" of any analyte is only a theoretical concept. The result obtained is an approximation or estimate of that value based on the method used to obtain it. Even a direct observation of a fresh, unstained drop of blood is biased by the method used to collect and handle it. For example, red cells, white cells, and platelets change shape and undergo various physiological processes as they are removed from the blood stream to be placed in contact with glass or other artificial substrates.

Descriptive statistics are a basis for characterizing analytical results. The following terms are part of the language for communi-

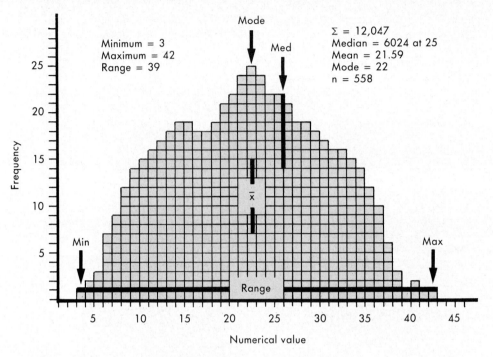

Fig. 29-3.   Descriptive statistics: characterizing sample or population data.
Minimum (min), maximum (max), range, mean (x̄), median (med) and mode of a hypothetical
sample.

cating the qualitative and quantitative nature of these characteristics.

DEFINITIONS OF DESCRIPTIVE TERMS

A **population** is an assembly or group of characters, values, or objects. The limits of the population must be specified, as in Fig. 29-1, but it is understood to contain all of the possible values of interest for a particular analysis (e.g., the hemoglobin values of children less than 12 years old in the southeast United States). In most cases, it is highly improbable that values for the entire population can be determined.

A **sample** is a subset of the population, selected either systematically (by some criteria or pattern) or randomly (all members of the population have an equal chance to be included) for testing. The sample, as mentioned in the definition of population,

can also be regarded as a population for sample derivation (e.g., hemoglobin determinations on black children with sickle cell anemia in Mississippi).

Although the group of values that comprises either a population or sample is defined somewhat arbitrarily (populations include an indeterminate number of different samples and subsamples), formal terms are used to describe characteristics or **attributes** of each group. A **parameter** is a formal attribute of a population (a theoretical value, unless the entire population can be measured); a **statistic** is a formal attribute of a sample. Examples of attributes include the average or mean value, the range and the standard deviation of values, the median, and the mode (Figs. 29-3 and 29-4).

The **maximum** value of a sample or population is the upper arithmetic limit that is

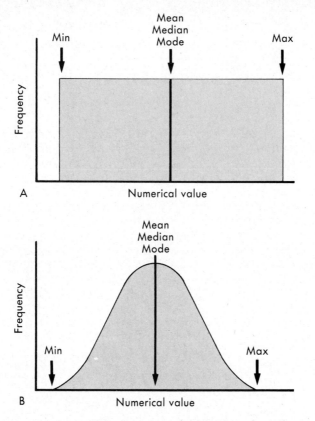

Fig. 29-4. Distribution curves and location of attributes.
A, Random or rectangular distribution. **B,** Normal distribution.

known (potential) or that is measured (realized in current sample). The **minimum** value is the lower limit, which may be a negative number, zero, or some positive value, depending on the analyte. The **range** of values is the inclusive set of data, cited as minimum to maximum (e.g., 8.0 g/dL to 18.4 g/dL) or as a single number or spread (10.4 g/dL in this example). A **distribution** of values is the relationship of the individual data points to each other throughout the range. Several types of distributions are described below.

The **mean** or arithmetic average is one measure of the central tendency of data points within a distribution of values. The

mean ($\bar{x}$) is calculated by adding the individual values (each x: $x_1, x_2, \ldots x_n$) and dividing the total (Σ x) by the number of observation (n):

$$\bar{x} = \frac{\Sigma x}{n}$$

The mid value, or **median,** of a distribution occurs where the number of values less than and greater than a numerical result are equal. It can be found by arranging the values from low to high and identifying the value that is midway between maximum and minimum (e.g., the 16th highest or lowest of 31 values or the mean of the 16th and 17th values of 32 values). The median can also be used to describe the central tendency of ranked (ordinal) data for comparison by nonparametric tests. The **mode** is the value represented by the most examples or the highest frequency of occurrence. Fig. 29-3 shows that the mean, median, and mode do not necessarily coincide.

The mean approximates the center of a distribution only if the values are distributed in a regular manner about the median. This does occur in a rectangular or **random distribution** (Fig. 29-4, *A*) in which all values over the possible range are equally likely to occur. Median and mean are equal and are easily defined as the mid-point of the range. There is no mode since all values, given a large number of measurements, should occur with equal frequency.

Most data in the real world reflects an optimum value, a point in the range of possible results that is most common or best suited for functional consequences (e.g.,

height and weight, hemoglobin concentration, blood cell count, prothrombin time). These absolute values are most commonly expressed as numbers and units, derived from the system used to measure them (centimeters, kilograms, g/dL, cells/µL, or seconds elapsed). Most data can also be *normalized* or converted to a range in which the minimum value represents 0% and the maximum value represents 100% of the range. If an optimum or common value occurs, most examples will be found near the midpoint of the range and a lower frequency of values occur at the extremes (Fig. 29-4, *B*). It can be empirically shown that most biological data, measured in absolute terms, fits a **normal frequency** or **Gaussian distribution curve** (Fig. 29-5). Simply stated, this means that most values in the range will occur near the central point of the range or that the median, mean, and mode will be about equal. The more values that

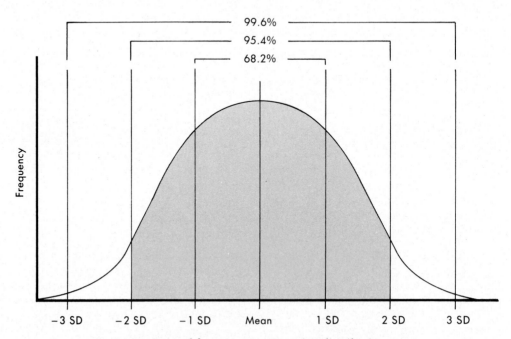

Fig. 29-5.   Normal frequency or Gaussian distribution curve.

are collected, the more apparent this distribution becomes (Fig. 29-6). The more replications in a sample series, the more confidence one can have that the values obtained will approximate the "true value" or theoretical mean of the population. Thus, the population mean (usually represented mathematically by the greek letter, μ) is the desired reference value that the sample mean ($\bar{x}$) is attempting to identify. Identification is facilitated by increasing sample size (the number of determinations or the total sampling interval) or increasing the method's precision so that variation about the sample mean decreases.

Some distributions show a greater frequency of values at certain points other than the median. A bias toward the minimum or maximum value may occur if a starting or ending point is the most likely event in a population. A distribution curve

of all the prothrombin time determinations in a laboratory would indicate a sharp increase from the minimum value, a peak in the normal range, and a long-tailed decrease to maximum values representing abnormal and anticoagulated patients (Fig. 29-7, *A*). Such a distribution is said to be "skewed to the left." Conversely, a frequency distribution of mean corpuscular hemoglobin concentration (MCHC) is "skewed to the right," indicating a long-tailed increase from minimum values to a narrow normal peak, followed by a truncated (cut-off) maximum: only so much hemoglobin can be packed into a red cell of a given volume (Fig. 29-7, *B*). Some distribution curves may display more than one peak or mode. Frequency plots of red cell volume in some anemias and in patients that have been recently transfused may reveal a **bimodal** distribution, indicating different cell popula-

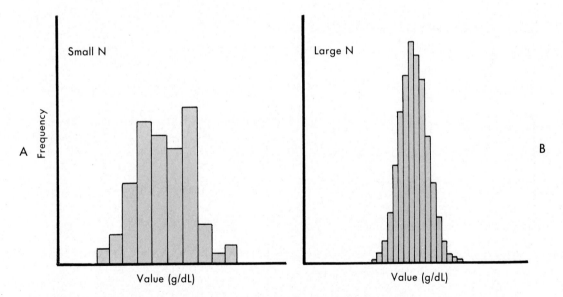

Fig. 29-6. Effects of sample size on distribution attributes.
A sample with a small number of values (**A**) may display a poorly-defined mean and mode. A larger sample of the same normally-distributed population (**B**) may show little increase in range relative to slope of modal peak. Sample mean is better defined and more representative of the population mean. Precision increases as definition of the central tendency increases.

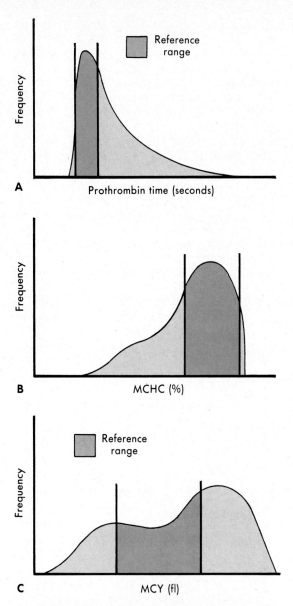

Fig. 29-7.   Other types of distribution curves.
A, Prothrombin time results, displaying skewing toward minimum values. **B,** Results for mean corpuscular hemoglobin concentration (MCHC), showing bias toward maximum values. **C,** A bimodal distribution of mean corpuscular volume (MCV) results in a patient with myelodysplastic syndrome.

tions (Fig. 29-7, *C*). Analysis of frequency histograms is an important component of the identification and enumeration methodology of automated cell counters (Chapter 26).

VARIATION AND DEVIATION

This is an imperfect world we live in and no technique, as wonderful as some of them may be, produces results that are 100% accurate. Human error, instrument error, physiological variation, and random events combine to insure that the results obtained in a laboratory procedure will show some variation. If the mean sample value $(\overline{x})$ is representative (accurate) of the population mean, then one can assess the extent to which individual determinations realize the mean. The difference between the sample mean and an individual value $(\overline{x} - x)$ represents the deviation from the desired result. Because some absolute values are large numbers and others are small, the amount of deviation is better expressed as a percent of the mean (a deviation of 10 from a mean of 100 is 10% but the same deviation from a mean of 1000 is only 1%).

Because confidence in results increases with reproducability, the average or mean deviation is a better statistic to evaluate variation than is any single difference. The statistic most often used is the **standard deviation** (represented by *s* for samples and by the greek letter σ for populations), which is based on a normal frequency curve (Fig. 29-5). A standard deviation represents an empirically-determined proportional difference of a value from the mean. When a large number of values are included in the sample, 68% of them will occur within one standard deviation below (−) or above (+) the mean, 95% of them will occur within two standard deviations and over 99% of them within three standard deviations. To put it another way, 19 out of 20 replicates of a particular test should fall within the values enclosed in the 2s limits and 1 of 20 (5%) will fall outside these limits by random error. It is important to emphasize that nonrandom errors produce additional deviations from a predetermined mean and that the normal distribution curve describes variation due to random error alone. The absolute values of deviation from the mean $(\overline{x} - x)$ are a combination of such random error and any other sources of variation that operate in the test system.

The calculation of standard deviation proceeds differently with manual or calculator application, but the fundamental formula is:

$$S = \sqrt{\frac{\Sigma(\overline{x} - x)^2}{n - 1}}$$

The deviations of each value from the mean are squared, eliminating positive and negative signs, and the squares are summed. If a *sample* standard deviation, particularly of small sample size n, is calculated, the sum of squares is divided by $n-1$, a correction for the number of values or *degrees of freedom* that have an impact on the distribution statistic. Calculation of the population standard deviation (σ) does not require this correction and the sum of squares is simply divided by n. The resulting statistic is termed the **variance** (s^2 for samples and σ^2 for populations). Taking the square root of the variance yields the standard deviation.

Since the absolute value of a standard deviation is only meaningful when compared with the absolute value of the mean, a ratio can be calculated so that s is expressed as a percent of x.

Coefficient of variation
(CV, in %) = standard deviation/mean $\times$ 100

This statistic provides a rapid method of comparing variability between analytes or methods having widely different mean values. The standard deviations are *relative* to the magnitudes of the means and this statistic is sometimes referred to as the *relative standard deviation (RSD)*.

How well does a sample standard deviation approximate a "true" or population SD? Tables of lower and upper confidence factors can be consulted that provide a means of calculating lower and upper limits for the standard deviation, **confidence limits,** based on the sample size:

Calculated SD $\times$ factor = confidence limit

These factors can be found in any statistics book (see list of Additional Readings for Section VI) and they provide a range of SD values in which the population SD should fall 95% of the time. The magnitude of the lower factor increases toward 1.0 and that of the upper factor decreases toward 1.0 as the sample size (degrees of freedom) increases. Confidence intervals are often cited by manufacturers and reagent suppliers as documentation of performance.

INFERENTIAL STATISTICS

Comparison of one sample with another or a sample with a population involves manipulations of the parameters previously described. Some tests, such as the *Chi-Square* or "goodness-of-fit" test examine how well a sample distribution approximates a theoretical or hypothetical distribution. Other tests, such as Student's t-test, compare two sample distributions to determine if they are significantly different. The statistical analysis assigns a **probability** (p) to the result, indicating the chance of a valid conclusion, based on numerical data alone. That is, statistical verification does not guarantee that two samples are different, the same, accurate or precise. It only guarantees that a probability (e.g., 95%) exists of the attempted comparison being valid.

Correlation is a technique that measures the degree of agreement between results obtained in two different samples. A correlation coefficient can be used to compare different methods of obtaining results (e.g., parallel testing on two lots of reagents) or results obtained by the same method at different times or places (two technologists, different shifts, or two laboratories).

The methods of inferential statistics are

beyond the scope of this book and they are obviously not confined to hematology, but the laboratory worker that is involved in research methodology or evaluation of new techniques and products would do well to obtain a background in statistical applications.

APPLICATION OF DESCRIPTIVE STATISTICS TO PATIENT TESTING

What are the normal values of an analyte for a population? What about a different population (older, younger, pregnant, etc.)? Collection and analysis of a sufficiently large number of blood samples from members of a healthy population (medical and nursing students are frequent "volunteers" for this noble endeavour) will produce data approximating the normal range for the analyte. If all of the data can be included on the basis of physiological normality of the donors, one can define a **reference range** that includes the mean value ± 2 standard deviations or 95% of the values. The remaining 5% of the data, lying outside the 2 SD limits, may well represent normal values, but these "outliers" can also be regarded as the result of random error. Again, a large sample size helps define the mean and the shape of the distribution curve so that the 95% limits can be clearly discerned.

This reference range can be used to identify individuals with test results above or below the 95% limits, but they should be applied only to individuals that are members of the same population from which the reference sample was drawn. Thus, if significant differences in the mean and distribution are identified with respect to a different donor population, a separate reference range (normal values) should be established. These differences are well established for red cell values in women versus men and for white cell counts in children of different ages.

When an individual test result lies outside of the reference range, is it due to random error or does the value reflect an abnormal physiological state? Replication of the test can help reduce the probability of the former (the odds of two sequential, independent determinations lying outside of two SD in the same direction = 0.025 × 0.025 = .000625 or 1 in 1600). Correlation with other test results and knowledge of the medical condition of the patient can also establish the validity of the result as abnormal.

APPLICATION OF DESCRIPTIVE STATISTICS TO QUALITY ASSURANCE

Standard deviations can also establish the performance criteria for an instrument and reagent system. Whether the data is accumulated and plotted manually or by an inbuilt computer, most QC applications analyze a sequential series of standard and control results to detect systematic errors. A chart typically displays the mean value and the 95% limits (± 2 SD) on the y or vertical axis and time or test sequence on the x or horizontal axis (Fig. 29-8). The values for that control or standard material are plotted for each sample run. About 1 in 20 determinations will fall outside of the 2 SD limits. The remaining values should occur about equally on both sides of the mean (Fig. 29-8, *A*). A **shift** in plotted values represents a sudden but consistent bias from the mean (Fig. 29-8, *B*). This can occur if a rapid deterioration in a reagent or the control material occurs of if an instrument component fails. A **trend** is a gradual change in a consistent direction from the mean (Fig. 29-8, *C*). Either change can be defined as a sequence of six or more values that occur on the same side of the mean, even though they may all occur within the 2 SD limits. Consistent deviations of these types can also be followed arithmetically by a **cumulative sum (CUSUM)** calculation. The deviation from the mean value is added sequentially and cumulatively to the previous days total deviation. Over a period of time, random deviation should cancel out and a net

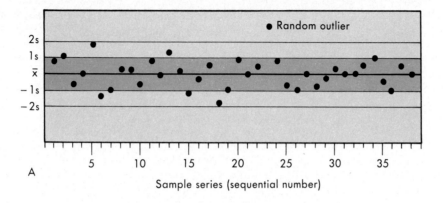

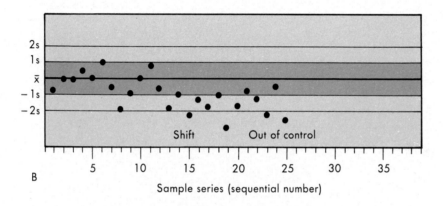

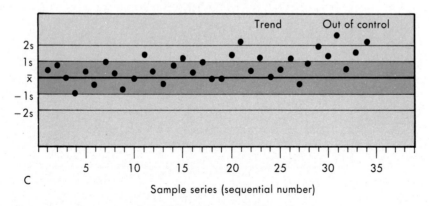

Fig. 29-8.   Graphs of sequential quality control data.
A, Results are in control, equally dispersed about the mean, 95% within 2 SD. **B,** A shift in control sample results is indicated by the sudden deviation from the mean. **C,** A trend of gradual deviation from the mean.

zero deviation should occur. A sequential run of six negative or positive differences indicates that a shift or trend has occurred. Parallel testing with a new control or use of new reagents can reveal error due to these materials. Rechecking instrument response (recalibration) may also be necessary. Manipulation or technique errors that occur consistently when certain laboratory personnel perform the procedure can be ascertained from daily logs.

Another QC technique uses a comparison between two independent control values run in concert (two samples by the same method or one sample by two methods). The mean and 95% limits for each sample form a square, one defining the vertical side and the other the horizontal side (Fig. 29-9). A diagonal line through the common position of the sample means defines a normal distribution for both samples. When the control sample values are plotted as an x,y pair, it is easy to detect errors that affect one control sample differently than the other because the points appear displaced from the diagonal line, even though they may well appear within the 2 SD limits. Shifts or trends away from the mean appear as localized clusters in the upper right or lower left corners. Unless the points are numbered, it is not obvious from the graph in what order the deviations appeared.

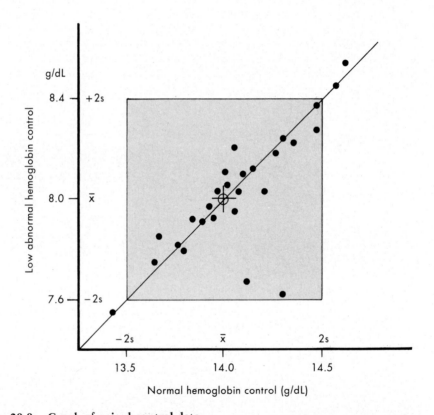

Fig. 29-9. Graph of paired control data.
The mean for each control sample, located in the center of the square, is indicated on an axis. The diagonal line is the theoretical base of normal distribution for the paired controls. Points deviating from the diagonal indicate a nonsystematic error affecting one sample preferentially. Points outside the square but on the diagonal are probably systematic (reagent or instrument).

The goal of quality assurance and statistical analysis is to identify and correct technical problems in the laboratory as they occur. The option of repeating erratic or questionable test results in a timely manner provides an extra measure of reliability and safety in the diagnostic regimen. Because of the complexity of processing a blood sample from collection to final reporting of results, a knowledge of potential errors and analytical control steps is essential. This knowledge is gained by thorough training and a solid theoretical base.

SUMMARY

- Quality assurance or quality control is a system of evaluations to document product reliability. For the clinical laboratory, the product is the analytical process and test results.
- A quality control system includes evaluations of instrument performance, reagent properties, the test procedure, technologist activity, and accuracy of data processing.
- Populations and samples are arbitrary defined in that all samples form subpopulations which can be sampled (subsampled). A continuum exists from the blood tissues of a large group of people to the individual cells comprising a differential count.
- Accuracy is the closeness of a sample value (result) to the population or desired value ("true" value). Precision is the reproducability of replicate determinations. Ideally, both are realized in a laboratory analysis.
- Standardization is a means of defining or establishing the performance criteria of a procedure. Preassayed sample values are correlated with instrument output or procedural results. Calibration establishes instrument performance on the basis of known physical properties, such as electronic frequency or electromagnetic spectrum emissions.
- Controls are samples with known contents that are run with unknown samples to verify procedural performance. The control may be preassayed to validate accuracy and precision or unassayed to validate precision only.
- Populations and samples can be described by mathematical attributes: parameters and statistics, respectively. Descriptive statistics of samples include measures of dispersion (range, maximum, and minimum), central tendency (mean, median, and mode), distribution (random, normal or Gaussian, bimodal, and skewed), and variation (variance, standard deviation, confidence limits, and coefficient of variation).
- Descriptive statistics can be used in inferential methods to compare sample means, distributions, correlate results, and test hypotheses. Results of inferential analyses are reported as probabilities of accepting or rejecting test hypotheses.
- Results of patient testing can be compared with reference values defined by means and standard deviations from tests of control populations. Two SDs define 95% limits of inclusion.
- Quality assurance also uses 95% limits about a mean to plot sequential data for control sample values. Deviations that represent systematic errors include trends and shifts of six or more values in a consistent direction from the mean value.

SUGGESTED READINGS—SECTION VI

Bauer JD: Clinical laboratory methods, ed 9, St. Louis, 1982, The CV Mosby Co.

Berner JJ: Effects of diseases on laboratory tests, Philadelphia, 1983, JB Lippincott Co.

Bessis M: Blood smears reinterpreted, Berlin, 1977, Springer International.

Bessman JD, Gilmer PR, and Gardner FH: Improved classification of anemia by MCV and RDW, Am J Clin Pathol 80:332, 1983.

Brown BA: Hematology: principles and procedures, ed 5, Philadelphia, 1988, Lea & Febiger.

Caalm RR: Reviewing the importance of specimen collection, J Am Med Technol 39: 297, 1977.

Caalm RR and Cooper MA: Recommended "order of draw" for collecting blood specimens into additive, Clin Chem 28:1399, 1982.

Cornbleet J: Automation in hematology-an overview, Lab Med 14:482, 1983.

Dacie JV and Lewis SM: Practical hematology, ed 6, New York, 1984, Churchill Livingstone, Inc.

Diggs LW, Sturm P, and Bell A: The morphology of human blood cells, ed 5, Chicago, 1985, Abbott Laboratories.

Dutcher TF: Automated leukocyte differentials: a review and prospectus, Lab Med 14:483, 1983.

England JM: Future needs and expected trends in peripheral blood cell analysis: erythrocyte histograms, Blood Cells 11:61, 1985.

Evans VJ: Platelet morphology and the blood smear, J Med Technol 1:689, 1984.

Fairbanks VF: Hemoglobinopathies and thalassemias: laboratory methods and clinical cases, New York, 1980, Thieme-Stratton.

Finley PR and Fletcher C: Laboratory tests in immune thrombocytopenia, J Med Technol 1:709, 1984.

Forman DT and Parker S: The measurement and interpretation of serum ferritin, Ann Clin Lab Sci 10:345, 1982.

Friedman EW: Reticulocyte counts: how to use them, what they mean, Diagn Med 7:29, 1984.

Harmening DH (editor): Modern blood banking principles and transfusion practices, ed 2, Philadelphia, 1989, FA Davis Co.

Hudson P, Shafer D, Belvedere D et al.: Troubleshooting coagulation screening test results, Miami, 1985, American Dade Education.

Kass L: Bone marrow interpretation, ed 2, Philadelphia, 1985, JB Lippincott Co.

Kupke, DR, Kather B, and Zeugner S: On the composition of capillary and venous blood serum, Clin Chem Acta 112:179, 1981.

Lenahan JG and Smith K: Hemostasis, ed 17, Morris Plains, NJ, 1985, General Diagnostics.

Lindenbaum J: Status of laboratory testing in the diagnosis of megaloblastic anemia, Blood 61:624, 1983.

Mielke CH Jr: Aspirin prolongation of the template bleeding time: influences of venostasis and direction of incision, Blood 60:1139, 1982.

Mielke CH Jr: Measurement of the bleeding time, Thromb Haemost 52:210, 1984.

O'Connor BH: A color atlas and instruction manual of peripheral blood cell morphology, Baltimore, 1984, William & Wilkins.

Pittiglio DH (editor): Clinical hematology and fundamentals of hemostasis, Philadelphia, 1987, FA Davis Co.

Poulsen KD: Controlling preanalytical variables in coagulation testing, J Med Technol 3:561, 1986.

Rosvoll RV, Mengason AP, Smith I et al.: Visual and automated differential leukocyte counts, Am J Clin Pathol 71:695, 1979.

Saunders AM: Sources of physiological variation in differential leukocyte counting, Blood Cells 11:31, 1985.

Sirredge MS and Shannon R: Laboratory evaluation of hemostasis and thrombosis, ed 3, Philadelphia, 1983, Lea & Febiger.

Stockbower JM and Blumenfeld TA: Collection and handling of laboratory specimens, Philadelphia, 1983, JB Lippincott Co.

Snyder EL and Falast GA: Significance of the direct antiglobulin test, Lab Med 16: 89, 1985.

Tietz NW (editor): Textbook of clinical chemistry, Philadelphia, 1986, WB Saunders Co.

Turgeon ML: Clinical hematology theory and procedures, Boston, 1988, Little, Brown & Co, Inc.

Triplett DA and Harms CS: Procedures for the coagulation laboratory, Chicago, 1981, American Society of Clinical Pathologists.

van Assendelft OW: Reference values for the total and differential leukocyte count, Blood Cells 11:77, 1985.

Waller KV and Bruzzese DB: Flow cytometry in the clinical laboratory, Lab Med 16:480, 1985.

Weisbrot IM: Statistics for the clinical laboratory, Philadelphia, 1985, JB Lippincott Co.

Weisbrot IM and Hollenberg CM: Platelet counting methods, Lab Med 11:307, 1980.

Glossary

absolute count Concentration of a cell type, expressed as number per volume of whole blood (e.g., $250 \times 10^3/\mu L$ or $250 \times 10^9/L$).

absorbance Optical density of a solution, a measure of the concentration of a color producing solute.

acanthocyte A spherical cell with uneven, spiny projections, seen in patients with some types of liver disease.

accuracy A comparison between a sample result and the target or population "true" value.

achlorhydria A lack of free hydrochloric acid in the stomach; adversely affects the transport and absorption of iron and vitamin B_{12} in the gastrointestinal tract.

acidophilic Attracted to or stained with the acid component of biological dyes (e.g., the eosin component of Wright's stain).

acid phosphatase An enzyme of platelets, leukocytes, and other tissues; activity within the cell can be used to identify lymphocytes and a particular isoenzyme (5) that is not inhibited by tartaric acid is characteristically found in the lymphocytes of hairy cell leukemia.

acquired A condition or disorder incurred from environmental factors or agents; not inherited.

acquired immunodeficiency syndrome (AIDS) A progressive, fatal collapse of the immune system caused by infection of T lymphocytes with a retrovirus, the human immunodeficiency virus (HIV).

activated partial thromboplastin test (APTT) A screening test using citrated plasma to evaluate the intrinsic and common pathway coagulation factors.

acute intermittent porphyria (AIP) An inherited deficiency of uroporphyrinogen I synthase of the heme synthesis pathway, producing accumulations of porphobilinogen in discrete attacks accompanied by neurological manifestations.

acute leukemia One of several forms of leukemia manifested by the presence of excess immature cells in the bone marrow and a rapid, often fatal, course. Peripheral blood cell concentrations may be increased, normal, or decreased, but blasts and other immature stages are predominate.

adenopathy A swelling or disease affecting glandular tissue.

ADP Adenosine diphosphate.

aggregation Clumping of cells or other particles (e.g., platelet aggregation in the formation of a hemostatic plug).

AHF Antihemophilic factor (factor VIII).

AIDS Acquired immunodeficiency syndrome.

AIHA Autoimmune hemolytic anemia.

Alder-Reilly anomaly The presence of large azurophilic inclusions in leukocytes, observed in association with certain hereditary disorders, such as the mucopolysaccharidoses.

alkaline phosphatase An enzyme present in many tissues, including granulocytes. Relative activity is used to distinguish chronic myeloid leukemia (low activity) from benign leukemoid reactions (high activity).

ALL Acute lymphocytic (lymphoblastic) leukemia.

allele An alternate form of a gene that encodes a phenotypic trait (e.g., *A*, *B*, and *O* are alleles of the ABO blood group gene). When the paired alleles of the homologous chromosomes are identical, the individual is homozygous (e.g., *AA*); when they differ, the individual is heterozygous (e.g., *AO*).

alpha chain A globin composing several forms of hemoglobin, specified by a gene on chromosome 16.

alpha granule A thin-walled organelle of platelets that contains any of several proteins (see Table 12-2).

alpha-2-macroglobulin A circulating glycoprotein that inhibits thrombin activity and therefore functions as a natural anticoagulant.

alpha thalassemia An inherited deficiency affecting the rate of alpha chain globin production.

AML Acute myelogenous leukemia.

AMP Adenosine monophosphate.

amplification Expansion of biological or chemical processes by recruitment or replication (e.g., induction of enzymatic activity by substrate changes and growth of tissues by the proliferation of specific cell precursors).

anemia Decreased delivery of oxygen to tissues (hypoxia) because of decreased red cell mass, decreased hemoglobin concentration, or the presence of an abnormal hemoglobin.

anisocytosis Red blood cells of increased variability (heterogeneous size) as seen on peripheral blood smears or as measured by mean cell volume (MCV) and calculated by distribution values (RDW).

ankyrin One of the cytoskeletal proteins underlying the lipid bilayer of red blood cells; serves as an attachment point for spectrin and the anion transport channel (band 3).

anomaly A condition or occurrence that is unusual or abnormal.

antibody A specific immunoglobulin produced by plasma cells in response to an antigen. Antibodies are capable of reacting with and neutralizing antigens, the so-called "humoral defense system."

anticoagulant A substance that prevents blood clotting. Most bind with or chelate calcium, others enhance the effects of natural, circulating anticoagulants (e.g., heparin potentiates antithrombin-III).

antigen A protein or other complex molecule of sufficiently high molecular weight that stimulates a specific immune response (antibody production) in a host.

antiglobulin test Use of an antisera against human immunoglobulin to detect antibodies in plasma/serum (indirect antiglobulin test, IAT) or antibodies coating red blood cells (direct antiglobulin test, DAT).

antithrombin III (AT-3) An alpha-2 globulin produced by the liver that circulates in the plasma and functions as a natural inhibitor of the coagulation cascade.

APC Antigen presenting cell, a macrophage.

aplastic An absence of growth or cellular proliferation (e.g., aplastic anemia: an absence of red cell production).

apoferritin A protein that combines with ferrous iron to form ferritin; regulates iron stores in the mucosal cells of the intestine.

apotransferrin A beta globulin that binds ferric iron and bicarbonate to form the plasma iron transport complex, transferrin.

APTT Activated partial thromboplastin time.

arachidonic acid A platelet metabolite that is mobilized from phospholipids during hemostatic activation; an intermediate in the formation of thromboxane and various prostaglandins. Also used as an aggregating reagent to test platelet function.

asynchrony Sequential, interacting events that are out of phase with each other (e.g., asynchrony of nuclear and cytoplasmic maturation in folate deficiencies).

ATP Adenosine triphosphate.

atypical lymphocyte An older term for reactive lymphocytes, cells responding immunologically to the presence of antigens, particularly viruses. Also generally refers to any lymphocyte that is larger or more basophilic than the small mature forms.

Auer rod Elongated, azurophilic rods composed of fused lysosomal granules, seen in the cytoplasm of myeloblasts, promyelocytes and monoblasts of patients with acute myelogenous leukemia.

AUL Acute undifferentiated leukemia. M1 of the FAB classification of acute leukemias.

autohemolysis Destruction of a person's red blood cells by his or her own serum, an indication of an autoimmune disorder.

autoimmune An immunological response to an individuals own tissues or antigens. Autoantibodies may be normal, benign and transient, or associated with pathological disorders.

autosome Any of the 22 pairs of chromosomes that are not sex-specific. Traits specified by autosomal genes can be inherited equally by males and females.

azurophilic Having an affinity for azure, the light-purplish blue component of dyes like methylene blue. Actually a misnomer, since the term is applied to granules that stain red to reddish-purple, such as the large granules of some lymphocytes and the primary granules of promyelocytes.

B cells B lymphocytes.

B lymphocytes Lymphoid cells that specialize in the humoral immune response; the precursors of plasma cells that produce antigen-specific immunoglobulins.

band 3 The electrophoretic designation for a major protein of the red cell membrane.

band 4.1 The electrophoretic designation for a major protein of the red cell membrane.

band cells (bands) The granulocyte stage in which the nucleus forms a "U" or curled rod prior to segmentation. Band neutrophils compromise about 1 to 3% of the peripheral leukocytes.

Barr body A small condensed mass of nuclear chromatin that represents the inactivated X-chromosome of females. Present in all somatic cells, but most readily demonstrated in segmented neutrophils, where it forms a drumstick-shaped projection into the cytoplasm in about 1 to 4% of the cells examined.

basophil A granulocyte that contains purple-blue organelles that contain heparin and vasoactive compounds. Basophils are mediators of anaphylactic hypersensitivity reactions (e.g., allergic reactions to wasp stings).

basophilia An absolute increase in the concentration of basophils in the peripheral blood, most often seen in chronic myelogenous leukemia.

basophilic Having an affinity for the basic component of chemical substances, such as biological dyes; attracting the purple-blue components of Wright's stain.

basophilic normoblast (prorubricyte) The second stage of erythrocyte maturation that is recognized by light microscopy on smears of marrow material. The first stage in which hemoglobin production occurs, as observed by electron microscopy.

basophilic stippling Round, dark-blue granules that appear in red blood cells on Wright-stained smears, associated with disturbances of heme synthesis (e.g., lead poisoning), many anemias, exposure to some drugs, severe burns, or septicemia. The granules represent precipitated ribosomes and mitochondria.

Bence-Jones protein A mixture of abnormal globulins (paraproteins) excreted in the urine, composed of lambda, kappa, or both, light chains. B-J protein precipitates when heated to about 56° C and redissolves at 100° C. This in-

complete immunoglobulin is most often seen in patients with multiple myeloma or other plasma cell disorders (e.g., heavy chain disease, macroglobulinemia).

benign A term used to describe disorders, conditions, or growths that progress slowly and that are not intrinsically life threatening. Contrasted with malignant conditions or growths, that are rapid, invasive, and often fatal. Benign tumors are usually solitary and do not reoccur if removed.

Bernard-Soulier syndrome (BSS) A rare hereditary bleeding disorder characterized by decreased platelet concentration and platelets of abnormally large size.

beta chain A globin chain of normal adult hemoglobin (Hb A).

beta thalassemia A hereditary disorder of hemoglobin synthesis due to reduced production of beta globin chains. Beta thalassemia minor results from the inheritance of one abnormal gene (heterozygote); beta thalassemia major results from the inheritance of two abnormal genes (homozygote)

bilirubin A product of heme degradation that is transported through the blood as a pigmented plasma protein and excreted in the urine and feces. Indirect bilirubin is a non-conjugated water-insoluble form; direct bilirubin is a water-soluble form that has been conjugated with glucuronide by the liver.

blast The first stage of a blood cell lineage that is morphologically identifiable with light microscopy and routine staining procedures.

blast crisis The terminal phase of leukemia that previously had been chronic or in remission, characterized by large numbers of blast cells in the marrow and peripheral blood.

blast transformation The process of maturation reversal in which a lymphocyte responds to the presence of a stimulating antigen by proliferating.

bleeding time (BT) An in vivo test of hemostatic function performed by timing the cessation of bleeding from capillary punctures. Most often used as a measure of platelet function.

Bohr effect The change in molecular configueration and oxygen affinity of hemoglobin that results in different ionic environments (e.g., higher pH of arterial blood results in increased oxygen binding). See oxygen dissociation curve.

bradykinin A plasma protein involved in the inflammatory response by increasing vascular permeability; a product produced from high molecular weight kininogen (HMWK) by the action of kallikrein during activation of the intrinsic coagulation pathway.

brilliant cresyl blue A so-called supravital dye used to precipitate and stain the ribosomal material of reticulocytes.

BSS Bernard-Soulier syndrome.

BT Bleeding time.

buffy coat The cloudy cream-colored layer that results from sedimentation or centrifugation of whole blood, containing leukocytes and platelets. Buffy coat preparations are used to prepare smears of concentrated white blood cells, especially when attempting to locate or identify cells of infrequent occurrence.

burr cell A common name for echinocytes.

burst forming unit (BFU) A primitive but committed erythropoietic stem cell, possibly the precursor of colony forming units (CFU-E) that precede pronormoblasts (rubriblasts).

Cabot ring A thin, large azurophilic loop or double loop (figure eight) found inside Wright-stained red blood cells. These inclusions are rare but they are most often associated with severe anemias or with myeloproliferative disorders, often in association with iron granules, basophilic stippling, and other signs of disturbed hemoglobin synthesis.

cAMP Cyclic adenosine monophosphate.

canalicular system Microtubules that connect the interior of the platelet with the outer surface, constituting part of the calcium regulating mechanism and serving as the conduit for release of ADP and other platelet products.

carcinoma A malignancy of epithelial tissue.

carrier An individual possessing a single abnormal gene (heterozygote state) for a recessive disorder or trait that may not be phenotypically expressed (e.g., females that "carry" genes for hemophilia, passing them on to some of their male offspring).

cathepsin A proteinase found in most cells, involved in autolysis of cells and tissues.

CBC Complete blood count.

cell-mediated immunity (CMI) The immunological response that involves the interaction of T lymphocytes and macrophages; the cellular mechanism type IV hypersensitivity.

cellularity The ratio of cellular to non-cellular elements in a tissue, usually expressed as percent cellularity.

ceruloplasmin A copper-containing glycoprotein that catalyzes the oxidation of ferrous iron, stored in mucosal cells, to ferric iron for transport in the plasma by transferrin.

CFU Colony forming unit.

Chédiak-Higashi syndrome A rare inherited disorder characterized by the appearance of large lysosomal granules and vacuoles in the cytoplasm of phagocytic leukocytes and other cells. Chemotaxis and microbial killing is impaired and the patient suffers from recurrent, eventually fatal, pyogenic infections.

chemotaxis The movement of an organism or cell, such as a phagocyte, toward or away from a source of chemical stimulation. A part of the inflammatory response, involving the reception and response of neutrophils and monocyte-macrophages to molecules from microorganisms and products of injured host tissue.

chromatin The stainable material of the cell nucleus, consisting of basic histones (basichromatin), condensed nucleoprotein (including DNA), and fine strands of parachromatin. Condensation increases with cell maturity, producing a darker color with Wright's and Giemsa stains.

chronic Describing a condition of long duration and gradual onset.

chronic granulomatous disease (CGD) A hereditary disorder, most often sex-linked, in which the enzymatic generation of lethal oxidants by neutrophils is defective, resulting in recurrent infections.

chronic leukemia Blood cell malignancies characterized by the appearance of increased concentrations of mature or moderately immature cells in the peripheral blood, often in greater numbers than in acute leukemic forms.

CLL Chronic lymphocytic leukemia.

clone A colony of genetically identical cells produced by replication from a single source cell or precursor. Clonal expansion describes the proliferation of a particular cell to form a dispersed or localized tissue, often at the expense of neighboring cells (e.g., leukemia, other malignancies).

CML Chronic myelogenous leukemia.

coagulopathy A disorder of the coagulation cascade, most often a quantitative or qualitative deficiency in one of the coagulation factors.

collagen A common protein of bone, cartilage, skin, and connective tissue. Collagen lines the blood vessels and its exposure during trauma activates platelets. An aggregating reagent for platelet function testing.

colony forming units (CFU) Hematopoietic stem cells that can be stimulated by growth promoting substances to proliferate and differentiate into colonies of a specific cell type (e.g., CFU-E, stem cells that will form colonies of erythroid precursors).

common pathway The final stages of coagulation, from the point of convergence of the extrinsic and intrinsic pathways (activation of factor X), to the formation of fibrin.

complement Circulating plasma proteins that are activated by the presence of foreign cells, such as microbes. Complement components (e.g., C3b, C5a) stimulate other processes of immunological defense, such as chemotactic responses, phagocytosis, and vasoconstriction. Antibodies to red cell antigens may activate complement and produce hemolysis.

congenital Existing from the time of birth, either as a genetic condition or one that is acquired during prenatal development.

contact coagulation factors Components of the early stages of intrinsic pathway activation: factors XI, XII, high molecular weight kininogen, and prekallikrein.

Coomb's test An older term for antiglobulin test, a means of detecting antibodies in plasma or on red blood cells. See antiglobulin test.

coproporphrinogen III An intermediate product in the synthetic pathway of heme.

Coulter principle A means of counting particles and measuring their size (volume) by the impedence change caused by the particle in a current conducting fluid (electrolyte). The operating basis of many blood cell counters, including Coulter Counter™, a specific commercial line of instruments founded by the developer of the impedence principle of particle counting.

coumarin One of several drugs used as an oral anticoagulant to provide long term therapy following heart attacks. Coumarin blocks the vitamin K-dependent synthesis of coagulation factors II, VII, IX and X. Dosage is monitored with periodic assays of the prothrombin time.

crenation Transformation of an erythrocyte from a biconcave disc to an echinocyte. Common in hyperosmotic solutions or during desiccation. See echinocyte.

CSF Colony stimulating factor; cerebral spinal fluid.

CV Coefficient of variation, a statistical parameter of population heterogeneity.

cyanmethemoglobin Oxidized hemoglobin combined with cyanide provided by Drabkin's solution during the measurement of whole blood hemoglobin concentration.

cyanocobalamin Vitamin B12, the extrinsic factor needed for nucleotidyl metabolism in maturing blood cells. Deficiencies result in megaloblastic anemia, a nuclear maturation defect.

cytoskeleton The microtubules and structural proteins that form the internal support network of the cell membrane.

cytotoxic T lymphocytes (T_c) Lymphocytes that can destroy immunological targets (e.g., tumor cells, cells infected with viruses) directly.

cyclooxygenase An enzyme in platelets that mediates the conversion of arachidonic acid to prostaglandins. Aspirin blocks cyclooxygenase activity, reducing or eliminating aggregation capability.

dacrocyte Tear-drop shaped red blood cell seen in myelofibrosis and other myeloproliferative disorders.

DAT Direct antiglobulin test.

degranulation Expulsion of granular contents from organelles by a cell or platelet, usually in response to a specific stimulus (e.g., release of hydrolases from eosinophilic lysosomes or heparin and vasoactive amines from basophils).

delayed hypersensitivity A synoym for type IV hypersensitivity or cell-mediated immunity, delayed in comparison to humoral reactions.

delta-aminolevulinic acid synthase The rate-limiting enzyme in the early stages of heme synthesis.

delta chain Globins that combine with alpha chains to form tetramers of hemoglobin A_2.

demarcation membrane The microtubular borders that delineate marginal zones of the megakaryocyte cytoplasm to become platelets.

dense bodies Platelet granules that contain ADP, serotonin, calcium, and other products; seen as thick-walled organelles by electron microscopy.

deoxyhemoglobin Hemoglobin that does not contain or carry oxygen.

Diamond-Blackfan syndrome A congenital red cell aplasia.

diapedesis Ameboid movement of blood cells across the vascular endothelium.

DIC Disseminated intravascular coagulation.

Di Guglielmo's syndrome See erythroleukemia.

2,3-diphosphoglycerate (2,3-DPG) A metabolite of glycolysis, 2,3-DPG combines with the beta chains of hemoglobin to decrease oxygen affinity, thus promoting oxygen delivery to the tissues.

discocyte The normal, biconcave disc-shaped erythrocyte.

disseminated intravascular coagulation (DIC) A state of hyperreactive hemostasis in which platelets and coagulation factors are consumed, leading to thrombosis and bleeding because of the presence of agents or substances that promote clotting (e.g., release of tissue thromboplastin from placental tissue during obstetric trauma; the action of some snake venoms).

DNA Deoxyribonucleic acid.

Döhle bodies Large basophilic (blue-gray) inclusions seen in the cytoplasm of neutrophils, associated with septicemia, chemical toxicity, and severe burns.

Donath-Landsteiner antibody An IgG antibody with biphasic temperature activity that is found in the plasma of patients with paroxysmal cold hemoglobinuria.

Downey cell An old term for one of several variants of reactive lymphocyte.

DPG Diphosphoglycerate.

drepanocyte Sickle cell, red blood cells with long thin forms that are sharply pointed at one or both ends, characteristic of sickle cell anemia.

dyserythropoiesis A condition of ineffective red blood cell production, characterized by morphological abnormalities of normoblasts, disturbed mitosis, and a peripheral anemia.

dysplasia Abnormal cell proliferation or tissue growth.

EBV Epstein-Barr virus.

ecchymosis A bruise or area of subdermal hemorrhage, often symptomatic of coagulopathies.

echinocytes Red blood cells with many blunt projections, resulting from exposure to hyperosmotic solutions or artificial surfaces, such as glass. Pathological forms are associated with uremia. Echinocytes contain adequate hemoglobin and the spiny knobs are regularly dispersed over the cell surface, unlike those of acanthocytes.

EDTA Ethylenediamine tetraacetate, an anticoagulant that binds calcium.

elliptocyte An elongated or oval erythrocyte (synonym: ovalocyte), resulting from a hereditary or acquired deficiency of an RBC membrane component.

Embden-Meyerhof pathway (EMP) Glycolysis, the anaerobic metabolism of glucose to lactic acid.

endoreduplication Nuclear lobe mitosis (endomitosis) in the early stages of megakaryocyte maturation, resulting in a polyploid cell (4N to 128N or more).

eosin The acidic component of Wright's stain, the orange component after which eosinophils are named.

eosinophil A mature granulocytic cell that responds to parasitic infections and allergic conditions; comprises about 1 to 4% of the peripheral leukocyte count. Granules stain a bright reddish-orange with Wright's or Giemsa stains.

epistaxis Nosebleed.

epsilon chain Globin found in embryonic hemoglobin produced by erythrocytes from the yolk sac.

Epstein-Barr virus (EBV) The causative agent of infectious mononucleosis and Burkitt's lymphoma.

erythroblastosis fetalis An old term for hemolytic disease of the newborn, based on the presence of numerous nucleated red blood cells in the neonate's peripheral blood.

erythrocyte sedimentation rate (ESR) A measure of the settling rate of red cells in plasma, reported in mm/hour. Used mainly to monitor inflammation and other changes in plasma proteins, ESR is also affected by red cell concentration, shape and size.

erythrocytosis Increased erythrocyte concentration in the peripheral blood.

erythroleukemia A form of acute myeloid leukemia (FAB type M6) characterized by immature erythroid and granulocytic elements (synonym: Di Guglielmos syndrome).

erythron The total erythroid mass, including normoblastic precursors of the marrow, circulating red blood cells, and cells present in the spleen and other tissues.

erythropoiesis The production of red blood cells.

erythropoietin A hormone produced mainly by the kidneys that responds to tissue hypoxia and regulates red cell production, rate of RBC maturation, and release of reticulocytes from the marrow.

ESR Erythrocyte sedimentation rate.

essential thrombocythemia An idiopathic increase in the production and concentration of platelets, a form of myeloproliferative disorder.

euglobulin A plasma protein fraction consisting of fibrinogen, plasminogen, and plasminogen activators.

extramedullary hematopoiesis Blood cell production occurring during the postnatal period outside of the medullary cavity of the bone marrow. Usually occurs in the liver and spleen as a result of severe anemia or as compensation for marrow disruption by fibrous tissue or tumor cells.

extravascular hemolysis Destruction of red blood cells outside of the blood vessels, usually by macrophages lining the sinuses of the spleen.

extrinsic coagulation pathway The clotting mechanism activated by tissue thromboplastin; factor VII and calcium are components.

FAB classification The French-American-British system for classifying acute leukemias and myelodysplastic syndromes, based on morphological and cytochemical findings.

Fanconi's anemia A hereditary hypoplasia and pancytopenia associated with numerous other abnormalities.

favism A hereditary sensitivity to the oxidizing effects of fava beans seen in persons, usually of Mediterranean origin, with a form of G6PD deficiency. Hemoglobin oxidation results in a severe hemolytic anemia.

FDP or fdp Fibrinogen (fibrin) degradation products.

FEP Free erythrocyte protoporphrin.

ferritin The major storage form of iron in tissues and in the developing normoblast.

ferrokinetics The metabolism and turnover dynamics of iron, including ingestion, absorption, transport, storage, utilization, and elimination.

fibrin The end product of coagulation, derived from the plasma protein, fibrinogen, by the action of thrombin. Fibrin forms a mesh to entrap blood cells, forming the visible clot.

fibrin(ogen) degradation products (FDP) Protein fragments enzymatically split from fibrinogen to form fibrin. Increased FDPs are seen in hypercoagulable states, such as disseminated intravascular coagulation.

fibrinogen A major plasma protein that is the substrate for thrombin action to form fibrin; coagulation factor I.

fibrinolysis Destruction of the fibrin clot by the action of plasmin.

fibrin stabilizing factor Coagulation factor XIII, stabilizes the fibrin polymer.

fibronectin A plasma protein that binds to damaged endothelial cells and exposed fibroblasts, involved in the adhesion of blood cells to surfaces.

fibrosis Increased proliferation of fibrous connective tissue. See myelofibrosis.

Fitzgerald factor High molecular weight kininogen (HWMK), one of the contact factors of the intrinsic coagulation pathway.

Fletcher factor Prekallikrein, one of the contact factors of the intrinsic coagulation pathway.

folate, folic acid A vitamin of the B complex provided by liver and green leafy vegetables, essential for nucleotidyl synthesis in blood cells; deficiencies result in megaloblastic anemia.

free erythrocyte protoporphyrin (FEP) The amount of protoporphrin remaining in the erythrocyte after heme synthesis ceases. A measure of effective hemoglobin production, FEP is complexed to zinc and is detectable by its fluorescence in ultraviolet light.

GALT Gut-associated lymphoid tissue.

gamma chain A globin that pairs with alpha chains to form tetramers of hemoglobin F.

gammopathy A disorder of immunoglobulin production in which a single clone of antibody producing cells proliferates, resulting in the appearance of a sharply defined protein spike in the plasma and urine (e.g., multiple myeloma).

Gaucher cell A large lipid-filled histiocyte seen in the bone marrow and spleen of patient's with Gaucher's disease.

Gaucher's disease A hereditary deficiency of the enzyme, beta-glucosidase, resulting in the accumulation of glucocerebrosides in histiocytes and macrophages; the disease is characterized by impaired development and early death of infants.

Glanzmann's thrombasthenia A hereditary hemostatic disorder in which platelets fail to respond to aggregating agents; clot retraction is also abnormal.

glucose-6-phosphate dehydrogenase (G6PD) The key enzyme of the hexose monophosphate shunt. Deficiencies result in the oxidation and precipitation of hemoglobin, producing a hemolytic anemia.

glycophorin One of several proteins of the red cell membrane, source of most of the negative surface charge that results in mutual repulsion of erythrocytes.

granulocyte A white blood cell that contains prominent cytoplasmic granules: neutrophils, eosinophils, basophils, and mast cells.

Hageman factor Coagulation factor XII, one of the contact factors of the intrinsic pathway.

hairy cell leukemia (HCL) A chronic form of lymphocytic leukemia characterized by mononuclear cells with filamentous pseudopods (synonym: leukemic reticuloendotheliosis).

haptoglobin A plasma protein, synthesized in the liver, that binds the alpha-beta dimers of hemoglobin. Depletion of haptoglobin is an indication of intravascular hemolysis.

Hb Hemoglobin.

HCL Hairy cell leukemia.

hct (HCT) Hematocrit.

heinz body Spherical inclusions of precipitated hemoglobin visualized with supravital stains near the outer periphery of the erythrocyte. Heinz body anemias result from a deficiency of enzymes that maintain reduced hemoglobin (e.g., G6PD, glutathione reductase, methemoglobin reductase).

hematocrit (HCT) The ratio of red cell volume to whole blood volume, expressed as percent.

heme The tetrapyrrole compound (protoporphrin) with a central atom of iron that comprises the oxygen-binding portion of hemoglobin. Synthesized in the mitochrondria and cytoplasm of developing erythroblasts.

heme-heme interaction The increase in oxygen affinity of the hemoglobin tetramer due to conformational changes associated with oxygen binding at each of the four heme groups.

Binding of the first molecule facilitates the uptake of additional oxygen molecules.

heme synthase The enzyme catalyzing the addition of iron to protoporphrin (synonym: ferrochelatase).

hemochromatosis A disorder of iron absorption or metabolism that results in the accumulation of excess iron in tissues, disrupting cardiac and hepatic function.

hemoglobin The intraerythrocytic, iron-containing protein that transports oxygen. Functions as a tetramer of four globin chains, each containing a heme moiety.

Hb A Adult hemoglobin, 94% to 98% of normal hemoglobin, consists of two alpha and two beta globin chains.

Hb A_2 A minor component (1% to 2%) of adult hemoglobin, consists of two alpha and two delta chains.

Hb Bart's An abnormal hemoglobin seen in neonatal alpha thalassemia (hydrops fetalis), consists of four gamma chains.

Hb F Fetal hemoglobin, major component during intrauterine development, up to 2% of adult total, consists of two alpha chains and two gamma chains.

Hb Gower Embryonic hemoglobin, produced in RBCs of the yolk sac, consists of two zeta and two epsilon chains (Gower 1) or two alpha and two epsilon chains (Gower 2).

Hb H An abnormal hemoglobin seen in severe alpha thalassemia, consists of four beta chains.

Hb Lepore An abnormal hemoglobin seen in thalassemia resulting from a mismatched crossover between the delta and beta gene regions of chromosome 11. Consists of two alpha and two beta-delta (fused) chains.

Hb Portland An embryonic hemoglobin, consists of two zeta and two gamma chains.

hemoglobinemia The presence of hemoglobin in plasma, a result of intravascular hemolysis.

hemoglobinopathy A hereditary disorder of hemoglobin structure caused by an amino acid substitution in a globin chain. Some result in severe anemias (e.g., sickle cell disease) while others are clinically benign.

hemolytic anemia Reduced peripheral red cell concentration due to increased destruction by one of several intravascular or extravascular mechanisms.

hemolytic disease of the newborn (HDN) Hemolytic anemia of fetal or neonatal red blood cells due to maternal antibodies resulting from previous isoimmune stimulation. Synonym: erythroblastosis fetalis.

hemolytic-uremic syndrome (HUS) A severe hemolytic anemia accompanied by renal failure, usually seen in young children who develop acute glomerulonephritis following gastroenteritis.

hemophilia One of several hereditary deficiencies of plasma coagulation proteins, resulting in a mild to severe bleeding disorder.

hemophilia A Classic bleeder's disease, a sex-linked deficiency of the coagulant component of factor VIII.

hemophilia B Christmas disease, a sex-linked deficiency of factor IX.

hemophilia C Parahemophilia, a deficiency of factor XI.

hemosiderin A storage form of iron, fine granules seen in the tissues only by electron microscopy.

HEMPAS *H*ereditary *e*rythroblastic *m*ultinuclearity (associated with a) *p*ositive *a*cidified *s*erum (test). Type II congenital dyserythropoietic anemia.

heparin An anticoagulant that combines with and enhances antithrombin III to prevent blood clotting. Used therapeutically to treat patients with thrombotic complications or to prevent thrombosis in patients with myocardial disease. Heparin sulfate is a natural coating of the endothelial cells of the capillaries.

hereditary spherocytosis (HS) A genetic deficiency of spectrin, the cytoskeletal protein of the red cell membrane, resulting in shortened survival and hemolytic anemia. Characterized by peripheral spherocytes and an increased osmotic fragility.

heterozygous Two dissimilar genes (alleles) at corresponding loci on homologous or paired chromosomes (e.g., the *A* and *B* genes, *AB* genotype).

histamine A vasoactive amine released by blood basophils and tissue mast cells when stimulated by IgE antibodies.

histiocyte Tissue macrophages that are immobile, serving a supportive or nutrional function.

HIV Human immunodeficiency virus.

HMS Hexose monophosphate shunt.

HMWK High molecular weight kininogen (Fitzgerald factor).

Hodgkin's disease A common type of malignant lymphoma, characterized by Reed-Sternberg cells in the marrow and spleen.

homozygous Two identical genes (alleles) at corresponding loci on homologous or paired chromosomes (e.g., inheritance of two *O* genes, *OO* genotype).

Howell-Jolly body Round blue-black inclusions of red blood cells seen on Wright-stained smears. H-J bodies are nuclear fragments (condensed DNA), normally removed by the spleen, but appearing in severe hemolytic anemias, in patients with dysfunctional spleens or after splenectomy.

HS Hereditary spherocytosis.

HUS Hemolytic-uremic syndrome.

hydrops fetalis An edematous state associated with severe alpha thalassemia in neonates.

hyperplasia Increased cell proliferation, usually a normal response to a physiological stimulus (e.g., erythroid hyperplasia in response to hypoxia).

hypersegmentation Increased lobulation of a granulocyte nucleus, seen in disorders of nuclear maturation, such as the megaloblastic anemias.

hypochromia Decreased hemoglobin content of red blood cells (low MCH, decreased pigment on smears).

hypoplasia Decreased cell proliferation, often due to toxic damage of stem cells or because of a lack of an essential nutrient.

hypoxia Decreased partial pressure of oxygen in tissues.

IAT Indirect antiglobulin test.

IDA Iron deficiency anemia.

idiopathic Unknown origin, cause not determined.

IF Intrinsic factor.

Ig Immunoglobulin (e.g., IgA, IgG).

IM Infectious mononucleosis; intramuscular.

immunoblast A proliferating B or T lymphocyte in response to an antigenic stimulus.

impedence counting See Coulter principle.

indices In hematology, referring to calculated values for red cell properties: mean cell volume (MCV), mean cell hemoglobin (MCH), and mean cell hemoglobin concentration (MCHC).

interferon Proteins secreted by cells that have been invaded by viruses, confers protection on noninfected cells.

interleukin (IL) An intracellular hormone secreted by lymphocytes or macrophages involved in cell-mediated immunity.

IL-1 A monokine produced by activated macrophages to stimulate T helper lymphocytes to proliferate (synonym: lymphocyte activating factor, LAF).

IL-2 A lymphokine secreted by activated T lymphocytes to promote T cell growth.

intravascular hemolysis Red cell destruction occurring within the blood vessels, liberating hemoglobin. Most commonly a result of antibody-mediated complement activation, toxic substances, or severe burns.

intrinsic coagulation pathway Utilization of the plasma contact factors, starting with the activation of factor XII, to initiate coagulation.

intrinsic factor (IF) A protein secreted by the gastric parietal cells that is required for the intestinal absorption of vitamin B-12. Pernicious anemia is a deficiency of intrinsic factor.

in vitro Outside of a living system, as in the laboratory or in an artificial container.

in vivo Inside a living organism, associated with the physiological system.

isoimmune An immune response (antibody production) directed against an antigen from a different individual of the same species.

ITP Idiopathic (immune) thrombocytopenic purpura.

IV Intravenous.

jaundice A yellow skin color due to increased bilirubin pigment; a result of liver damage (e.g., hepatitis) or due to acute intravascular hemolysis.

kallikrein The activated contact factor, derived from prekallikrein, in the intrinsic pathway of coagulation.

kappa chain One of two light polypeptide chains that comprise immunoglobulins, produced by plasma cells.

karyotype A pattern analysis of chromosomes and banding patterns, obtained from mitotically active cells at metaphase. The cell nucleus is photographed and dispersed chromosomes are paired and examined for abnormalities.

keratocyte Red blood cells with one or two large pointed projections or "horns."

kernicterus The accumulation of bilirubin metabolites in the central nervous system, resulting in mental retardation or death of infants with hemolytic disease of the newborn. Can be treated by exchange transfusion to lower bilirubin concentrations.

kinin Plasma peptides involved in the inflammatory response (e.g., bradykinin).

Kleihauer-Betke test A test for the presence of fetal hemoglobin in red blood cells, based on the resistance of Hb F to acid elution. Detects and semiquantifies fetomaternal bleeds.

lambda chain One of two light polypeptide chains that comprise immunoglobulin, produced by plasma cells.

LAP Leukocyte alkaline phosphatase.

large granular lymphocyte (LGL) A lymphocyte with sky blue cytoplasm containing several large azurophilic granules. Some of these have been identified as natural killer (NK) cells.

LCAT Lecithin-cholesterol acyl transferase, an enzyme that mediates exchange of plasma and membrane cholesterol fractions.

LDH Lactic dehydrogenase, one of several isoenzymes found in a variety of tissues, including red blood cells.

leptocyte A thin (flattened) hypochromic erythrocyte, most often seen in patients with liver disease.

leukemia A malignant proliferation of one or more white blood cell lines. See **acute leukemia** and **chronic leukemia.**

leukocyte alkaline phosphatase (LAP) An enzyme found in granulocytes that mediates phosphate transfer. A cytochemical procedure for determining relative enzyme activity and differentiating leukemia (low activity) from leukemoid reactions (high activity).

leukocytosis Increased white blood cell concentration of the peripheral blood.

leukopenia Decreased white blood cell concentration of the peripheral blood.

LUC Large unstained cell, identified on histographs from automated differential counters.

Luebering-Rappaport pathway An associated reaction of the glycolytic pathway that generates 2,3-diphosphoglycerate, essential for inhibiting oxygen-hemoglobin interaction.

lymphadenopathy Disease or disorder involving the lymphnodes, usually producing a visible swelling or change in mass.

lymphoma A localized, malignant tumor of lymphoid tissue.

lysosomes The granules of white blood cells that contain acid hydrolases and other enzymes associated with intracellular digestion of microbes.

macrocyte Large (> 100 fL) erythrocyte in the peripheral blood.

macroglobulinemia Excessive quantities of large molecular weight immunoglobulins in the plasma associated with plasma cell dyscrasias.

macrophage Large mononuclear phagocyte that migrates through the tissues or becomes localized in specific organs (synonyms: reticuloendothelial cells, histiocytes); blood monocytes are the immature forms of macrophages.

major basic protein (MBP) A dominant component of the large crystalloid granules of eosinophils.

malignant An invasive, rapidly progressive neoplasm; cancerous.

marginal pool The neutrophils that adhere to the vascular endothelium, comprising 40 to 60% of the circulating neutrophils but not routinely included in peripheral white cell counts.

mast cells Tissue basophils, containing histamine, heparin, and most of the other chemical constituents of blood basophils.

May-Hegglin anomaly A hereditary disorder characterized by large platelets, thrombocytopenia, and the presence of large basophilic inclusions in leukocytes, resembling Döhle bodies.

MCH Mean corpuscular (cell) hemoglobin.

MCHC Mean corpuscular (cell) hemoglobin concentration.

MCV Mean corpuscular (cell) volume.

MDS Myelodysplastic syndrome.

M:E ratio Myeloid to erythroid cell ratio of the bone marrow, a relative index of blood cell production, normally about 2.5 to 5:1.

megakaryocyte (MKC) Large polyploid cells of the bone marrow that produce platelets by demarcation of cytoplasmic fragments.

megaloblast An abnormally large erythroblast that results from a nuclear maturation defect, most commonly associated with folate or cobalamin deficiency.

metastatic The capability of changing locations, referring to the migratory and invasive nature of some malignancies (e.g., carcinomas).

methemalbumin The combination of heme and albumin resulting from intravascular hemolysis.

methemoglobin Oxidized hemoglobin, heme contains ferric iron.

methemoglobin reductase pathway (MRP) Associated with glycolysis, enzymatically maintains hemoglobin in a reduced state. MRP deficiency results in a Heinz body anemia.

methylene blue The basic, blue-colored component of Wright's stain. A general biological dye, a component of many stains.

microcyte Small (< 80 fL) erythrocyte in the peripheral blood.

MKC Megakaryocyte.

MM Myeloid metaplasia; multiple myeloma.

monoclonal antibody A specific immunoglobulin or antibody derived from a single genetic line of plasma cells. Plasma cells are fused with immortal cancer cells, forming a hybridoma that assures production of large quantities of antibody for reagent purposes.

monocyte A large mononuclear phagocyte of the peripheral blood; the immature stage of macrophages.

MPV Mean platelet volume.

mRNA Messenger ribonucleic acid.

multiple myeloma A plasma cell malignancy resulting from the proliferation of a single cell (monoclonal); the production of large amounts of immunoglobulin, identified by serum and urine electrophoresis as sharp spikes (M components or M proteins).

myeloperoxidase An enzyme present in granulocytes and monocytes. A cytochemical technique for identifying immature cells of the myeloid and monocytoid lines.

myelodysplastic syndrome (MDS) Abnormal maturation and production of one or more marrow cell types, often associated with a type of refractory anemia. Some of the changes are pre-leukemic and the syndrome terminates in a myeloproliferative disorder.

myeloid metaplasia (MM) A myeloproliferative disease characterized by displacement of marrow hematopoietic elements by fibrous connective tissue (myelofibrosis) and a progressive pancytopenia; loss of marrow blood cell production may be compensated by extramedullary hematopoiesis.

myeloproliferative disorder Abnormal proliferation of one or more bone marrow cell lines, including fibrous connective tissue.

NBT Nitroblue tetrazolium.

N:C Ratio of nucleus to cytoplasm areas.

neonatal The period of life from birth to six weeks of age; the newborn infant.

neoplasm New growth, a tumor or abnormal proliferation of cells.

neutrophil The mature stage of the phagocytic granulocyte that comprises 40 to 75% of the peripheral leukocyte count. Characterized by a segmented nucleus, made up of 3 to 5 lobes, and a pinkish to beige cytoplasm containing faint granules.

Niemann-Pick disease A lipid storage disease of macrophages (histiocytes) caused by a deficiency of sphingomyelinase.

nitroblue tetrazolium test (NBT) A dye reduction test for neutrophil function, the ability to generate oxidative products during the respiratory burst. Used to screen for NADPH oxidase deficiency, as in chronic granulomatous disease.

normochromic Red blood cells with normal hemoglobin concentration, having a small area of central pallor on blood smears.

normocytic Red blood cells of normal size or volume (85 to 95 fL).

nRBC or NRBC Nucleated red blood cell; erythroblast.

nucleoli The basophilic areas of the nucleus that are rich in RNA, especially prominent in immature and mitotically active cells.

opsonin A plasma protein or other substance that enhances phagocytosis of microbes and other antibody-coated targets. Opsonization is part of the inflammatory response, involving the complement cascade.

orthochromic normoblast Metarubricyte, the last nucleated red blood cell stage.

osmotic fragility A test to determine the ability of red blood cells to withstand hypo-osmotic solutions. Cells with membrane defects (e.g., hereditary spherocytosis) have increased osmotic fragility or less ability to withstand water influx.

ovalocyte Egg-shaped or elliptical cells, most often associated with megaloblastic anemia (macroovalocyte) or hereditary elliptocytosis. See elliptocyte.

oxygen dissociation curve The relationship between oxygen saturation of hemoglobin (affinity) and partial pressure of oxygen (availability).

oxyhemoglobin The oxygenated form of hemoglobin.

PAGE Polyacrylamide gel electrophoresis.

pancytopenia Decreased concentrations of all blood cells, indicative of generalized bone marrow failure or aplastic anemia.

Pappenheimer body Iron containing granules in peripheral red blood cells that are seen with Wright's stain because the iron is aggregated with mitochondria and ribosomes. Associated with disorders of hemoglobin synthesis and dyserythropoietic syndromes.

parenteral Administration of a drug or substance by the intravenous, intramuscular or intradermal route; bypassing the processes of ingestion and absorption.

paroxysmal nocturnal hemoglobinuria (PNH) A chronic form of hemolytic anemia in which red blood cells are sensitive to small decreases in pH.

PAS Periodic acid-Schiff.

PCL Plasma cell leukemia.

PCT Prothrombin consumption test.

PCV Packed cell volume, hematocrit.

PDW Platelet distribution width.

Pelger-Huët anomaly A benign hereditary condition characterized by decreased segmentation and increased symmetry of the granulocyte nuclei, particularly evident in neutrophils. The morphological abnormality is not accompanied by functional problems.

periodic acid-Schiff (PAS) A cytochemical technique used to demonstrate carbohydrates in blood cells and to stain electrophoretic bands of membrane constituents.

pernicious anemia (PA) A form of megaloblastic anemia, a nuclear maturation defect caused by a deficiency of intrinsic factor; IF is necessary for vitamin B12 absorption.

petechiae Pin point red-purple spots on the skin and mucosal surfaces caused by capillary bleeding, most often associated with thrombocytopenia or disorders of platelet function.

PF3 Platelet factor 3, the phospholipid component of the platelet membrane that exhibits procoagulant activity during the coagulation process.

phagocyte A leukocyte capable of ingesting microbial organisms, normally applied to neutrophils and monocytes, but eosinophils and lymphocytes also have limited phagocytic abilities.

Philadelphia chromosome (Ph¹) A translocation from chromosome 22 to chromosome 9 (92% of Ph¹) or another chromosome, seen in the myeloid precursors of most patients with chronic myelogenous leukemia.

phospholipid A major constituent of cell membranes and the substrate on platelets for activation of clotting factor complexes.

PK Prekallikrein; pyruvate kinase.

plasma cell, plasmacyte A mature B lymphocyte that is specialized for antibody (immunoglobulin) production; rarely found in the peripheral blood.

plasmin A proteolytic enzyme that breaks down fibrin, generated by the activation of the plasma precursor, plasminogen.

platelet The cytoplasmic fragments of megakaryocytes, circulating as small discs in the peripheral blood, that initiate hemostasis by forming an adherent plug at the site of hemorrhage. Platelets also contribute to the coagulation cascade and help maintain the endothelial lining of the blood vessels.

PNH Paroxysmal nocturnal hemoglobinuria.

poikilocytosis Variability in red blood cell shape.

polychromatophilia Increased numbers of peripheral red blood cells that have a basophilic (blue-gray) tint on Wright-stained smears, indicating the presence of cytoplasmic RNA. Many of these cells prove to be reticulocytes when stained with supravital stains.

polycythemia Increased concentration of cells in the peripheral blood; as commonly used, it refers to increased erythrocyte concentration.

polycythemia vera A myeloproliferative disorder, an autonomous increase in erythrocyte production and concentration, usually accompanied by hyperplasia of other blood cell lines.

polymorphonuclear (PMN) Referring to a leukocyte with a segmented nucleus. ie., a mature granulocyte, especially a neutrophil.

porphobilinogen (PBG) An intermediate product of heme synthesis.

porphyria A hereditary or acquired disorder resulting from disturbed heme synthesis in which porphrin metabolites are excreted in high concentrations and accumulate in tissues.

PPP Platelet poor plasma, supernatant from plasma centrifuged at high speed to remove platelets.

precision A measure of reproducability in a series of repeated assays of the same sample; low coefficient of variation, ability to duplicate a test result.

prekallikrein (PK) Fletcher factor, one of the circulating contact factors of the intrinsic coagulation pathway.

preleukemia A syndrome of hematopoietic abnormalities that often preceeds the appearance of typical leukemia. Many of these changes are classified as specific types of myelodysplastic syndrome.

primary granules An older term for the non-specific, azurophilic granules that are prominent in promyelocytes. Identifiable as lysosomes in various leukocytes.

pronormoblast Rubriblast.

prostaglandin One of several fatty acid compounds that can stimulate contraction of smooth muscle. Prostaglandins are metabolic products of the arachidonic acid pathway in platelets.

protamine sulfate A reagent used to detect fibrin monomers, especially those formed during hypercoagulation states; a drug used to counteract intravenous heparin and decrease the clotting time.

protease An enzyme that splits proteins.

protein C A plasma protein that interacts with tissue plasminogen activator in the fibrinolysis system.

protein S A plasma protein that is a cofactor for the activation of protein C in the fibrinolytic pathway.

prothrombin Coagulation factor II, produced by the liver and vitamin K-dependent.

prothrombin time (PT) A test of extrinsic and common coagulation pathway integrity, used to monitor the dosage of oral anticoagulants.

PRP Platelet rich plasma.

Prussian blue stain Potassium ferrocyanide reacts with iron deposits to produce the blue-green pigment, ferric ferrocyanide to identify siderocytes and sideroblasts as well as iron deposits in marrow and other tissues.

PT Prothrombin time.

PTT Partial thromboplastin time.

purpura Darkened areas of the skin, mucosal membranes, and various tissues caused by bleeding; a characteristic of platelet disorders and some coagulopathies.

pyknotic A nucleus with very condensed chromatin, usually referring to a degenerating leukocyte or to the nuclei of metarubricytes just prior to expulsion.

pyridoxal phosphate An active form of vitamin B_6, a cofactor in the synthesis of delta aminolevulinic acid in the heme synthesis pathway.

pyruvate kinase (PK) A key enzyme in the Embden-Meyerhof pathway (glycolysis); deficiencies of PK can result in a hemolytic anemia.

RBC Red blood cell; red blood cell count.

RDW Red cell distribution width, a measure of cell size variation or anisocytosis.

reactive lymphocyte A mature lymphocyte that is responding to antigen stimulation. Some are larger than the typical small cells, others are basophilic and have features of immaturity (synonyms: Downey cell, atypical lymphocyte, virocyte, immunocyte).

Reed-Sternberg cell A large malignant macrophage or histiocyte seen in the spleen and bone marrow, specifically associated with Hodgkin's disease.

refractory A term used to indicate a lack of response to therapy (e.g., refractory anemia).

RES Reticuloendothelial system.

respiratory burst The rapid uptake of oxygen by phagocytes associated with the generation of lethal oxidants used during intracellular microbicidal activity.

reticulocyte The first non-nucleated red cell stage, identified by precipitable ribosomal material with supravital stains.

reticulofilamentous substance The precipitated ribosomal material seen in reticulocytes after exposure to supravital stains, such as brilliant cresyl blue.

ringed sideroblast An erythroblast containing excess iron deposits associated with the perinuclear mitochondria, forming a dense ring of Prussian blue positive granules. Indicative of sideroblastic anemias due to disrupted heme synthesis.

ristocetin An antibiotic used to test platelet aggregation, especially useful for diagnosing von Willebrand's disease.

RNA Ribonucleic acid.

Romanowsky stain A biological stain composed of methylene blue or its deriviatives and a counterstain, such as eosin (e.g., Wright's stain, Giemsa stain, May-Grunwald stain).

rouleaux Red cells that align face to face in columns, resembling a "stack of coins"; enhanced by increased plasma protein concentration, especially in inflammatory states and in hypergammaglobulinemias (e.g., multiple myeloma).

RPI Reticulocyte production index.

rubriblast Pronormoblast.

rubricyte Polychromatophilic normoblast.

runner's anemia Anemia developed by long distance runners and other athletes involved in some types of strenuous exercise of long duration, due to chronic gastrointestinal blood loss and accompanying iron deficiency.

sarcoma Malignant, often metastatic, growth of connective tissue (muscle, bone, lymphoid).

Schilling test A means of determining cobalamin (vitamin B12) absorption using a radioactive oral dose and measuring urinary excretion. Can be given with and without intrinsic factor to diagnose pernicious anemia.

schistocyte, schizocyte A split or fragmented red blood cell, very irregular in shape, associated with microthromboses, prosthetic heart valves, and severe hemolytic states.

SD Standard deviation.

SE Standard error.

sequestration Concentration of cells or platelets in a tissue or organ, especially the spleen.

serotonin A vasoconstrictor carried by platelets and released during aggregation (synonym: hydroxytryptamine).

sex-linked Genes that are associated with the X chromosome; females can be homozygous or heterozygous for a trait, whereas males are hemizygous, either having a single copy of the gene or none.

Sézary syndrome An infiltration of the skin by Sézary cells, large lymphocytes with cleaved nuclei and scant cytoplasm.

sialic acid A constituent of the red cell membrane, source of the erythrocyte's negative charge.

sickle cell A crescent-shaped erythrocyte with sharp ends produced as a result of hemoglobin S polymerization in patients with sickle cell disease.

sickle cell anemia Homozygous state for the presence of genes coding for Hemoglobin S; the sixth position of the beta chain contains valine instead of glutamic acid. A severe hemolytic anemia, found almost exclusively in black people. The heterozygous state (sickle cell trait) has minimal clinical manifestations.

sideroblast An erythroblast containing excess iron stores.

sideroblastic anemia (SA) An anemia characterized by disrupted heme synthesis, iron accumulation, and the presence of marrow sideroblasts.

siderocyte An erythrocyte containing excess iron granules.

SLE Systemic lupus erythematosus.

smudge cell A leukocyte that is damaged during preparation of wedge smears, usually because the cell has increased mechanical fragility (e.g., leukemic lymphocytes).

spectrin A major cytoskeletal protein of the red cell membrane.

spherocyte A round (spherical) erythrocyte, usually a result of excess water influx. Microspherocytes are seen in severe burn victims. Hereditary spherocytosis is a membrane defect. Spherocytic change preceeds cell lysis.

sphingomyelin A lipid component of cell membranes.

splenomegaly Enlarged spleen, a finding in several types of malignancies, platelet disorders, and hemolytic anemias.

stem cell A general term referring to relatively undifferentiated blood cell precursors. Totipotential, multipotential (pluripotential), and unipotential stem cells possess increasing degrees of commitment to a particular cell lineage.

stomatocyte An erythrocyte with a large slit or "mouth" in the central region of the disc.

substitution study In coagulation testing, a means of determining a factor deficiency by performing a prothrombin or partial thromboplastin test using aged serum or absorbed plasma, each of which lacks specific factors.

suppressor T lymphocyte A mature lymphocyte that inhibits immune responses, especially in B lymphocytes.

systemic lupus erythematosus (SLE) An autoimmune disease, most common in young adult women, associated with increased IgG production against cellular DNA, a progressive anemia and thrombocytopenia, and the development of glomerulonephritis.

TAR baby syndrome Thrombocytopenia with absent radii, a congenital abnormality affecting limb development, the heart, and megakaryocyte production.

target cell An erythrocyte with a central color spot in the area of pallor, resembling a target (smear) or peaked hat (three dimensional); synonym: codocyte. Seen in many hemolytic anemias, especially sickle cell, Hb C disease, and thalassemia.

TdT Terminal deoxyribonucleotidyl transferase, a DNA polymerase present in early lymphocyte stages, used as a marker to identify lymphoblastic leukemias.

telangiectiasia The presence of abnormal coils or loops in small blood vessels that appear as small red lesions on the skin or mucous membranes.

thalassemia One of several hereditary disorders in which globin chain production is greatly diminished. Accumulation of the chains not affected stimulates phagocytic destruction in the spleen and a severe hemolytic anemia in the major (homozygous) forms of the disease. Most commonly seen in oriental peoples from southeast Asia and from peoples of the Mediterranean region.

thrombin The activated form of factor II that acts as a serine protease to cleave fibrinogen and form fibrin. A reagent used to test platelet aggregation.

thrombocyte A general term for platelet, more commonly used for non-human species.

thrombocythemia An increased concentration of peripheral blood platelets, most often used in disorders that are idiopathic or have autonomous mechanisms (essential thrombocythemia, a myeloproliferative disorder).

thrombocytopathy A platelet disorder.

thrombocytopenia A decreased concentration of peripheral blood platelets.

thrombocytosis Increased platelet concentration, most often a benign response to increased demand or turnover.

thrombosis The formation of blood clots.

thrombosthenin A contractile protein of platelets, responsible for clot retraction and platelet shape change.

thromboxane A platelet metabolite of the arachidonic acid pathway, stimulates platelet aggregation and vasoconstriction.

thymosin Thymic hormone, secreted by the thymus to stimulate the growth of secondary lymphoid tissue

TIBC Total iron binding capacity, equivalent to the plasma transferrin concentration.

t-PA Tissue plasminogen activator, a natural substance produced in the vascular endothelial cells that activates plasminogen to form plasmin, the protease that dissolves fibrin clots. Available as a commercial product to manage thrombotic disorders and complications.

transferrin The plasma protein that transports iron, measured as the total iron binding capacity or TIBC.

tRNA Transfer ribonucleic acid.

TTP thrombotic thrombocytopenic purpura.

urobilinogen (UBG) A colorless metabolite of bilirubin formed by intestinal bacteria. Increased quantities in the urine and stool are associated with hemolytic anemias.

uroporphrinogen (UPG) An intermediate product of heme synthesis.

von Willebrand's disease One of several forms of hereditary deficiency of the factor VIII component (vW factor) that mediates interactions between platelets and the subendothelium. Characterized clinically as a mild to severe bleeding disorder and in the laboratory by the absence of ristocetin-induced platelet aggregation.

vWD von Willebrand's disease.

vWF Von Willebrand's factor, the component of factor VIII synthesized by the vascular endothelial cells.

WAIHA Warm autoimmune hemolytic anemia, referring to activity of the antibody at 37° C.

Waldenström's macroglobulinemia A plasma cell malignancy that results in an increased concentration of plasma immunoglobulins.

WBC White blood cell; white blood cell count.

Wiskott-Aldrich syndrome A hereditary disorder characterized by small platelets, bleeding tendencies and recurrent pyogenic infections.

zeta chain A globin chain found in embryonic hemoglobin.

zymogen The inactive or circulating form of an enzyme, such as a plasma coagulation factor.

Appendixes

APPENDIX A: UNITS OF MEASUREMENT

Length

1 inch (in) = 2.54 centimeters (cm)
1 centimeter (cm) = 0.394 inches (in)
1 Angstrom (Å) = 0.1 nanometers (nm)
1 micrometer (μm) = 10,000 (10^4) Angstroms (Å)

Volume

1 quart (qt) = 32 ounces (oz) = 0.946 Liters (L)

1 Liter (L) = 1.06 quarts (qts) = 33.81 ounces (oz)
1 microliter (μL) = 1.0 cubic millimeter (mm^3)
1 milliliter (mL) = 1.0 cubic centimeter (cm^3)

Mass

1 ounce (oz av) = 28.35 grams (g)
1 pound (lb) = 16 ounces (oz av) = 454 grams (g)
1 kilogram (kg) = 35.27 ounces (oz) = 2.2 pounds (lbs)

APPENDIX B: REFERENCE VALUES FOR HEMATOLOGY

	Neonates	Children	Adults Male	Female
Erythrocyte evaluation				
Red blood cell count ($10^6/\mu$L)	4.8-7.0	3.8-5.4	4.2-6.0	3.8-5.4
Hemoglobin (g/dL)	16-23	10-15	13-17	12-16
Hematocrit (% of blood volume)	50-70	32-44	38-50	36-46
Mean corpuscular volume (fL)	95-120	75-88	85-95	
Mean corpuscular hemoglobin (pg)	36-40	25-29	27-31	
Mean corpuscular hemoglobin concentration (g/dL or %)	30-34	31-35	32-36	
Reticulocyte count (% of RBCs)	1.0-5.0	0.5-1.5	0.5-1.5	
Erythrocyte sedimentation rate (mm/hour)			0-10	0-20
Hemoglobin electrophoresis (% of total hemoglobin):				
Hemoglobin A	15-40		96-99	
Hemoglobin A2	0.2-2.5		0.3-3.5	
Hemoglobin F	60-85		0.0-2.0	
Methemoglobin (% of total)			0.0-1.0	
Serum iron (μg/dL)	90-200		70-180	60-180
Iron binding capacity (μg/dL)	200-350		250-450	

Appendix B, cont'd

	Neonates	Children	Adults Male	Female
Transferrin saturation (%)	60-80		20-50	15-50
Serum ferritin (μg/L)	100-240		20-300	10-120
Red cell folate (ng/mL of RBCs)			150-450	
Serum folate (ng/mL)			2.0-10.0	
Plasma vitamin B12 (pg/mL)			150-500	
Red cell 2,3-DPG (μmol/g hemoglobin)			13-17	
Glucose-6-phosphate dehydrogenase (U/mL of RBCs)			3.3-4.8	
Pyruvate kinase (U/g hemoglobin)			12-18	
Free erythrocyte protoporphyrin (μg/dL of RBCs)			15-80	
Erythrocyte coproporphyrin (μg/dL of RBCs)			0.5-1.5	
Copper (μg/dL of red cells)			90-150	
Serum haptoglobin (mg/dL)			100-400	
Plasma hemoglobin (mg/dL)			0.0-1.0	
Osmotic fragility (% normal saline)				
Not incubated			0.40-0.45	
Incubated			0.45-0.55	
Hemoglobin oxygen affinity, P_{50} (mm Hg)	17-21		25-29	
Leukocyte evaluation				
White blood cell count (10^3/μL)	10-25	5-15	4-11	
Differential WBC count (%)				
Segmented neutrophils	40-75	35-65	45-70	
Band neutrophils	5-14	1-5	1-5	
Lymphocytes	20-40	25-75	20-45	
Monocytes	2-10	3-9	2-8	
Eosinophils	0-5	0-5	0-5	
Basophils	0-2	0-2	0-2	
Absolute eosinophil count (per μL)	20-1000	40-650	50-300	
Leukocyte alkaline phosphatase (score, in Kaplow units)			40-150	
Hemostasis evaluation				
Platelet count (10^3/μL)	100-350	150-400	150-400	
Bleeding time (minutes)				
Ivy			2-6	
Simplate			3-10	
Simplate, after aspirin			4-21	
Platelet factor 3 availability (seconds)			30-60	
Plasma platelet factor 4 (ng/mL)			0-10	
Plasma beta-thromboglobulin (ng/mL)			15-70	
Thrombin generation time (minutes)			15-30	
Fibrinogen (mg/dL)			150-400	
Plasminogen, fluorogenic substrate (CTA U/mL)			2.4-3.8	

The reference values in the table have been compiled from several sources. Considerable variation exists between laboratories and test systems, therefore these reference ranges should be used as a guide and not as determinants of "normal" or "abnormal" levels for a particular analyte. Some values for children change dramatically with age. Those listed are for children 3 to 6 years of age. Reference ranges in relation to specific procedures can be found in the readings cited in Section VI. Results of most tests for coagulation factors are reported as "percent of normal activity" when the patient is compared to a normal control plasma. Ranges of 50% to 150% are considered normal. Screening tests, such as the prothrombin time and activated partial thromboplastin time, are reported in seconds but the normal ranges depend on the specific reagent test system used. The times are only meaningful in comparison to the control values.

APPENDIX C: SELECTED SOURCE MATERIAL FOR HEMATOLOGY

Professional organizations

American Association of Blood Banks (AABB)
1117 North 19th Street, Suite 600
Arlington, VA 22209

American Medical Technologists (AMT)
710 Higgins Road
Park Ridge, IL 60068

American Society of Clinical Pathologists (ASCP)
2100 West Harrison Street
Chicago, IL 60612

American Society for Medical Technology (ASMT)
2021 L Street NW, Suite 400
Washington, DC 20036

Periodicals

Acta Haematologica. Basel, W. Germany: S. Karger

American Journal of Hematology. New York: Alan R. Liss

American Journal of Pediatric Hematology/Oncology. New York: Masson Publishers, Inc.

Blood. Orlando, Fla: Grune & Stratton

Blood Cells. New York: Springer International

Blut. Berlin: Springer-Verlag

British Journal of Haematology. Oxford: Blackwell Scientific Publishers

Clinical and Laboratory Haematology. Oxford: Blackwell Scientific Publishers

Clinical Laboratory Science. Washington, DC: American Society for Medical Technology

Experimental Hematology. New York: Springer-Verlag

Folia Haematologica. Leipzig (DDR): Akad. Verlag Geest. & Portig K.-G.

Haematologia. Utrecht (Netherlands): Ynu Science Press

Haematologica. Rome: II Pensiero Scientifico Editore

Hemostasis. Basel, W. Germany: S. Karger

Journal of Leukocyte Biology. New York: Alan R. Liss

Laboratory Medicine. Chicago: American Society of Clinical Pathologists

Leukemia Research. Oxford: Pergamon Press

Nouvelle Revue Française d'Hématologie. Berlin: Springer International

Progress in Hematology. Orlando, Fla: Grune & Stratton

Progress in Hemostasis and Thrombosis. Orlando, Fla: Grune & Stratton

Scandinavian Journal of Haematology. Copenhagen: Munksgaard

Seminars in Hematology. Orlando, Fla: Grune & Stratton

Seminars in Thrombosis and Hemostasis. New York: Thieme-Stratton

Thrombosis and Haemostasis. Stuttgart: Schattauer

Thrombosis Research. New York: Pergamon Press

Year Book of Hematology. Chicago: Year Book Medical Publishers, Inc.

Index

Italics indicate illustration.
t indicates table.